The Complete Tex
Holistic
Self Diagnosis

- Simple easy to use methods for non-professional and professionals

- Find the cause of a disease in less than a minute

- Take control of your health

- Many easy physical examinations that reveal disease

- Many Illustrations, Charts, Tables, and easy Chemical Test

- Learn many body symptoms of sickness

- You will identify the cause of an illness

- You can Prevent disease and Stop illness

LLAILA O. AFRIKA

Other books by the author:
- African Holistic Health
- Vitamins and Minerals from A to Z
- Raising Black Children
- Melanin
- The Gullah
- Nutricide

Llaila has a line of specialty disease remedy Supplements. To order Supplements, Telephone Health Consultations, Health and Science classes, Lectures, DVD's, and CDs contact:

Llaila Afrika
P.O Box 501274
Indianapolis, Indiana 46250
Email: Llailaafrika@juno.com
Online classes: drafrikaonline.com
Official Website: llailaafrika.com

Holistic Therapies and Education Center
P.O Box 501274
Indianapolis, Indiana 46250
Copyright 9 July 2013
ISBN978-0-9896906-0-7

All rights reserved. No part of this book may be reproduced in any form, or by any means including, non-print, electronic, mechanical, photocopying, or stored in a retrieval system without permission in writing from the author except by a reviewer who may quote a brief passage to be included in a review.

Production
Melanie D. Stevenson

Cover Design
Llaila O. Afrika

All Illustrations
Llaila O. Afrika

Manufactured and Printed in the United States of America

Disclaimer

The author disclaims any liability caused by the direct or indirect use or misuse of the information in this book. None of the information is meant to take the place of an accredited license medical health practitioner.

Introduction

Readers of this book will become aware of the many ways the body reveals an illness. Let Holistic Diagnosis help you to discover the cause of a disease. Diagnosis will no longer be a secret that is reserved for scientist and medical practitioner. And, those that are practitioners will gain more skills for diagnosing.

This book has many diagnosis methods. Choose a diagnosis method that is easy and comfortable for you to use. You can stay with one method and add others later. If you try to learn all the methods you may feel overwhelm. Some methods are easier than others while others present a challenge. Children and parents can learn many methods. Diagnosis skills will help you to gain the ability to investigate disease causes and prevent, avoid and overcome illness.

There are many subjective and objective types of diagnosis methods because people have different learning styles and types. The subjective (symptom) diagnosis requires observation with touch (palpatory), sight (ophthalmic), smell (olfactive) and hearing (auditory). The objective (signs) diagnosis use numbers to evaluate temperature, blood pressure, pulse rate, respiratory rate, pH (potential of hydrogen) and breathe hold time. The objective measures of chemical home test in this book are easy to perform and it does not require a chemistry background. The many subjective and objective diagnosis choices allow you to have different ways to arrive at a precise cause of a disease plus having different choices does not confine you to one method.

Many of the diagnosis methods in this book are derived from traditional medical practices and ancient traditions (accepted practice). Keep in mind that modern science is theory (belief unproven) based science. Modern science normal standards and scientific values for health and disease established for signs (objective measures) and symptoms (subjective measures) were never based upon a science of facts and non-beliefs. The traditional modern disease calibration classification standards used random people that were not tested for disease and their health status was not assessed. The random selected people used to set the normal standards for disease and wellness did not have similar ages, diets, lifestyles, jobs, medical histories, and weight or height. Also they may have had undiagnosed diseases. These people's sign and symptoms are used to set todays standards. This is not scientific but accepted in modern traditional medicine. Modern medicine has its tradition of using theories. Theories give a focus for ideas; however, a theory is a belief and guess, which relies upon the creativity of a scientist. A belief or guess is not scientific. The many theories used in science would be better taught in a philosophy class. It is unfortunate that theories are often accepted as scientific facts. Some of the theories are Electron Orbital, Free Radical, Anti-oxidant, Free Trait, Relativity, Space/Time, Left Hemisphere and Right Hemisphere of the Brain, Speed of Light, Determinism, Centrifugal, Catharsis, Orchid, Big Bang, Evolution, String, and Gravity etc. Both traditional medicine and modern medicine rely on their accepted practice (traditions). This book presents both traditions without prejudice. Both traditions have their limitations, range of use and unique languages. You should not feel uneasy or threaten of the diagnosis (unique languages). The purpose of language is to communicate to you an understanding of diagnosis.

In this book there are many diagnosis methods that do not require computer programs or many science gadgets. This allows you to use them without electricity or reliance on technologies, so you can freely use them in any place in the world. I have used these methods on my clients for many years with good results. The diagnosis skills in this book will enable you to see the human body as a dictionary that reveals the specific cause of disease. Without diagnosing skills many people buy remedies as if they are blindfold or go from one health practitioner to another searching for the solution to their illness. When you use diagnosis skills you can make intelligent choices of remedy solutions because you understand how the body uses symptoms and signs to tell you what is wrong. Use Holistic Diagnosis skills to claim your right to know what is going wrong in the body. You should not be a prisoner of diagnosis ignorance. Holistic Diagnosis gives you the right to claim power over illnesses and own you right to be healthy.

I wrote this book in 1990. It has had many challenges to get published. Publishers got me to sign with them with the promise to publish the book but never presented to me a final copy to approve. I contact many artists that assumed they could do medical illustrations and they could not. Their prices were too expensive and in the 1990s usually wanted to charge $50.00 to $70.00 per illustrated page. The artist prices caused many publishers to see the book as too expensive to produce. Finally, out of Frustration I did all my illustrations. I had not done art or illustrations in about 30 years. My artistic skill level is not precise. I humbly ask my deceased art teacher not to get out his grave to complain about the illustrations. He always would say the power of a graphic artist is in the ability to master straight and curved lines and brush strokes. It seems that this book had its own "Rites of Passage", rhythm, trials and tribulations, pregnancy and birth. My wife Melanie volunteered to type the text and scan illustrations. This required her to learn many computer programs and to become a computer geek. She invested tons of hours of energy and love into the book. Without her this book would still be in my closet crying to be born. Melanie is a Licensed Medical Practitioner (does not prescribe drugs, or treat STD's) and has used and taught many of the diagnosis methods in this book. We suggest you use the methods in this book to heal yourself and help others.

Llaila Afrika
Indianapolis, Indiana

About the Author

Llaila (la-ee-la) Afrika is a holistic health practitioner. He has been in the health profession for over 40 years. His background includes working as a social worker, psychotherapist, group facilitator, community organizer, nurse, and naturopath. Llaila has a Doctorate in Naturopathy diploma and is a Certified Addictionologist, Certified Acupuncturist, Massage Therapist and a licensed Traditional Healer in Ghana, Togo, and Benin. He is essentially self-taught in holistic sciences. Llaila is an author, teacher, lecturer, practitioner, and historian.

Llaila lectures and teaches certification classes with his wife Dr. Melanie Stevenson. The classes are of a wide variety such as Holistic Nutritional Counselor, Anatomy and Physiology, Massage, Needle-less Acupuncture, Ethical Midwifery, Hypnosis, Holistic Nutrition, Holistic Sex and Relationship, Holistic Skin Care and Analysis, Touch Diagnosis, Holistic Diagnosis etc.

Table of Contents

Introduction	I
About the Author	III
How to Do a Self-Diagnosis	XVII
Diagnosing Instructions	1
Health Assessments	2
Health Assessments	3
Self-Diagnosis Steps	4
Holistic Body	5
Organ Regions of the Body	6
Human Development – Skin Layers	7
Embryonic Body	8
Embryo Energy	9
Energy Meridians (Acupuncture Highways)	10
Energy Centers	10
Embryo Position	11
Circadian Rhythm and Organs	12
Energy Transformation Movement	13
Male/Female Principle	14
Male/Female Principle	15
Male/Female Principle Chart	16
Sympathetic (Male Principle)/ Parasympathetic (Female Principle) Actions	17
Physical Aspects Influenced by the Parasympathetic Nervous System (Female Principle)	18
Female Principle/Parasympathetic Dominant	19
Female Principle/Parasympathetic Characteristics	20
Physical Aspects influenced by the Sympathetic Nervous System (Male Principle)	21
Physical Aspects Influenced by the Sympathetic Nervous System (Male Principle)	22
Male Principle/Sympathetic Metabolizers	23
Male/Female Principle Chart	23
Personality Diagnosis	24
Extrovert and Introvert Personality Traits	25
Personality Styles and Types Diagnosis	26
Learning Style	27
Digestion	28
Location of Metabolism of Food Types	30
Digestion, Urine and Saliva Flow Chart	31
Stomach	32
Ulcers	33
Ulcer Symptom Chart	33
Stomach Hernia	34
Variations in "Normal" Stomach	34
Stomach and Esophagus	35
Body Fat and Food Cravings	36
Music and Disease	36
Food Combining Chart	37
Digestion Time of Food Combinations	38
Digestive System's Circadian Rhythm	38
Colon/Body Connection	39
Unhealthy colon	39

- *Average Mineral Loss in Vegetables--- Due To Cooking* 40
- *Body's Energy and Food* 40
- *Mineral Relativity Wheel* 41
- *pH Range of Acceptance* 42
- *Digestive Enzyme Points* 43
- *Digestive Enzymes* 44
- *How to Test Tryptophan* 45

Nose 46
- *Nose Types* 47
- *Nose Examination* 48
- *Nose* 48
- *Various Nose Forms* 49
- *Side of the Nose* 50
- *Height of the Nose* 51
- *Tip of the Nose* 51
- *Nose Massage* 52

LIPS 53
- *Lips* 54
- *Forms of the Mouth* 54
- *Forms of Lips* 55
- *Lips Correlation to the Body* 56
- *Shape of the Mouth* 57
- *Central Part of Lips* 57
- *Size of the Mouth* 58
- *Swollen Lips* 59

FACE 60
- *Racial Facial Types* 61
- *Face Development* 62
- *Face Reveals* 62
- *Cute Face* 63
- *Head Shape* 64
- *Adult Head Chart* 64
- *Birth Canal* 64
- *Face Pressure Points* 65
- *Amino Acids Points on Face* 66
- *Face Chart* 67
- *Development of Systems in Embryo* 68
- *Face Shapes* 69
- *Systems* 70
- *Face, Planets, and Disease* 71
- *Face and Zodiac Signs* 72
- *Regions of the Forehead* 73
- *Facial and Bone Deformities* 74
- *Face* 75
- *Face Changes/Bodily Degenerating* 76
- *Types of Facial Deformities* 77
- *Measurement of Neck* 78
- *Thyroid Massage* 79

Face Type (Zodiac) and Health Problems 80
- *Aries (March 21- April 19)* 81
- *Taurus (April 20- May 20)* 82
- *Gemini (May 21- June 20)* 83

v

- Cancer (June 21- July 22) 84
- Leo (July 23- August 22) 85
- Virgo (August 23- September 22) 86
- Libra (September 23- October 22) 87
- Scorpio (October 23- November 21) 88
- Sagittarius (November 22- December 21) 89
- Capricorn (December 22- January 19) 90
- Aquarius (January 20- February 18) 91
- Pisces (February 19- March 20) 92

Face Types (Planets) and Health Problems 93
- Sun 94
- Moon 95
- Mercury 96
- Venus 97
- Mars 98
- Jupiter 99
- Saturn 100
- Uranus 101
- Neptune 102

Eyes 103
- Eyeball, Iris and White Part of Eyes 104
- Size of the Eyeball 104
- Eye Expansion 105
- Regions of the Sclera (white part of eyes) 106
- Sclera and Body 107
- Eye Skeletal Chart 107
- Male and Female Principle 108
- Eyes and Eyebrows 109
- Pupil Size Distortion and Pupil Asymmetry 110
- Pupil Size 110
- Eyes by the Numbers 111
- Left Eye Numbers 112
- Right Eye Numbers 113
- Eye Sclera 114
- Iris 115
- Vein Types in Sclera 116
- Vessels on the White of the Eye 117
- Vein Shapes Indicate Illness 118
- Sclera 119
- Pupil 119
- Iris Indicates Disease 121
- Iris 122
- Inside (underside) the Eyelid 123
- Eye Blinking 123
- Arcus Senilis 124
- Eyelash Types 125
- Color Around the Eyes 125

Eye Exercise and Massage 126
- Eye Exercise 127
- Eye Stimulation Massage 128
- Eye Exercise Chart Guide 129
- Eye Exercise Chart 130

Hair 131
Hair Chart 132

Ear 133
Ear and Body 136
Ear Chart 137
Ear Position and Shape 138
Ear Angles 139
Sounds 140

Cheeks 141
Cheeks 142

Teeth 143
Teeth 144
Tongue Exercise and Gum Massage 144
Teeth Deformities 145
Teeth and the Body 146
Unnatural Tooth Gaps Exam 147
Children's Primary Teeth and Growth 148
Adult Teeth and Growth 148

Tongue 149
Tongue Diagnosis 150
Tongue and Organs 150
Description of Tongues 152
Tongue Shapes 153

Disease And Taste 154
Disease and Taste 155

Fingers And Fingernails 156
Curvature of fingers 157
Finger Placement 158
Fingertip Conditions 158
Nail Diagnosis 159
Fingernail Diagnosis 160
Shape and Size 161
Finger Analysis 162
Fingernail Form 163
Fingertip Forms 164
Twelve Types of Fingernails and the Zodiac 165
Zodiac and Body 166
Planets and Fingers 167
Finger Shapes 168
Fingers 169
Finger Spaces 170
Color of the Center of the Palm 171
Points at the Base of the Palm 172
Finger Regions 173
Space Between Fingers 174
Webbed Fingers 174
Long and Short Finger 175
The Wrist 176

Fingers And Planets 177
2nd- Finger Saturn 180
3rd Finger (Sun) 182

VII

    4th- Finger (Mercury) *184*
    Fingers and Emotions *186*

Palms of Hand **190**
    Hands *191*
    Lines in the Hand *192*
    Hand (Palm) Moisture *193*
    Hand Temperatures *194*
    Hands *195*
    Fingers, Relationship to Systems, and Organs *197*
    Mounts *198*
    Palm Line and Age *199*
    Hand Acupuncture Meridian Points *200*
    Pulse (Palpitation) Diagnosis *201*
    Normal Pulse *201*
    Pulse Divisions *202*
    Factors that influence a Pulse Reading *203*
    Pulse and Disease *203*
    Pulse and Organ Problems *204*
    Disease Pulse Readings *204*

Feet **205**
    Feet *206*
    Feet, Toes, and Ankle Correlation *207*
    Feet, Glands, Lower Blood Pressure *208*
    Feet Indications *209*
    Foot Pressure Points *210*
    Two Diagnosis Points on the Foot *210*
    Length of Toes *211*
    Callouses *212*
    Toe Nail Color *213*
    Toes and Body Functions *214*
    Foot Colors and Disease *215*
    Acupuncture Meridian Points on Lower Leg and Foot *216*

Body's Effect on Shoes and Feet **217**
    Diagnoses Using Shoes *218*
    Position of Feet *219*
    Angle of Feet *220*

Acupuncture **221**
    Acupressure Finger Position *222*
    Organ Energy Points *223*
    Amino Acid Points *224*
    Acupressure/Acupuncture Points on the Body *225*
    Acupuncture/ Acupressure Meridian on Body *226*
    Points on Body Chart *227*
    Points on Body *228*
    Organ Zones on Body *229*
    Melanin Energy Lines and The Pulses *230*
    Acupuncture Points *231*
    Acupuncture (acupressure) Points *232*
    Abdominal Section *233*
    Organ Areas *234*
    Disease and Body Areas *235*
    Disease and Leg Hair *236*

Handwriting Diagnosis..*237*
How to Do a Writing Diagnosis..*237*
Letter Size..*237*

SEX ORGANS..**240**
Female Genitals (Side View)..*240*
Male Genitals (Side View)..*240*
Female Sex Organs...*241*
Male Sex Organs..*242*
Sexual Response..*243*
Rhythm Theory...*243*
Sexual Response Time..*244*
Intercourse Position..*245*
Types of Sexual Intercourse Positions..*246*
Sex Response..*247*
Sex Organs and Your Body...*248*
Female Hormones and Glands..*249*
Fibroid Tumor..*250*
Female Warning Signs for Cancer..*251*
Enlarge Prostate..*252*
Female Sexual Process (6 Erections)..*253*
Vagina Organ Zones...*254*
Zodiac Vagina and Acupressure Points..*255*
Breast Shape..*256*
Breast Areola...*257*
Breast Exam While Standing...*257*
Penis / Organ relationship...*259*
Penis and Testicles Sexual Process..*260*
Reduce Sexual Arousal...*262*
Inguinal Hernia..*263*
Test For Prostate...*263*
Test the prostate gland by palpating; insert your lubricated glove with index finger into the rectum. On the anterior (front) rectum wall (skin) slightly pass the anorectal (ring) then palpate the prostate. The gland should feel smooth, rubbery and is the size of a walnut...............................*263*
Sexual Energy Center (Acupuncture Meridian Point)..*264*
Sexual Regeneration Orgasm..*265*
Orgasm Chart..*266*
Sex Organs and Your Body...*267*
Sexual Hormonal Rhythm Method..*268*

HEALING AND DISEASE SEX POSITIONS..**269**
Sexual Positions...*270*
Nutritional Disorders Diagnosis...*278*

Body Posture Diagnosis...**279**
Posture Against Gravity...*280*
Postural Alignment...*281*
Posture Misalignment...*282*
Posture Needy and Rigid Types...*283*
Female Pelvis...*284*
Locked Knees...*285*
Grounding..*287*
Displacement..*288*
An Overburdened Individual..*289*
Pelvis Misalignment..*290*
Normal Belly (abdominal)..*291*

Abnormal Belly (Abdominal) 292
Left-Right Split Posture 293
Head and Neck 294
Pelvis Angle 295
Burdened Posture 296
The Rigid Type 297
Posture Rules 298
Posture Do's and Don'ts 299
Shoulder Angles 300

Anatomy And Body Types **301**
Torn Ligaments Symptoms 302
Muscles, Deep Layer, Front View 303
Muscles, Deep Layer, Back View 304
Muscles, Superficial Layer, Front View 305
Muscles, Superficial Layer, Back View 306
Skeleton 307
Bones Of The Foot, Right Inside View 308
Bones of The Hand, Right Palm 309
Skeleton, Front View 310
Skeleton, Back View 311
Skeleton, Side View 312
Muscle Exercise 313
Back Muscles and Exercise 314
Muscle of the Hand, Palm View 315
Muscle of the Foot, Outer View 316
Muscles of the Foot, Inner View 316
pH and the Body 317
pH of Fluids and Tissues 317
Fluids in the Body 318
Body Types 319
Lymphatic System, Blood System 321
Organs 322
Nervous System, Endocrine Glands 323
Brain Centers 324
Brain Parts 325
Gland and Organ Test 326
Backbone (vertebrae) and Illness 328
Spinal Column 329
Organs and Feelings 330

Abdomen **331**
Abdomen and Organs 332
Abdomen 333
Abdomen Test 334
Abdominal Measurement 335
Umbilicus 336
Abdominal Measurement 337

Childhood and Adult Disease Symptoms and Signs **338**
Childhood Disease Symptoms 339
Delivery of Baby Affects Emotions 346
Diaper Rashes 347
Fevers in Children and Adults 348
Skin Eruptions in Children and Adults 349
Sleeping Disorders of Children 350

Test for Disease, Examinations, and Symptoms 351
    Abdomen Palpation Exam 352
    Aneurysms in Blood Vessels Test 352
    Aortic Aneurysm in the Abdomen 352
    Appendicitis Symptoms 352
    Astigmatism Test 353
    Auditory Nerve Test 354
    Dominant Eye Examination 355
    Blind Spot Test 355
    Test Procedure 355
    Facial Nerve and Blinking 356
    Phlebitis Symptoms 356
    Phlebitis Test 356
    Blockages in Vein 356
    Plaque Test 357
    Position Sense Test 357
    Position Arm Test 357
    Position Leg Test 357
    Pupillary Eye Reflex Test 357
    Rheumatoid Arthritis Symptoms 357
    Rib Fracture Test 357
    Scoliosis Test 358
    Slipped Disc Test 358
    Back Problems 359
    Bilateral Muscle Strength Test 360
    Breast Exam 360
    Fractured (Broken) Collarbone Test 360
    Fractured Limb Signs and Symptoms 360
    Gallbladder Symptoms 360
    Glossopharyngeal Nerve Test 361
    Gum Disease Signs 361
    Hearing and Loss Test 361
    Indication of Hearing Loss 361
    Hearing loss Test 361
    Hypoglossal (Tongue) Nerve Test 362
    Kidney Pain and Kidney Stones Test 362
    Large Intestine Examine 363
    Liver and Gallbladder Exam 363
    Lumber Lordosis Test 363
    Spine Exam 363
    Lung Vital Capacity and Peak Air Flow Test 364
    Match Test 364
    Lymph System Test 364
    Neck Lymph Nodes Exam 364
    Malocclusion (improper bite) Test 364
    Minimum Strength and Flexibility Test 364
    Motor Functioning 365
    Movement Sense Test 365
    Muscle Spasm Symptoms 365
    Myasthenia Gravis Test 365
    Tooth Nerve Damage 365
    Oculomotor (Eye) Nerve Test 365
    Olfactory (Smell) Nerve Test 366
    Optic Nerve and Eye Movement Test 366

Osteoarthritis Symptoms *366*
Overactive Thyroid Test *366*
Sensation in the Throat (Vagus Nerve) Test *366*
Scrotum, Testicles, and Inguinal Exam *367*
Small Intestine Exam *367*
Spinal Accessory Nerve Test *367*
Sport Injuries *367*
Stereognostic (Decoding) Sense Test *367*
Stomach Exam *367*
Stroke Symptoms *368*
Strabismus Eyes *368*
Superficial (Slight) Pain Sensation Test *368*
Tactile (Touch) Sensation Test *368*
Throat and Tonsils Exam *368*
Tendinitis Symptoms *370*
Tooth Sensitivity Test *370*
Underactive Thyroid Test *370*
Testing Procedure *370*
Visible Field Test *371*
Test Procedure *371*
Blood Pressure Interpretation *372*
How to use the Blood Pressure and Pulse Table *373*
Blood Pressure Chart *373*
pH Test Procedure *374*
pH Test *374*
How to Read Symptoms *374*
pH Disease Progression *374*
Multistix 10SG Test Procedure *374*
Multistix Urinalysis 10SG (SG=Specific Gravity) *375*
Interpretations *376*
Pulse Pressure *378*

Blood Test Interpretation **379**
Glucose *380*
Sodium *380*
Potassium *380*
Magnesium *381*
Chloride *381*
Blood Urea Nitrogen (BUN) *381*
Creatinine *382*
BUN/Creatinine Ratio *382*
Uric Acid *383*
Phosphorus *383*
Calcium *383*
Albumin *384*
Globulin *384*
Albumins and Globulin Ratio *385*
Alkaline Phosphatase *385*
SGPT/ALT & SGOT/AST *385*
GGT (Gamma-Glutamyl Transerase) *386*
LDH (Lactate Dehydroenase) *386*
Total Protein *387*
Iron *387*
Ferritin *387*
Triglycerides *388*

XII

Cholesterol *388*
LDL Cholesterol (Low Density Lipoproteins) *388*
HDL (High Density Lipoprotein) *389*
Cholesterol/ HDL Ratio *389*
CO2 (Carbon Dioxide) *389*
White Blood Cell (WBC) *390*
Neutrophils *390*
Monocytes *390*
Lymphocytes *391*
Eosinophils *391*
Red Blood Cells (RBC) *391*
Hemoglobin *392*
Hematocrit *392*
Reticulocyte Count *392*
Platelets (Thrombocytes) *393*
MCV (Mean Corpuscular Volume) *393*
MCH (Mean Corpuscular Hemoglobin) *393*
Thyroid Function *393*
T3 (Tri-Iodthyronine) *394*
T7 (FTI-Free Thyroxine Index) *394*
T3 Uptake *394*
TSH (Thyroid Stimulating Hormone) *394*
ESR (Erythrocyte Sedimentation Rate) *395*

Test (Nutrients, Biochemical Actions) 396

Breathe – Hold Test *397*
Pulse Challenge Food Sensitivity Testing *397*
Diet /Pulse Record *398*
Pulse Testing Individual Foods *398*
Diet /Pulse (3-day test record) *398*
Acid-Alkaline Imbalance Interpretation *399*
Respiratory Rate *400*
Urine Vitamin C Test *400*
Lingual Ascorbic Acid Test (Lingual-C) *401*
Iodine Patch Test *402*
Functions of Iodine *403*
Iodine Patch Test Form *403*
Zinc Challenge *405*
HCl (Hydrochloric Acid) Challenge Test *405*
Hypochlorhydria (low hydrochloric acid) *406*
HCl Challenge Test *407*
Basal Body Temperature Test *408*
Basal Body Temperature Test *409*
Bowel Transit Time *410*
Bile Transit Time Instruction for Self-Testing *413*
Respiratory Rate *414*
Increased Respiratory Rate (hyperventilation) *414*
Decrease Respiratory Rate *414*
Metabolic pH Assessment *414*
2° Buffering Systems *415*
Oxidata Free Radical Test *416*
High Increase In Oxidative Stress *417*
Oxidative Stress and Free Radicals *418*
Endogenous causes of free radicals *418*
Exogenous causes of free radicals *418*

Assessment of Acid/Alkaline Imbalances	419
Breathe holding time and respiration rate	419
Urine pH and Salivary pH	419
Breathe –Hold Test	419

Directions for Test 420

Lingual Ascorbic Acid Test	421
Dr. Bieler's Salivary pH Acid Challenge Test	421
Zinc Taste Test	421
Dr. Kane's Mineral Assessment Test	421
Urine Specific Gravity Use Multistix 10 SG Test	421
Urine Sediment Test	421
Calcium Phosphate Sediment	422
Urine pH Using pH Meter	422
Urinary Adrenal Test For Urinary Chloride	422
Urine Calcium Test	422
Gastro Test For Determining Stomach pH	422
Uric Acid Sediment	423
Calcium Oxalate Sediment	423
Oxidata Free Radical Test	423
Iodine Patch	423

Interpretations of Test Information 424

Metabolic pH Assessment	425
1°Buffering -- /the Bicarbonate Buffering System	425
1° Buffering System	427
Determination of Patterns of Acid/Alkaline Imbalance	428
Acid/Alkaline Assessment	429
Assessment	430
Calcium and Mineralization	431
Macronutrient Improper Digestion Patterns	432
Urine Bilirubin with Urine Urobilinogen levels	432
Acidic Urine – Urine pH < 6.4	433
Alkaline Urine – Urine pH> 6.8	433
Alkaline Saliva	433
Acidic Saliva	434
Commonly Used Chemical Notations	434
Common Signs and Symptoms of Acidosis and Alkalosis	435
Causes Of Respiratory Acidosis and Alkalosis	436
Causes of Metabolic Acidosis and Alkalosis	437
Salivary pH	438
Findings in Patterns of Acidosis and Alkalosis	438
Urine pH: >6.8	439
Subsequent Urine Samples	440
Alkaline Urine – Urine pH: >6.8	440
Urine pH: 5.65—6.8	440
Acidic Urine – Urine pH<6.4	440
Salivary pH	441
Alkaline Saliva	442
Acid Saliva	442

Medical Astrology 443

How to Do Your Astrology Chart	444
Anagrams	445
Zodiac Signs and Symbols	446
Element Evaluation	447

Quality Evaluation 447
Health House/ Planet Indicators 448
Glands and Signs 448
Rulers of the Houses 449
Triplicities Kinds of Houses 450
Quadruplicities Kinds of Houses 451
Aspects PLANETS DEGREES APART) 452
Moon Aspects 455
Mercury Aspects 456
Venus Aspects 457
Mars Aspects 458
Jupiter Aspects 459
Saturn Aspects 460
Uranus Aspects 461
Neptune Aspects 462

Houses of Zodiac 463
Ruling Planets 464
House of Zodiac 465

Zodiac Profiles 466
Aries (Born between March 21 – April 19) 467
Taurus (April 20 – May 20) 468
Gemini (May 21 – June 20) 469
Cancer (June 21 – July 22) 470
Leo (July 23 – August 22) 471
Virgo (August 23 – September 22) 472
Libra (September 23 – October 22) 473
Scorpio (October 23 – November 21) 474
Sagittarius (November 22 – December 21 475
DUALITY   Masculine 475
Capricorn (December 22 – January 19) 476
Aquarius (January 20 – February 18) 477
Pisces (February 19 – March 20) 478
Planet and Herbs 479

Medical Astrology Guidelines 480
Sun Health Profile 481
Sun In Signs 481
Sun in Houses 485
Moon Health Profile 486
Body Parts Ruled 487
Moon In Signs 487
Moon In Houses 490
Mercury Health Profile 491
Mercury In Signs 492
Mercury In Houses 493
Venus Health Profile 494
Venus In Signs 495
Venus In Houses 496
Mars Health Profile 497
Mars In Signs 498
Mars In Houses 499
Jupiter Health Profile 501
Jupiter In Signs 502
Jupiter In Houses 503

XV

Saturn Health Profile *504*
Saturn In Signs *505*
Saturn In Houses *506*
Uranus Health Profile *508*
Uranus In Signs *509*
Uranus In Houses *510*
Neptune Health Profile *511*
Neptune In Signs *511*
Neptune In Houses *512*
Pluto Health Profile *514*
General House Health *514*
Planets Afflicting Ascendant *516*
Very Poor Health Indications *516*
Signs of Long And Short Illness *516*
Ascendant And Descendant Health Profile *517*

Medical Abbreviations **535**
Medical Abbreviations *536*

Systems and Diseases **540**
System & Diagnosis *541*

Disease Analysis Charts **553**
Cardiovascular Disorders *554*
Blood Disorders *555*
Endocrine Disorders *556*
Heart Failure *557*
Joint Disorders *558*
Nervous System Disorders *561*
Disorders of the Urinary System *562*
Digestive System Disorders *563*
Nutritional and Metabolic Disorders *564*

Supplies **577**

Index **580**
Suggested Reading *584*

How to Do a Self-Diagnosis

Diagnosing Instructions

The body uses changes on the outside skin quality (eyes are a type of skin) and hair quality and quantity to indicate changes on the inside skin such as organs and parts. Any inconsistency on the outside indicates an inconsistency on the inside.

When examining and assessing changes in the body's health look for inconsistency such as:

1. Texture Changes; dry, smooth, rough, oily, tenderness to touch, rashes
2. Integrity Changes: bumps, cyst, sores, scratches, cold, hot, slight warmth, or cool skin areas, edema (swelling puffiness)
3. Color Changes: dark or light areas, redness, blotches, paleness
4. Hair Change: (on the head, body, eyebrow, eye lashes)—thinning, short or long areas, split ends, curliness, limpness, coarse, fine, dry, oily, discoloration
5. Note the Acupuncture Meridian and or Point: changes in the skin, hair, and/or muscle soreness, tension, flaccid, and rigidness on an organ, or system acupuncture meridian point.
6. Anatomical Irregularities such as misalignments, structural change: irregular widths and lengths increase or decrease in size and shapes of bones and muscles (not due to body building), posture changes.

Health Assessments

Health Assessments

The health assessment is holistic (spirit, mind, emotions, and body). Each section of the body can have factors that may have caused an illness. The part (lower, middle, upper) that has more physical abnormalities (inconsistencies) than another part is the primary one focused upon for treatment.

Holistic Health Chart

Mind (Lower)	**Lower Area**	**Middle Area**	**Upper Area**
Physical trauma that affect area	Sex organs, bladder related to kidneys, rectum related to intestine, lymph glands, nerves, back	Liver, gallbladder, pancreas, spleen, large and small intestines, digestion, nerves, lumbar and thoracic spine	Brain, lungs, heart, glands, cervical
Body (Middle)	**Past Events**	**Present Events**	**Future Events**
Excessive use, under use, unresolved issues, emotional injury	Unhealed past painful or unhappy social or emotional event that has distorted ones ability to live.	Present emotional behavior and or lifestyle have distorted the ability to interpret reality.	Distorted perception and conception of future creates painful and unhappy emotions.
Spirit (Upper)	**Creating your Spirit**	**Moving your Spirit**	**Spiritual Purpose**
	Lack of understanding or use of spiritual intelligence, searching for right path in life	Not achieving movement toward goals to satisfy spiritual needs	Inadequate or lack of serving God's purpose for your existence. Identify and knowing the reason why you were created?
Trimesters (three month segments)	**First** (three months)	**Second** (three months)	**Third** (three months)
Stress during prenatal growth	Bonding and/or Reattachment problems	Identity and/or Competence problems	Concern and/or Intimacy problems
Enzyme/System (weak, stressed or impaired)	Lipase, Digestion System	Amylase, Nervous System	Protease, Circulatory System

Self-Diagnosis Steps

1. Select a part of the body to examine. Use the illustrations, charts and or tables related to body sections.
2. Locate the Lower, Middle, and Upper sections of that body part.
3. Look for inconsistencies in the sections.
4. Identify which section (Lower, Middle, Upper) has the most inconsistencies.
5. Examine at least four parts of the body (looking for inconsistencies). You can examine more.
6. You can choose an objective test such as a pH Test and or Multistix 10SG test or the Blood Pressure Pulse Table. Objective test are not mandatory.
7. Identify the numbers on the objective test that are the furthest away from normal. Relate the numbers to an organ system and body section.
8. Use the results of the subjective examination and objective pH, Multistix 10SG and/or Blood Pressure Pulse Table to identify the cause of the health problem or disease.

Holistic Body

Organ Regions of the Body

The body was once an undifferentiated mass (an egg). All parts of the body were related to each other and specialization of parts of the egg produce organs and limbs. When parts of the egg began to separate and form organs and parts, the nerves related to those specific organs remained attached and grew longer. The nerves never lost their connection to the nucleus and/or central nervous system.

The three mayor divisions of the body are A= Upper Region, B= Middle Region, C= Lower Region. Spiritual Regions are A= Spiritual Purpose, B= Will your Spirit, C= Create Your Spirit. Holistic Regions A= Spirit, B=Mind, C=Body. Prenatal (before birth) Gestation Regions A= Third Trimester, B= Second Trimester, C= First Trimester.

Any inconsistency of skin integrity (discoloration, skin eruptions, excessive hotness or coldness, rashes, scratches) or slow blood refill when finger pressure is applied and then released) or pain, soreness or sensitiveness to touch, indicates that the organ related to that region is in a dis-ease condition or having problems.

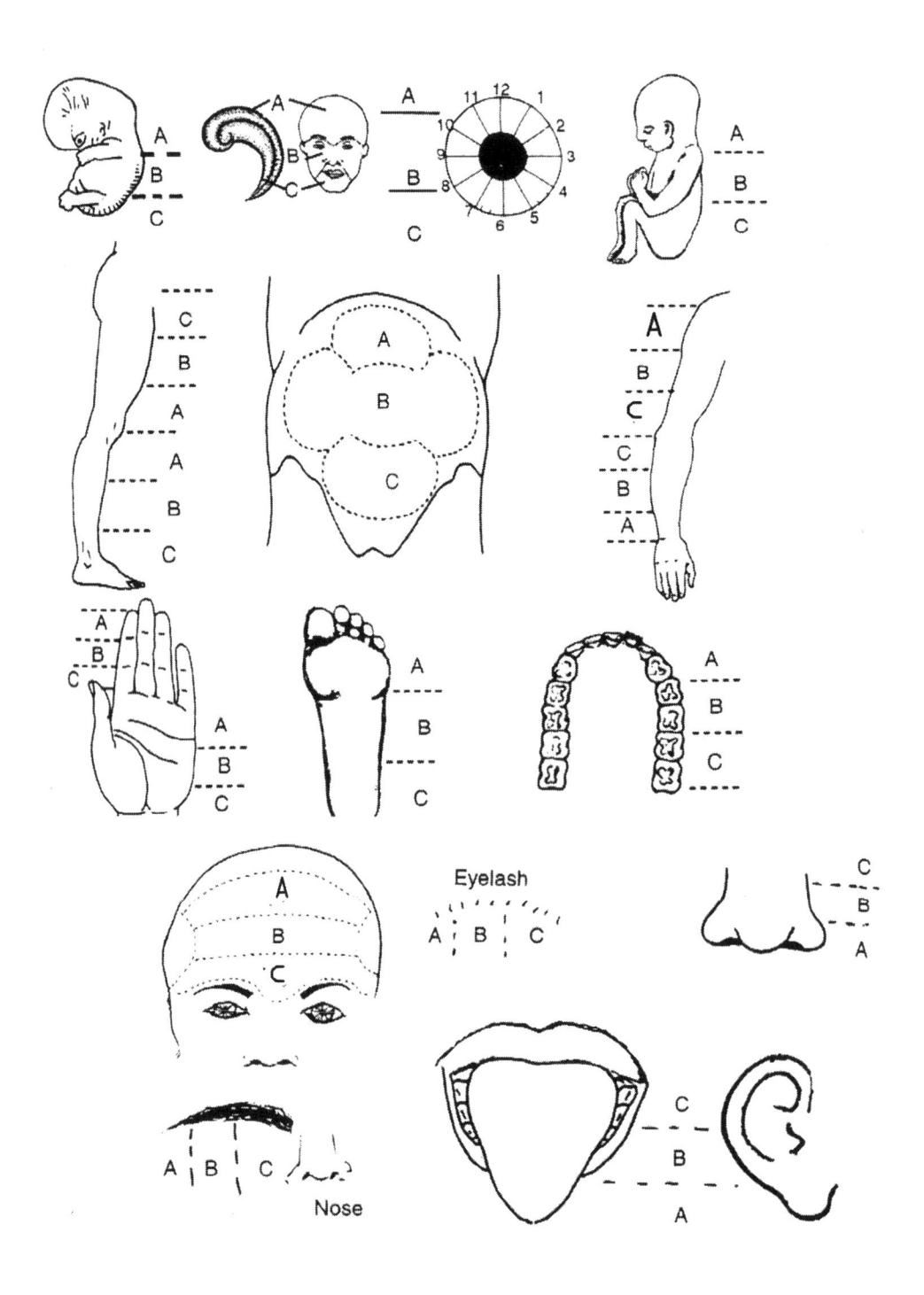

Human Development – Skin Layers

The body developed from one cell that became many types of skin (derma), each particular organ and bodily part developed from that derma layer. Consequently, organs and parts share a common derma ancestry and have a biochemical and DNA relationship, which can cause them to share disease. A disease to an organ or system affects all parts developed from that skin (derm) layer.

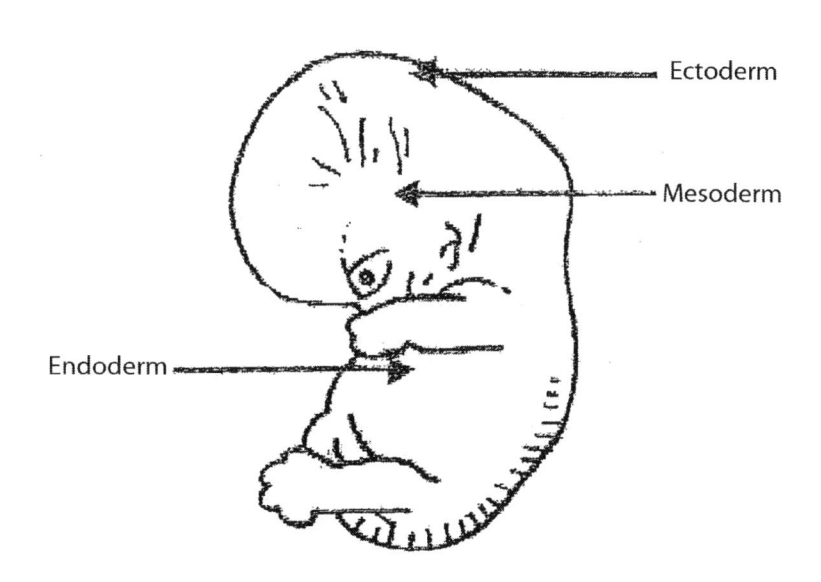

Types of Skin Layers

Mesoderm
Pineal Gland (melanin), brain, spinal cord, heart, muscle, cartilage, kidney, sex organs, bones, lymph
Ectoderm
Bladder, mouth, urethra, lens cornea, nasal cavity, skin
Endoderm
Liver, pancreas, lungs, thyroid

Embryonic Body

The Male Principle is expressed by the neurons of the brain, blood, which is red and active. Under the Female Principle is the Glia cells of the brain, lymph, which is clear and gathers the used body fluid from the periphery and moves back to the heart. These systems are distributed (Female), and gathering (Male).

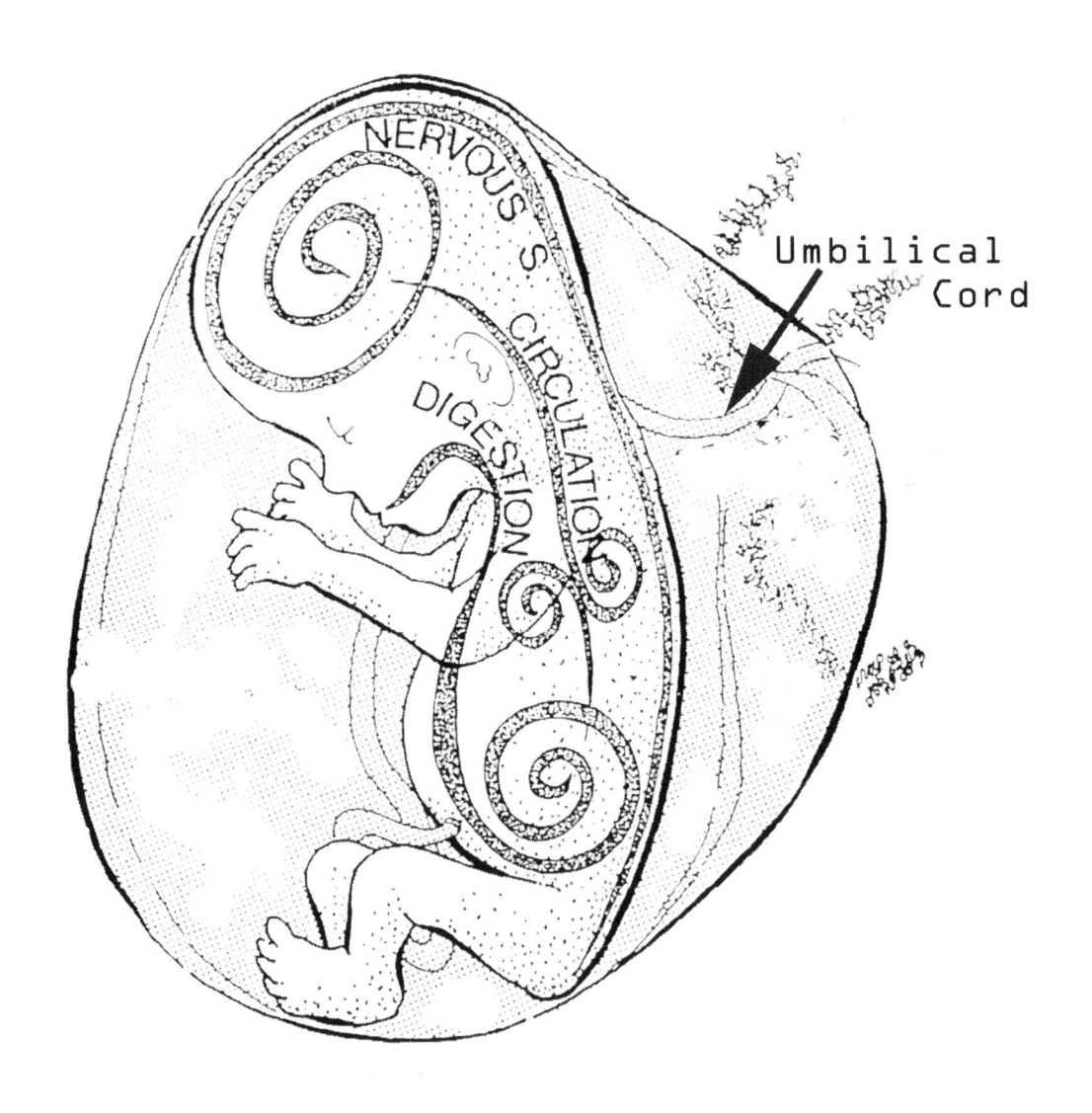

The position of the three major systems in the embryo

Embryo Energy

Embryonic Formation of Organs and Extremities (Arms and Legs)

Embryonic Formation of the Systems

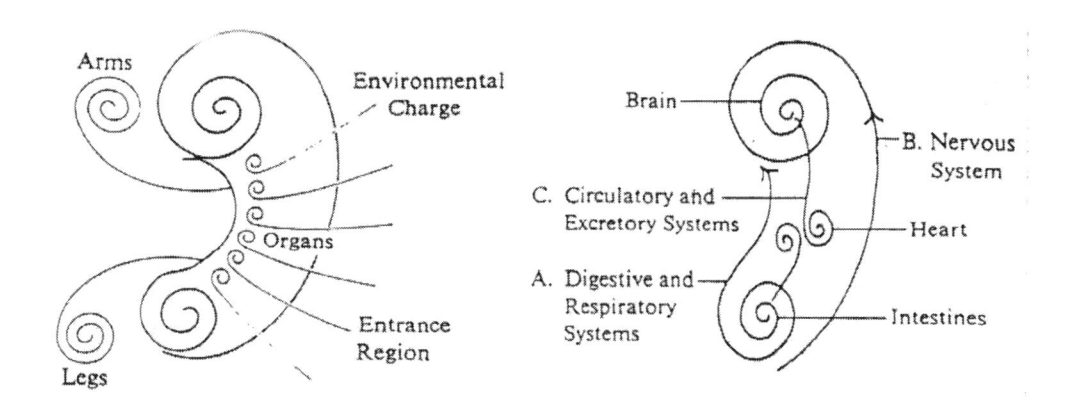

These electromagnetic and biochemical spirals develop into organs and functions, and move upward and downward in direction. Electromagnetic and biochemical energy is stimulated and moves outward toward the peripheral parts of both sides of the embryo. Electromagnetic and biochemical energy moves inward and downward toward the central part of the embryo. These energies form outer spirals, upper spirals, and lower spirals, and develop as arms and legs. Accordingly, electromagnetic and biochemical currents running through the arms and legs in the form acupuncture (meridians) energy highways.

Energy Meridians (Acupuncture Highways)

Male Principle (Compacted) Organs
Female Principle (Slow) movement
Lungs
Spleen and Pancreas
Heart
Kidneys
Circulation
Liver
Glia cells of brain

Female Principle (expanded) Organs
Male Principle (active) Movement
Large Intestine
Stomach
Small Intestine
Bladder
Metabolism
Gall Bladder
Neuron cells of the brain

Arms	Legs
Lung Meridian	Spleen Meridian
Large Intestine Meridian	Liver Meridian
Circulation Meridian	Stomach Meridian
Metabolism Meridian	Gall Bladder Meridian
Heart Meridian	Bladder Meridian
Small Intestine Meridian	Kidney Meridian

Energy Centers

In the body there are the Male and Female Principles energies–front (Female Principle), solid (Male Principle), liquid (Female Principle), and air (Male Principle) are all taken in by the front systems (digestive and respiratory). They are part of the back system (nervous). Food is classified acid under the Male Principle, is drawn downwards spirally and radiates from the center. Magnetic/Electrical energy, which classified alkaline under the Female Principle, tends to go upwards, in a spiral motion, to the brain. The two regions are the "Solar Plex" and the "Third Eye".

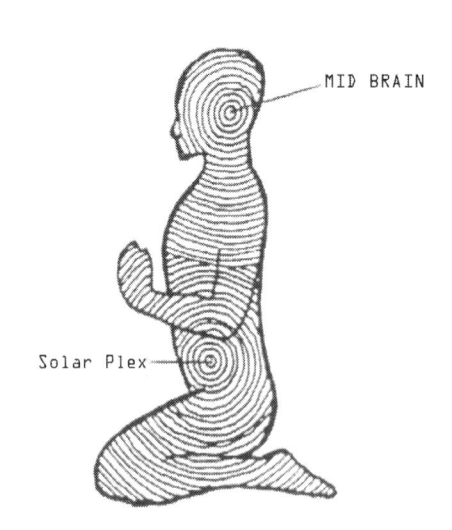

The circulatory, digestive and nervous systems concentrate at the mouth. This section is the most concentrated and Male Principle. The Male Principle can gather and take in. Whether the section of the mouth is Female or Male is the determining factor of each individual's personality or spirituality. This section indicates the body's individuality and functioning.

Embryo Position

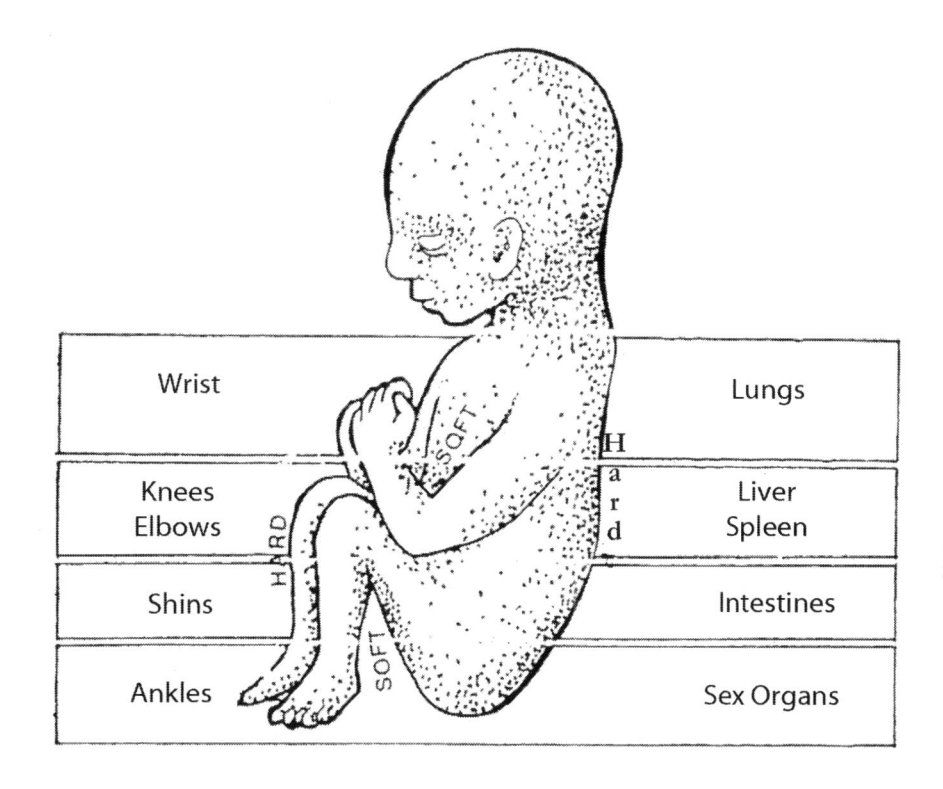

Wrist	Lungs
Knees / Elbows	Liver / Spleen
Shins	Intestines
Ankles	Sex Organs

The internal organs are related to the embryonic developmental position of the arms and legs. The ankles and buttocks are related to organs in that section (sexual organs). The middle section of the legs is related to the digestive organs. The section around the elbow and knees are related to the liver, spleen and pancreas. The hands developmental position was organs in that section (lungs). The hands were folded across the face. After birth, the arms hang at the sides and take on a relationship to organs in that section. The wrist section begins to relate to the sexual functions. If the wrist is stiff, it can indicate the sexual section is blocked, or rigid. If the wrist is flexible, the sexual organs are functioning well. If the wrist holds the hand in a limp position the sex organs are weak or deteriorating.

Circadian Rhythm and Organs

The circadian (circle, cycle) rhythm of organs indicates the optimum energy producing and cleansing time for an organ. When an organ is stressed, weak, ill, deteriorating, and /or malfunctioning the individual either feels their best or worse at that time.

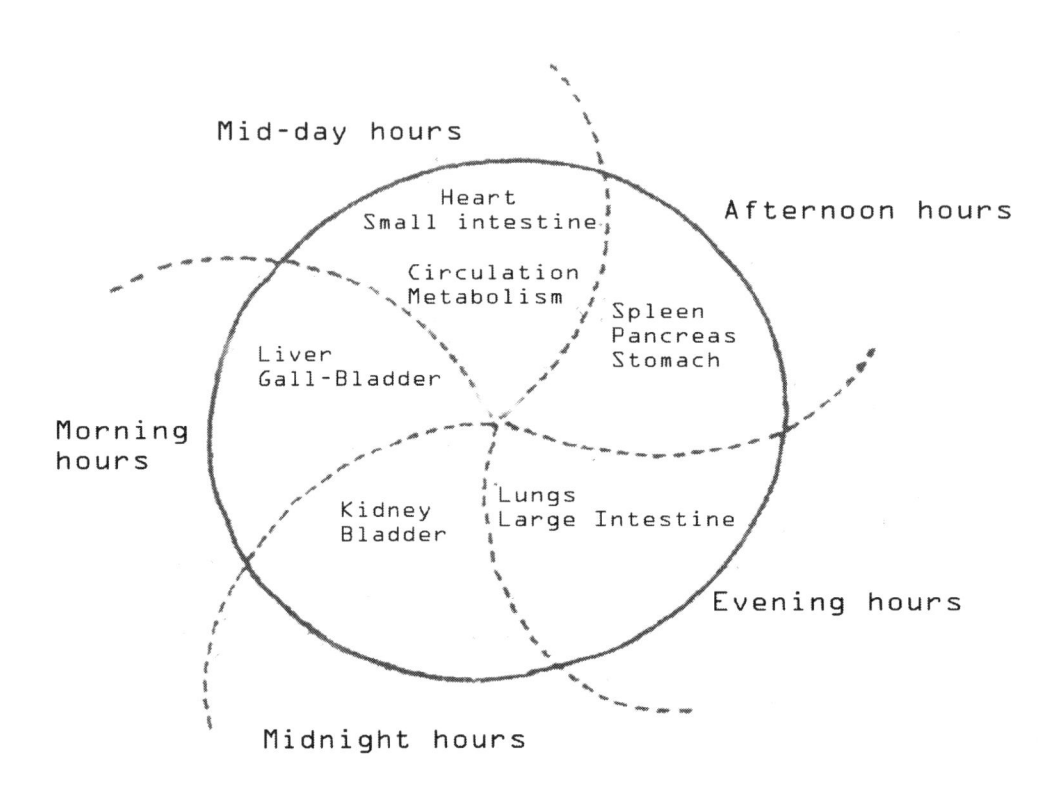

```
                    Mid-day hours
                       Heart
                       Small intestine      Afternoon hours
                       Circulation
                       Metabolism
                                      Spleen
                                      Pancreas
                       Liver          Stomach
                       Gall-Bladder
Morning
hours
                       Kidney    Lungs
                       Bladder   Large Intestine
                                              Evening hours

                    Midnight hours
```

Organ Function Cycle (24 Hour)

1 AM LIVER (LV)
3 AM LUNGS (LG)
5 AM LARGE INTESTINE (LI)
7 AM STOMACH (ST)
9 AM SPLEEN (SP)
11AM HEART (HT)
1PM SMALL INTESTINE (SI)
3PM BLADDER (BL)
5 PM KIDNEY (KD)
7PM METABOLISM (M)
9PM CIRCULATION (C)
11PM GALL BLADDER (GB)

Weight of Organs (not a complete listing)

The Liver and Brain each weigh approximately 1.45 kilograms (3 pounds). The Lungs weigh approximately 450 grams (1 pound), which is equal to the weight of a soccer ball (450 grams) and a little less than the weight of a basketball (624 grams). The Stomach and Spleen each weigh approximately 170 grams (6 ounces), which is the weight of a pool (billiard) ball that is 160 grams (5 ounces). The Eyeball weighs 25 grams (1 ounce), which is half the weight of a tennis ball (2 ounces = 58 grams). The Skin weighs 9 pounds.

Energy Transformation Movement

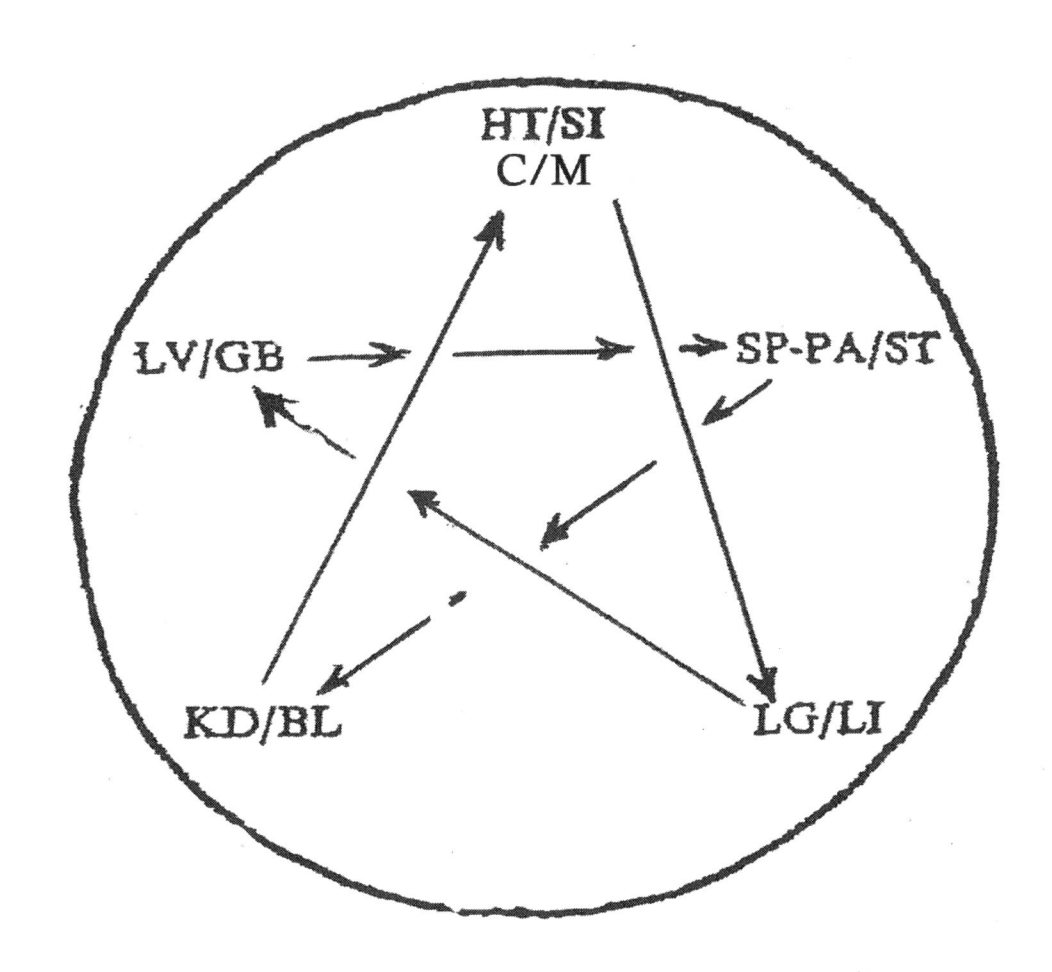

Sympathetic, (Contracted, Male Principle)	Parasympathetic (Expanded, Female Principle)
LV/ GB-Liver and Gallbladder	SP-PA/ST- Spleen, Pancreas, and Stomach
HT//SI Heart and Small Intestine	LG/LI Lungs and Large Intestine
C/M Circulatory and Metabolism	KD/BL- Kidneys and Bladder

Male/Female Principle

Male/Female Principle

The Self Diagnosis methods help you to understand that the body has rigid fixed biochemical, pH, hormonal, psychological, spiritual, and electrical responses. The actions and reactions are bipolar (Male Principle, Female Principle). The body will not simultaneously have both responses together. The body will not breath in oxygen (inhale) and breath out carbon dioxide (exhale) at the same time. It will make a choice to do one or the other and never both. The autonomic nervous system is bipolar (Male and Female Principle). It will not completely turn on the sympathetic nervous system (Male Principle) and the parasympathetic nervous system (Female Principle) simultaneously. This is a fixed rigid rule of the body. The body will not let a woman be simultaneously half pregnant and half not pregnant. The body will not allow you to be sick and healthy simultaneously or have cancer that is sleep in the body and yet not have cancer. The body chooses one or the other. Therefore, you are pregnant or not pregnant, dead or alive, sick or healthy and have cancer or do not have cancer.

Whenever there is a choice between an action or reaction the body will choose either the Male Principe or Female Principle. When pinpointing the cause of the disease you should identify the body's biochemical response as the Male or Female Principle. For example, you have a choice between two body fluids urine and saliva. Urine is destroyed liquid food nutrients (liquid left after metabolizing food, juice, and or water) while saliva is a fluid enzyme used to nourish the body. The Male Principle is associated with waste, destruction, analytical thinking (breaking rationales apart) and action. Consequently, urine is Male. There is over activity (hyper=action) and under activity (hypo=relaxation). Therefore, hyperactivity is Male and hypoactivity is Female. Further, the heart has an action phase (systolic) and a resting phase (diastolic). The systolic is Male and diastolic is Female. There are two jawbones and two eyelids. The upper eyelid and lower jawbone moves more (Male) than the lower eyelid, and upper jaw (Female). Once a bodily action and/or reaction is classified as Male all the factors in the category Male are included such as pH acid, insulin hormone, burning of starch, focusing on the future life, moving (will) the spirit, left Hemisphere of the brain etc.

All health and disease action and reactions of the body are bipolar and holistic. Each action and reaction requires a change in the ratio of elements, vitamins, minerals, amino acids, fats, proteins, neurotransmitters, enzymes, hormones, and chemicals in the body. A change in the body's elements that make bio-chemicals has an effect on the brain's elements that make thoughts emotions and spirit vitality. Consequently, looking at all the factors in the category Male and Female Principles gives you a holistic picture of the biochemical elements that make behavior and physiological functions.

The science of biology and chemistry uses numbers and letters (mathematics) to talk about facts, and beliefs (theories). People and scientist use Logic/Rationales (mathematics) to explain Emotions (theories) and use Emotions (beliefs) to explain Logic (surveys, statistics, and polls which is Mob Rule). The Male Principle is used to explain the Female Principle and the Female Principle is used to explain the Male Principle. The mathematical language is another way of talking. Numbers translated into words. For example, the potential of Hydrogen (pH) is evaluated with a pH test. Consequently, the number 6.0 means Acid and the number 7.0 means alkaline. The holistic translation of 6.0 means acid, sympathetic stress, insulin, left hemisphere of the brain, mental focus on the future, the burning of starches, moving the spirit negatively toward your purpose, systolic and the Male Principle. Numbers are generated by using biochemical test and are objective measurements. The Multistix 10SG (SG=Specific Gravity) is an objective test that generates numbers. In Science the biochemical language of High Specific Gravity, Hemolyzed Blood and High Turbidity is another chemical method of saying Male Principle. There are many different words (languages) used to say Male or Female Principles. The changing from one word to another does not change the physiological processes. For example "breath-in", inhale, inspiration and aerobic while "breath-out" words are exhale, expiration and anaerobic. The words change the process remains the same.

Male/Female Principle Chart

There are many different words used to describe and define the body's various biochemical, physiology, hormonal, and psychological actions and reactions. Below is a brief list of those different words:

The Male Principle	The Female Principle
Go	Stop
Sympathetic	Parasympathetic
Acid (fast moving)	Alkaline (slow moving)
Vertical	Horizontal
Destruction	Construction
Catabolic	Anabolic
Anaerobic	Aerobic
Systolic	Diastolic
Melanin insufficient	Melanin deficient
High specific gravity	Low specific gravity
Hemolyzed	Non-hemolyzed
Action	Relaxation
Future	Past
Left brain (Rationale, Analytical, Realistic)	Right brain (Emotional, Harmonizer, Idealistic)
Lower jaw	Upper jaw
Incisors	Molars
Think 1st, Feel 2nd	Feel 1st, Think 2nd
Contraction	Expansion
Constipation	Diarrhea
Insulin	Glucagon
Carbohydrates	Fats
Urine - waste	Saliva – enzymes
Bright colors	Dark colors
Objective	Subjective
High turbidity	Low turbidity
High pulse	Low pulse
Science	Art
Salt	Sugar
Vagina	Penis
Fight/Flight	Tend/Befriend
Oxidant (oxidize)	Antioxidant
Extroverted	Introverted
Neurons of brain	Glia cells of brain
Acetylcholine	Dopamine
Explicit	Implicit

Sympathetic (Male Principle)/ Parasympathetic (Female Principle) Actions

One part of the biochemical/reactions is on standby (low energy state) while the other is active.

Sympathetic	Parasympathetic
H+	OH-
Calcium: Potassium	Potassium, Sodium, Magnesium
Adrenal Medulla: Thyroid	Pancreas Tail: Pancreas Head
Hypothalamus: Pineal	Thymus: Parotid
Testosterone: Progesterone	Estrogen
G.I. Sphincters	G.I. Lumen motility: G.I. secretion & salivary glands
Sphincter of Vater	Gall Bladder & Bile Ducts
Liver glycogen mobilization	None
Respiratory center	Bronchial muscles & glands
None	Nasal & Pharyngeal secretion
None	Larynx
Myocardium	None
Vasomotor activity (constriction and dilation)	None
Pupil dilators: muscles of Muller (exophtalmous)	Pupil constrictors: muscles of the iris: muscles of accommodation: levator palpbrae (exoptholmous)
None	Lacrimal secretion
Prostate: Cowpers and Bartholins	Prostate: Cowpers and Bartholins release of secretion
Penis Flaccid	Penis Erection
Vagina Muscles Active	Vaginal Muscles Inactive
Bladder trigonum and sphincters: urethra	Bladder wall
Pilomotor activity: sweet secretory activity	None
None	Histamine

Sympathetic	Parasympathetic
Pulse increased	Pulse decreased
Respiratory rate increased	Respiratory rate decreased
Systolic BP & pulse pressure increased	Orthostatic failure of systolic BP & pulse pressure
Pupil large	Pupil small
Oliguria	Polyuria
Temperature increased	Temperature decreased
Cold sweats on hands or, cold dry hands	Hands warm and dry
Tremors	Cough reflex easily stimulated
Nervous tension: insomnia	Nervous tension: depression
Dry mouth	Saliva quality increased
None	Tear quality increased
Exophtalmous	Enophtalmous usual: exophtalmous with irritation if cranial nerve III (e.g. from exophthalmic goiter) which results in contracture of the levator pulpebrae
Glucose increased	Glucose decrease (or increased)
WBC decreased	WBC increased
Low resistance to infection, Rheumatoid Arthritis	Osteoarthritis
Poor circulation associated with vasoconstriction	Poor circulation associated with decreased pulse pressure
Indigestion: ulcers, gall bladder or bowel problems	Indigestion: ulcers, bowel problems, colitis
Food allergies	Allergies, asthma
High energy	Low energy
Pathological Disintegration	Pathological Hyperplasia

Physical Aspects Influenced by the Parasympathetic Nervous System (Female Principle)

RIGHT BRAIN: intuitive and special capacities

HYPOTHALAMUS: anterior medial

POSTERIOR PITUITARY GLAND: produces two hormones, controls metabolism, blood pressure, kidney function, smooth muscle action

PINEAL GLAND: is responsive to light, reproductive cycles and pigment

PAROTID GLANDS: helps conserve DNA material, stimulates parasympathetic organs and glands

PARATHYROIDS: Parathyroid hormones releases calcium from bones

TONSILS: immune system organ, infection warning system

THYMUS: immune system organs

LUNGS: carbon dioxide, oxygen and waste gases exchange from blood

LIVER: energy storage, food processing, detoxification,

GALLBLADDER: bile storage

ADRENAL CORTEX: outer produces several hormones; controls swelling, inflammation, sodium potassium balance: glucocosticoid stimulate production of carbohydrates fom proteins

STOMACH: produces hydrochloric acid for digestion

PANCREAS: stimulated by vagus nerve, produces digestive enzymes: carbohydrate metabolism

SPLEEN: immune system organ, blood regulation

DUODENUM: first part of small intestine: contains opening of pancreatic duct and absorption

SMALL INTESTINE: digestion and absorption

LARGE INTESTINE: B vitamins manufactured, water absorbed

APPENDIX: immune system organ, regulates blood cell production

Female Principle/Parasympathetic Dominant

Dominant types tend to have many of these symptoms such as:

Craving for acid foods	Fast, strong digestion
Alcoholism (because alcohol raises blood sugar)	Diverticulosis
Alkalosis	Drooling
Allergies	Dropsy
Excessive appetite	Drowsiness
Arthritis (osteoarthritis, hypertrophic)	Eczema
Asthenia (weakness)	Edema
Atherosclerosis	Emphysema
Asthma	Energy gain after eating
Loss of control of bladder	Energy loss after sweets
Blackouts	Fatigue
Bloating	Good fat metabolism
Low blood pressure	Foul smelling gas
Easy bowel movements	Gingivitis
Bone breaks	Growling gut
Brucellosis (fever)	Bleeding gums
Colds, flu, gripe	Receding gums
Cold sores, fever blisters	Oily hair
Mucous colitis	Hay fever
Chronic cough	Headaches, eyestrains
Cough up mucous	Slow healing bones
Cramps	Hepatitis
Dandruff	Hernia
Dermatitis	Herpes simplex
	Herpes zoster (shingles)
Diarrhea	Hiccups

Female Principle/Parasympathetic Characteristics

Tend to have many of these symptoms:

Extremely sluggish	Very enlarged, round chest
Actions are relaxed, calm, firm, and positive	Ruddy complexion, good face color
Desires to be cautious	Often feel sad or dejected
Slow to make decisions	Very good digestion
Crave butter/fatty foods like cream sauce	Above normal appetite
Difficulty in holding urine	Crave salty food
Bowel movements easy to start	Crave fatty meats
Slow breathing rate	Dreams are vivid and often in color
Frequently coughing up mucus	Recall most dreams
Frequent deep cough	Not much "get up and go"
Eyes look sunken in	Fall asleep quickly
Oily skin	Urinate several times a day
Feel better after eating at bedtime	Gums dark pink or bluish
Eating fruits causes jitters	Excessive saliva
Feel better and satisfied when eating meat	Strong hunger pains
Emotional stability	Intestines rumble and growl a lot
Marked endurance	Eyestrain causes headache
Intensely dislike exercise	Hard to get going in the morning
Thin, scanty eyebrows	Seldom gets angry
Droopy or soggy eyelids	Energy is elevated after eating
Very little fear	Dreams frequently

The most often needed nutritional support for the parasympathetic type includes Vitamin E and niacinamide, pantothenic acid, choline, inositol, calcium, phosphorus, calcium ascorbate, bioflavo comples, zinc and RNA.

Female Principle/Parasympathetic
Dominant Metabolizer:

Histamine reactions (redness caused by histadine)	Good oxygen metabolism
Hives	Post nasal drip
Hoarseness	Good protein metabolism
Hydration	Psoriasis
Hypoglycemia	Pyorrhea
Vital infections	Sexual problems, impotence
Intermittent claudication (limping)	Itching skin
Jittery feeling	Sleepwalking
Leg ulcers	Sluggish
Leukemia	Sneezing attacks
Leucopoenia (low white blood cells)	Stomach pain, excessive hydrochloric acid
Lymphoma (tissue growth in lymph)	Telangiectasis (sores of vascular)
Melanoma (tumor)	Tingling in extremities
Nausea from eye strain	Duodenal ulcer
Obesity	Urinary incontinence
Osteoporosis	Sudden urge to urinate
Perondontoclasia (inflamed degenerating gums)	Ease in focusing eyes
Strong reaction to poison ivy, poison oak	Warts
Phlebitis (inflamed veins)	

Physical Aspects influenced by the Sympathetic Nervous System (Male Principle)

LEFT BRAIN: verbal and analytical capacity

Posterior Lateral HYPOTHALAMUS

THALAMUS: switchboard to higher brain centers

ANTERIOR PITUITARY GLAND: works in balance with thyroid, adrenal and gonads: the following hormones:
1. GH (growth hormone): bone and general body growth, physical shape
2. TSH (thyroid stimulating hormone); stimulates formation and growth of thyroid gland
3. ACTH (adrenal cortex stimulating hormones): stimulates formation of adrenal cortex hormones
4. LH, FSH, beta-LPH

THYROID: produces thyroxin, increases activity of cells, regulates metabolism and calcitonin for depositing calcium in bones and tissues

HEART

ADRENAL MEDULLA: (inner) produce adrenaline, controls 'fight or flight' reaction

KIDNEYS
URETER
OVARIES
UTERUS
BLADDER
PROSTATE
URETHRA
TESTES

Genito –URINARY SYSTEM:
Kidney, Bladder, Urethra, Ureters

REPRODUCTIVE SYSTEM:
Ovaries, Uterus, Testes, Prostate

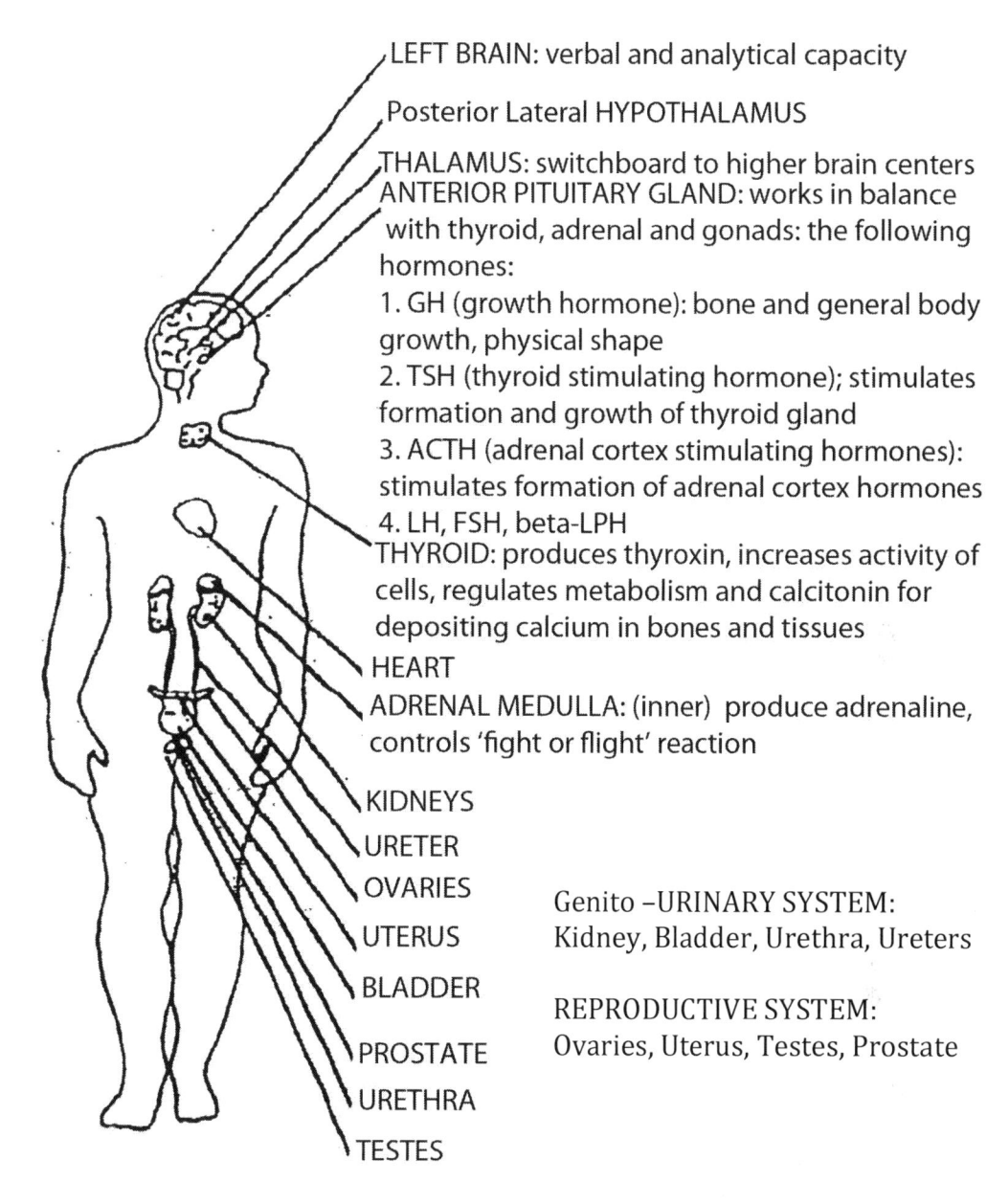

Sympathetic Anatomy

Skeletal system	Ligaments, connective tissue
Muscle system	Arteries
Cardiovascular system	Veins
Neuromuscular system	Capillaries
Urinary system	Calcium metabolism
Reproductive system	

Physical Aspects Influenced by the Sympathetic Nervous System (Male Principle)

Dominant types tend to have many of these signs and symptoms such as:

Tends to make decisions	Enjoy vegetables
Actions usually abrupt	Food eaten before bedtime interferes with sleep
Extremely active	Enjoys exercise
Angers easily	Thick eyebrows
Usually underweight	Sleep difficulties
Rapid breathing	Eyelids are open wide
Irregular breathing	Strong emotions
Outward eye protrude	Increase sexual desire
Soles of feet soft and no callous	Fingernails have many cross-ridges
Thin, flat chest	Gag easily
Bowel movements normally light in color	Skin easily forms "gooseflesh"
Increased ability to concentrate high	Dry mouth
Craves sweets, fruits	Tendency to have colds
Seldom depressed	Poor gum circulation
Fatty or oily foods dislike	Severe indigestion
Weak dreams if any	Impatient, irritable
Poor dream recall	Firm muscle tone
Seldom dream	Pupils of eyes usually large
Energetic	Unexpected noise
Dry hair	Thick, ropy saliva
Dry skin	Skin usually soft and feels velvety
Very jumpy and nervous	

Male Principle/Sympathetic Metabolizers

Tend to have these physical problems

Cystitis (inflamed bladder)	Kidney infections
Dehydration	Kidney stones
Diabetes	Night restless in legs
Slow digestion	Dry mouth
Dizziness	Myocarditis
Earache	Nephritis
Easily upset emotionally	Nervous strain
Lack of endurance	Numbness, nerve damage
Low energy reserve	Poor oxygen metabolism
Epilepsy	Unusual sensitivity to pain
Cool extremities	Pellagra (vitamin B3 deficient)
Dry eyes	Peyronie's disease (hardening of the penis skin)
Slow fat metabolism	Photophobia
Food feels heavy in stomach	Pneumonia
Function well in hot weather	Poor protein metabolism
Febrile diseases	Fast pulse
Chokes easily	Purpura (hemorrhage into skin)
Sweet smelling gas	Rheumatic fever
Glossitis	Sensitivity to light
Goiter	Sensitivity to shots
Gout	Dry, Thick skin
Halitosis	Sour stomach
Dry light, ribbony stools	Gastric ulcers
Little sweating	Uremia (kidney does not excrete nitrogenous substance)
Pearly white teeth	Frequent urination
Tinnitus (ringing in ears)	Varicose veins
Tonsillitis	Vincent's infection (mouth sores, swollen lymph)
Muscle tremors	
Difficulty in focusing eyes	

Male/Female Principle Chart

Principle	Blood Pressure	Fluid	pH	Pancreas Hormone	Food	Time	Spirit
Male	Systolic	Urine	Acid	Insulin	Starches	Future	Move
Female	Diastolic	Saliva	Alkaline	Glucagon	Fats	Past	Create

Brain/Hemisphere

Male-Left Hemisphere	**Female-Right Hemisphere**
Neuron brain cells	Glia brain cells

Personality Diagnosis

Extrovert and Introvert Personality Traits

The category that has the most traits identifies a personality characteristic.

Extrovert	Introvert
Socializer	Loner
Needs increase emotional and intellectual stimulation	Decrease (very little) emotional and intellectual stimulation
For Extrovert to understand an Introvert add emotions to their words	For an Introvert to understand an Extrovert subtract emotions out of their words
Noise/Music increase awareness	Noise/ impairs awareness
Acts then Thinks	Thinks then Acts
Thinks out loud (talks to self)	Thinks introspectively (quiet)
Confronts conflict	Avoids conflict
Multitasker	Single Tasker
Quick to make decisions	Slow to make decision, increases accuracy
"What is" are concerns	"What if" are concerns
Brain's Back Insula Lobe integrates Occipital, Parietal and Temporal Lobes	Brain's Front Insula Lobe evaluates negative and positive aspects of other lobes input
Less saliva secreted when lemon juice placed on tongue	Increase Saliva
Cingulate Gyrus Fork (variety, new experiences, quick stimulation)	Left Mid-Cingulate (analytical, evaluate, concentrate)
Temporal Lobe (signal motor area to move body, short term memory)	Frontal Lobe (abstract, processes long term memory)
Hypothalamus (evaluates and acts upon emotions)	Thalamus (selects emotions to act upon)
Long nerve Allele requires increase stimulation for response	Short nerve Allele less stimulation required
Uses Brain Stem, Limbic System in cognitive ability (past and present emotions/thought)	Uses Brain Stem, Limbic System and Neocortex (past, present and future thought/emotion)
Desires Dopamine to regulate behavior emotion, Dopamine Regulating (DRD4) gene	Desires Serotonin to regulate behavior/emotions. Serotonin Regulating (SERT) gene
Tendency for eyes to dilates more when stimulated	Tendency for less dilation of eyes
Tendency for less sweating from physical/emotion stimulation	Increase sweating
Uses mostly Brain's Neuron cells	Uses mostly Brains Glia cells

Personality Styles and Types Diagnosis

A person tends to use a mixture of styles and types but will dominate in a specific one.

Thinking Styles

Style	Tendency	Speech	Dominate Words	When Conversations dominate in Different Thinking styles
Realistic	Focus upon immediate problems or issue	Uses descriptive words and short or direct statements	"Everybody knows that,". " Its obvious that…."	Tends to get agitated, appears rigid
Critical/Analytical	Focus upon structured, rational sequential ideas to support their opinion	Uses organized and extended statements	"It stand s to reason…" "If you look at it logically.."	Tends to withdraw and becomes aloof. Emotionless facial expression, seems non-involved
Harmonizer	Focus on others feelings, ideas concepts, opinions eliminates contradictions	Uses statements to explain different points of views	"On the other hand.." "That's not always true.."	Tends to make others opinions foolish and makes fun of others ideas. Seems to be a troublemaker
Idealistic	Focus on purpose, and goals. Desires perfect emotions, behaviors, social situations and /or society.	Uses indirect questions, talks about values and feelings	"It seems to me…" "Don't you think"?	Tends to appear hurt. Sound resentful and disappointed

Listening Styles

Style	Listening Preference
Information	Listens to gather information. Does not have a goal or focus for information. Collects data but fails to organize it. In conversation uses information to get attention or appear smart.
Enhancer	Listens for beneficial or valuable ideas that can improve their life or help others. Favors information that can solve social or medical problems.
Critical	Listens to criticize opinions of others mistakes in logic or debatable issues or ideas or points of disagreement. Tends to criticize the speaker.

Learning Type

Type	Definition	Statements /Phrases
Visual	Tends to use words that are associated with sight (seeing)	"I don't see the point", "Is it clear", "See what I am saying", "That idea is foggy", "See it my way"
Rhythm/Touch	Tends to use words that are associated with physical activities, the sense of touch and taste	"Touchy subject", "That hurt my feelings", "I don't feel that", "That moved me", "Do you feel me",
Auditory	Tends to use words that are associated with sound	"That was a blast", "Shoot, I missed that", "That sounds stupid", "That gave me a buzz"

Learning Style

Style	Description
Random	They tend to switch/skip to one idea or activity before completion of first task. They seem to have an accidental process and lack a define plan. They start and stop task and multitask. Conversations change focus or topic in mid sentence.
Sequential	They tend to follow a series of step-by-step arrangements or procedures. They start a task and finish it, then start another task. Conversations are orderly and focused on one subject at a time.
Abstract	They require written instructions or a brief description to understand a task. They tend to use one idea/metaphor to represent another statement. Their statements can seem irrational and meaningless.
Concrete	They tend to require ideas or instructions to relate to actual events, specific real objects, places, and things. They require physical description or a picture to understand a task.

Digestion

Digestive System

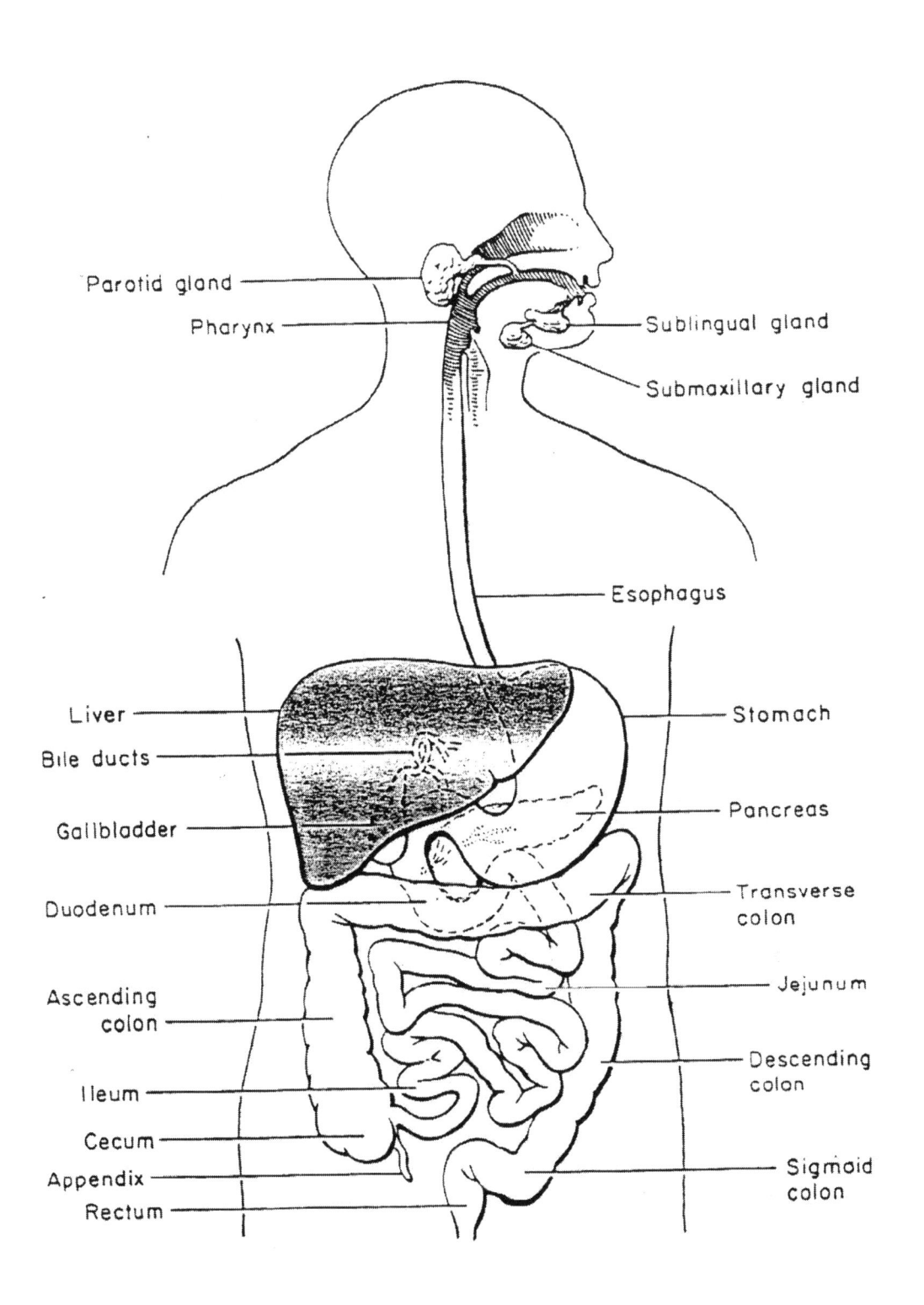

Location of Metabolism of Food Types

The darken areas indicate metabolism location

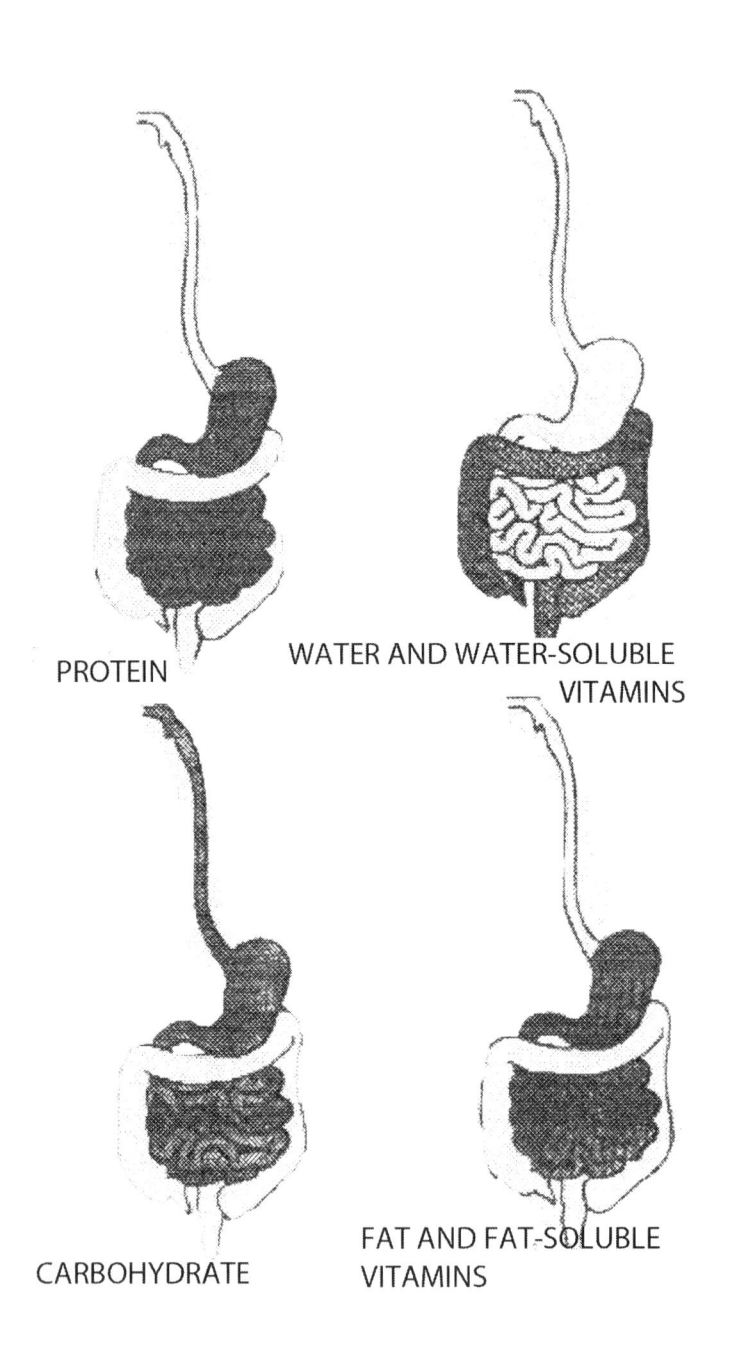

PROTEIN

WATER AND WATER-SOLUBLE VITAMINS

CARBOHYDRATE

FAT AND FAT-SOLUBLE VITAMINS

Digestion, Urine and Saliva Flow Chart

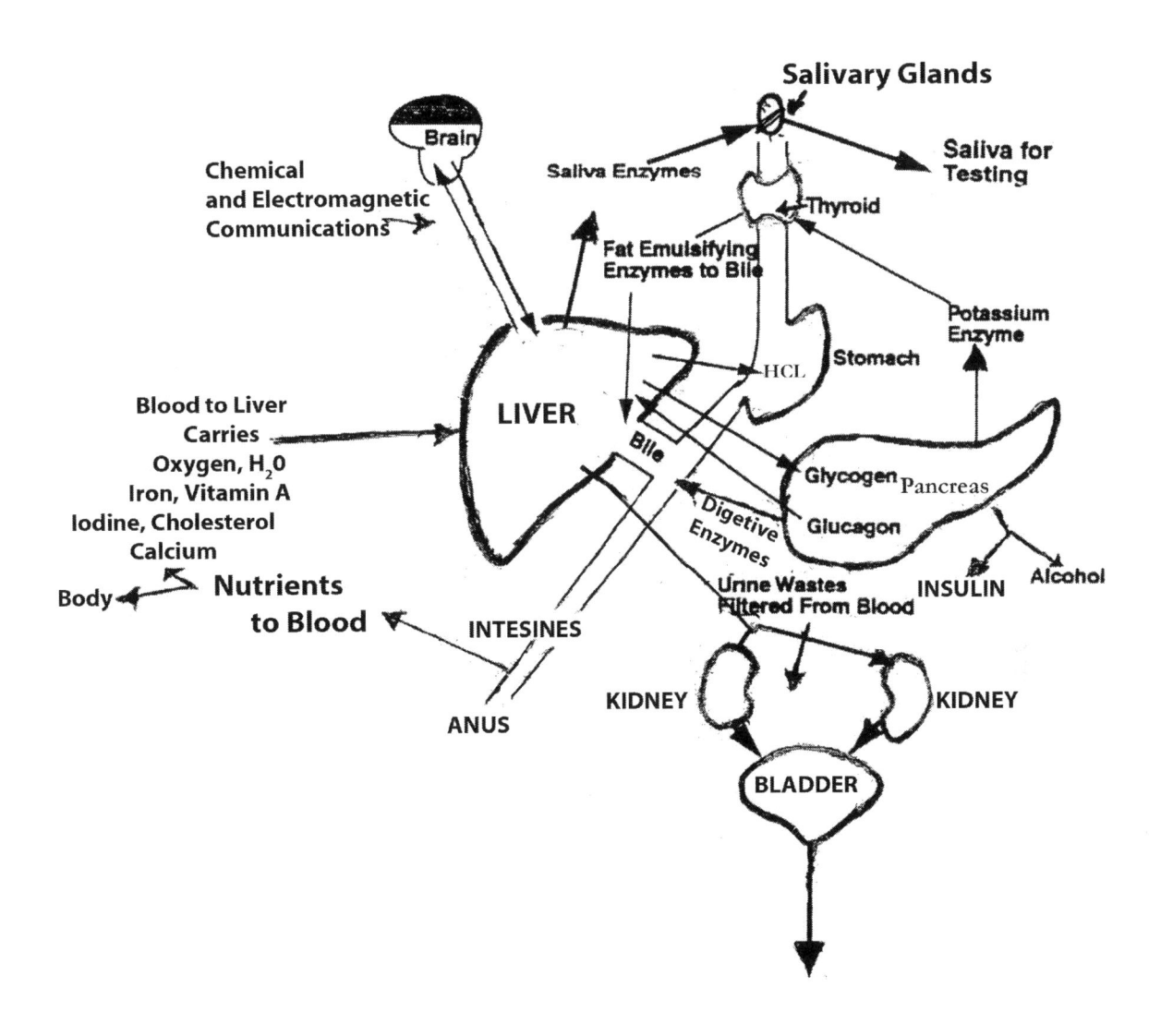

Salivary Glands

- Saliva Enzymes
- Saliva for Testing
- Thyroid
- Brain
- Chemical and Electromagnetic Communications
- Fat Emulsifying Enzymes to Bile
- HCL
- Stomach
- Potassium Enzyme
- Blood to Liver Carries Oxygen, H_2O, Iron, Vitamin A, Iodine, Cholesterol, Calcium
- LIVER
- Bile
- Glycogen
- Pancreas
- Digetive Enzymes
- Glucagon
- INSULIN
- Alcohol
- Body
- Nutrients to Blood
- INTESINES
- ANUS
- Urine Wastes Filtered From Blood
- KIDNEY
- KIDNEY
- BLADDER

31

Stomach

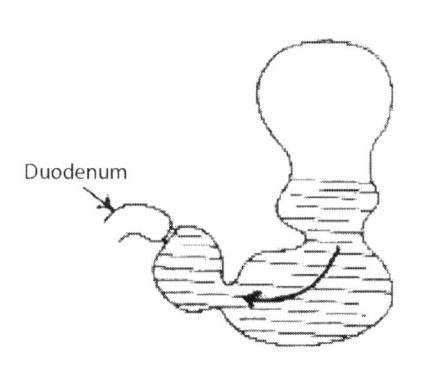

Hypotonic Stomach: bent stomach, slack, collapsed in area, expanded lumen. The function is slow-down hyposensitivity, inefficient hypomotoricity, more than 3 finger widths. The hypotonic stomach usually has a bent to hooked form, is sunken, and has an enlarged stomach bubble with a dull (poor tone) percussion sound. A weak stomach may require irritants (pepper, mustard etc.) and /or the pressure of a stomach full of food in order to force food movement in the intestine. Food stays in it too long. Because of the sunken shape, the movement of food to the duodenum is less efficient.

Atonic stomach: Prolapse (slack) ptosis often into the minor pelvis, sluggish, inefficient function, and large stomach bubble with splashing sounds "splashy stomach". The atonic stomach lack of muscular tone can extend into minor pelvis. The stomach has reduced sensitivity and motoricity, which causes food to remain for a long time in the "stomach sack", where it ferments, rots and decomposes. Percussion and gastric succession yield – due to almost total lack of tone- back and forth slushing of food and waste cause splashing sounds.

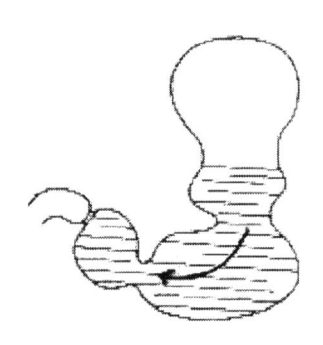

Normotonic Stomach: Bullhorn shape, optimal efficient function, normal volume, stomach bubble precursory 3 finger widths high, weak tympany.

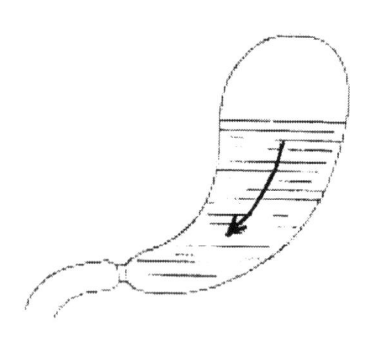

Hypertonic Stomach: Contracted shape, narrowed lumen, can tolerate small food portions at mealtime, food move fast (quick evacuation). Has a reduced amount of space with decreased curvature and reduced lumen. This causes smaller amounts of food to be tolerated at a time. Food evacuation is hypermotoric (accelerated). Stomachs can have mixed shapes stomachs with partially superimposed hypertonicity, conditioned by inflammatory processes: gastritis, gastroduodentitis, ulcers, and malignancies with concomitant gastritis. The stomach, with metallic percussion sounds, painful when percussed and gastric succession combined with muscle tension can be hypertonic.

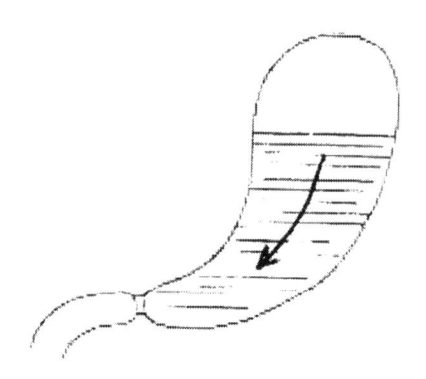

Ulcers

Sites of Ulcers:

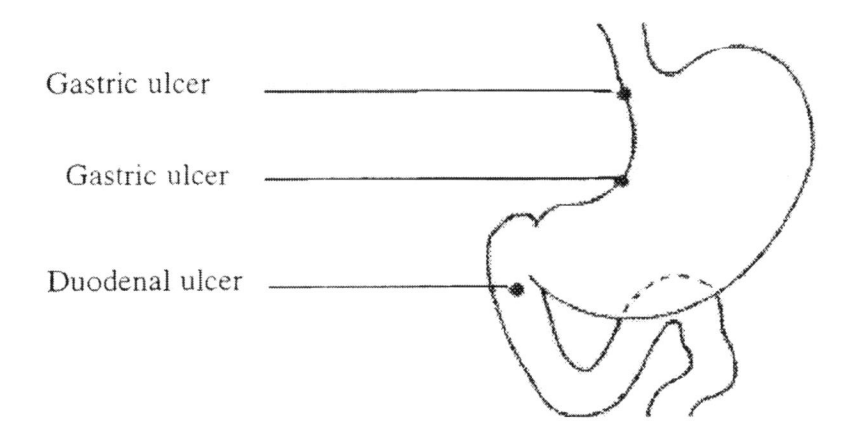

Gastric ulcer ⎯⎯⎯⎯⎯⎯⎯→

Gastric ulcer ⎯⎯⎯⎯⎯⎯⎯→

Duodenal ulcer ⎯⎯⎯⎯⎯⎯→

Ulcer Symptom Chart

Ulcers	Duodenal	Gastric
Pain Occurs:	Before meals or 2 to 2 ½ hours after meals	½ to 2 hours after meals
Do you feel better by eating?	Yes	Sometimes
Vomiting?	Rare	Common
Appetite?	Good	Fair

Stomach Hernia

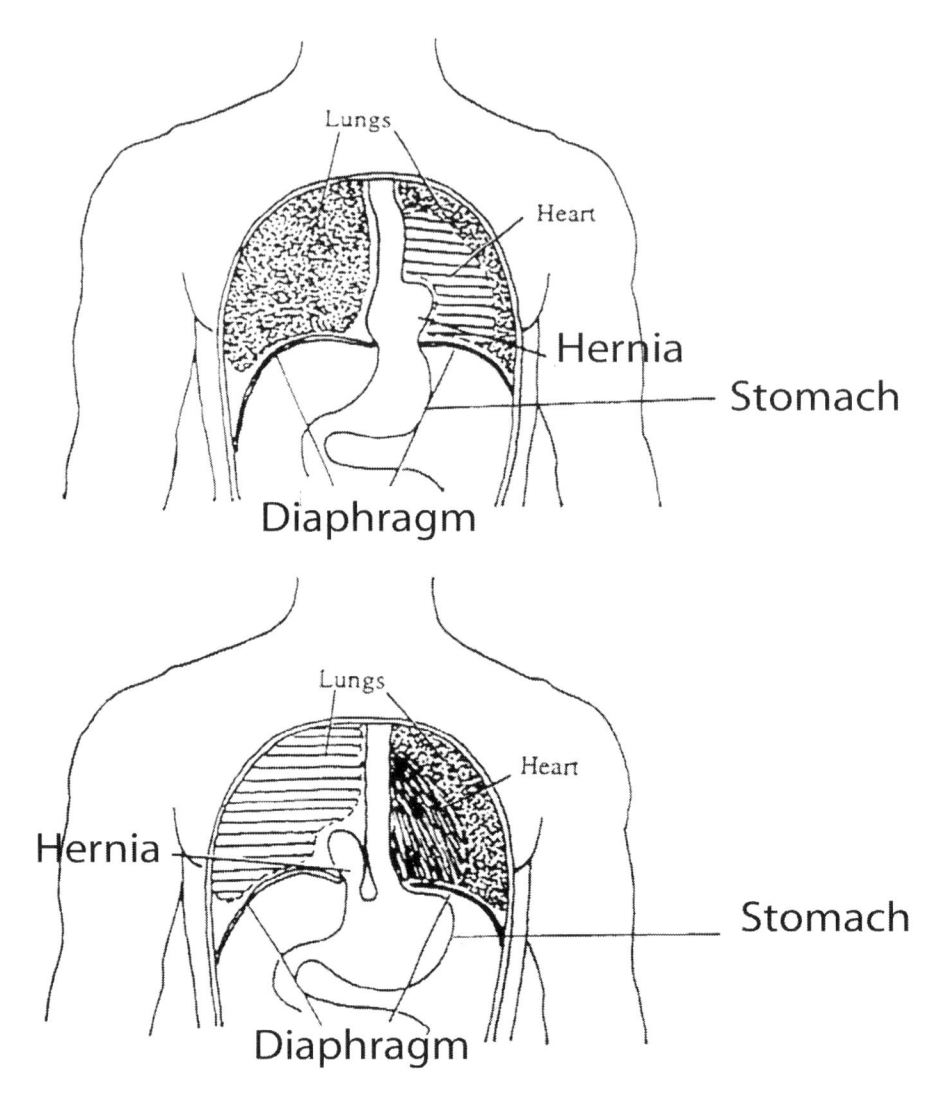

Variations in "Normal" Stomach

All stomachs do not have "J" shape or the same location.

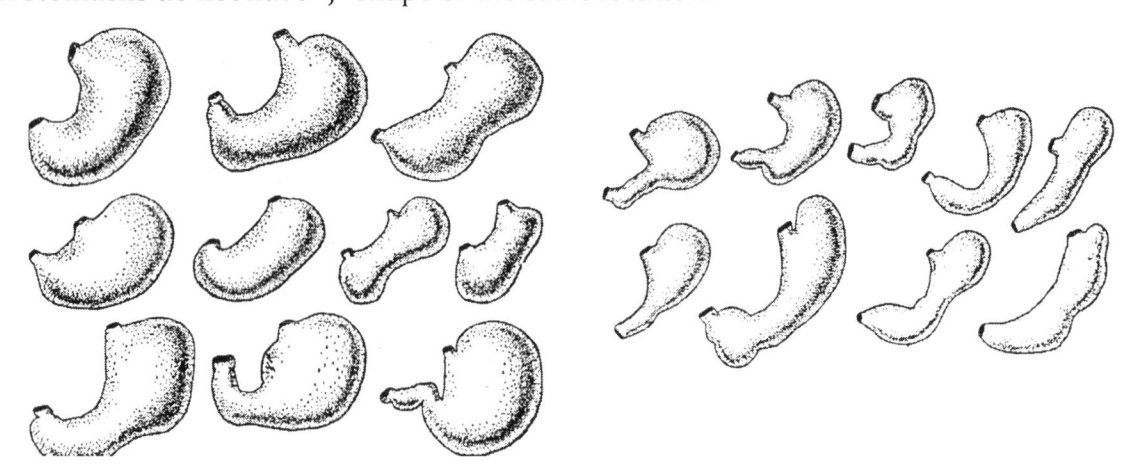

34

Stomach and Esophagus

The trachea (windpipe) is a cartilaginous tube that can be felt in the front part of the neck. It carries air to the lungs. The esophagus is a muscular tube that moves food from the mouth to the stomach. It is located behind the trachea and in front of the vertebrae bones of the neck. It cannot be felt.

In adults the esophagus goes through the diaphragm at the level of the xiphoid process (breastbone) and turns to the left for about an inch and enters the stomach.

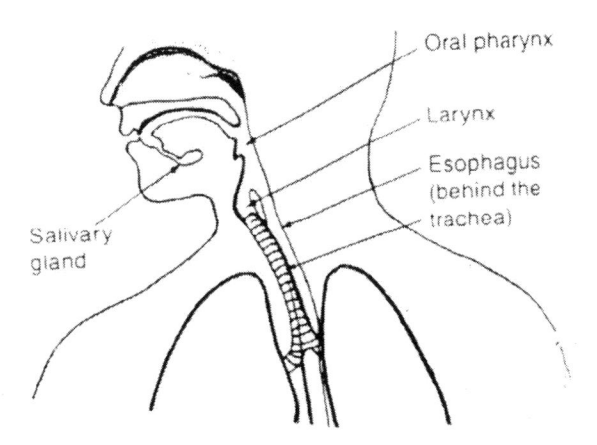

Body Fat and Food Cravings

Dominancy	Fat Location	Herbs to Decrease Craving	Stress Reaction	Food Cravings	Body Type	Work Habits	Diseases
Thyroid	"spare tire" Fat pouch in front abdomen	red raspberry, chickweed, fenugreek seeds.	nervous irritable	Starches, Sweets, coffee	Tall, long limbs	intense spurts of energy then exhaustion	allergies, skin problems, colds, flu, infection
Gonadal	"rear end" buttock fat	red clover, chickweed	frustration	fats, spices, salt	pear-shaped	calm, even energy all day	lumpy breasts
Adrenal	"beer belly" abdomen area	parsley, chickweed	aggravation	meat, potatoes, eggs, alcohol, vinegar	solid	workaholic	vascular disease
Pituitary	"baby fat" generalized fat all over	Fenugreek seeds, chickweed	anxious unfocused "spacy"	fruits, dairy products	child's body shape, big head	procrastination	allergies

Music and Disease

The musical notes are related to the anatomy and physiology of the body. Musical notes indicate a health problem as well as a disease. There are only seven notes in music. Each of the notes can be either sharp (slightly higher sound) or Flat (slightly lower sound) or sound natural (neither sharp or flat). A person tends to subconsciously choose instrumental and vocal melodies that use a specific note more than other notes. It is the specific note that the person likes which can identify a health concern. A musician or a computer program can identify the note that appears the most in a person's favorite tunes.

Music Note	Indication
C	Liver, kidney, reproductive system, lower abdomen, pancreas, intestine
D	Digestion, respiratory system, pituitary, adrenal, bladder, cerebrum, nose
E	Pancreas, diabetes, rectum, neck, cerebellum, throat, prostate, ovary
F	Nervous system, circulation, heart, sciatica nerve, fallopian tubes, thymus, buttocks, thigh
G	Immunity, stress, skin, knees, teeth, bones
A	Ear, nose, emotions, parathyroid, ankles, spleen, lower leg
B	Feet, pineal gland, breast, veins, arteries, stomach, brain stress, moods

Food Combining Chart

One type of food at a meal is ideal for the easiest and best digestion. Combinations of several foods at a meal should be according to the chart below. A meal should not consist of more than four food types.

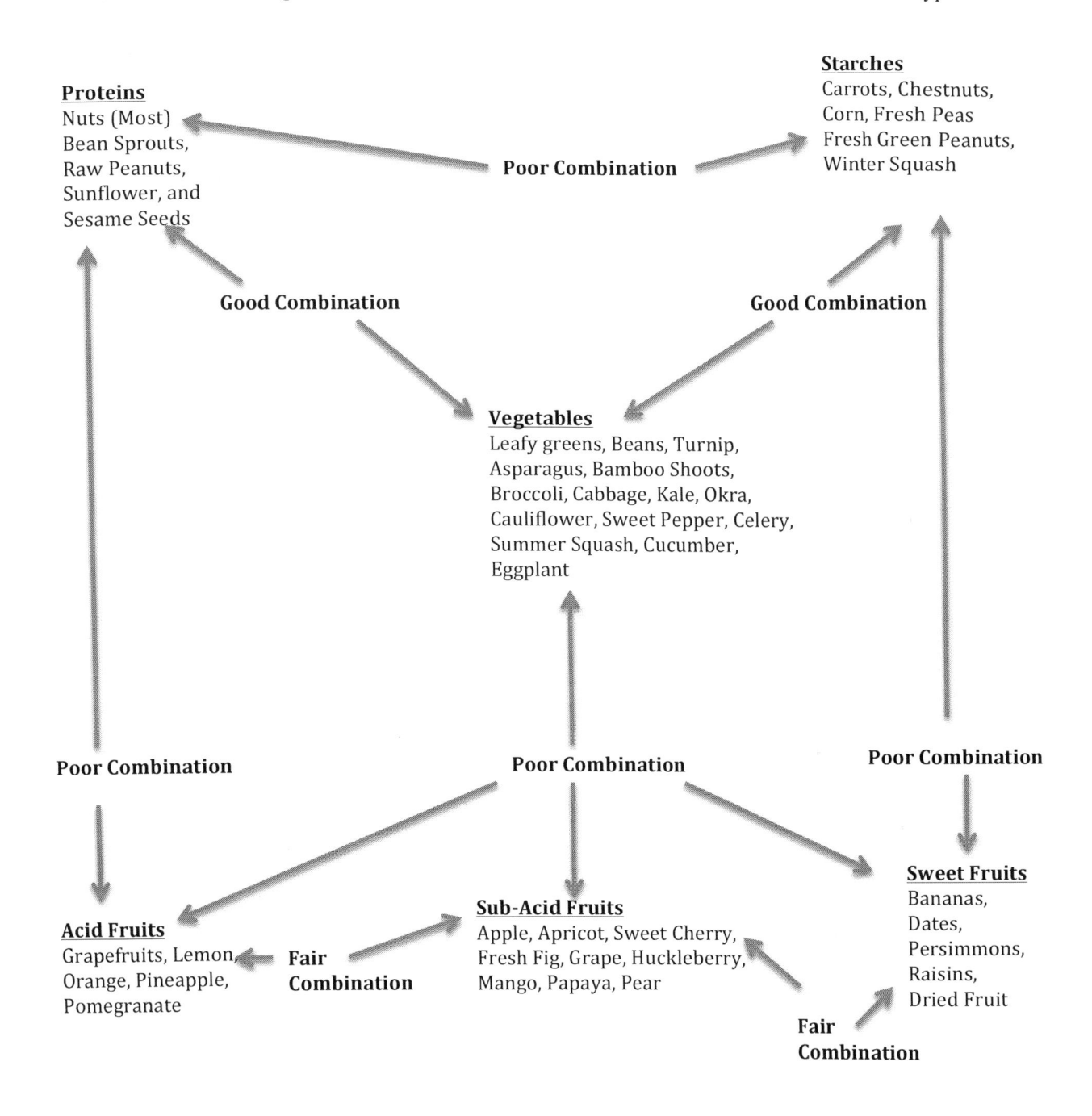

Proteins
Nuts (Most)
Bean Sprouts,
Raw Peanuts,
Sunflower, and
Sesame Seeds

Starches
Carrots, Chestnuts,
Corn, Fresh Peas
Fresh Green Peanuts,
Winter Squash

Proteins ← Poor Combination → Starches

Proteins → Good Combination → Vegetables ← Good Combination ← Starches

Vegetables
Leafy greens, Beans, Turnip,
Asparagus, Bamboo Shoots,
Broccoli, Cabbage, Kale, Okra,
Cauliflower, Sweet Pepper, Celery,
Summer Squash, Cucumber,
Eggplant

Poor Combination (Proteins ↓ Acid Fruits)
Poor Combination (Vegetables ↓ Sub-Acid Fruits)
Poor Combination (Starches ↓ Sweet Fruits)

Acid Fruits
Grapefruits, Lemon,
Orange, Pineapple,
Pomegranate

Sub-Acid Fruits
Apple, Apricot, Sweet Cherry,
Fresh Fig, Grape, Huckleberry,
Mango, Papaya, Pear

Sweet Fruits
Bananas,
Dates,
Persimmons,
Raisins,
Dried Fruit

Acid Fruits ← Fair Combination → Sub-Acid Fruits → Fair Combination → Sweet Fruits

Avocados, rich in fat, are best combined with green vegetables. Tomatoes are best eaten with more starchy vegetables and proteins. Sweet fruits should not be eaten with protein, vegetables or starches.

Digestion Time of Food Combinations

Salad or raw vegetables	2 hours
Properly combined meal, without flesh	3 hours
Properly combined meal, with flesh	4 hours
Any improperly combined meal	8 hours

Hours	Foods
1¼	Parsley
1½	Lemon, agar, Irish moss
1¾	Avocado, grapes, mango, olive (fresh), raspberry
2	Blueberry, sweet cherry, grapefruit, orange, raisin, coconut milk, artichoke, beet greens, garlic, potato, tomato, brown rice
2¼	Fig, (fresh) pear, pineapple, strawberry, asparagus, carrot, cauliflower, lettuce, iceberg, romaine
2½	Blackberry, date (dried), fig (dried), gooseberry, peach, fresh almond, dandelion greens, leeks, mushrooms, okra, lima beans, white rice
2¾	Apple, fresh apricot, fresh currant, peach, dried plum, watermelon, chestnut, coconut meat, fresh pecan, pignolia, beets, dock (sorrel), summer squash, wheat bran
3	Banana, guava, lime, prune, dried beechnut, filbert, walnut, broccoli, common cabbage, Swiss chard, sweet corn, endive (escarole), kohlrabi, rhubarb, spinach, winter squash, white bean, lentil, soybean, wheat germ
3¼	Cranberry, cantaloupe, casava melon, olive oil, pomegranate, cashew nut, coconut meat, celery, cucumber, onion, sweet green pepper, pumpkin, radish, rutabaga, sweet potato, turnip greens, watercress, snap bean, cowpea, fresh peanut, millet
3½	Safflower seed oil, sesame seed oil, celery, eggplant, mustard greens, parsnip, pea, dried soybean oil, rye grain
3¾	Persimmon, quince, red cabbage, barley, wheat grass
4	Brussels sprouts, horseradish, turnip

Digestive System's Circadian Rhythm

Process	Time
Appropriation (eating & digestion)	12 noon – 8 p.m.
Assimilation (absorption & use)	8 p.m. – 4 a.m.
Elimination (of body waste)	4 a.m. - 12 noon

Colon/Body Connection

The colon (large intestine) can have sensitive, sore, ballooned, twisted, impacted, gas filled, blocked, inflamed and prolapsed areas that can cause an unpleasant sensitization or feel lumpy when palpated (pressed/rubbed). Areas that have lost their skin integrity or natural shape are related to bodily functions/organs that can cause nutrient deficiencies, malfunctions, and result in an illness.

Healthy Colon

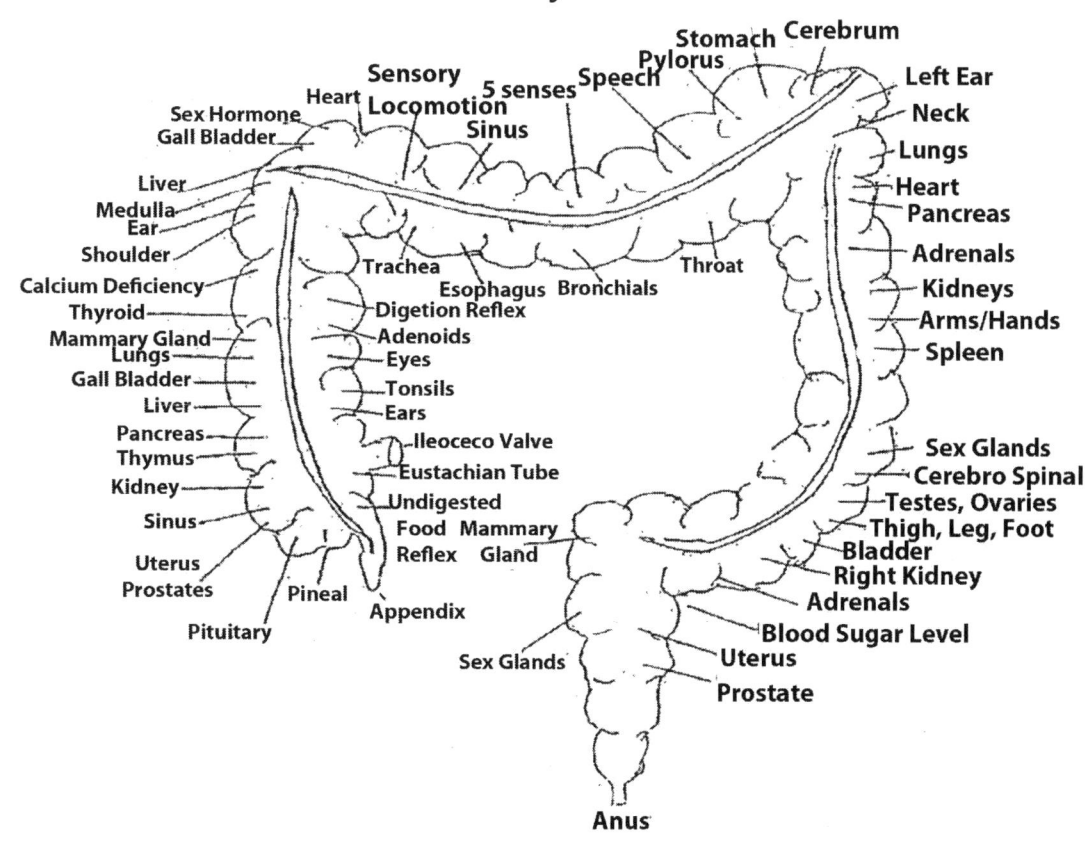

Unhealthy colon

The pictures of colons below are the average conditions caused by processed food, lack of adequate raw foods in the diet and/or wrong food combination.

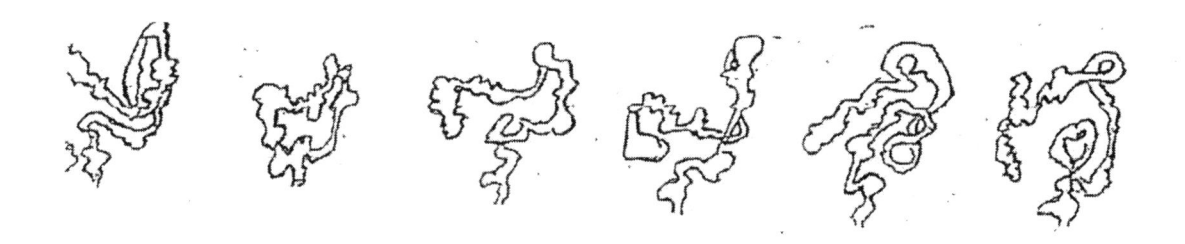

Average Mineral Loss in Vegetables--- Due To Cooking

Mineral	Mineral Loss Due To Boiling
Iron	48.9%
Magnesium	46.4%
Phosphorous	44.7%
Calcium	31.0%

Body's Energy and Food

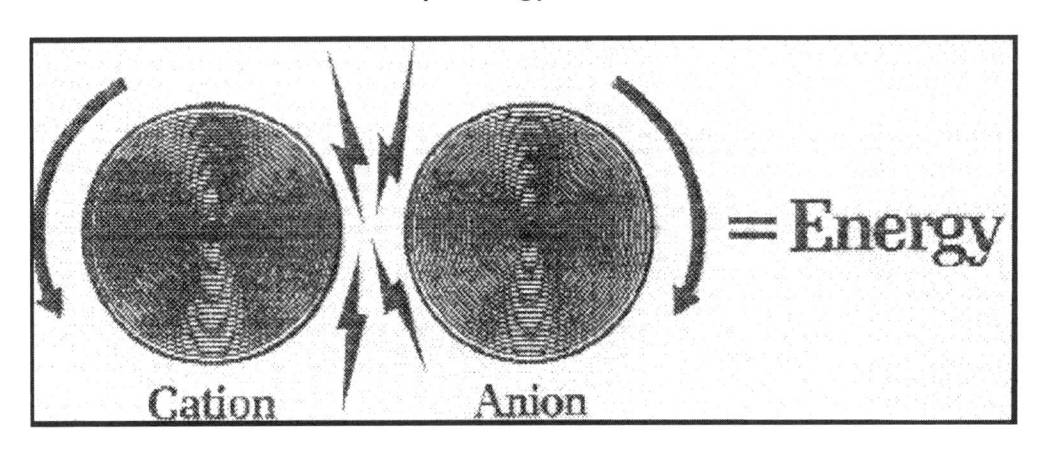

Ions are elements that have an electrical charge.
Ions can be Cation or Anion.
The Anion orbits in a clockwise direction.
The Cation orbits in a counter- clockwise direction.
The resistance between these two forces creates energy,

ANION
An alkaline substance.

CATION
An acid substance.

Food does not give you energy. Food stimulates the spinning of the Cation and Anion. The spinning of the elements in the body causing energy.

Mineral Relativity Wheel

Minerals work in ratio relationships with each other. To identify the minerals that work together, pick a mineral, and then look for the longest and shortest line connecting to another mineral. For example, if Calcium is to be utilized properly in the body, it must be in relationship with Manganese (Female shortest line connected to a mineral), and Magnesium (Male longest line that connects to a mineral). If Calcium is cooked it becomes coarse and too hard and partially unusable in the body. This decreases the efficient use of Manganese and Magnesium because the mineral ratio is violated.

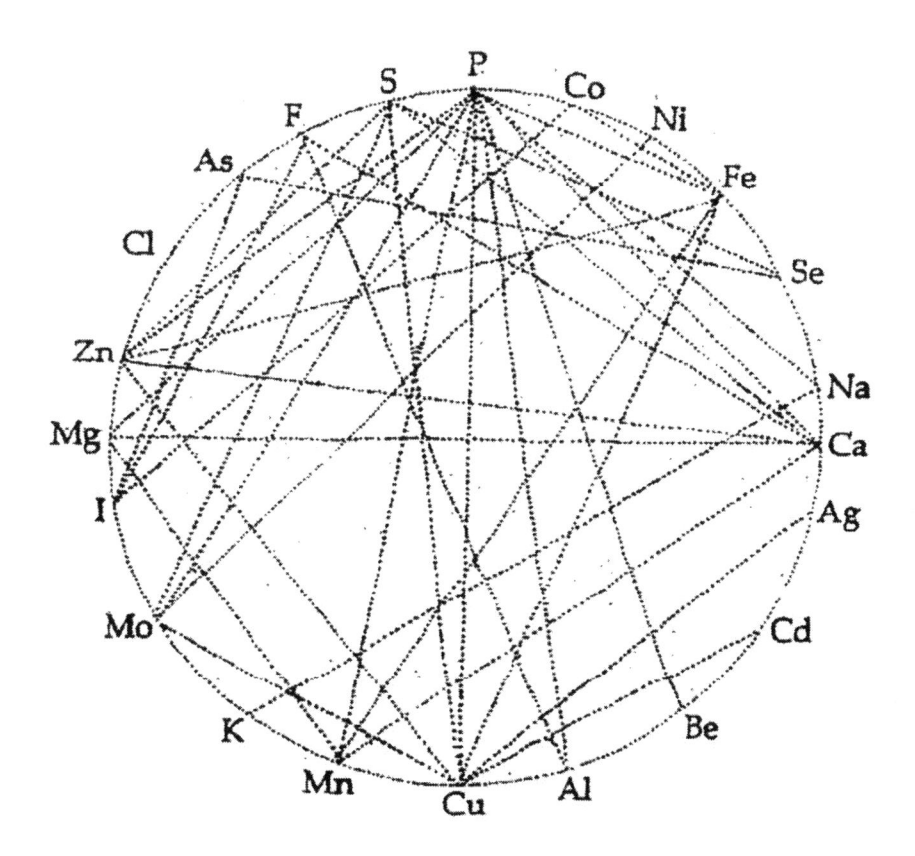

Aluminum - Al	Fluorine - F	Potassium – K
Arsenic -As	Iodine - I	Selenium – Se
Beryllium - Be	Iron - Fe	Silver – Ag
Cadmium - Cd	Magnesium - Mg	Sodium - Na
Calcium - CA	Manganese -Mn	Sulfur – S
Chlorine – Cl	Molybdenum - Mo	Zinc - Zn
Cobalt - Co	Nickel – Ni	
Copper – Cu	Phosphorus - P	

pH Range of Acceptance

The potential (p) of Hydrogen (H) indicates acid or alkaline. pH is an electrical (ion) measurement. The body is slightly acid 6.4. Therefore, a pH number less than 6.4 is considered acid, while a pH higher than 6.4 is considered alkaline. At 6.4 the pH can swing through the 5.4 to 7.6 range similar to a pendulum. At 6.4 the circadian rhythm allows minerals to be absorbed.

How to Read the Chart

If a person has a pH 6.0 follow the broken vertical line down to the broken horizontal line at chromium, then follow the broken horizontal line across (transverse) to Cobalt and then follow the broken vertical line upward to 7.0. The elements from 6.0 to 7.0 will be absorbed (accepted). The elements less than 6.0 and greater than 7.0 will not be accepted. The 6.0 do not allow the circadian rhythm to swing like a pendulum and absorb all the minerals.

Range of Elements Acceptance Chart

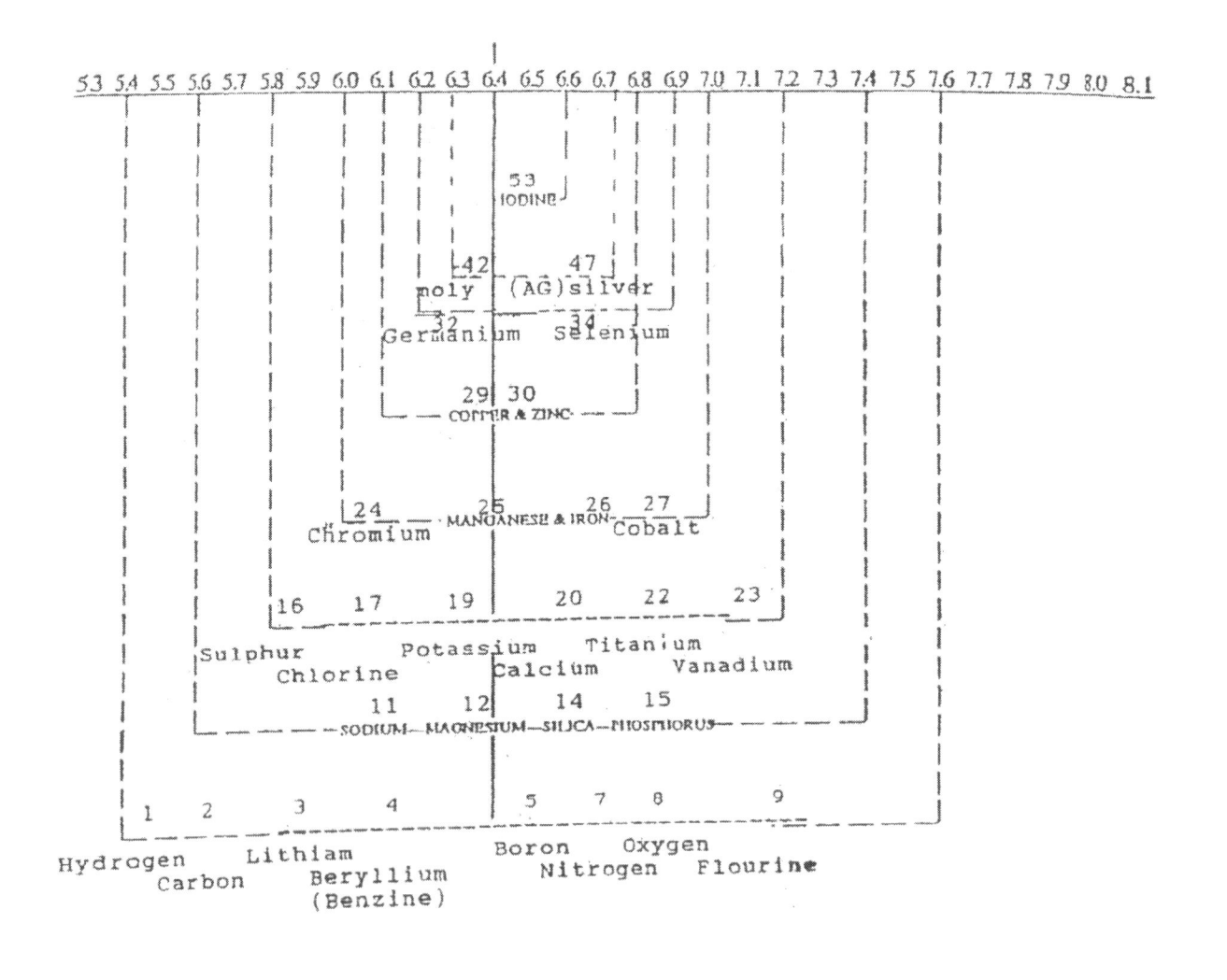

5.3 5.4 5.5 5.6 5.7 5.8 5.9 6.0 6.1 6.2 6.3 6.4 6.5 6.6 6.7 6.8 6.9 7.0 7.1 7.2 7.3 7.4 7.5 7.6 7.7 7.8 7.9 8.0 8.1

53 IODINE

42 poly | 47 (AG) silver
32 Germanium | 34 Selenium
29 30 COPPER & ZINC

24 Chromium | 25 26 MANGANESE & IRON | 27 Cobalt

16 17 19 20 22 23
Sulphur Potassium Titanium
Chlorine Calcium Vanadium
11 12 14 15
SODIUM MAGNESIUM SILICA PHOSPHORUS

1 2 3 4 5 7 8 9
Hydrogen Lithium Boron Oxygen
Carbon Beryllium Nitrogen Flourine
(Benzine)

Digestive Enzyme Points

If the enzyme meridian points are sensitive to touch, have discoloration, dryness, oiliness, texture change, bumps, and/or rashes on the point this can indicate a problem with that enzyme. Always look for inconsistencies in skin, hair, eyes, lips, teeth, tongue, nails etc. An inconsistency on the outside of the body indicates an inconsistency inside the body.

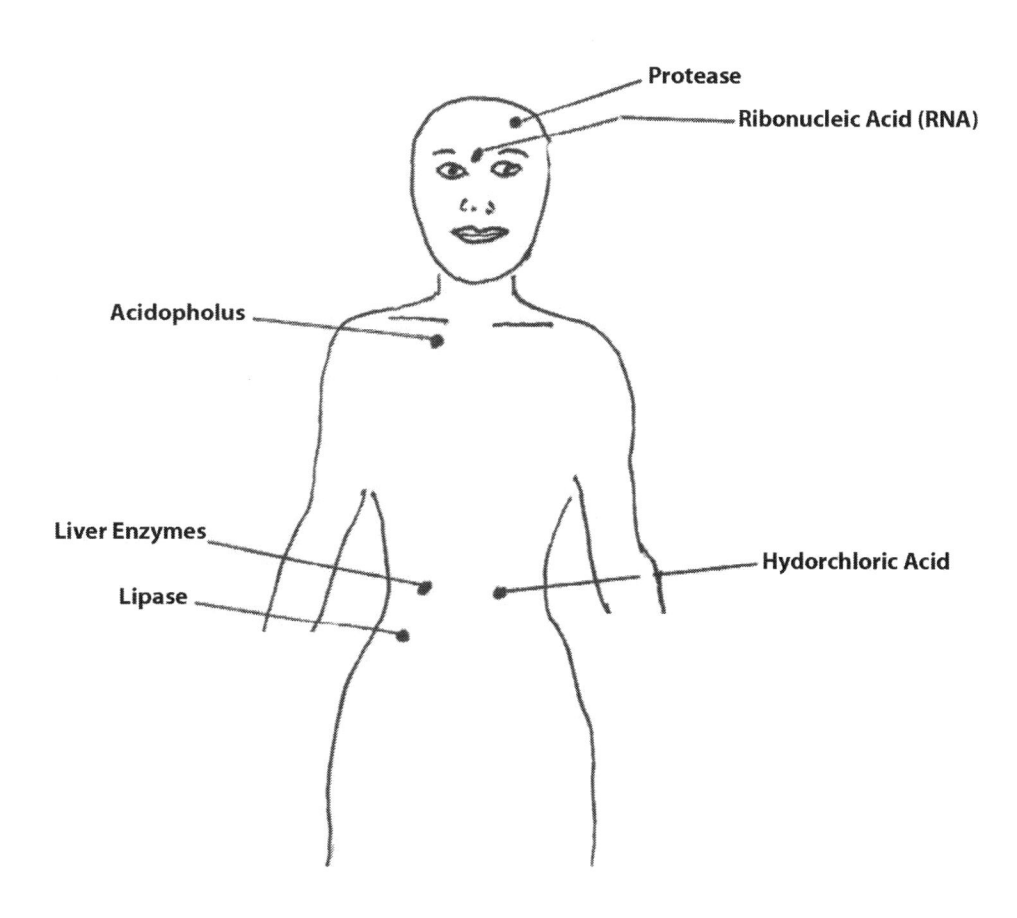

- Protease
- Ribonucleic Acid (RNA)
- Acidopholus
- Liver Enzymes
- Lipase
- Hydorchloric Acid

Digestive Enzymes

The enzyme acupuncture meridian point for Digestion is located 1 to 1½ inches to the right of the center of the body on the lower border of the rib cage.

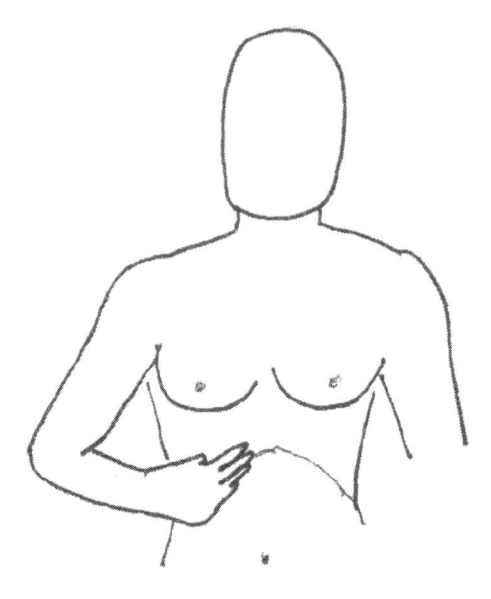

The Ribonucleic Acid meridian point is located on the bridge of the nose between the eyebrows.

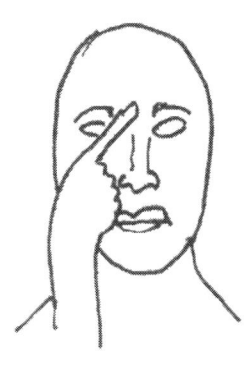

The Lipase meridian is located 2 to 2½ inches to the right of the center of the body.

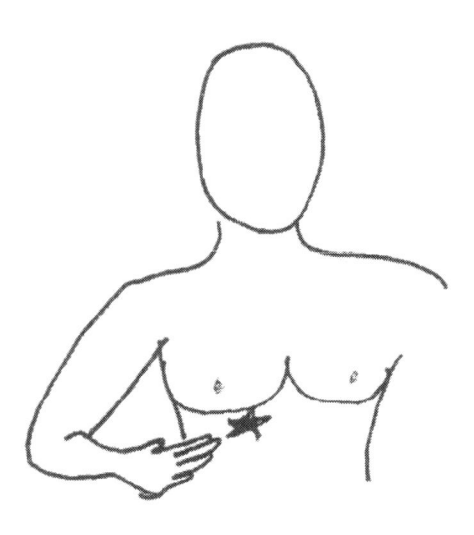

How to Test Tryptophan

The test of Tryptophan is done by placing the Tryptophan capsule or pills in one hand, and then place that hand in a fist position onto the Solar Plexus area while extending the other arm to be used for testing. When the proper dosage of Tryptophan pills is in the hand, the other arm will become rigid when the tester (another person) presses down on the arm. The nerve center located in the back of the neck can be used for testing. If the nerve center seems weak after placing the fingers at the back of the neck and a tester (another person) presses down on an extended arm, increase the dosage until the arm is rigid. Test by placing the pill in the palm, while touching the fingers to the back of the neck and the tester pushes down on the extended arm. Add or subtract the quantity of dosage until the amount that makes the extended arms rigid. When you find the dosage (quantity of capsules/pills) needed, you have reached the treatment level for the therapeutic minimum/maximum for the condition.

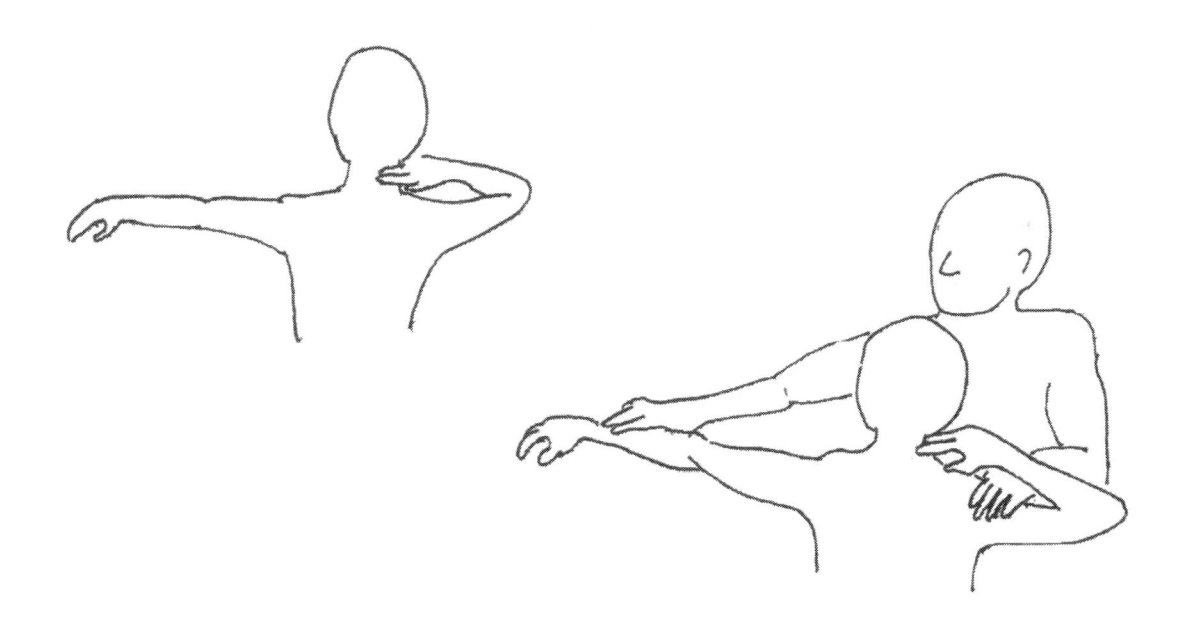

Nose

Nose Types

The nose indicates the nervous, circulatory, and digestive system. The type of nose, size, shape, color, and other characteristics indicate health conditions. The shape of the nose indicates the quality of emotions, mental, and physical health.

Nose Types

Normal

Straight and Long

Large

Short and Flat

Nose Examination

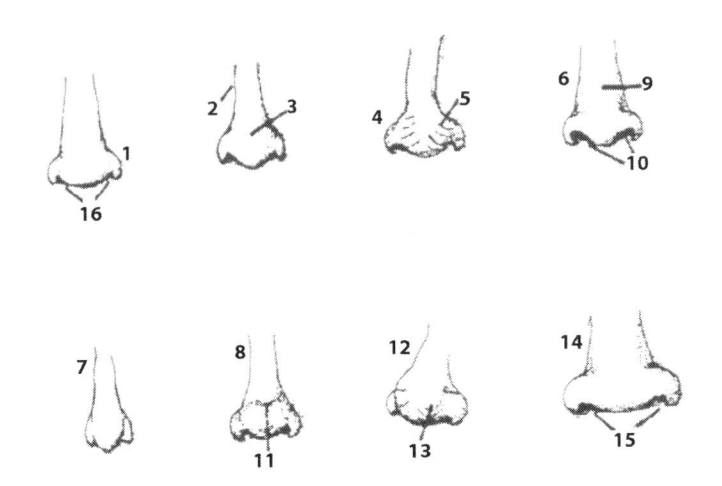

Nose

Type	Symptom
1. Pale nose	Anemia
2. Non-Symmetrical Nose Shaft	Heart problems on corresponding side
3. Nose with darken complexion	digestive tract and gland problem
4. Crooked Bridge & Shaft	scoliosis
5. Veins dark on nose	heart problems, acidic condition, low oxygen, mineral imbalance
6. Long & Large Nose	eating disorder, congestion in heart
7. Narrow	physical weakness
8. Hard Bulbousness	heart problems, fat accumulation, rheumatism of the heart
9. Dark Nose	mucous congestion, degenerated blood
10. Flare Nostrils	inner vitality, high reserve energy, good immunity
11. Cleft	heart murmur
12. Swelling	enlarged heart, mucus congestion
13. Dark blood Vessels at Tip	high blood pressure
14. Flat & Wide	physical vitality, minerals stable, strong lungs
15. Large nostrils	good respiratory system

Nose Examination:
Soft and watery appearance – heart problems, excess mineral waste
Oily and shiny – liver problems, glands congested, fat metabolism weak
Thickening of, or pain in Nostrils – stagnated processed oils, on the inside of nose: heart problems,
Dry nostrils – dehydrating food consumption, potassium deficiency
Sneezing – excess mucus waste, cellular congestion
Mucus dripping out of nose – mucus and waste congestion

Various Nose Forms

Crooked nose toward right

Crooked nose toward left

Tip of nose pointing toward front

Drooping nose

Eagle nose

Nose with upward tilted tip

Cleft nose

Swollen nose

Hardening nose

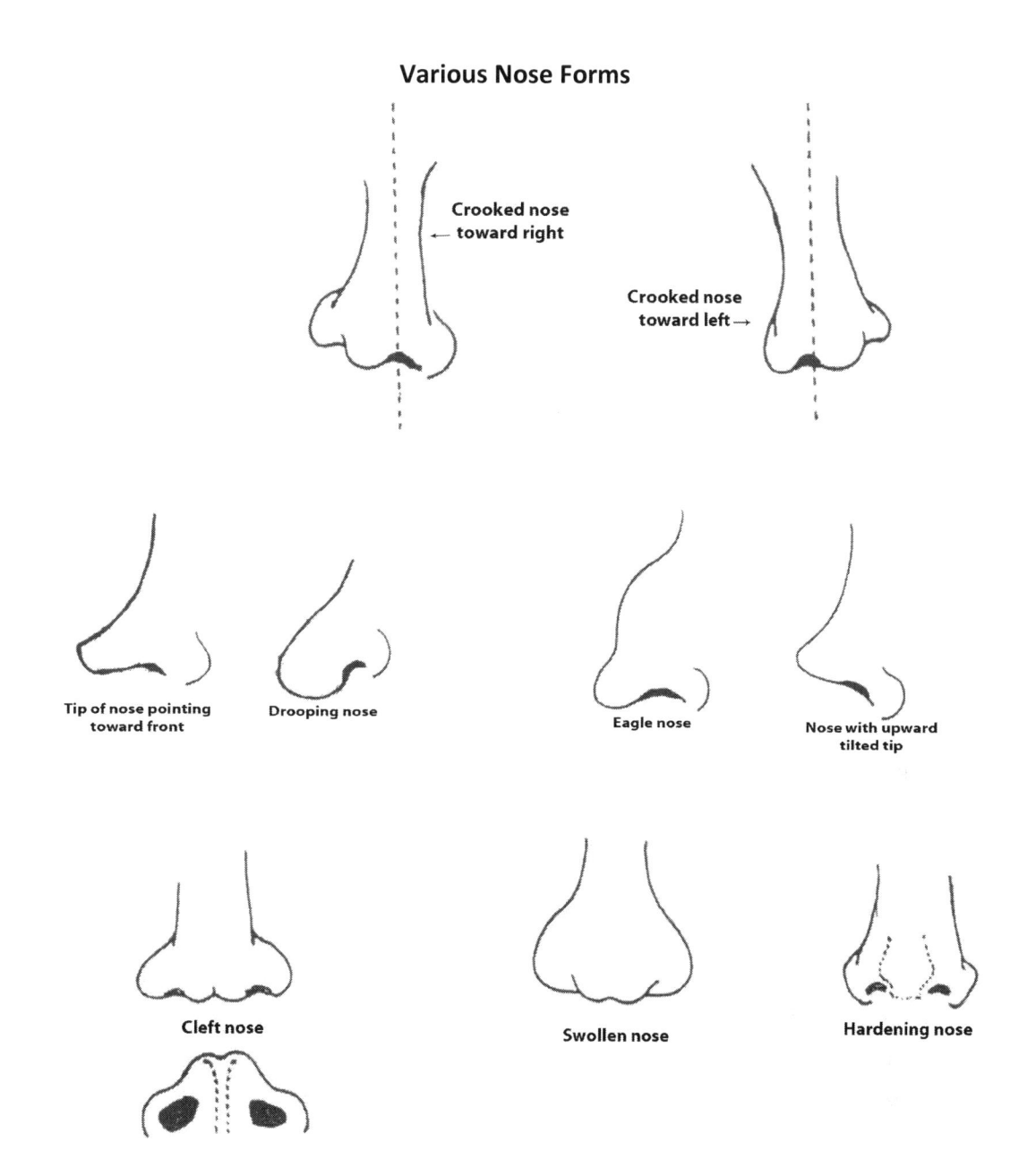

Upward-tilted tip of the nose indicates a tendency toward shortsightedness, good deductive thinking and rigidity in understanding or accepting ideas. Parasympathetic stress

Drooping nose indicates kidneys, and heart problems. May tend to have reproductive problems.

High, rounded shape indicates a tendency to be self-centered, hyperactive, Aggressiveness tendencies. It can indicate a mineral deficiency.

Cleft nose when the tip of the nose has a split or an indentation, this can indicate a nutritional imbalance, embryonic pituitary stress, heart arrhythmias, or heart murmur.

Swollen nose indicates problems with the circulatory and excretory system.

Hardening at the tip is caused by the intake of cooked and/or processed saturated animal or vegetable fat (oils). This can indicate hardening of the arteries, muscles, heart, liver, kidneys, spleen, uterus, and prostate gland problems. This may indicate a heart attack or stroke tendency.

Side of the Nose

The raised, bony areas on the sides of the nose indicate imbalanced thinking and/or middle organ problems. If these areas are less pronounced, there is more of a tendency toward clear balanced thinking.

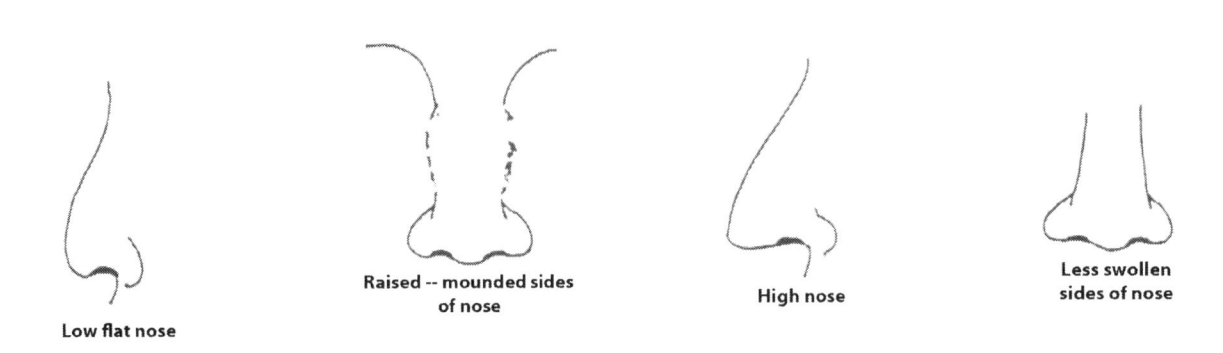

Low flat nose

Raised -- mounded sides of nose

High nose

Less swollen sides of nose

Nostrils

Well-developed nostrils can indicate, aggressiveness, determination, bold courage, and strong character (see Male Principle); less developed nostrils indicate sensitivity, gentleness, and a nurturing character (see Female Principle).

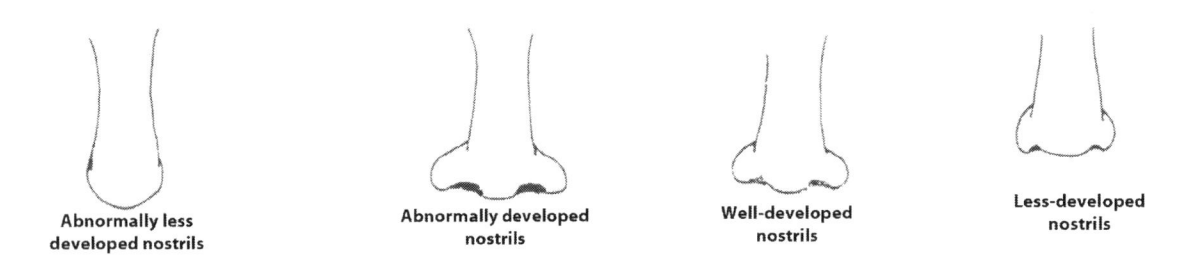

Abnormally less developed nostrils

Abnormally developed nostrils

Well-developed nostrils

Less-developed nostrils

Height of the Nose

A high nose indicates a tendency to be proud, fertility problems, aggressive, competitive, and discriminating. A lower or flatter nose indicates a tendency to be more generous, passive, humanistic, accommodating toward others, and can let emotions dominate.

Extremely short and flat nose

Extremely high and long nose

Tip of the Nose

When the tip of the nose hangs down slightly and it partially covers a section of the nostril, it indicates a tendency toward nervousness, emotional sensitivity and unstable emotions. When the nose is shaped so that the two nostrils can be clearly seen from the front; it indicates unstable or random thinking and shifting character logic.

Nose hanging down

Two nostril holes can be seen

Nose Massage

The nose indicates the condition of the lungs. If the spots are sensitive or inconsistent in skin condition it is symptoms of respiratory problems, runny nose and blocked sinuses. The health of the lungs can be maintained by stimulating certain spots around the nose. These are spots, that stimulate the meridians that supply the nose and surrounding areas with energy, and stimulate continual flow of air through the nasal and sinus passages. This exercise can be done as many times a necessary to help correct sinus or nasal problems.

1. Using the tip of the index or the second fingers of each hand, press down on the three points.
2. Begin at the base of the nose and press these points for about ten seconds. Then rub these points briefly.
3. Next, press the points midway up on either side of the nose for about ten seconds. Then rub briefly.

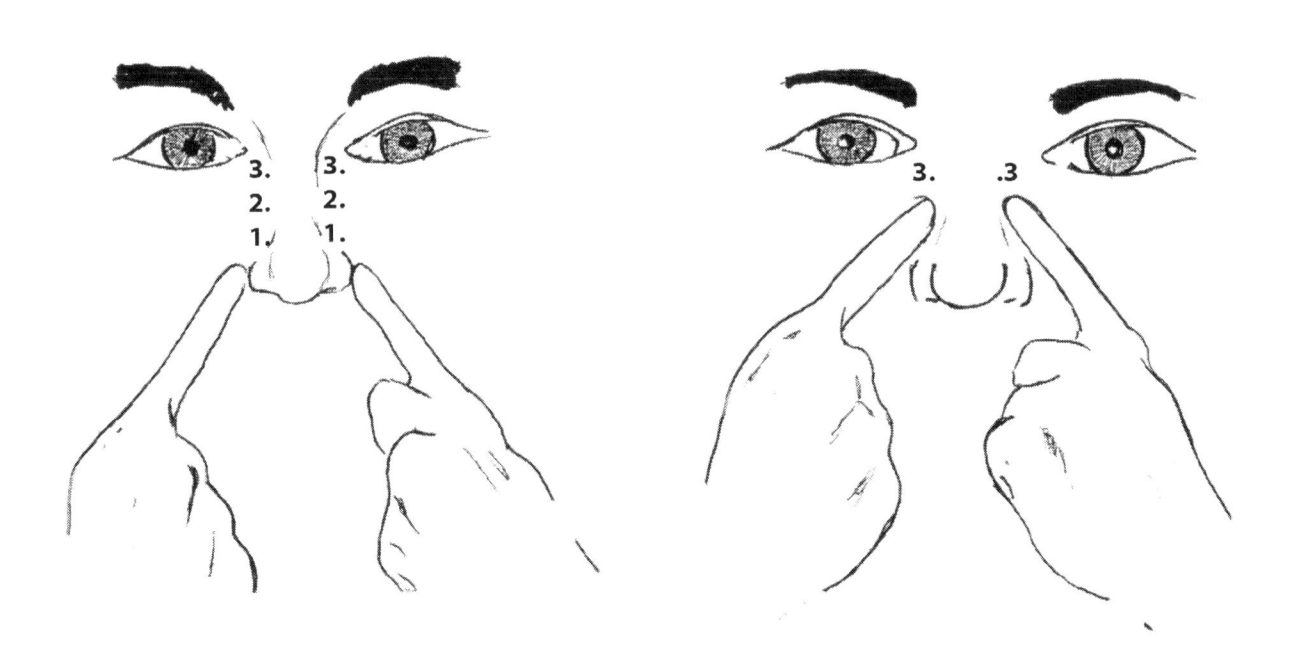

LIPS

Lips

Inconsistent skin color, texture, deep vertical and or horizontal wrinkles in an area point to the organ that is malfunctioning. Dry or cracked lips indicate dehydration of the digestive tract. Pale lips are symptomatic of anemia. Dark spots are a sign of indigestion and/or worms in the colon. Herpes blisters or ulcers on the lips indicate impurities. Tremors of the lips are a sign of anxiety, stress, tension, or fear.

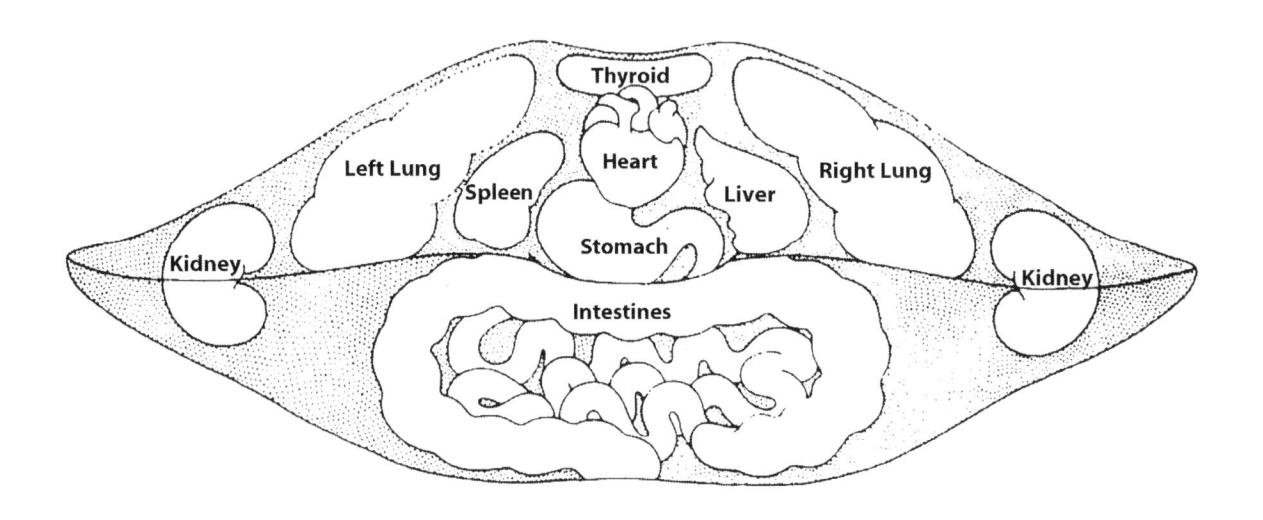

Forms of the Mouth

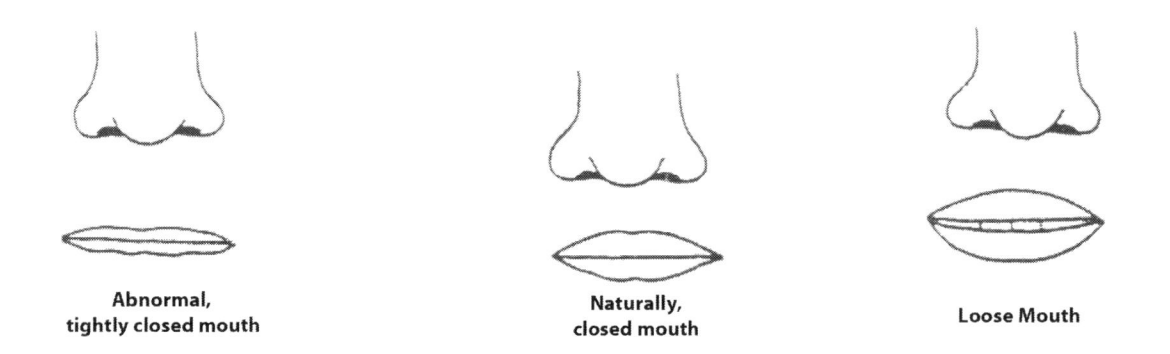

Abnormal, tightly closed mouth

Naturally, closed mouth

Loose Mouth

54

Forms of Lips

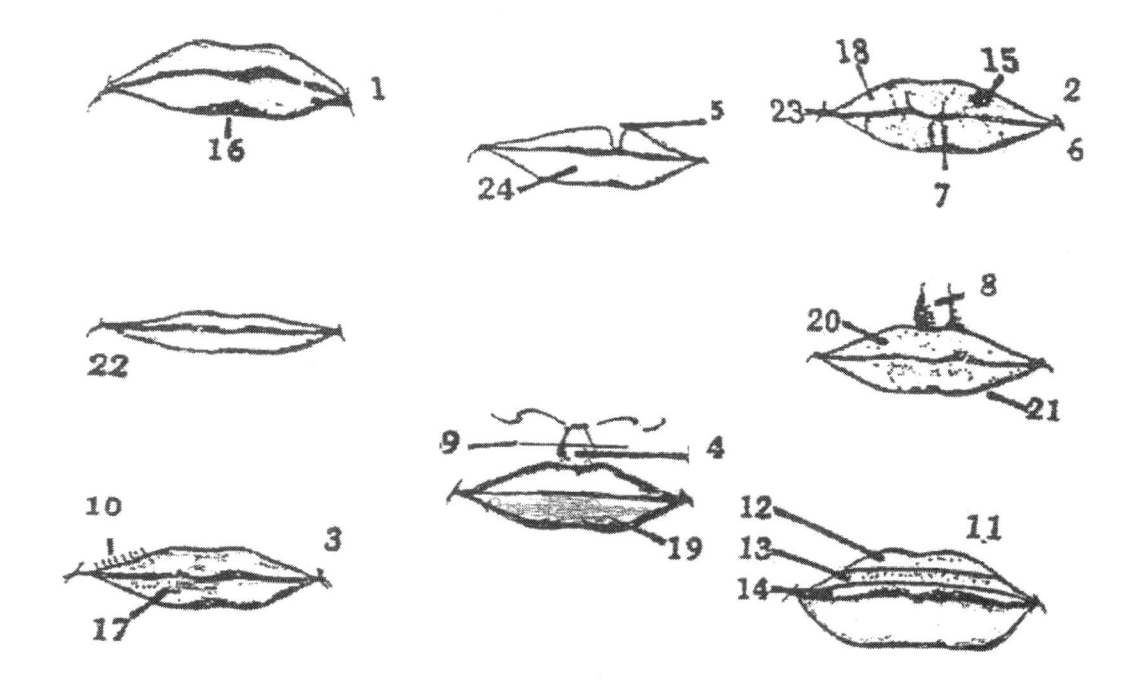

1.	Downturned Corners	Intestinal hardening, arteriosclerosis
2.	Thick Lips	Strong vitality, good immunity
3.	Swollen Lips	Digestive system congested, weakness
4.	Shallow Cleft Above Lip	Sexual organs weak
5.	Cleft Pallet or Hair Lip	Tendency to eat concentrated sweeteners
6.	Small Wrinkles on Lip	Weak digestion, diarrhea, fast transit time
7.	Cracked Lips	Large intestine & lung diseases
8.	Deep Cleft Above Lip	Increased sexual desire
9.	Horizontal Line Above Lip	Sexual organs diseased
10.	Wrinkles Above Lip	Sexual organs dehydrated
11.	Top Area, Upper Lip	Upper stomach
12.	Middle Area, Upper Lip	Middle stomach
13.	Lower Area, Upper Lip	Duodenum
14.	Sores	Stagnation, ulceration related to area
15.	Outward Swelling Lower Lip	Constipation, colon congested and hard
16.	Spots on Lip	Intestinal sores
17.	Peeling Lips	Intestinal wall deteriorating
18.	Bright Red	Inflammation of liver, hemorrhoids
19.	Purple Lips	Not enough oxygen, toxins in blood
20.	White Around Lips	Anemia
21.	Tight Lips	Intestines & vagina dehydrated
22.	Cracked or Blistered at Corners	Ulcer or colitis condition
23.	Pale	Weak lungs, anemia

Lips Correlation to the Body

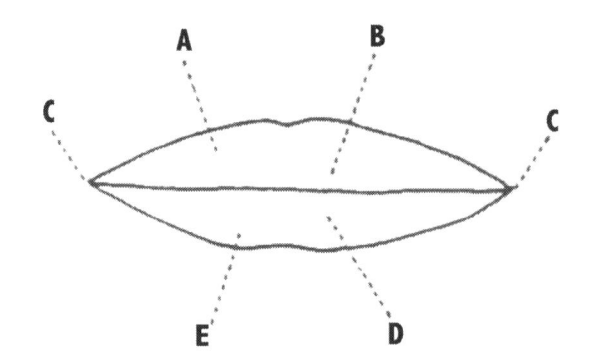

A.	Esophagus area
B.	Stomach area
C.	Duodenum area
D.	Small intestine area
E.	Large intestine area

Whitish patches:
Excessive amounts of dairy foods and processed hydrogenated oils, and animal fats are being discharged. Indicates problems with digestive, respiratory, and lymphatic functions.

Yellowish brown shade:
Indicates a diet of meat poultry and eggs, dairy products (yogurt, cheese), and cook saturated fats. The liver and the gallbladder are stressed.

Dark purplish spots:
This indicates high amounts of carbon dioxide in blood in the section of the body and/or digestive tract that corresponds to the area of the mouth where the spots appear.

Black spots:
Excessive refined carbohydrates, processed sugar products; concentrated sweeteners (i.e. syrups, honey) cause kidney and urinary problems. These spots appear when processed oils, and hardened fats accumulate in the digestive tract.

Closed mouth and loose mouth:
A mouth that is naturally closed indicates a normal nervous system, normal digestive and respiratory functions. A mouth that is tightly closed indicates liver, gallbladder, or kidneys problems caused by consumption of salts, meat, fried foods, white sugar, concentrated sweeteners, poultry, eggs and dairy products.
A loose mouth indicates digestive, respiratory, excretory, nervous, deterioration caused by consumption of sugars and other concentrated sweeteners, legal and illegal drugs, as well as food addiction.

Swollen Lips: indicate digestive disorders. A swollen upper lip indicates stomach and digestion problems. A swollen and expanded lower lip indicates indigestion, gas production, worms, constipation, and diarrhea. If the swollen and expanded lower lip is wet, the intestinal disorder is accompanied with diarrhea. If the central part of the lips is not clearly formed it indicates weakness of the heart, small intestines, sexual functions, the stomach, pancreatic functions, and indigestion.

Square mouth:
If the corners of the mouth appear like the angles of a square when the mouth is wide open or when laughing it indicates a diet of processed foods, cooked animal flesh, dairy products and improperly combined foods during embryonic development.

Shape of the Mouth

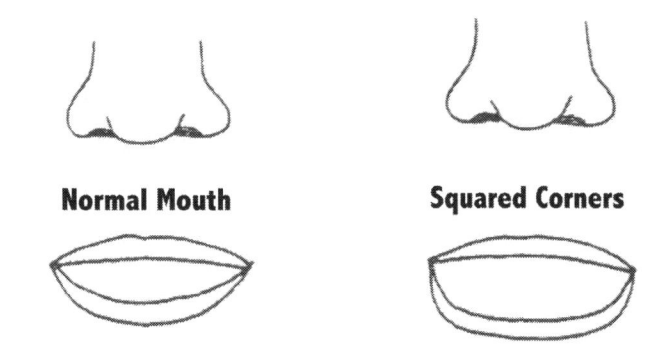

Normal Mouth **Squared Corners**

Central Part of Lips

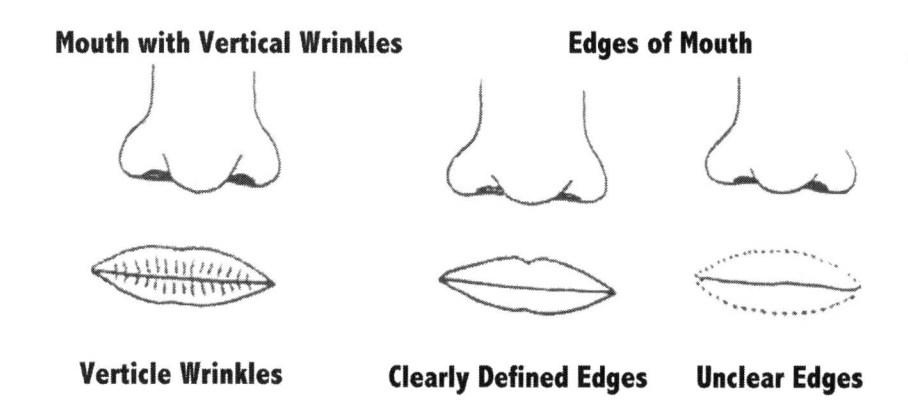

Mouth with Vertical Wrinkles   **Edges of Mouth**

Verticle Wrinkles   **Clearly Defined Edges**   **Unclear Edges**

Vertical wrinkles:
On the lips indicate hormone problems and deterioration of sexual functions. Wrinkles can indicate dehydration, and consumption of dehydrating foods such as sodas, mineral water, coffee, alcohol, salt, fried, baked, or toasted foods, processed starches, legal and illegal drugs.

Clearly Defined Edges on Mouth:
A mouth with clearly defined edges indicates a balanced diet. A mouth with a unclear edges can be caused by weakness in the digestive and excretory functions.

Clearly shaped lips:
The central part of the lips is clearly shaped it can indicate a balanced diet during the embryonic period as well as healthy heart, small intestine and sexual organs.

Size of the Mouth

A mouth larger both in horizontal width and vertical height reflects a diet of vegetables and vegetable fats (oils), and fruits, during the prenatal growing periods. The peripheral parts of the body have good circulation such as the skin and muscles. The internal organs such as the heart, liver, spleen and small intestine have good immunity.

Mouth larger in horizontal width but not in vertical width

Mouth larger in both horizontal and vertical width

Mouth larger in vertical width but not in horizontal width

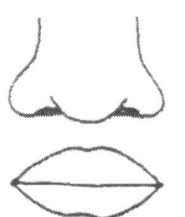

Lower Lip:
The lower lip indicates the condition of the small and large intestines and lower digestive tract. The inner area of the lower lip relates to the condition of the small intestine, and the peripheral areas relate to the large intestine.

Upper Lip:
The upper lip indicates the condition of the stomach and upper part of the digestive tract. The inner part of the upper lip corresponds to both upper and lower ends of the stomach. The peripheral areas of the upper lip correspond to the middle region of the stomach.

General Conditions:
The size of the mouth, including its horizontal width and breadth, and vertical fullness, indicates the functioning of the body and internal organs, immunity and digestive tract.

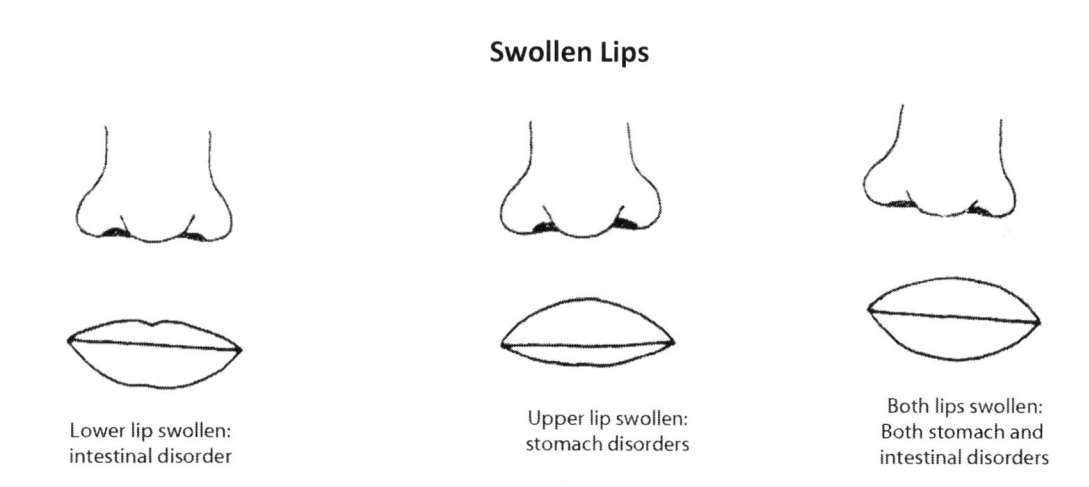

Swollen Lips

Lower lip swollen: intestinal disorder

Upper lip swollen: stomach disorders

Both lips swollen: Both stomach and intestinal disorders

Crust at corner of Lip:
Crust produced at the corners of the mouth indicates a diet high in animal protein, cooked processed oils and fried foods. This disorder occurs in the duodenum and related area. A yellowish color crust indicates that the excretion of bile from the liver and gallbladder is abnormal. It can indicate a diet of a high amount of processed saturated fats, fried foods, meat, poultry, eggs, cheese, fish, seafood, and combing meat with starches.

Corners of Lips:
The corners of the lips indicate the duodenum and the middle region of the digestive tract. The right corner relates to the duodenum's reaction to bile secretion from the liver and gallbladder. The left corner relates to pancreatic secretions.

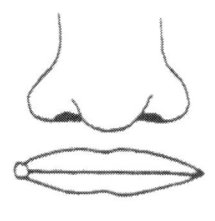

Crust formation at the corner of mouth

FACE

Racial Facial Types

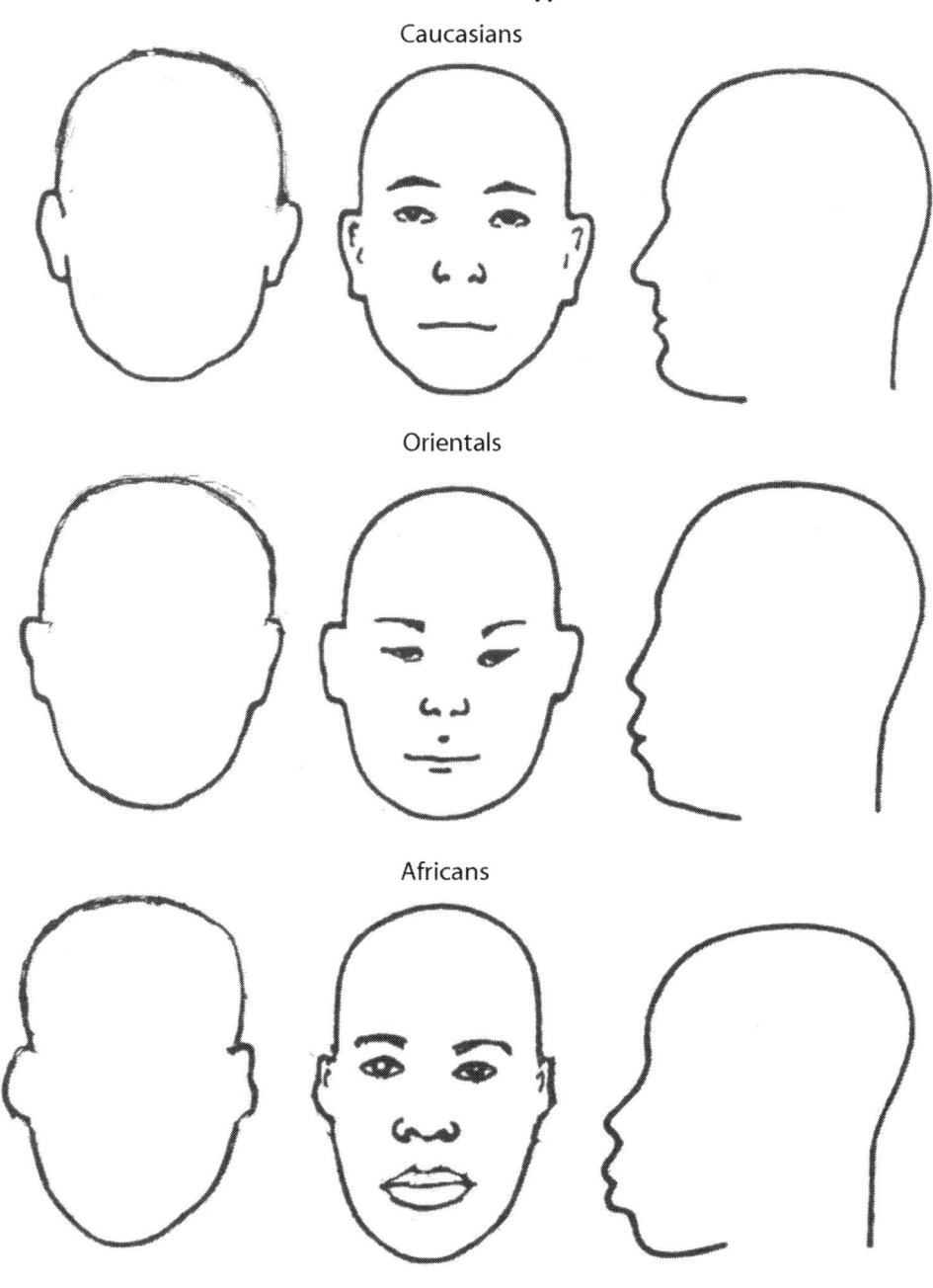

Caucasians

Orientals

Africans

Body on the Face

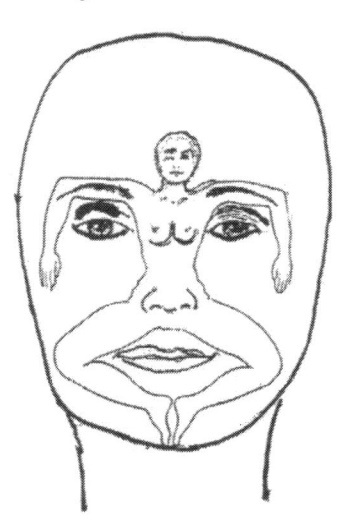

61

Face Development

These are the three stages in the development of the face in the embryo.

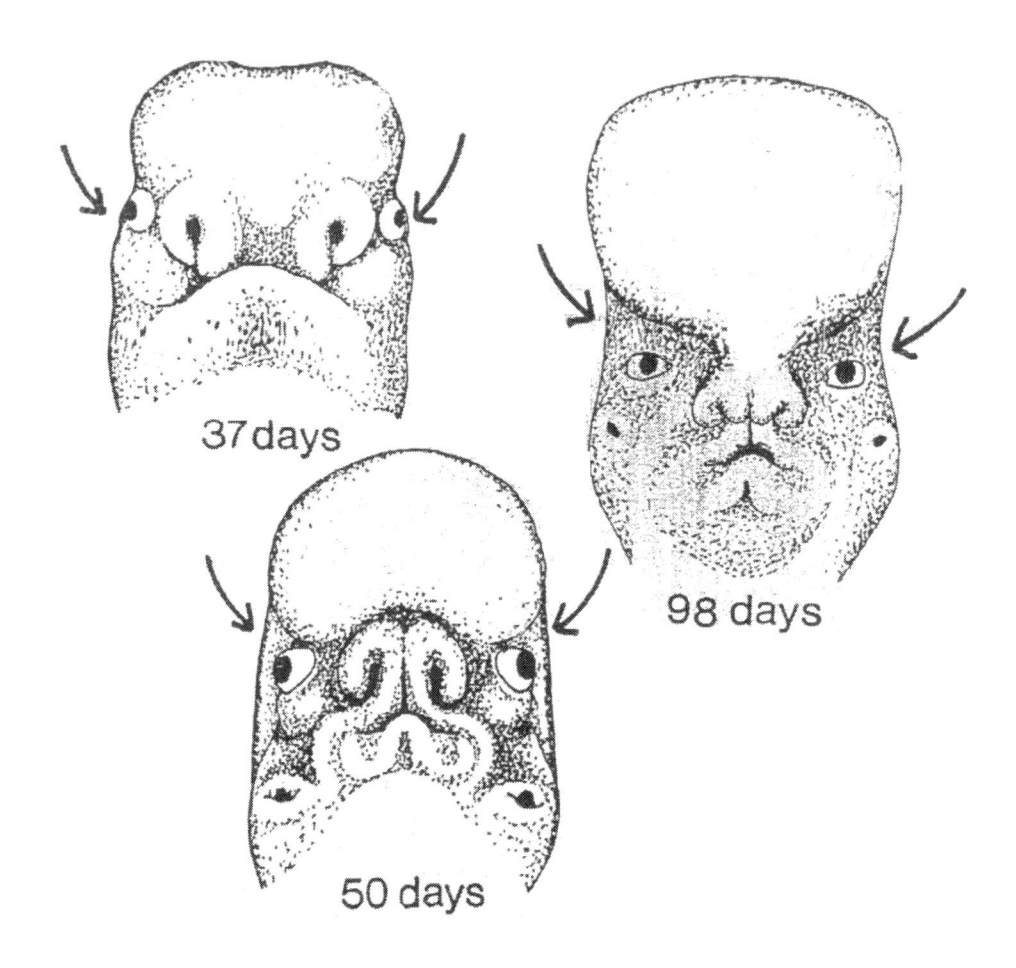

37 days

50 days

98 days

Face Reveals

1.) The face reveals accidents or severe trauma, lower organ weakness, and a passive person (see Female Principle).   2.) The face reveals aggressive or violent tendency, and upper organ weakness (see Male Principle).

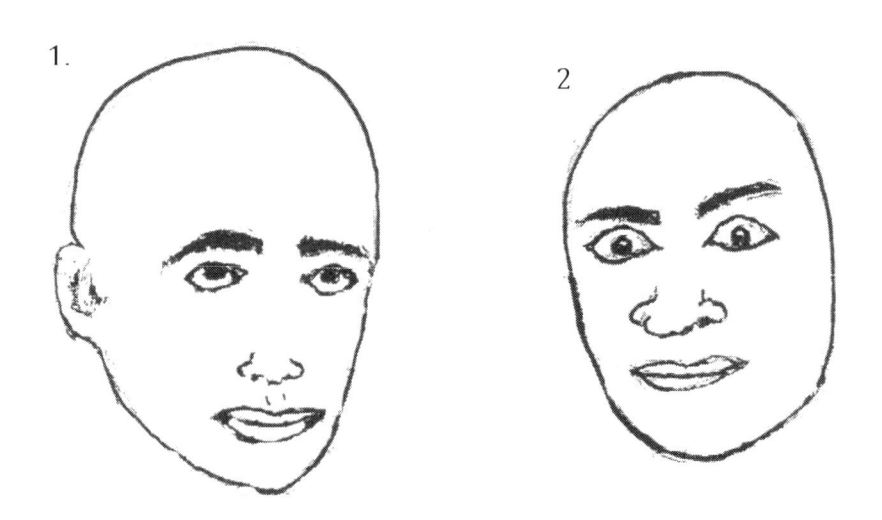

Cute Face

A cute face has youthful infantile features such as clear complexion, long eyelashes, smooth baby-like skin, no wrinkles, symmetrical features, round and clear eyes, forehead round, and small mouth etc. Animal infants also have large eyes, small mouth, round faces, and foreheads and small ears. An attractive face usually means sexually appealing such as moving lips as if kissing or simulating oral sex, blinking long eyelashes while looking at a person's genitals, breathing in a sexual rhythm manner while talking. A beautiful face is defined by culture. For example, the ancient Greeks considered shaved eyebrows (ex. painting of Mona Lisa) and small ankles beautiful, other cultures consider long hair as beautiful, sculpture facial hair (mustache, beard), sculpture head of hair (hair cut) of men as beautiful, authoritative voice, a man's strong look into women's eye as a sign of beauty. Women with long eyelashes, breast, and/or buttocks are viewed as attractive.

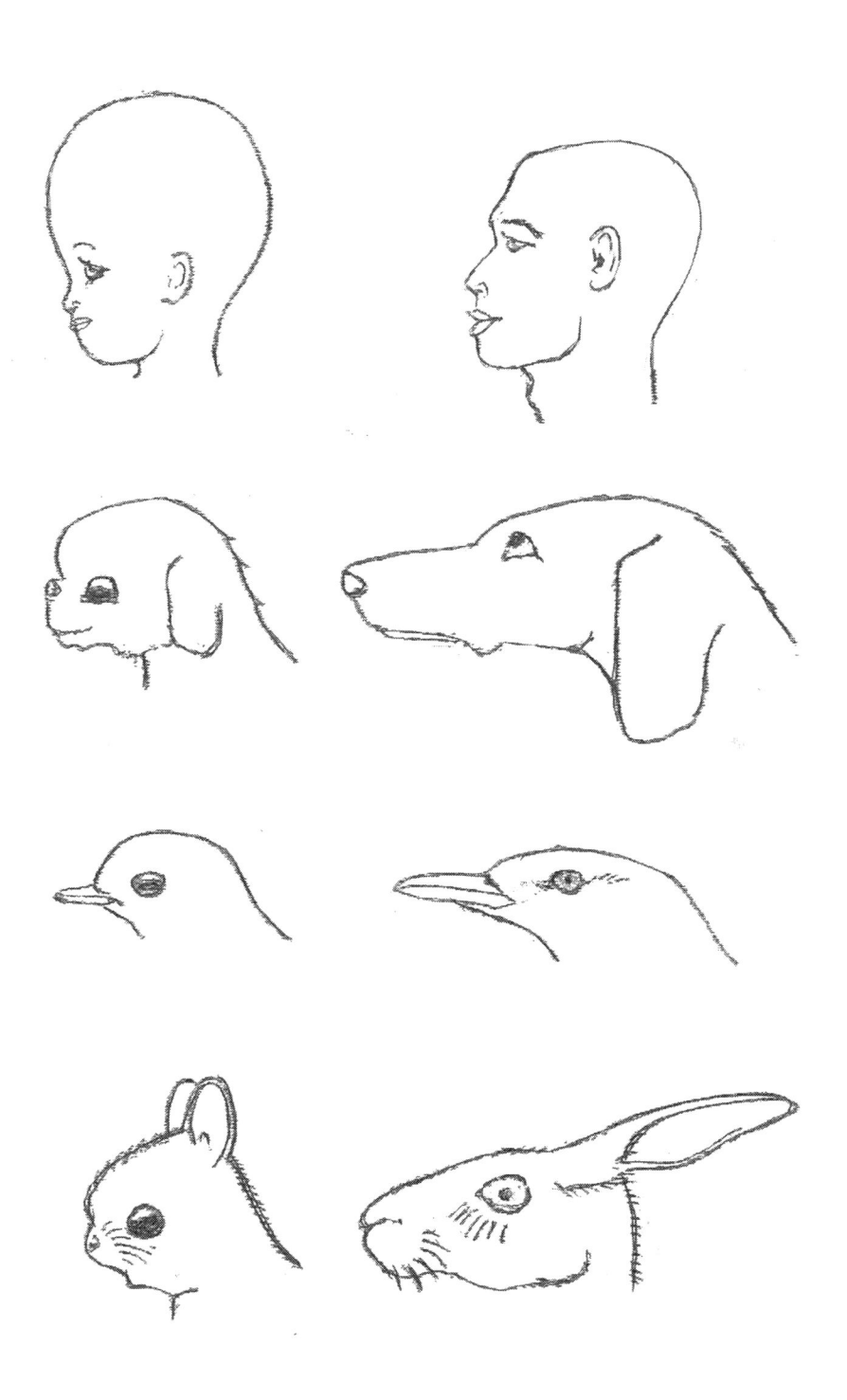

Head Shape

The adult head (skull) shape is formed (molding) by the first part of the infant's flexible bones of the skull that moved through the mother's pelvic bones. At birth the flexible skull bones (frontal, parietal, occipital) are compressed together by the mother's pelvic bones and muscle contractions. Eventually the skull bones harden (ossification) indicating the position of the skull coming through the birth canal.

Adult Head Chart

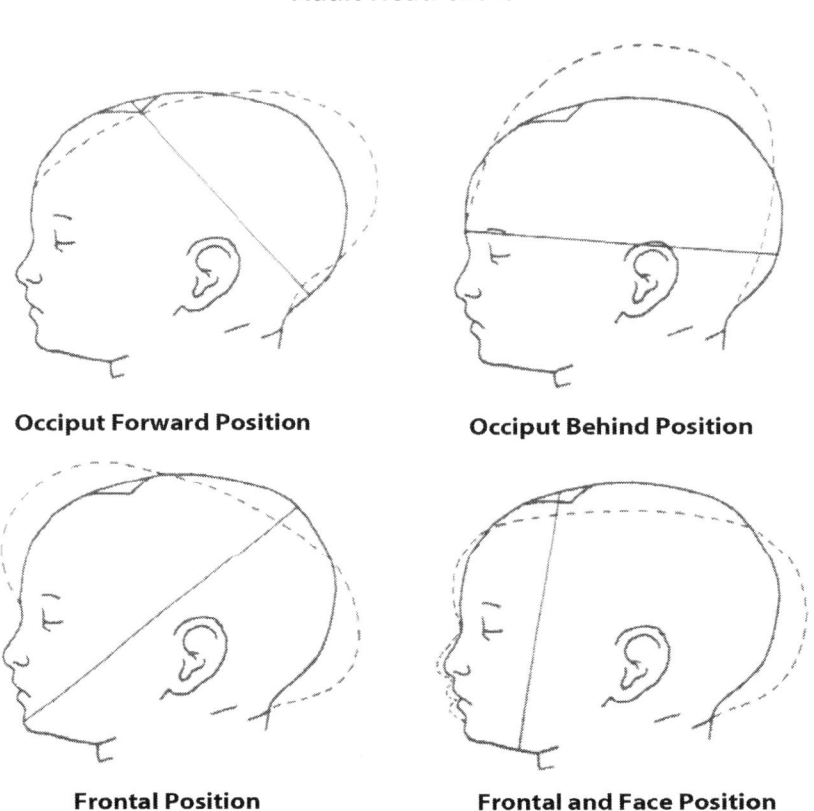

Occiput Forward Position

Occiput Behind Position

Frontal Position

Frontal and Face Position

Birth Canal

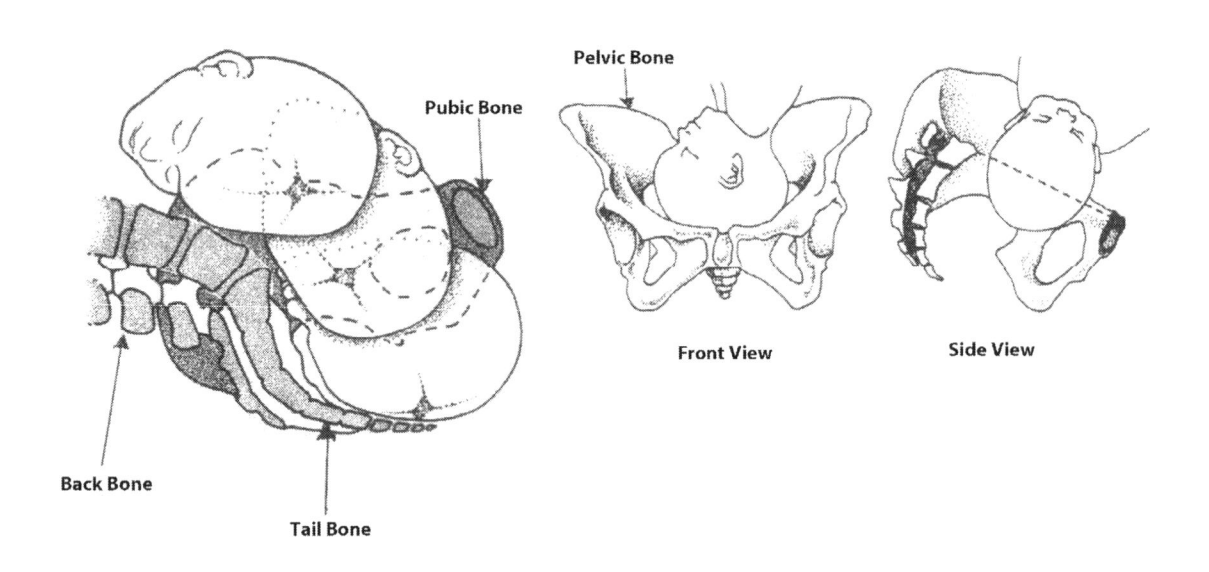

Pubic Bone

Pelvic Bone

Front View

Side View

Back Bone

Tail Bone

64

Face Pressure Points

Any inconsistency of the skin, or if the points feels sensitive when touched indicates a problem with an organ or part of the body.

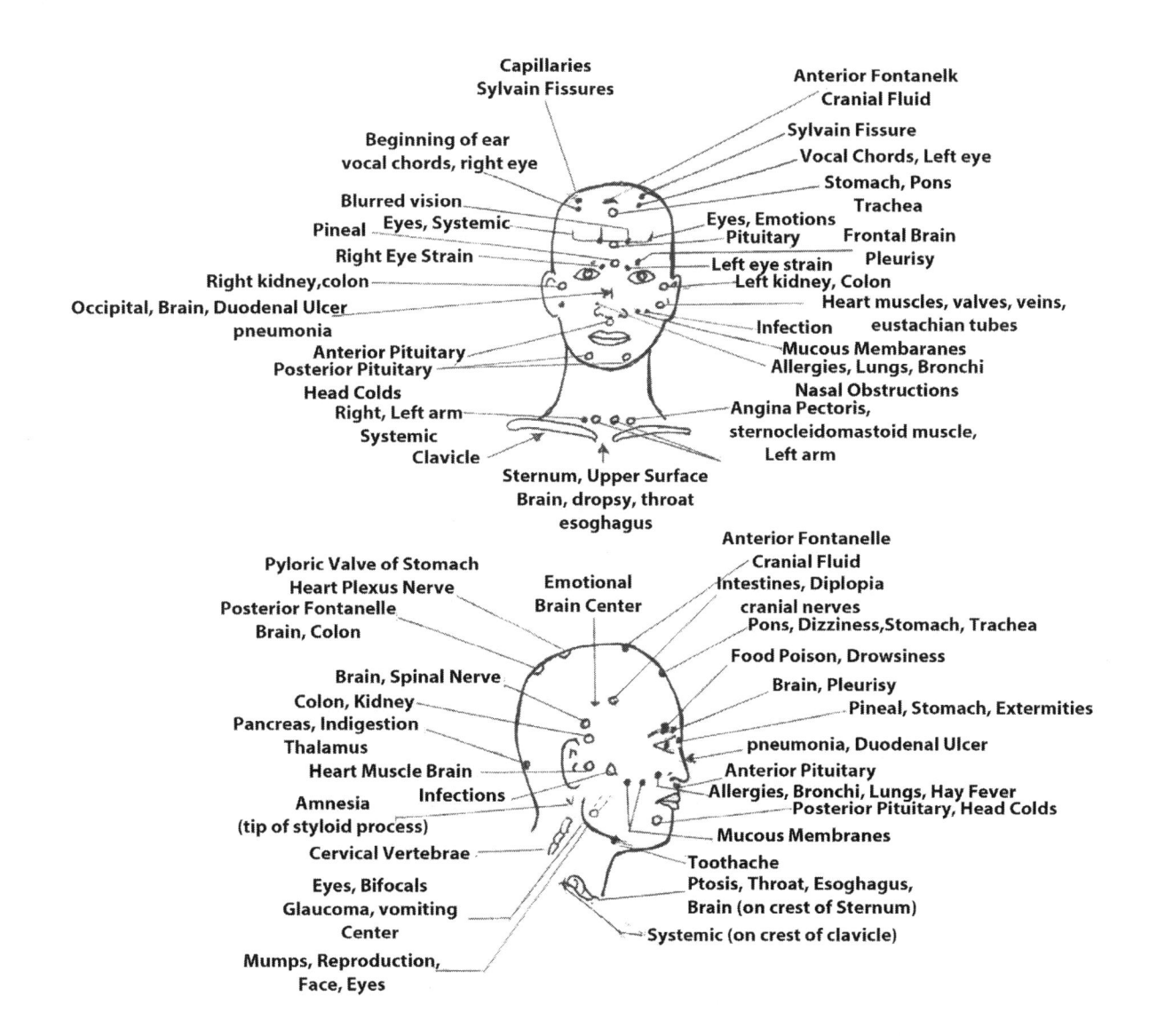

Front view labels:
- Capillaries
- Sylvain Fissures
- Anterior Fontanelk
- Cranial Fluid
- Beginning of ear vocal chords, right eye
- Sylvain Fissure
- Vocal Chords, Left eye
- Stomach, Pons
- Blurred vision
- Trachea
- Pineal
- Eyes, Systemic
- Eyes, Emotions
- Pituitary
- Frontal Brain
- Right Eye Strain
- Left eye strain
- Pleurisy
- Right kidney, colon
- Left kidney, Colon
- Occipital, Brain, Duodenal Ulcer
- Heart muscles, valves, veins, eustachian tubes
- pneumonia
- Infection
- Anterior Pituitary
- Mucous Membaranes
- Posterior Pituitary
- Allergies, Lungs, Bronchi
- Head Colds
- Nasal Obstructions
- Right, Left arm
- Angina Pectoris, sternocleidomastoid muscle, Left arm
- Systemic
- Clavicle
- Sternum, Upper Surface Brain, dropsy, throat esoghagus

Side view labels:
- Pyloric Valve of Stomach
- Heart Plexus Nerve
- Emotional Brain Center
- Anterior Fontanelle
- Cranial Fluid
- Posterior Fontanelle
- Intestines, Diplopia
- Brain, Colon
- cranial nerves
- Pons, Dizziness, Stomach, Trachea
- Brain, Spinal Nerve
- Food Poison, Drowsiness
- Colon, Kidney
- Brain, Pleurisy
- Pancreas, Indigestion
- Pineal, Stomach, Extermities
- Thalamus
- pneumonia, Duodenal Ulcer
- Heart Muscle Brain
- Anterior Pituitary
- Amnesia
- Allergies, Bronchi, Lungs, Hay Fever
- Infections
- Posterior Pituitary, Head Colds
- (tip of styloid process)
- Mucous Membranes
- Cervical Vertebrae
- Toothache
- Eyes, Bifocals
- Ptosis, Throat, Esoghagus,
- Glaucoma, vomiting
- Brain (on crest of Sternum)
- Center
- Systemic (on crest of clavicle)
- Mumps, Reproduction, Face, Eyes

65

Amino Acids Points on Face

These points are the same on both sides of the face.

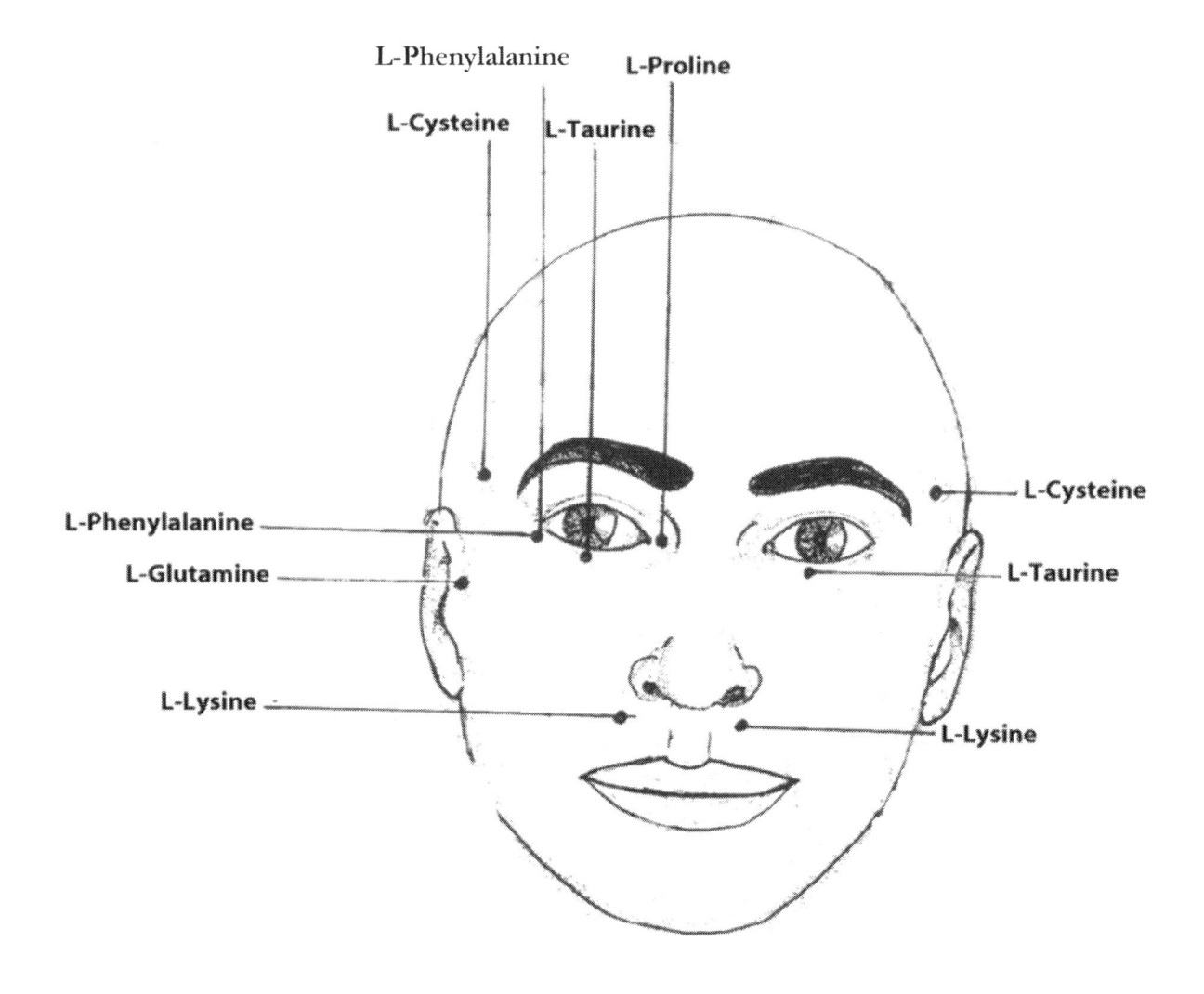

L-Phenylalanine
L-Proline
L-Cysteine
L-Taurine

L-Cysteine
L-Phenylalanine
L-Taurine
L-Glutamine
L-Lysine
L-Lysine

Any inconsistency of the skin on a point or if the point feels sensitive to touch or if there is a weak muscle test indicates problems with that amino acid.

Face Chart

Any inconsistency in the skin in an organ area indicates problems with that organ.

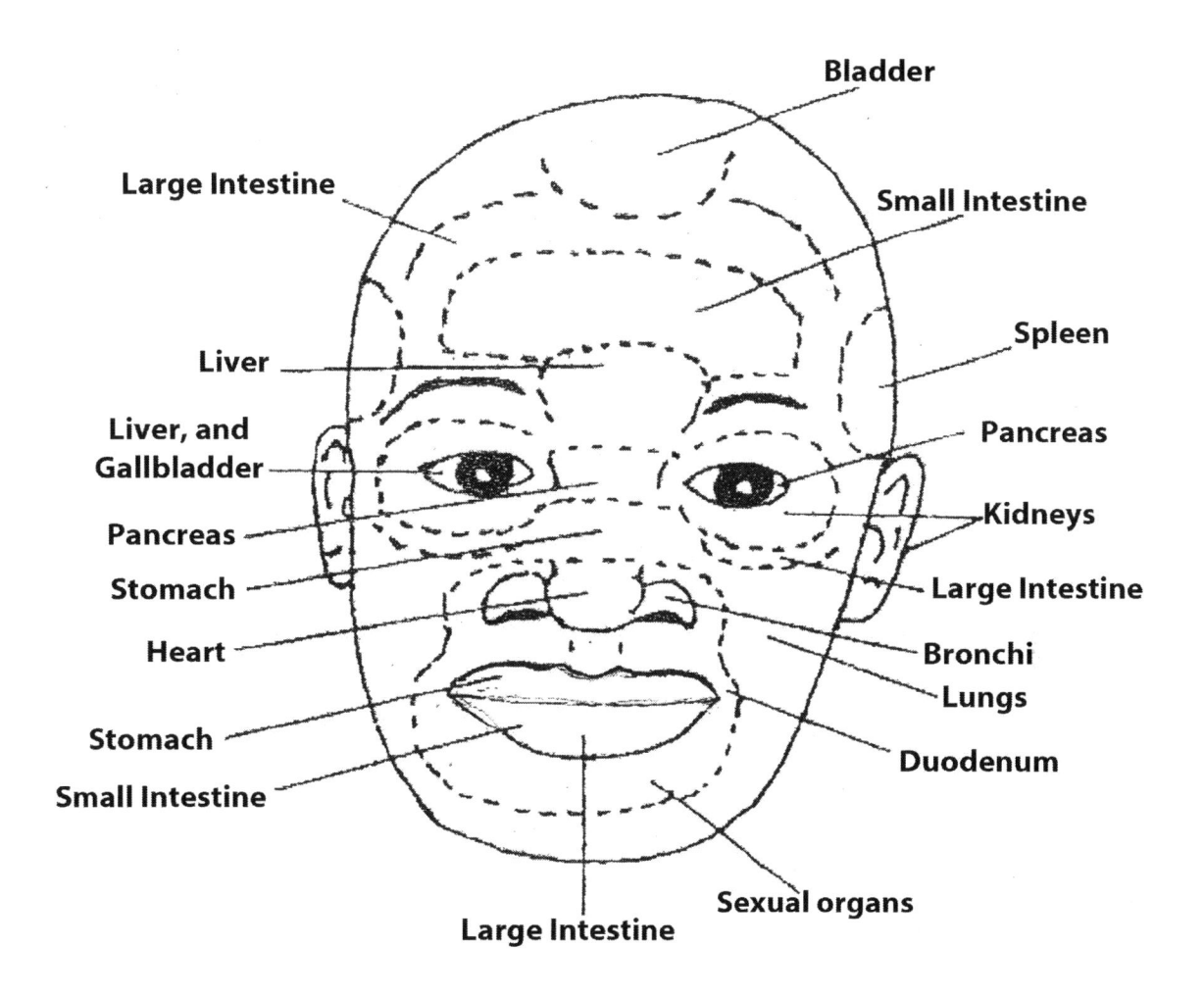

- Bladder
- Large Intestine
- Small Intestine
- Liver
- Spleen
- Liver, and Gallbladder
- Pancreas
- Pancreas
- Kidneys
- Stomach
- Large Intestine
- Heart
- Bronchi
- Lungs
- Stomach
- Duodenum
- Small Intestine
- Sexual organs
- Large Intestine

Development of Systems in Embryo

Any high inconsistency of the skin in a Trimester skin area indicates spiritual, emotional, mental, and or nutritional stress in that embryonic trimester.

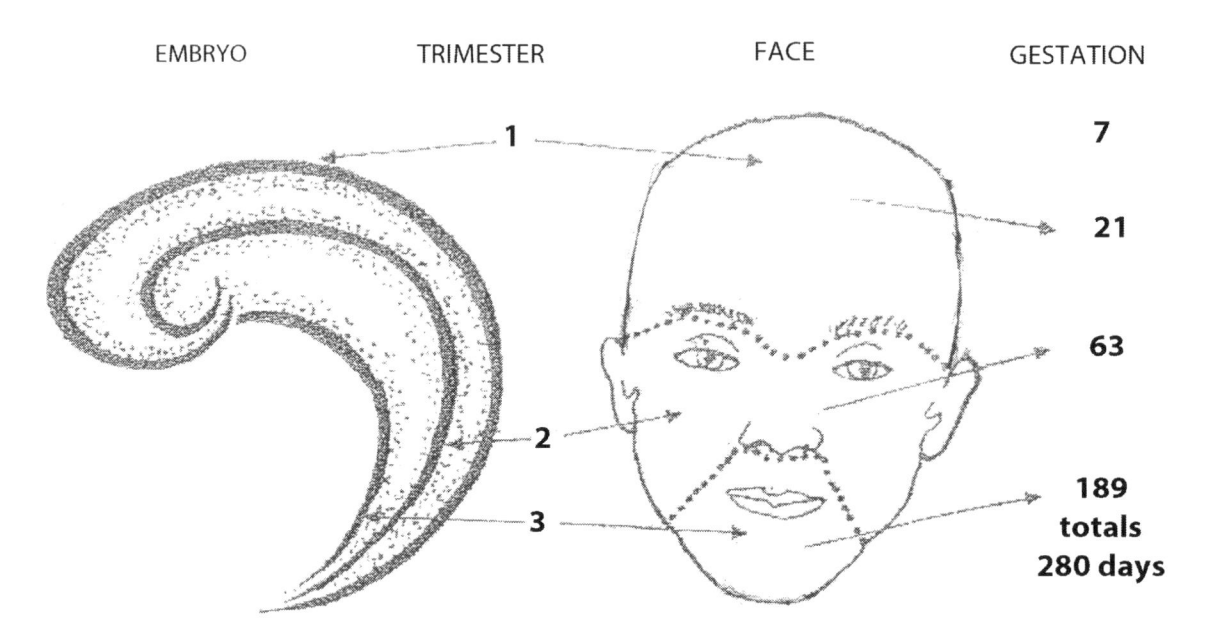

EMBRYO   TRIMESTER   FACE   GESTATION

1 — 7
21
63
2
3 — 189 totals
280 days

Head/Buttock Correlation

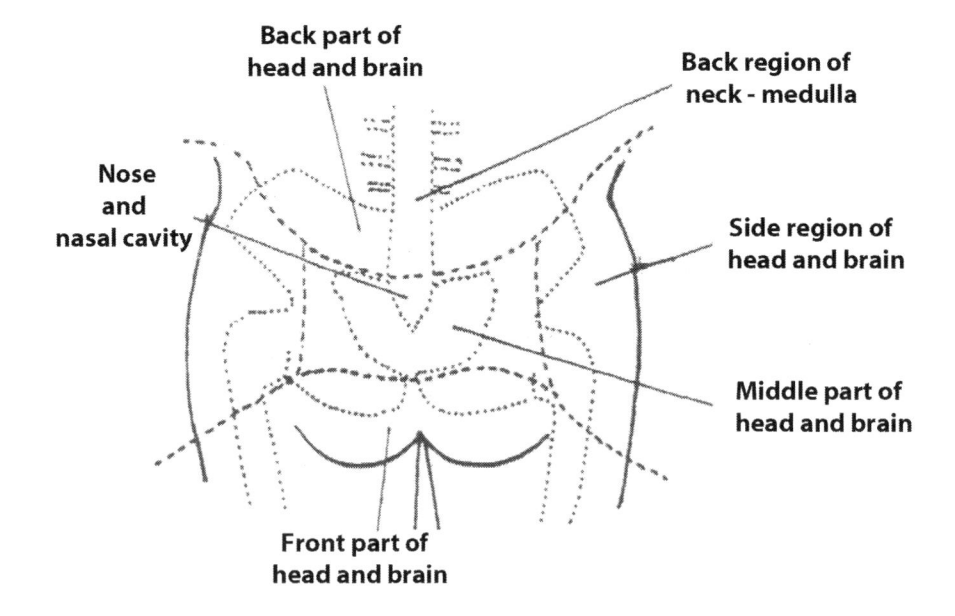

- Back part of head and brain
- Back region of neck - medulla
- Nose and nasal cavity
- Side region of head and brain
- Middle part of head and brain
- Front part of head and brain

68

Face Shapes

Children primarily focus on the Width Height Ratio (WHR). WHR is the space from the upper lip to the eyebrow. If the width is wider than the height distance it indicates the Male Principle/Extrovert personality. If the Height distance is taller than the width of the face it is the Female Principle/Introvert/Nurturing personality. The children prefer the Female Principle.

Type A is steady, realistic, and practical. **Type B** is more romantic and emotional, sentimental, and idealistic. **Type C** tends to be an analyzer, thinker, and intellectual. **Type D** is active, a do-er.

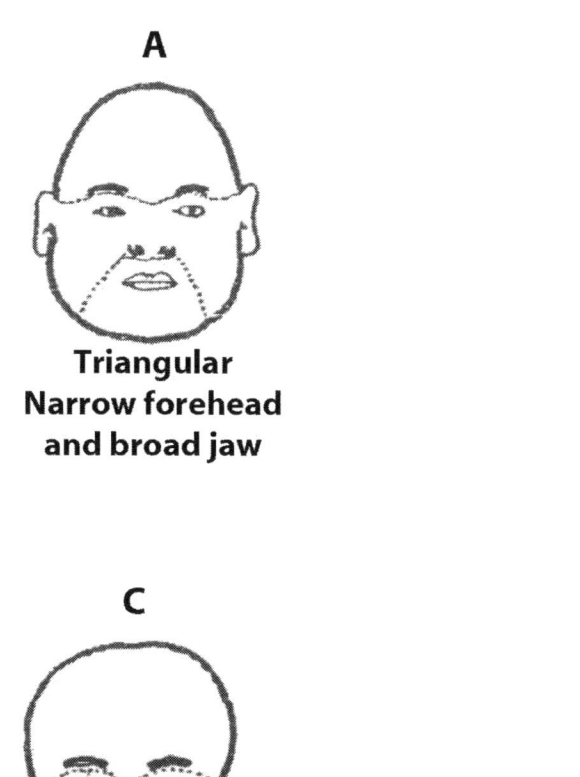

A

**Triangular
Narrow forehead
and broad jaw**

B

**Long or
Oval**

C

**Triangular
Broad forehead,
and narrow jaw**

D

Round

Systems

The area with the most inconsistency of skin can indicate problems with that system.

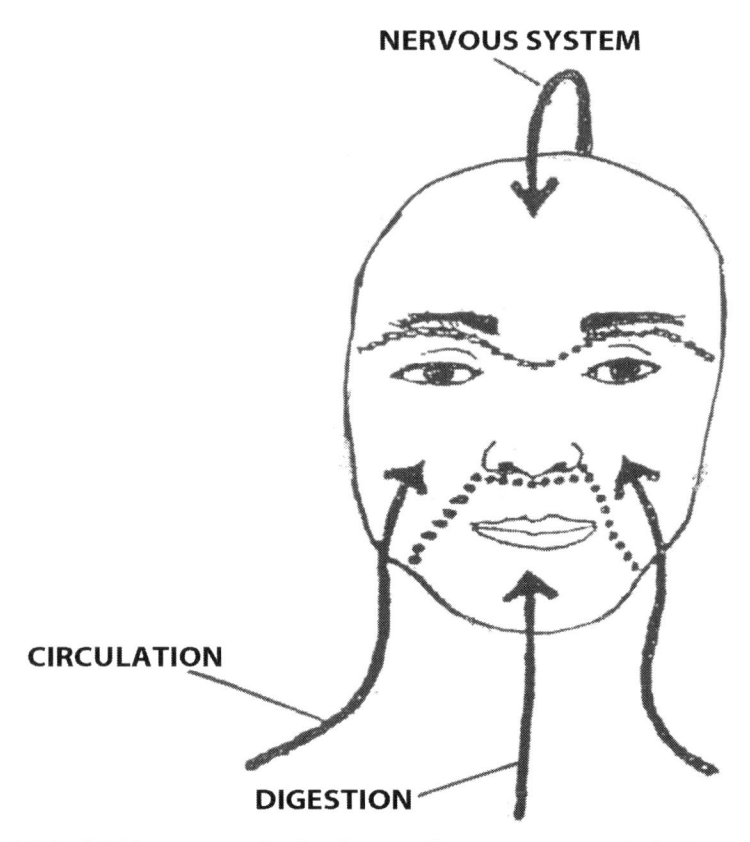

NERVOUS SYSTEM

CIRCULATION

DIGESTION

The nose and nasol-labial folds serve as the dividing markers. **Areas 1** include the cheeks, lips, jaw, and mouth. **Areas 2** include the right side of face from forehead to nasol-labial fold, which includes the right eye and eyebrow, the right forehead, and the area beneath the eyes. **Area 3** includes the same structures area as 2, only on the left side. **Area 4** includes the area between the eyebrows and forehead.

Areas on the Face

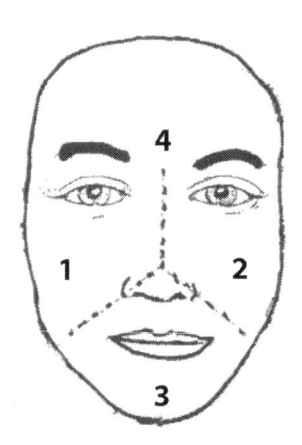

Face, Planets, and Disease

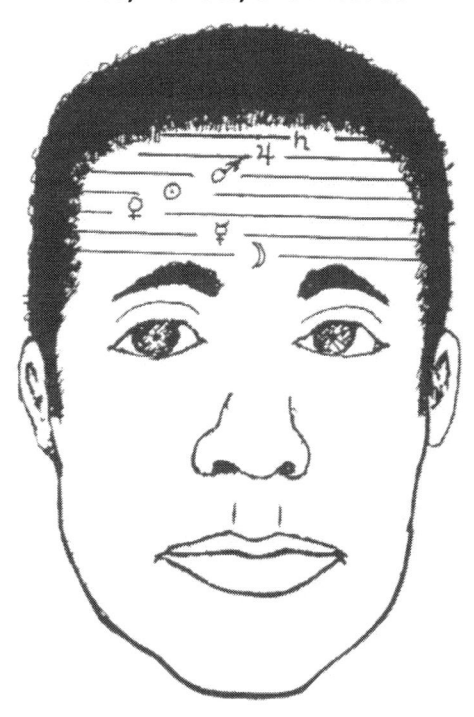

The forehead has areas that correspond to planets. Inconsistency in the skin indicates problems with corresponding planet's symptoms.

Planets	Symptoms
Sun ☉	Heart disease, artery and vein weakness
Moon ☽	Inflammation of mucous membranes, edema, dehydration
Mercury ☿	Neuritis, respiratory diseases
Venus ♀	Throat infections, thyroid imbalance, kidney problems
Mars ♂	Swelling and inflammation, fevers, infections, accidents hemorrhage and blood disease
Jupiter ♃	Liver diseases (hepatitis), pancreatic disease (hypoglycemia, diabetes), obesity, tumors, cysts, warts
Saturn ♄	Arthritis, rheumatism, fractures, spinal ailments, dental problems, skin diseases, gall stones
Uranus ♅	Cramps, spasm, shocks, paralysis, epilepsy, muscle problems, radiation toxicity
Neptune ♆	Hallucinations, alcoholism, addictions, toxic conditions, schizophrenia, undiagnosed diseases, reactions to synthetic chemicals and hormones
Pluto ♇	Disease of the reproductive organs, degenerative diseases, weak tissue

Face and Zodiac Signs

The face has areas that correspond to zodiac signs. Each side of the forehead has different signs while each side of the cheeks; chin, as well as the neck have the same sign. A change in color (darkness, lightness), blotchiness, rash, oiliness, dryness, slight temperature variation (cold or warm areas) and/or skin eruptions in a sign indicates emotional, mental and or physical stress, weakness, or a disease with the body part that the sign represents.

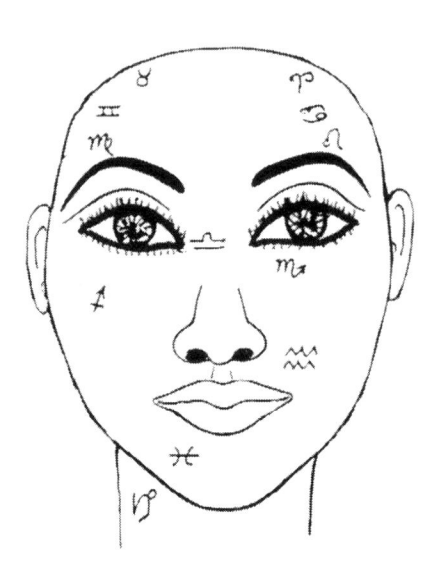

Aries	♈	Head, face, cerebrum, eyes, nose, pituitary
Taurus	♉	Neck, throat, cerebellum, mouth, tonsils, vocal cords, thyroid
Gemini	♊	Arms, shoulders, lungs, fallopian tubes
Cancer	♋	Stomach, breasts, arteries, diaghragm, uterus, veins
Leo	♌	Cardiac region, spleen, heart
Virgo	♍	Small intestine, pancreas, lower abdomen
Libra	♎	Small of back, adrenal, kidneys, bladder
Scorpio	♏	Pelvis, reproductive organs, gonads, colon, rectum
Sagittarius	♐	Thighs, hips, buttocks, liver, sciatic nerve
Capricorn	♑	Knees, bones, gall bladder, teeth, cartilage
Aquarius	♒	Calves, ankles, bladder, retina of eyes, parathyroid
Pisces	♓	Feet, circulation, pineal, lymphatic system

Regions of the Forehead

A. **Lower region** - Digestive and respiratory systems
B. **Middle region** - Nervous system
C. **Upper region** - Circulatory and excretory systems
D. **Temples region** - spleen, pancreas (Left temple), liver and gall bladder (Right Temple)

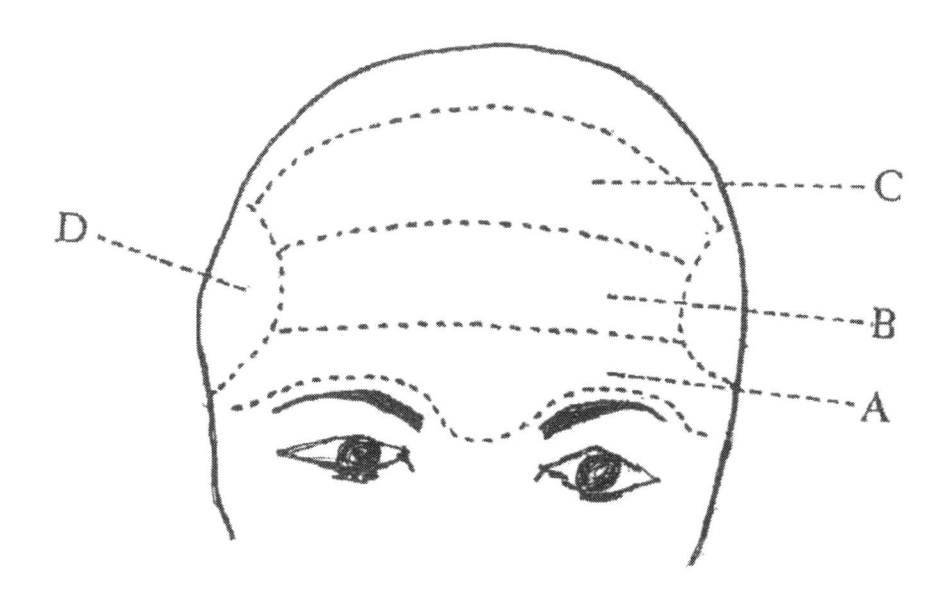

There can be up to 3 horizontal deep, long or broken lines on the forehead of skin inconsistency (color, texture, oily, dry, bumps) that can indicate problems in a system and/or organ. Pimples indicate fat deposits and liver problems.

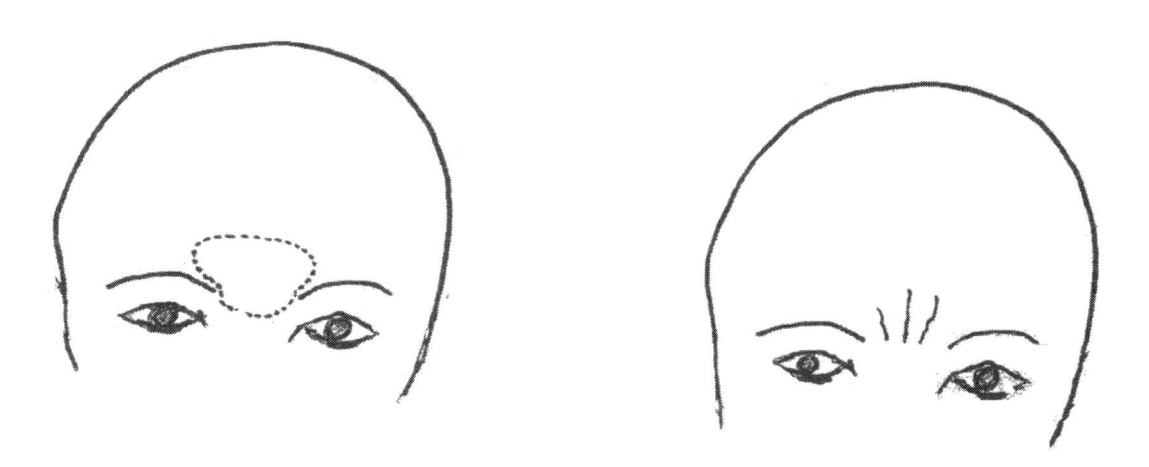

There can be vertical wrinkles between the eyes that indicate liver problems. Mentally the wrinkles can indicate rigidity, emotional issues, short temper and/or unstableness.

Facial and Bone Deformities

Normal bone structure, showing width through all parts of face and wide spacing between eyes

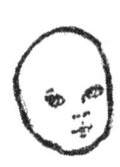

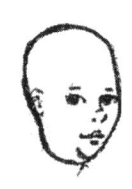

Underdevelopment through lower third of face

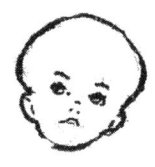

Abnormal overgrowth of cartilage-like base of bone above ears

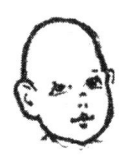

Underdevelopment, especially through upper third of face

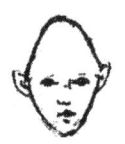

Stunted growth of entire skull, allowing inadequate space for brain

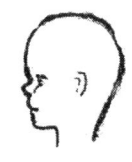

Normal Profile

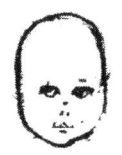

Abnormal bone structure eyes too close together and too deeply set

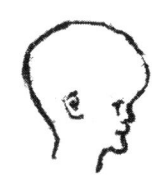

Underdevelopment through center third of face

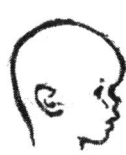

Abnormal, bulging forehead

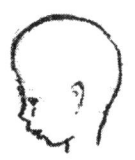

Underdevelopment through upper two-thirds of face

Underdeveloped chin

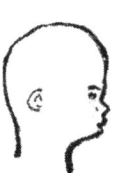

Buck teeth, resulting from faulty bone growth

Face

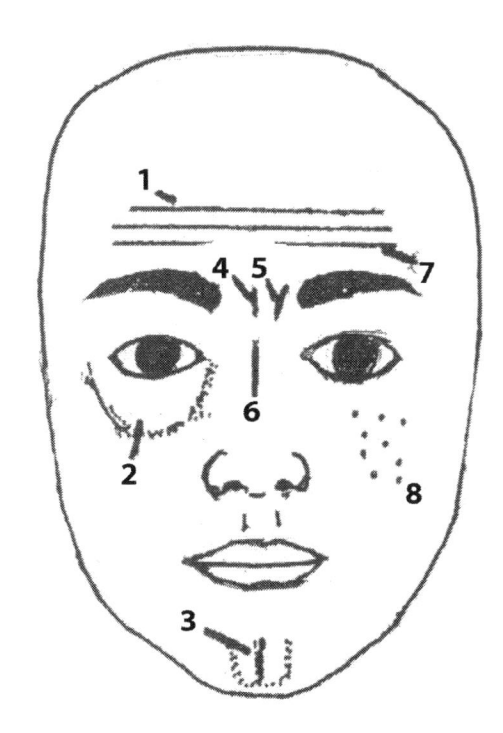

1. **Parallel Horizontal Lines on Forehead or Under Eyes** – edema, nerve and lung issues, excess liquid, overeating, kidney disorder, intestinal problems.
2. **Large, Low Bag Under Eyes** – overeating, intestinal problems
3. **Cleft Chin** – contraction during birthing, stress reaction
4. **Vertical Line Between Eyes** – spleen disorder
5. **Vertical Line Above & to Sides of Nose** – excess sodium chloride, protein foods, liver disorder
6. **Horizontal line on Bridge of Nose** – excess protein, liver problems
7. **Chaotic Horizontal Lines on Forehead** – stress, anxiety, brain disorder, Mental Problems
8. **Pimples** – fermentation in intestines, constipation
    - Swollen Area Between Nose & Lip – mucous congestion in stomach, spleen, pancreas
    - Acne or Pockmarks – excess chemicals, drugs, concentrated sweeteners
    - Horizontal Lines – excess liquids, concentrated sweeteners, Edema
    - Vertical Lines – excess sodium chloride and protein
    - Vertical Line Above & to Side of Nose (caused by puffiness) – excess concentrated sweeteners, constipation, liver problems

Face Changes/Bodily Degenerating

The following Face changes indicate the overall health progressively getting worse (degenerating).

Normal

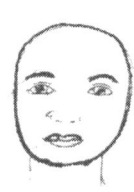

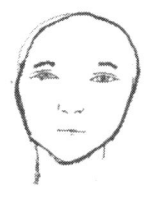

Spastic

Round (Rotunda) Type

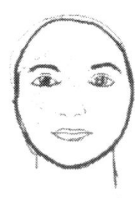

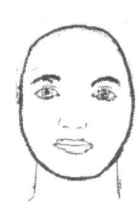

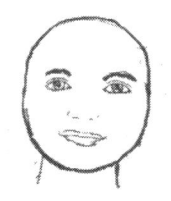

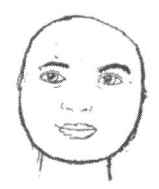

Drying Up (Atroph Plana) Type

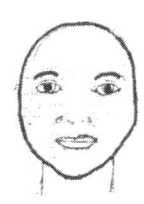

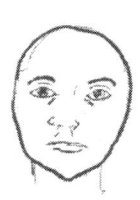

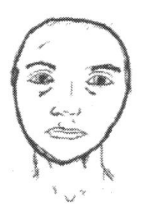

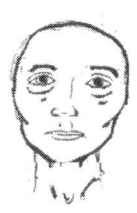

Types of Facial Deformities

Line (Atroph Striata)

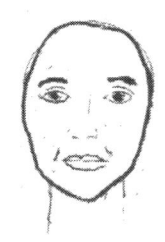

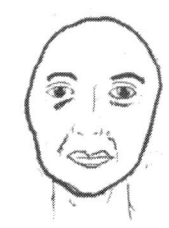

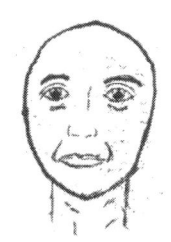

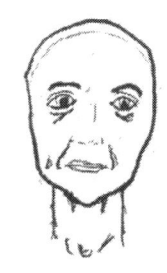

Wrinkle Dry (Atroph Plic. Plic.)

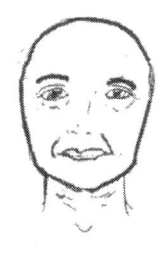

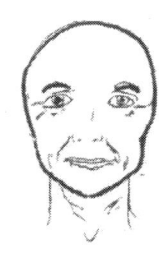

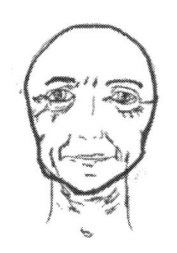

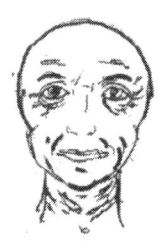

Folding (Plicata)

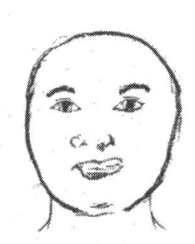

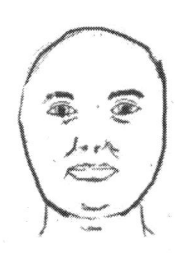

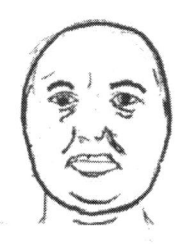

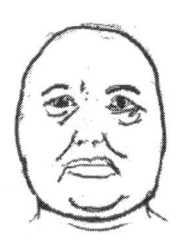

77

Measurement of Neck

The normal length of the front (ventral) and back (dorsal) of the neck is 4 fingers widths.

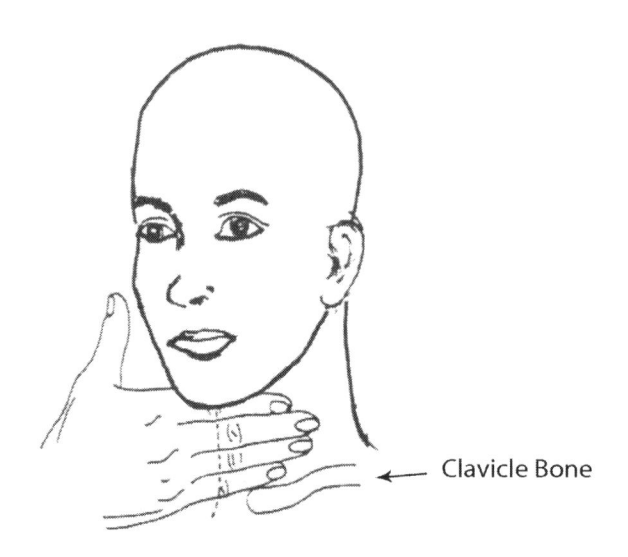

← Clavicle Bone

Neck Lengths

Different Neck Lengths (NL) as a result of digestive disturbances.

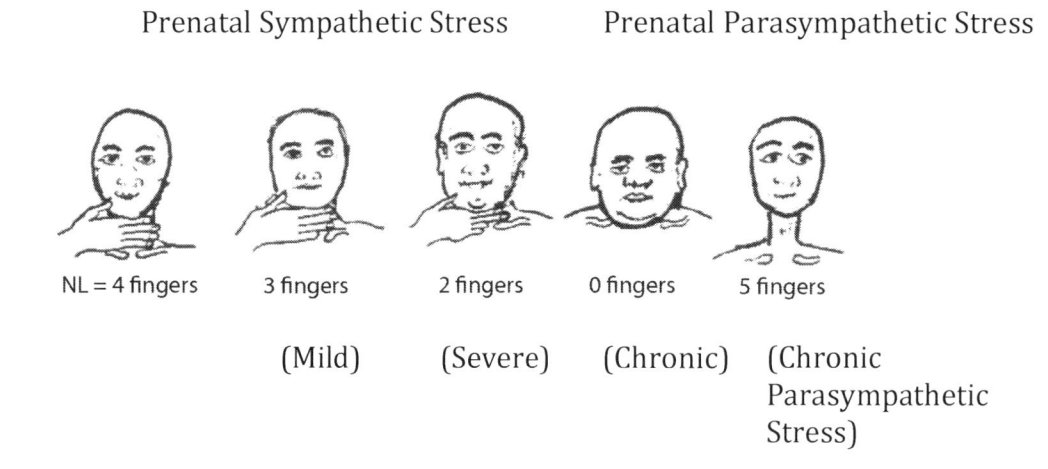

Prenatal Sympathetic Stress   Prenatal Parasympathetic Stress

NL = 4 fingers   3 fingers   2 fingers   0 fingers   5 fingers

(Mild)   (Severe)   (Chronic)   (Chronic Parasympathetic Stress)

Thyroid Massage

The thyroid gland influences the rate of metabolism. A massage of the thyroid area will help it to function. Metabolism will be increased along with the elimination of poisons and toxins. Digestion and absorption of nutrients will be enhanced. Inconsistency of the skin or sensitivity to touch can indicate thyroid problems.

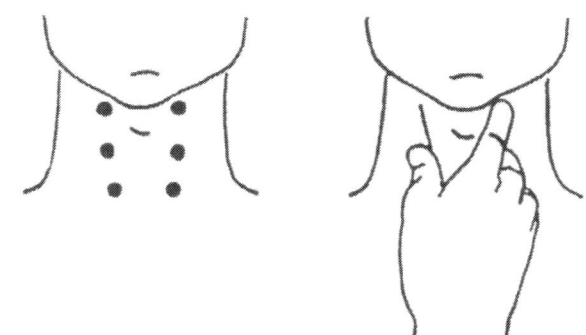

Face Type (Zodiac) and Health Problems

A zodiac facial structure can have many of the features and problems listed but not necessarily include all of them.

Aries (March 21- April 19)

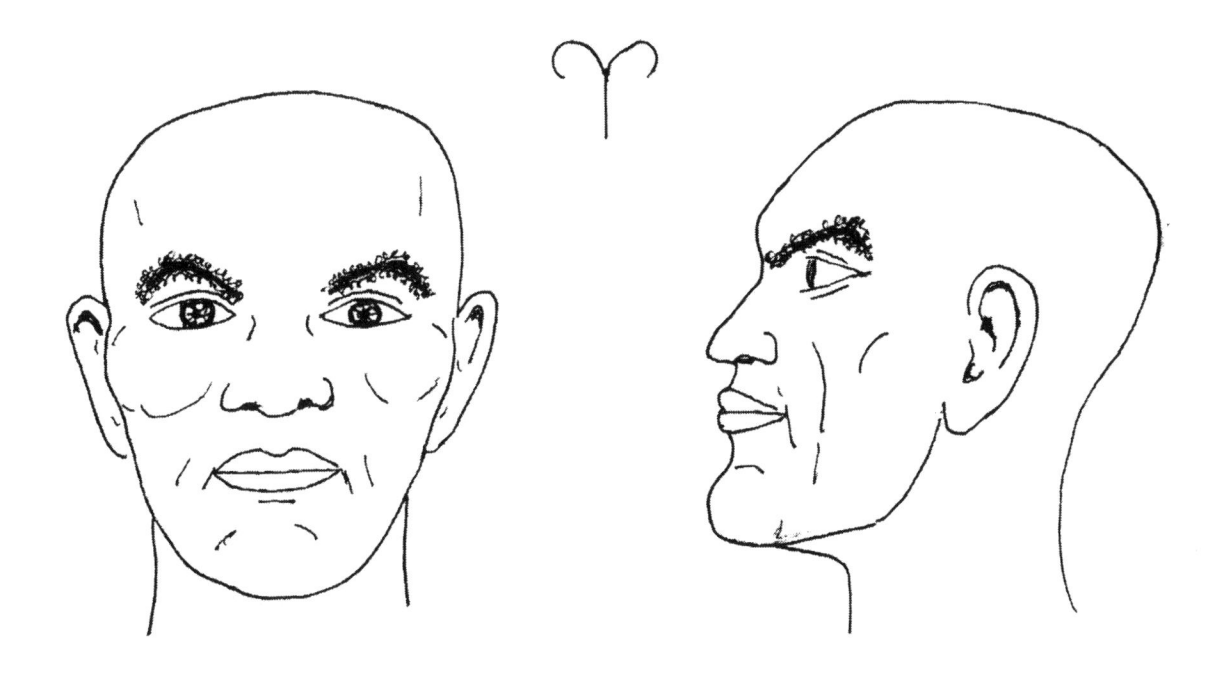

Features

Bony angular face; protruding long chin; large ears with long lobes; pronounced lower forehead; lines around mouth, bushy eyebrows that curve up; Tend to have mental problems, headaches, minor injuries to head and face; and physical problems with cerebrum, eyes; nose; and pituitary.

Taurus (April 20- May 20)

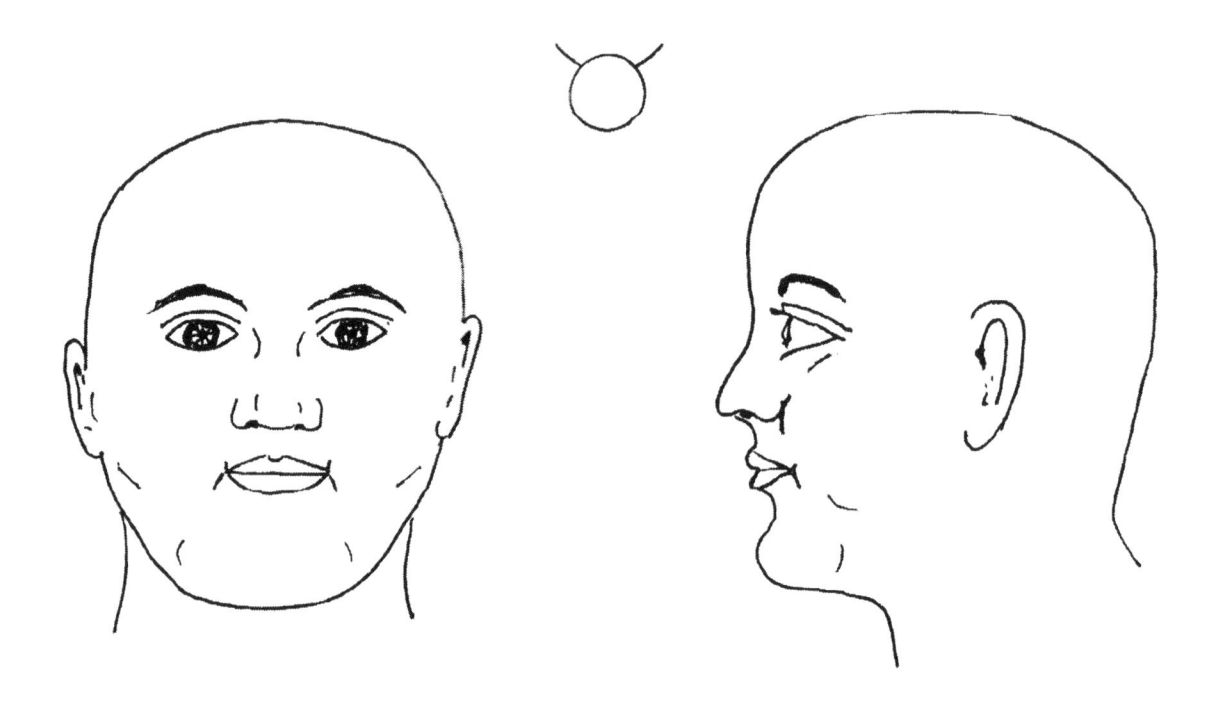

Features

Soft full face; heavy jaw; short nose; good voice; rounded high forehead; slightly protruding eyes; full lips and nostrils; soft hair; Tends to have problems in neck areas, laryngitis, sore throat, thyroid problems, colds, flu, vocal cords, tonsils, and brain's cerebellum.

Gemini (May 21- June 20)

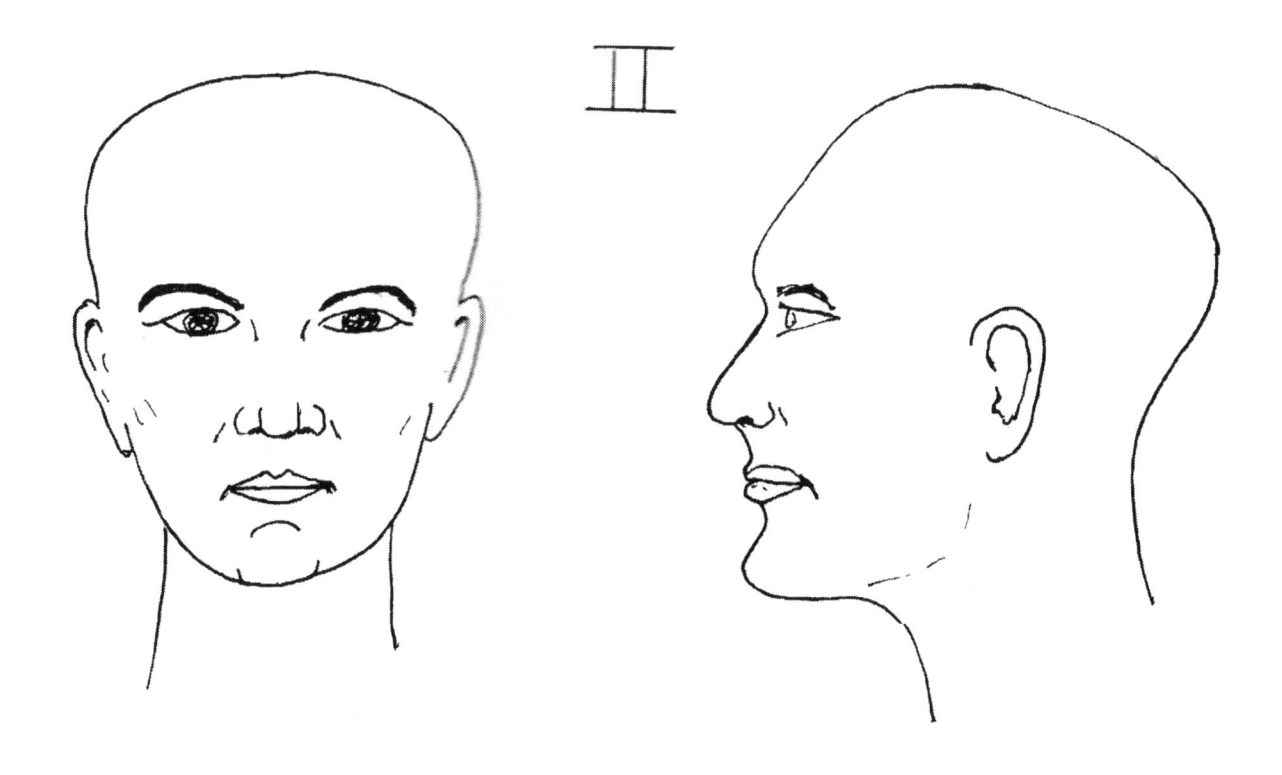

Features

Receding forehead wide at top; protruding chin; narrow mouth; long head narrow between ears; quick eye movements; Tend to have problems with arms, shoulders, and hands, can have respiratory diseases and problems with bronchitis, fallopian tubes, and testicles.

Cancer (June 21- July 22)

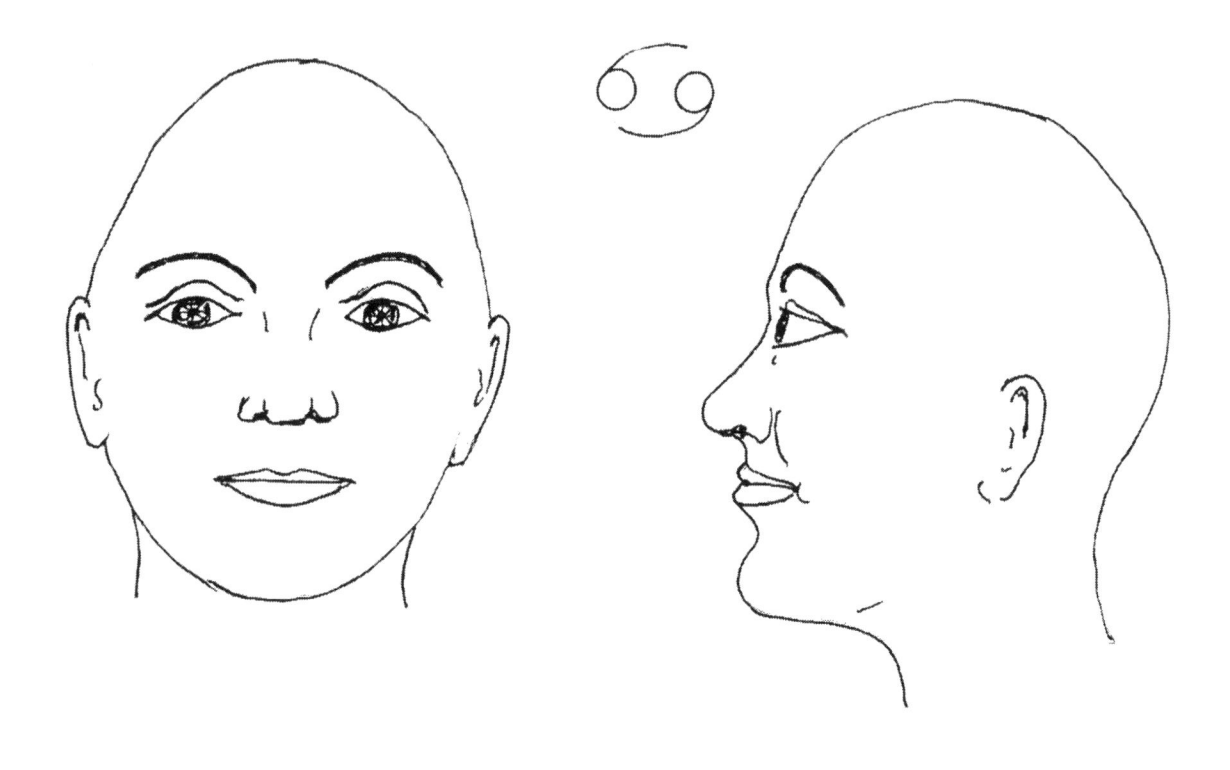

Features

Egg shaped face; head wide between ears; round chin; upper head narrow and high; high forehead; protruding eyes; heavy upper eyelids; fleshy middle face; skin loose in texture; Tend to have breast, stomach, uterus, veins, arteries, sex hormone, and digestive problems; Emotions can cause physical problems, and tends to medicate emotions by over eating.

Leo (July 23- August 22)

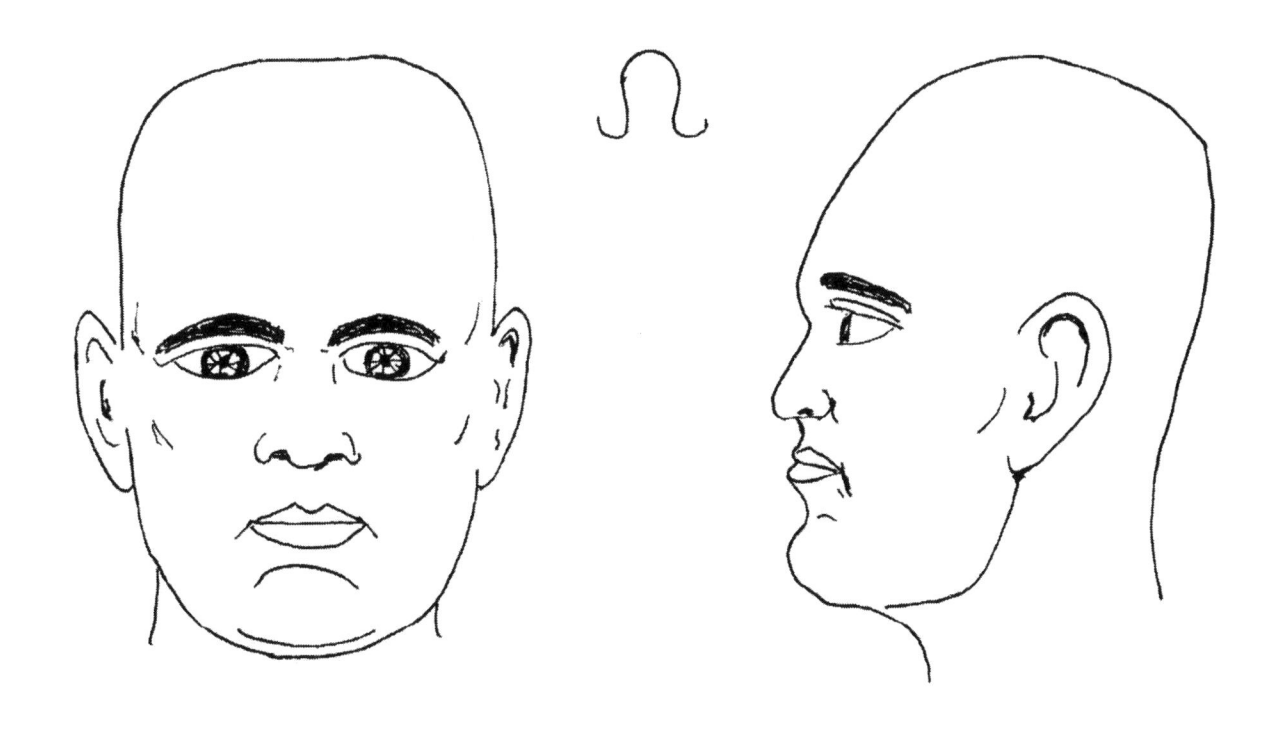

Features

Prominent cheek bones; heavy jaw and full chin; protruding lower lip; mouth corners firm; large ears, high forehead and head; back of head flat; large neck; penetrating eyes; Tend to have problems with back, spine, heart, spleen, and emotional stresses.

Virgo (August 23- September 22)

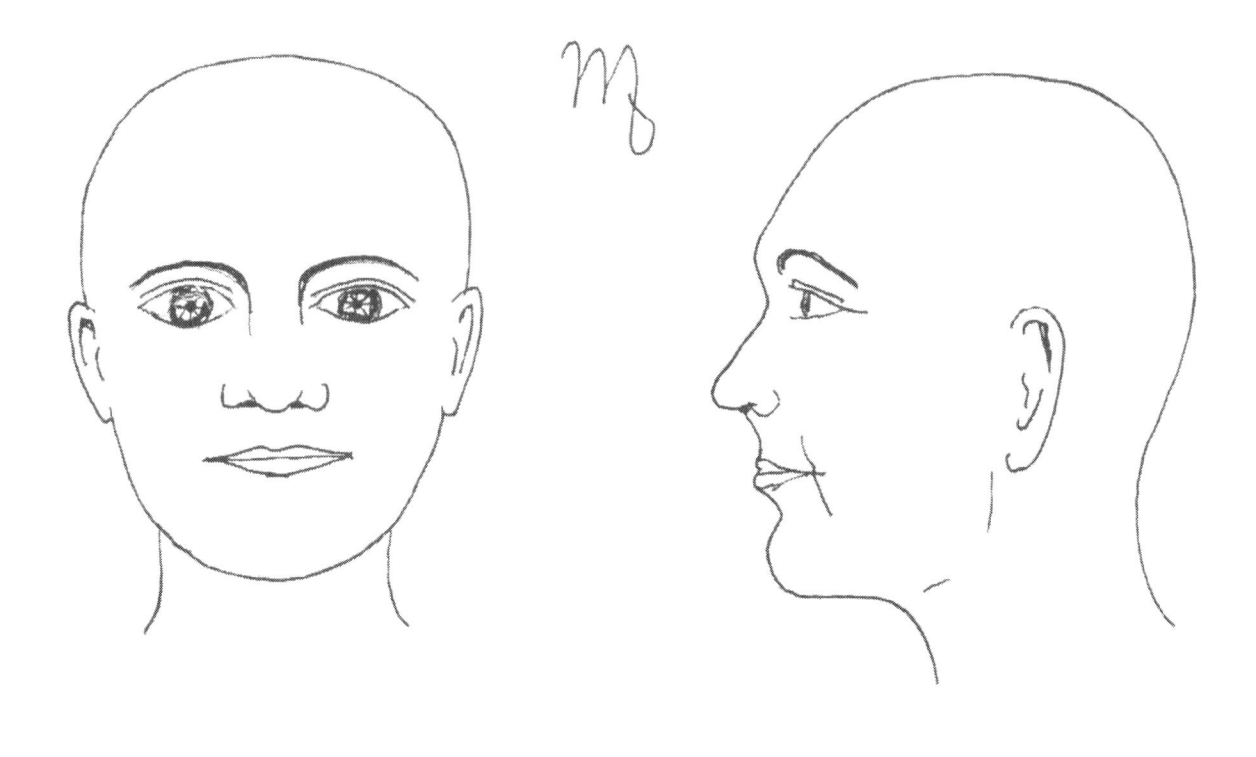

Features

High even forehead with full base; well formed face; finely shaped mouth; wide nose; analytical facial appearance; Tend to have problems with stress, nervous system, lower abdomen, pancreas, and intestines, susceptible to ulcers.

Libra (September 23 - October 22)

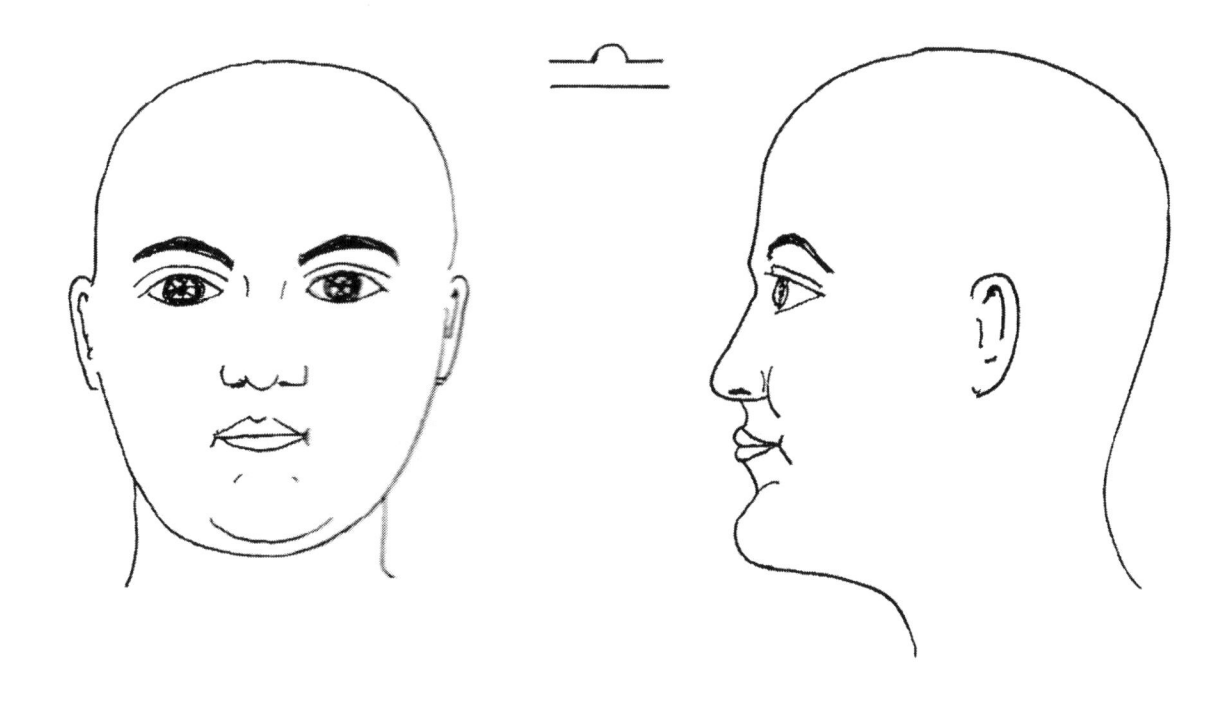

Features

Full rounded forehead; oval face, finely curved mouth with soft lips; graceful body figure; Tend to have lower back (Lumbar), kidney disease, back strain, adrenals, and bladder problems.

Scorpio (October 23- November 21)

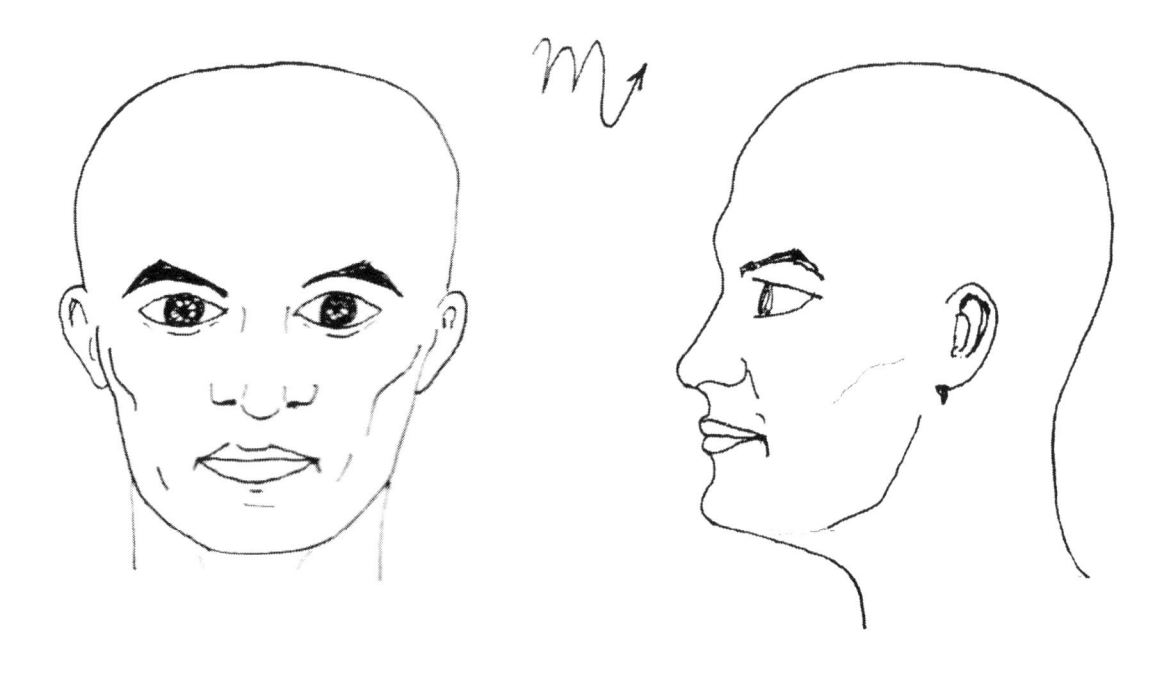

Features

Broad forehead; prominent cheek bones; small ears; strong jaw; round tip of nose; Tends to have urinary, colon, rectum, pelvis, and genital problems; venereal disease and reproductive diseases; Emotions can cause disease and exhaustion.

Sagittarius (November 22- December 21)

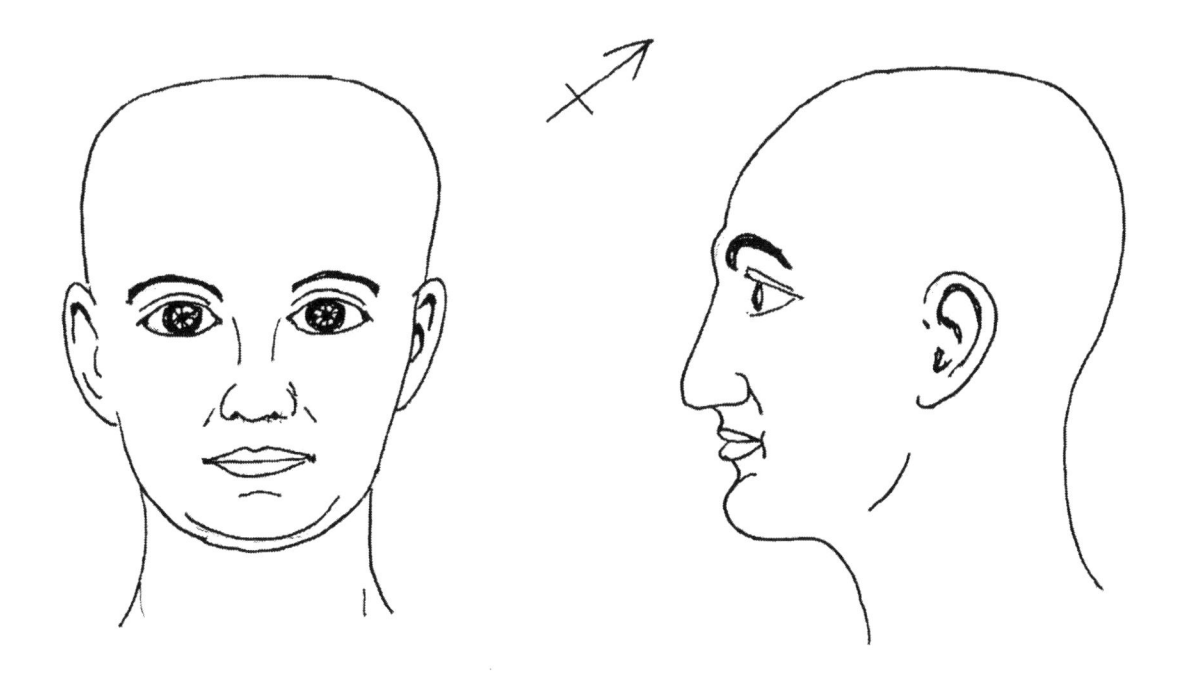

Features

Large eyes; round forehead; high head, full in back; long nose; Tends to have problems with hips, thighs, liver, and sciatic nerve. Susceptible to hepatitis and chemical abuse (i.e. alcohol, caffeine, nicotine, drugs).

Capricorn (December 22- January 19)

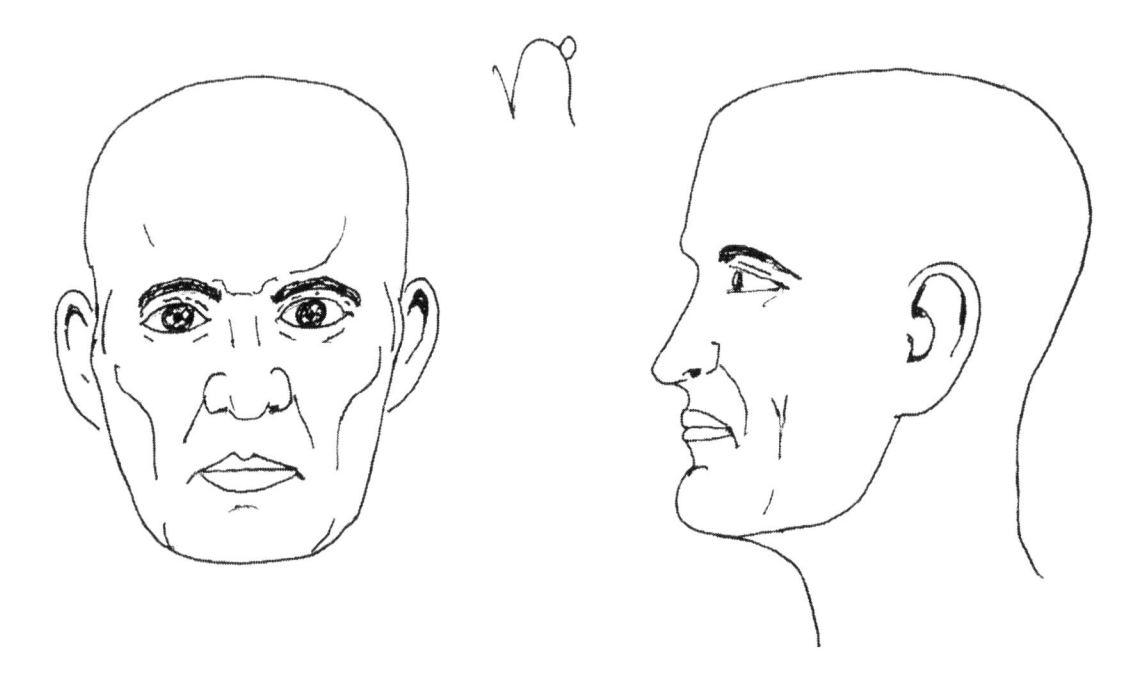

Features

Developed forehead especially above the root of the nose and the upper corners; narrow mouth; protruding lower lip; firm chin; steady look with eyes; Tends to have problems with knees, joints, bones, rheumatism, cartilage, teeth, gallbladder.

Aquarius (January 20- February 18)

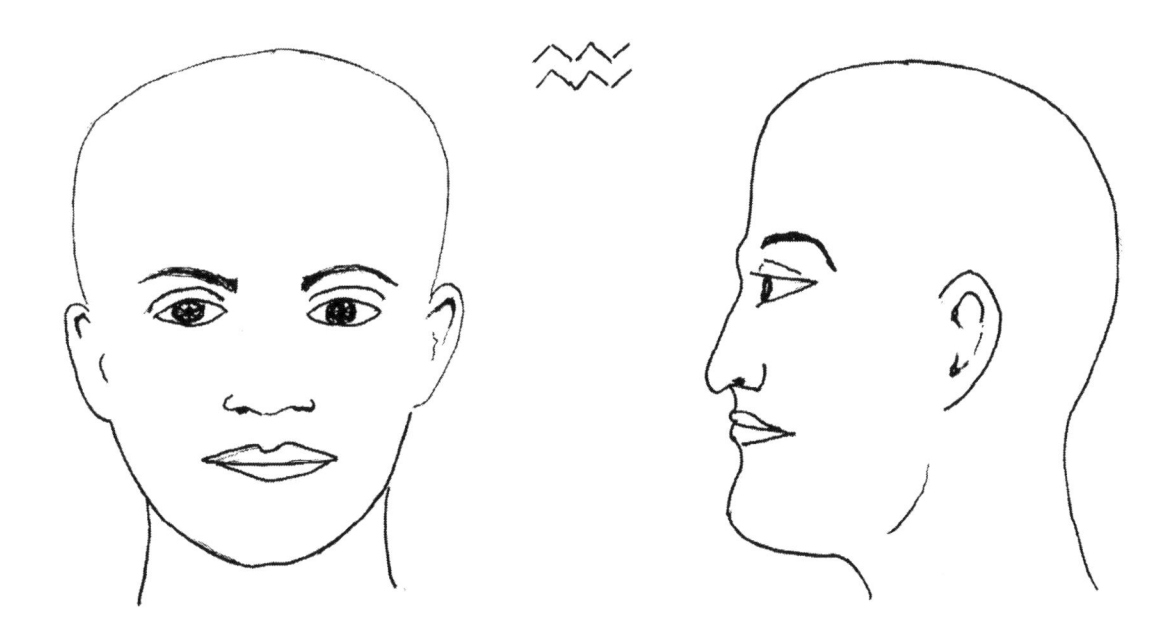

Features

Front of head developed, the upper part of head flat, lower back of head, full soft upper eye lids; firm mouth; Tends to have problems with circulatory system, shins, ankles, hardening of arteries, varicose veins, parathyroid, retina of eyes and bladder.

Pisces (February 19- March 20)

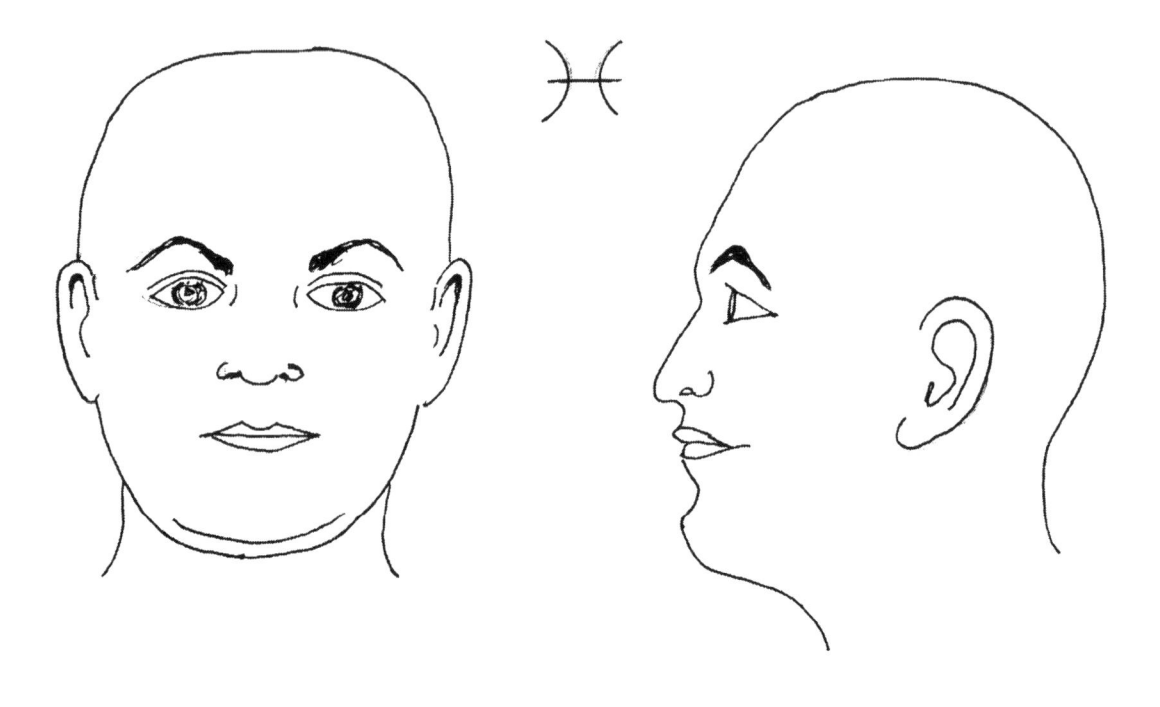

Features

High head; forehead wide at center of base; slightly receding upper forehead; full wide and soft middle part of the face; lower part of face full; double chin, dreamy type eyes; Tends to have problems with feet, susceptible to chemical abuse (i.e. alcohol, drugs); problems with lymphatic system, and circulation.

Face Types (Planets) and Health Problems

This applies to those born with a planet in their Zodiac Sign as well as the ruler of their Zodiac sign. Planet types tend to have most of the features and various combinations of features but not necessarily all features.

Sun

Features

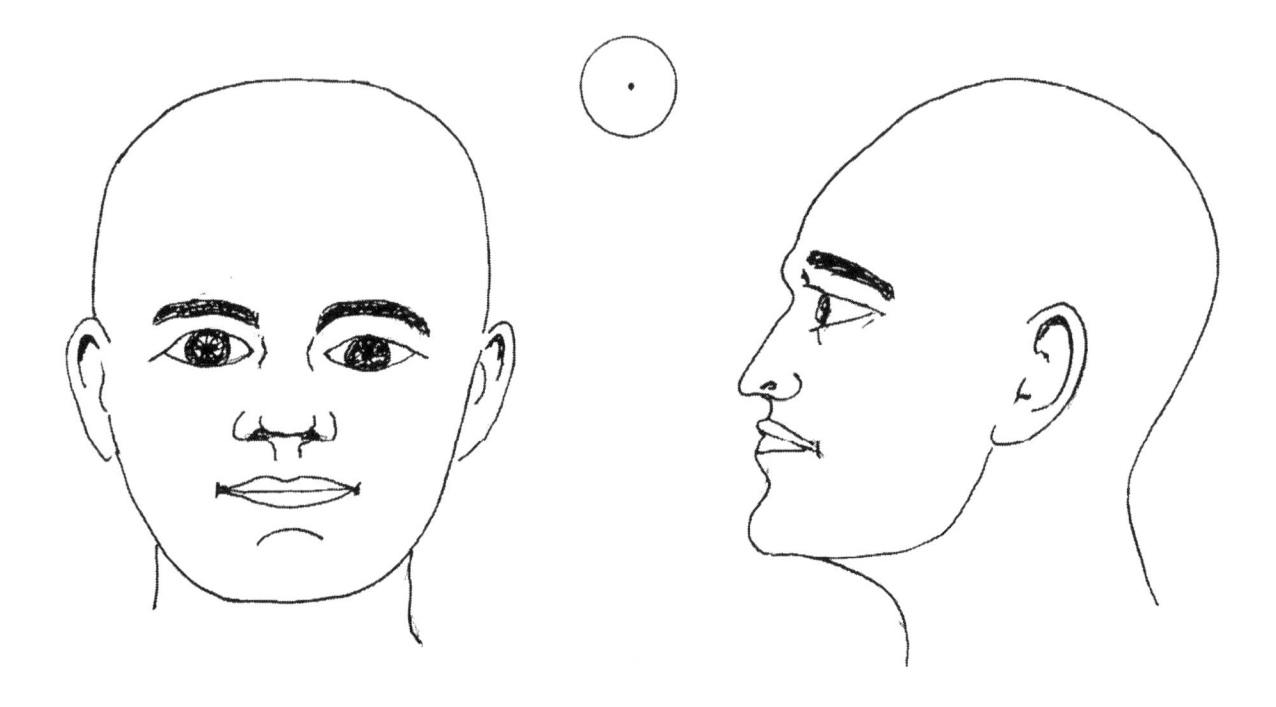

Rounded forehead; active facial muscles can make expressions; penetrating bright eyes; fine hair; tends to get angry with self for being ill; likes to control treatment process; Tends to have heart disease, Congestive Heart Failure, clogged heart arteries, and/or artery and vein weakness.

Moon

Features

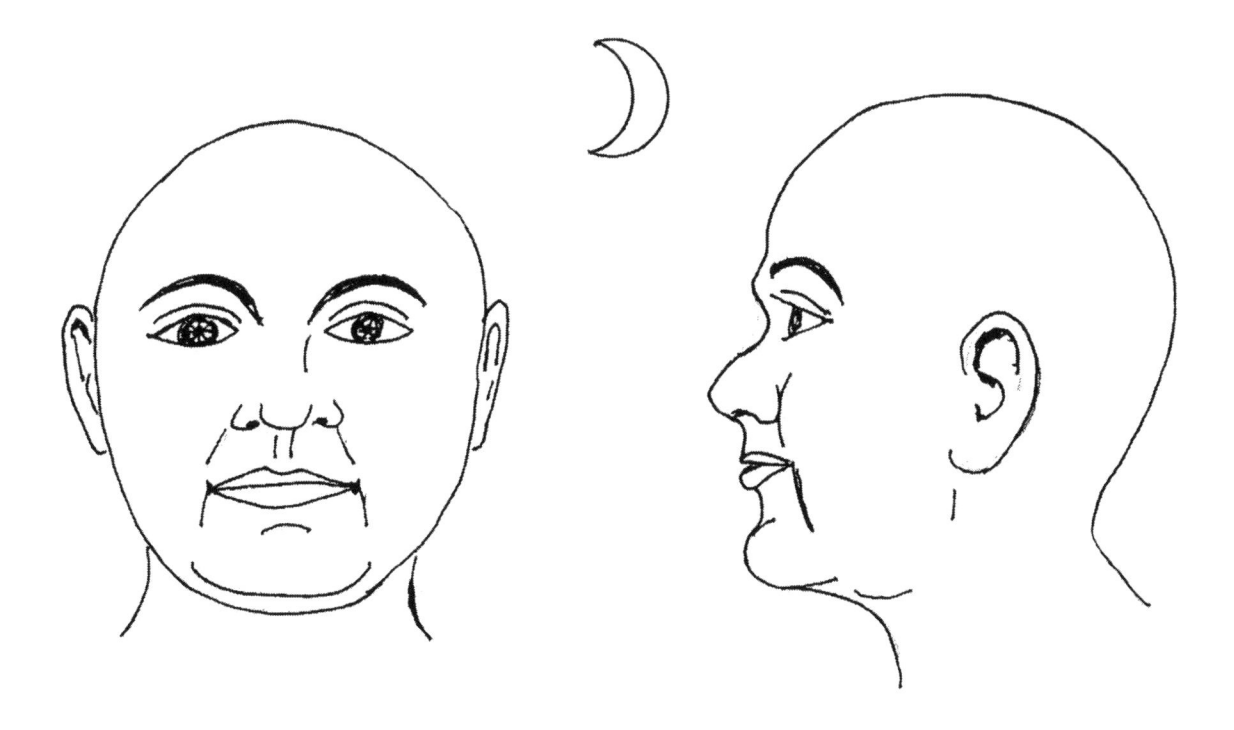

Broad face; rounded lower forehead, soft central part of face; round head; round chin; concave nose; inconsistent in following remedies; emotionally changes from one health protocol to another, emotions can cause illness and can be psychic; Tends to have inflammation of mucous membranes, imbalance of electrolytes (edema, dehydration), digestive problems, and/or electrolyte stress.

Mercury

Features

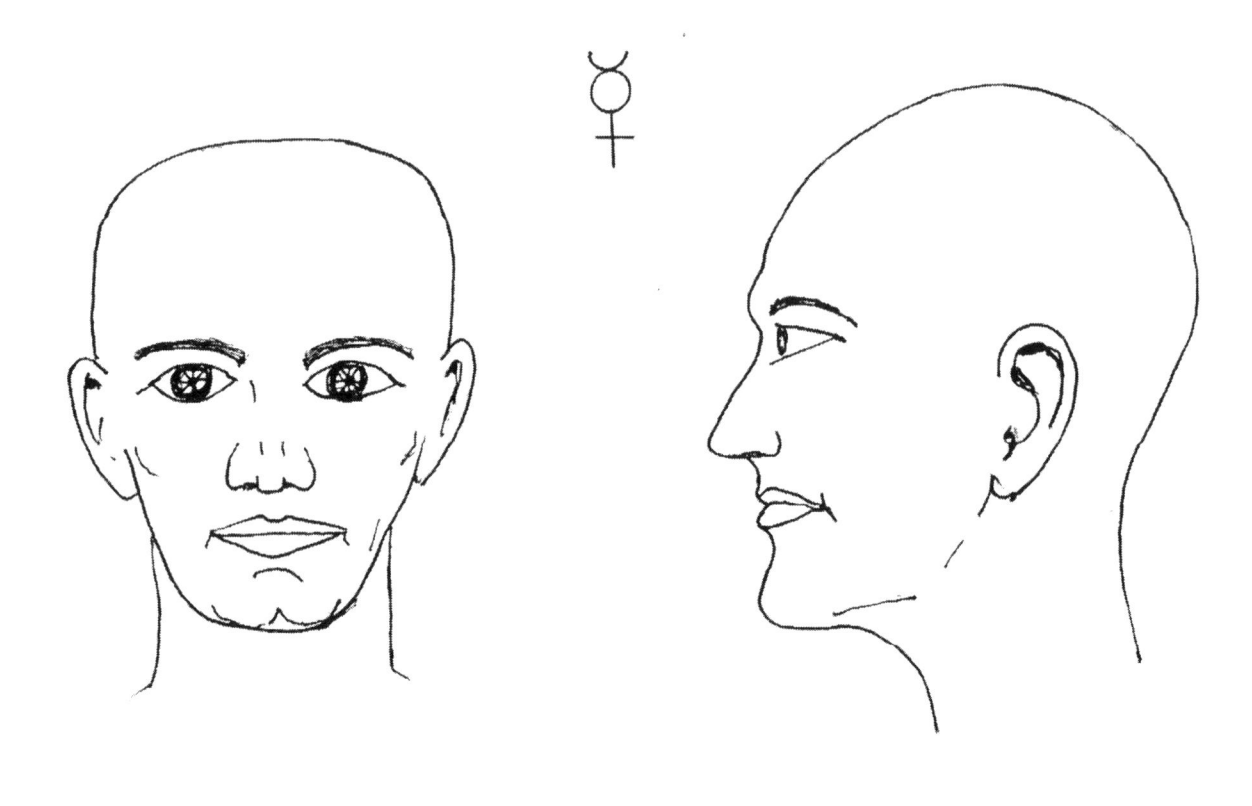

Upper forehead recedes with sides well developed; lower part of middle forehead pronounced, fine features, long nose, penetrating look, likes to read about health, and approaches disease logically; Tends to over research, thinks excessively then follows treatments, and sometimes their intelligence blocks following treatment. Tends to have neuritis and/or respiratory ailments.

Venus

Features

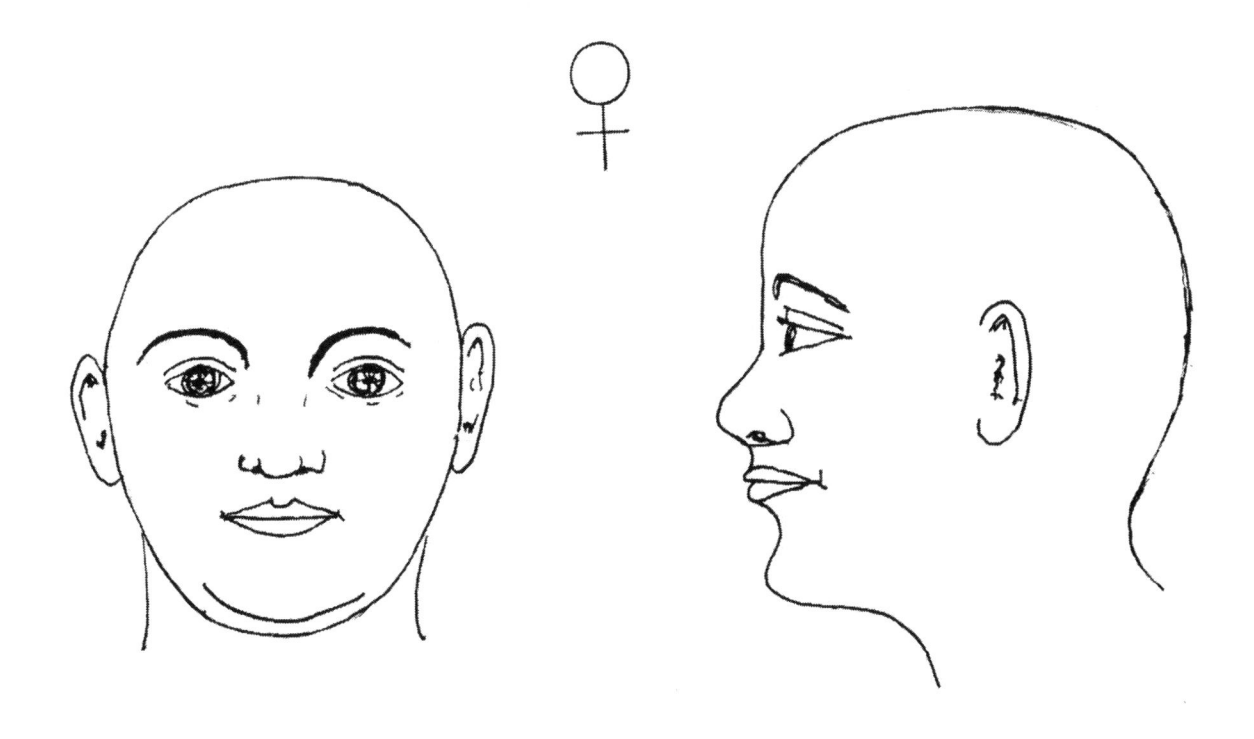

Oval face; soft eyelids; bright eyes, expression appears friendly, easily adjust to health protocols, emotionally sensitive about health, emotions can cause physical illness and can be psychic; Tends to have throat infections, thyroid problems, and/or Kidney problems.

Mars

Features

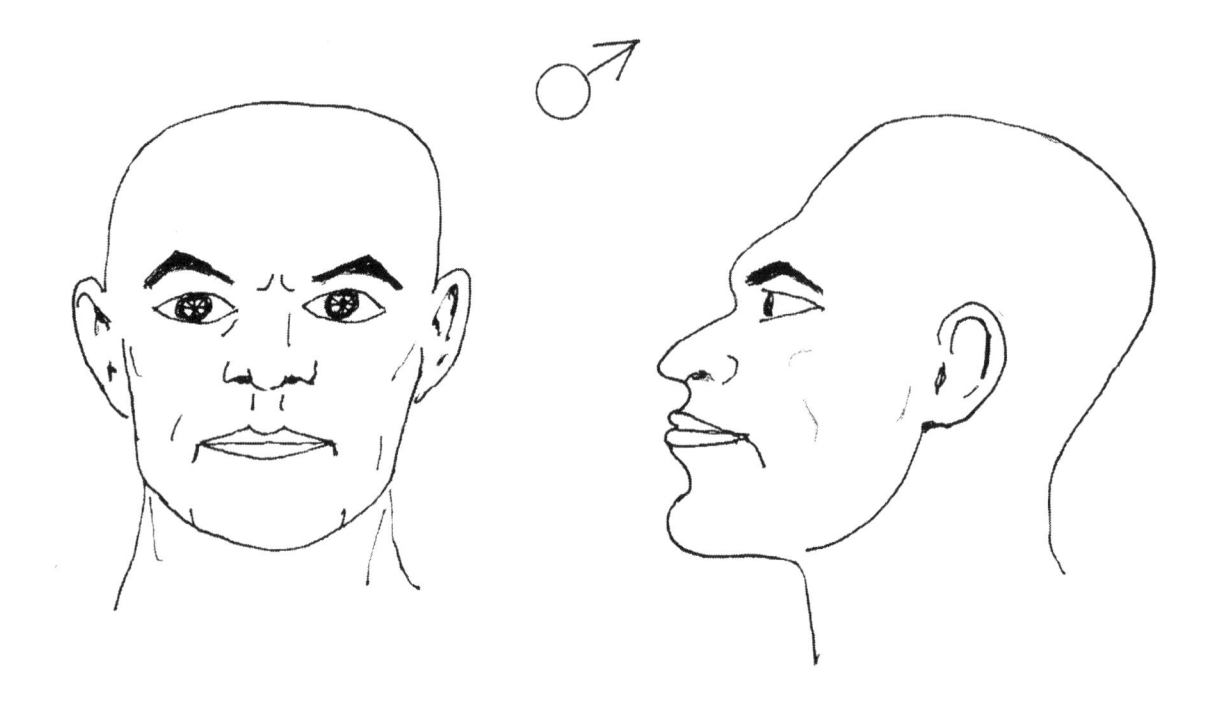

Protruding jaw; big chin, prominent cheekbone, slightly bulging and angular forehead, long head, low hairline, can be inconsiderate of their health, and will be aggressive when seeking remedies. Tends to have swellings, fevers, infections, accidents, blood diseases, hemorrhages, and/or accidents that harm the body.

Jupiter

Features

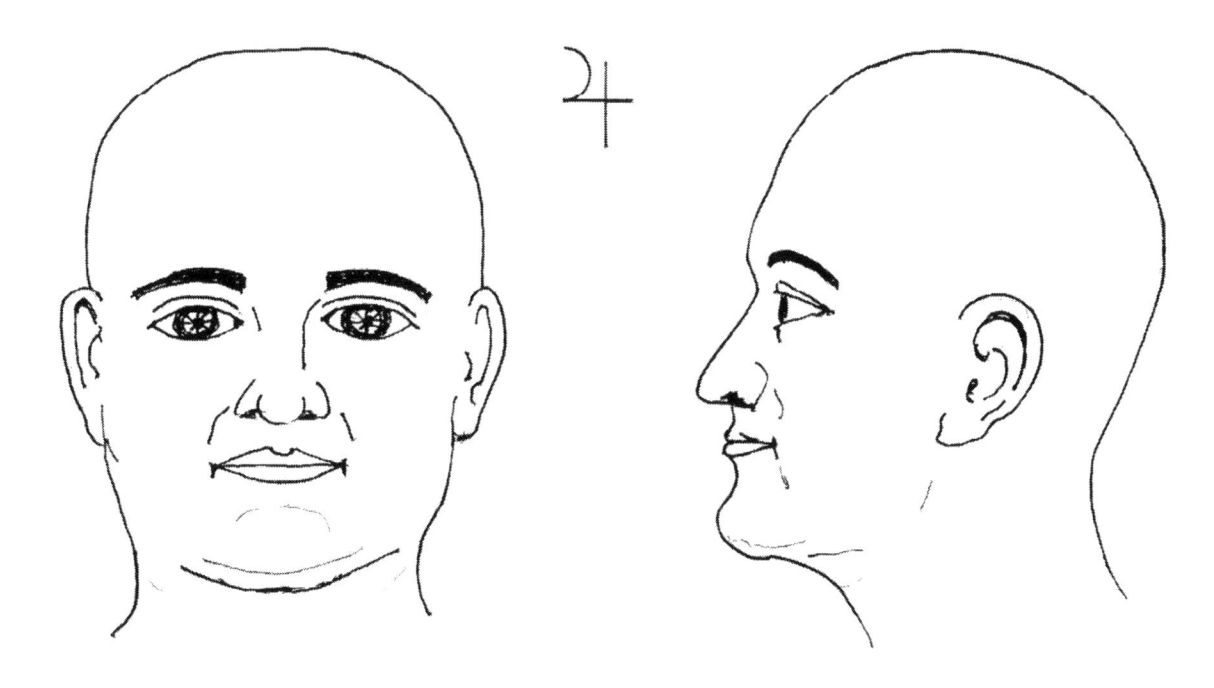

High forehead; wide, large and full upper part of head, nose is well developed, central and lower face is full; double chin, tends to believe in various health remedies, knowledgeable about health, needs nurturing during healing, tends to have liver disease, hypoglycemia, diabetes, obesity, tumors, cyst, pancreatic disease, and/or warts.

Saturn

♄

Features

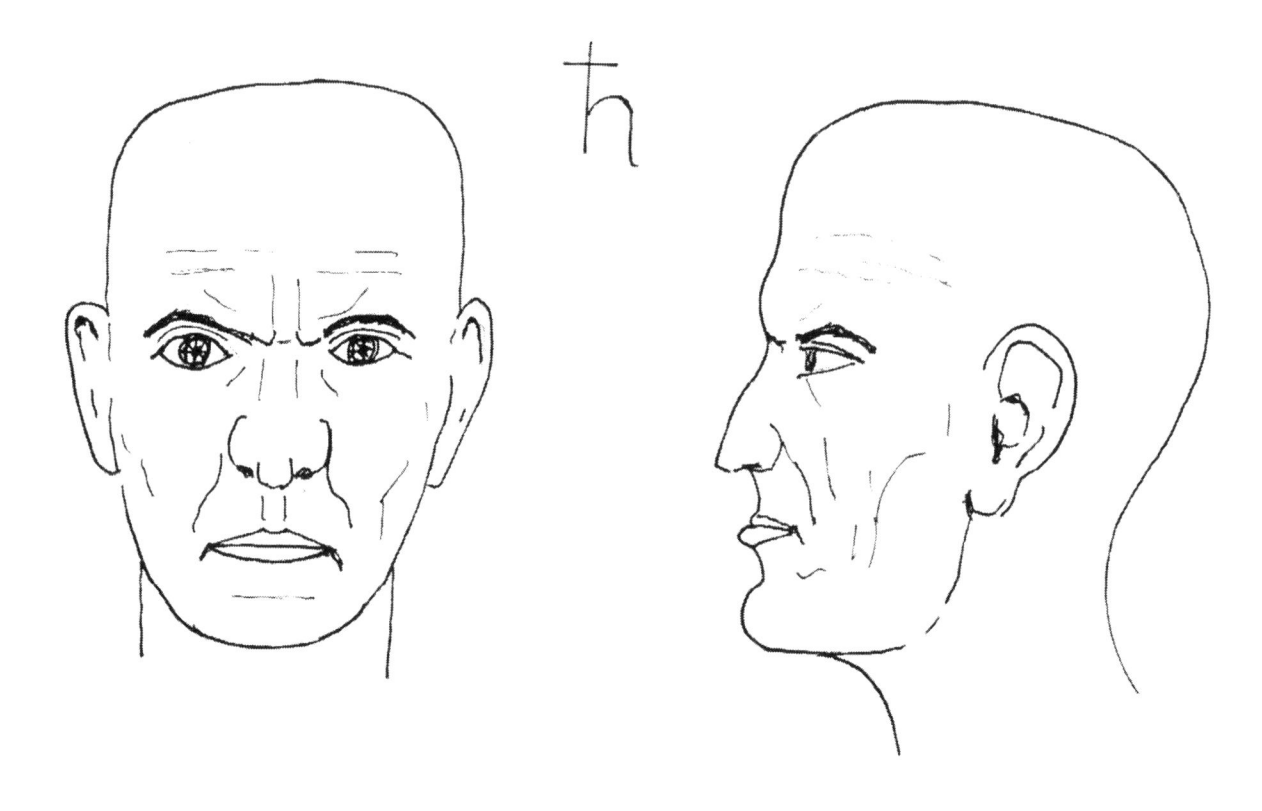

Deep set eyes; overhanging brows, forehead wrinkled but well developed in upper portion and above root of nose; deep indentation at root of nose, lines or wrinkles on cheeks, narrow mouth; protruding lower lip and chin; mouth turns downward at corners, Tends to be stubborn and does not change bad health habits to good health habits easily, worries about health, may not tell the truth about severity of an illness, will work seriously on health if motivated, Tends to have arthritis, rheumatism, fractures, gall stones, spinal ailments, dental problems, skin disease, and/or liver problems.

Uranus

Features

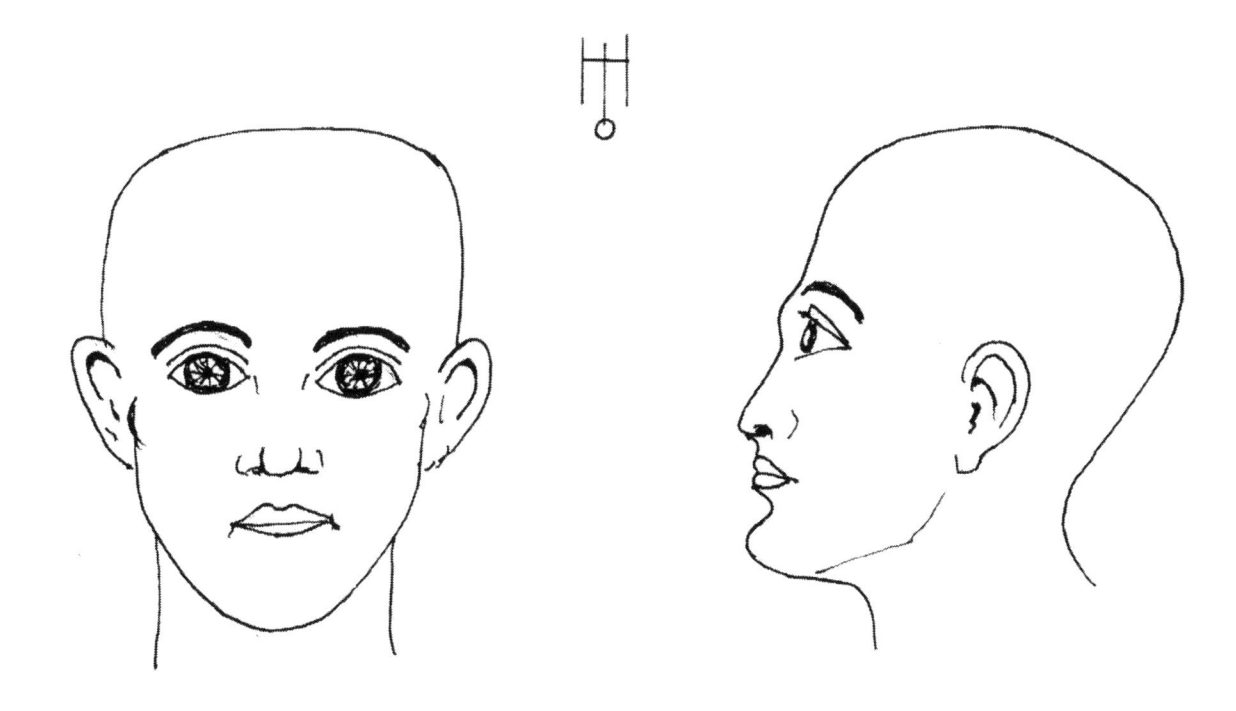

Shining eyes; penetrating look; nose usually broad at the root near eyes; part of face above eyes well developed; broad cheek bones, fine hair, illness seems to start suddenly and emotionally upsets them, they will comply to treatments and improvise and explore remedies. Tends to have cramps, spasms, shocks, epilepsy, paralysis, nerve damage, radiation poison and/or muscle problems.

Neptune

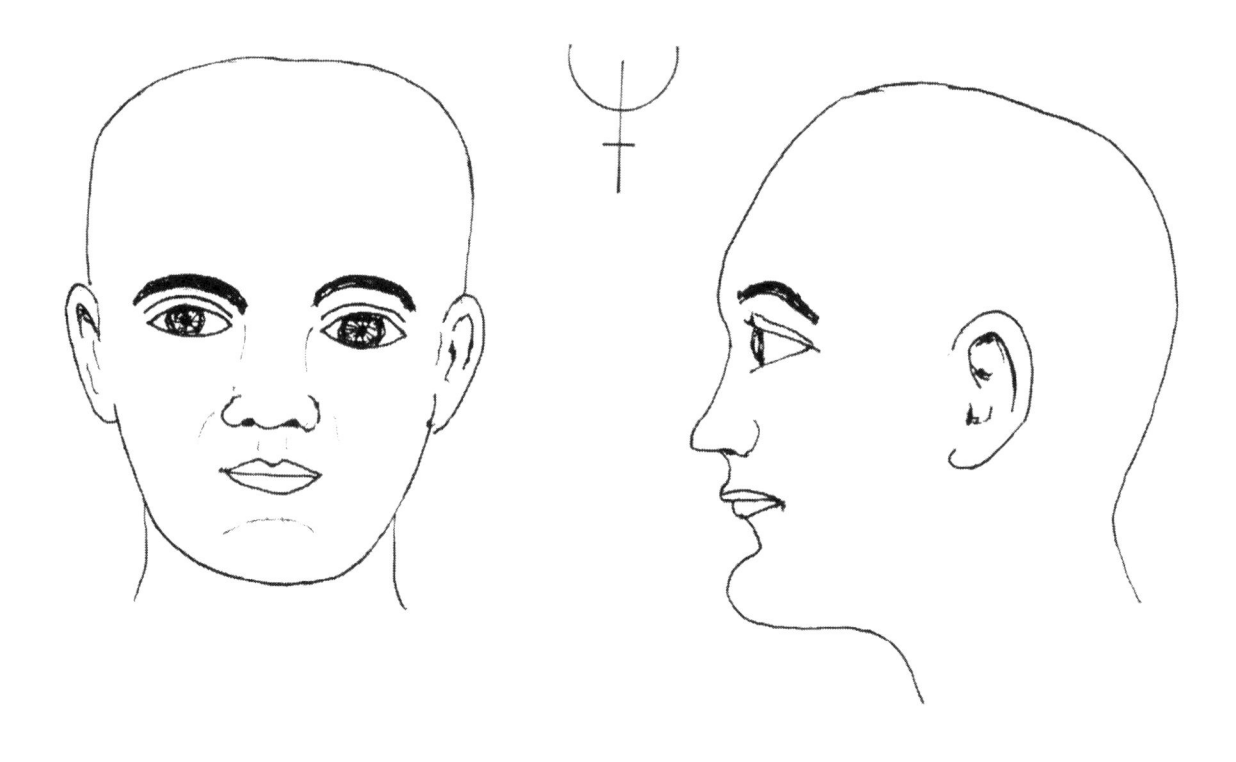

Features

High cranium; wide and well developed forehead, eyes appear to conceal something, fine well formed central part of face, soft flexible face muscles, oval face, and soft hair. Tends to follow Female Principle (Parasympathetic illness) and have mental and emotional problems, addictions, obscure diseases and/or abuses chemicals.

Eyes

Eyeball, Iris and White Part of Eyes

The eyeballs are part of the nervous system, and indicate the physical, mental, emotional and spiritual functions.

Eyeball Size

The eyeballs change in size due to the type of diet (junk vs. health food) as well as according to age. During infancy and early childhood, the eyeballs are comparatively small, and they expand as growth progresses.

Expansion and Contraction of the Eyeball and Lens

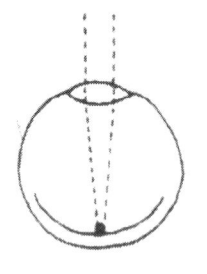

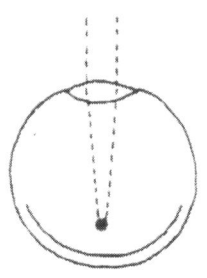

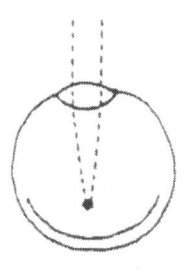

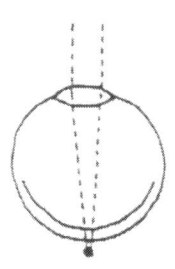

Normal Eyeball

Expanded eye-ball causing nearsightedness

Contracted lens causing near sightedness

Contracted eyeball, causing farsightedness

Size of the Eyeball

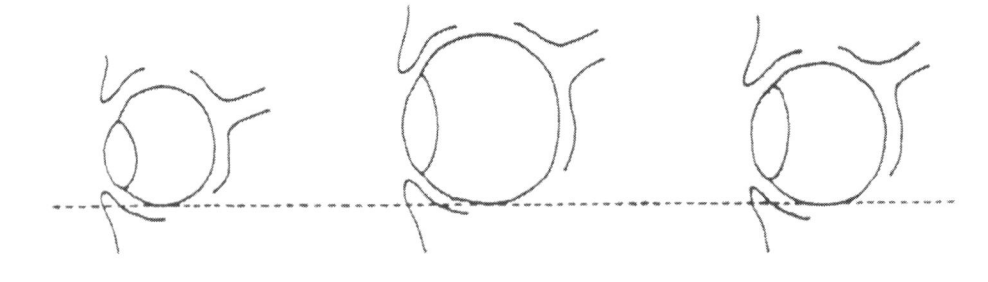

Smaller eyeballs during infancy and childhood

Normal eyeballs during adulthood

Contracted eyeballs during old age

Eye Expansion

When the eyes have horizontal expansion it indicates acidic condition. When horizontal expansion occurs, the eyesight changes. The distance between the lens and the retina is altered, producing near-sightedness.

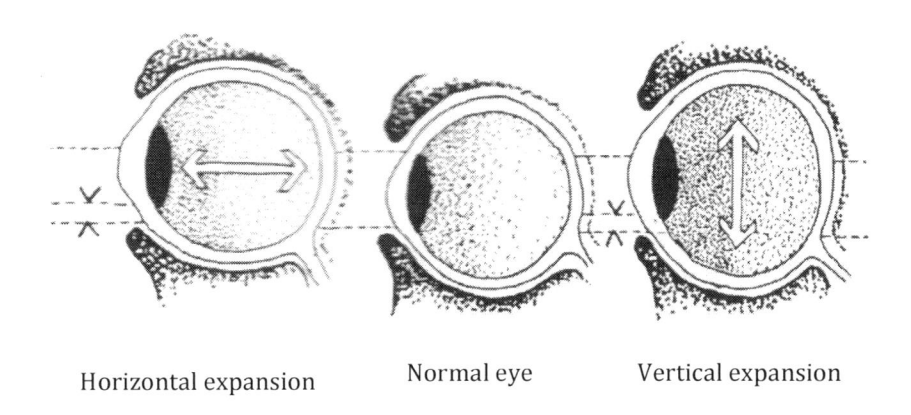

Horizontal expansion   Normal eye   Vertical expansion

Round Eyes and Thin Eyes
Women tend to have rounder eyes. Eyes that are round indicate a parasympathetic tendency. Eyes that are narrow and thin indicate a sympathetic tendency.

Cross Eyes
Eyes rotate on a vertical axis as a result of muscle contraction of the eyes. If the eyes go in opposite direction, the cause is the consumption of excess acidic food, drugs and/or acid (toxic) environment.

Extraocular Eye Muscles
The movements they produce and their
Cranial Nerve (N) Supply

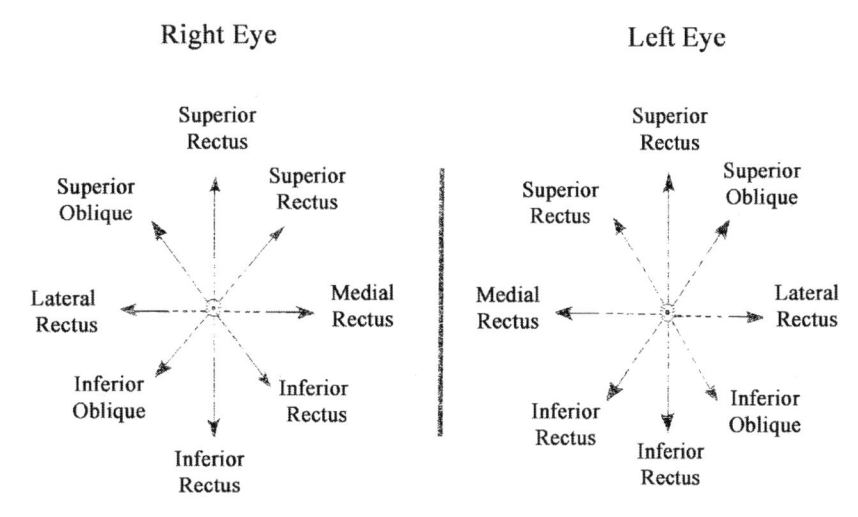

Right Eye

- Superior Rectus
- Superior Oblique
- Superior Rectus
- Lateral Rectus
- Medial Rectus
- Inferior Oblique
- Inferior Rectus
- Inferior Rectus

Left Eye

- Superior Rectus
- Superior Rectus
- Superior Oblique
- Medial Rectus
- Lateral Rectus
- Inferior Rectus
- Inferior Oblique
- Inferior Rectus

Regions of the Sclera (white part of eyes)

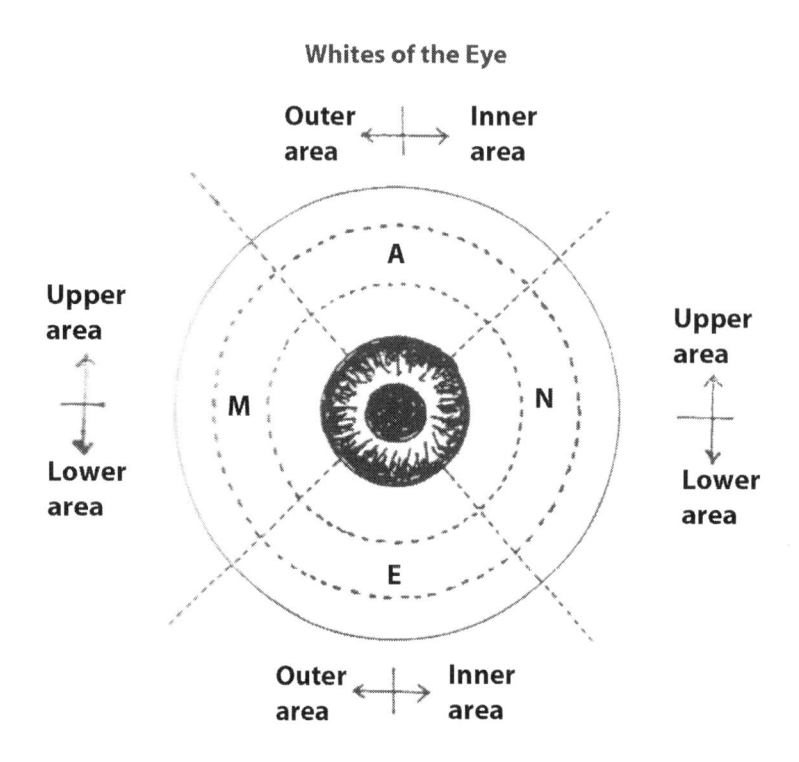

Whites of the Eye

```
         Outer  |  Inner
         area  ←→  area

              A

Upper                    Upper
area                     area
 ↑                        ↑
 ↓    M         N         ↓
Lower                    Lower
area                     area

              E

         Outer  |  Inner
         area  ←→  area
```

A—Upper regions of body

M—Middle front regions of body

E—Lower regions of body

N—Middle back regions of body

Outer dotted circle section- Digestive and respiratory functions

Inner dotted circle are section- Circulatory and excretory functions

Iris and pupil- Nervous functions

Inner part of white- Compacted organs (Male Principle) in each section

Outer part of white- Expanded organs (Female Principle) in each section

Veins, discoloration and spots in areas indicate disease and/or malfunction in the organs or part of the body that corresponds to the area.

Sclera and Body

Area of the White	Part of the Body
Upper area	The brain, upper back, face, neck, chest, lungs and heart.
Middle area	The stomach, duodenum, spleen, pancreas, liver, middle back, gallbladder and kidneys.
Lower area	The small and large intestines, lower back, bladder, reproductive organs and buttocks.

Eye Zones Areas

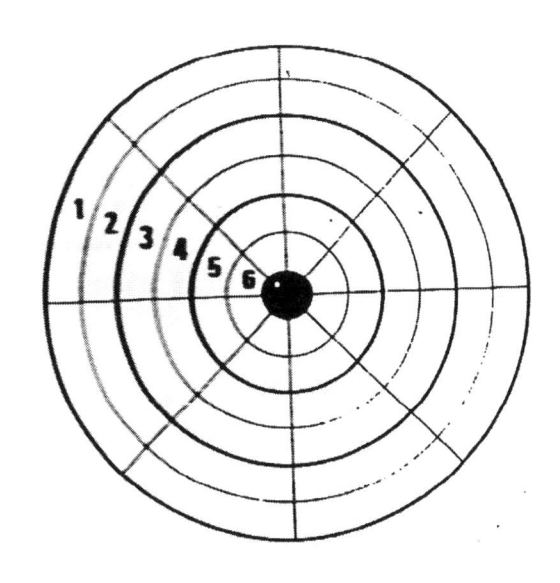

1. Skin
2. Bones
3. Muscles
4. Blood
5. Intestines
6. Stomach

Eye Skeletal Chart

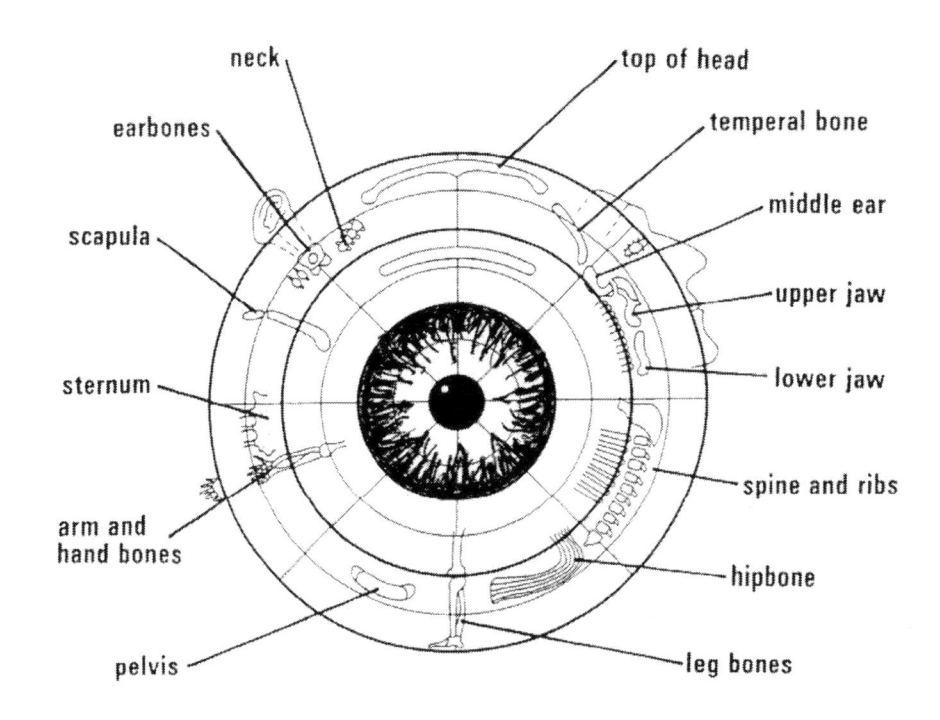

neck
top of head
earbones
temperal bone
scapula
middle ear
upper jaw
sternum
lower jaw
spine and ribs
arm and hand bones
hipbone
pelvis
leg bones

Male and Female Principle

The Sclera of the Eyes

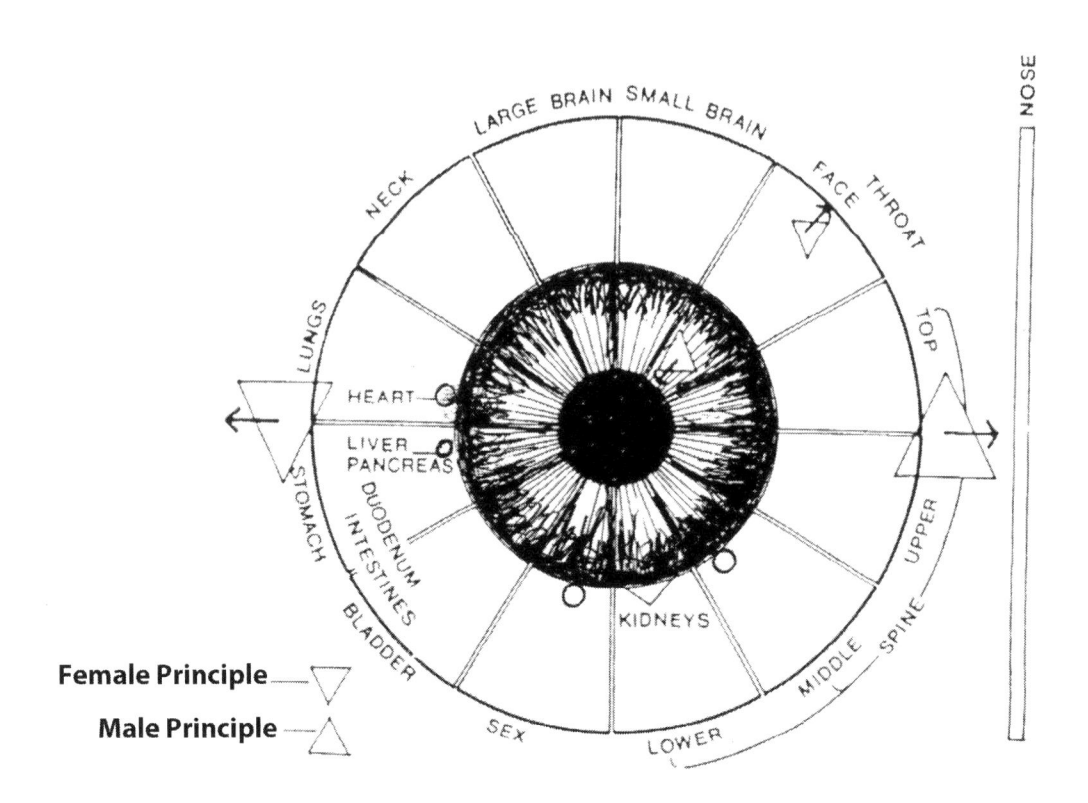

The eye sclera (white part of eye) is divided into Female and Male Principle sections. The Male section is those closer to the nose and those in towards the center of the eyeball (iris). The most Male section corresponds to the most Male parts of the body (the back). The Female areas of the eyeball are those towards the outside of the face toward the ears and the periphery of the eyeball. The most Female areas correspond to the soft parts of the body (the front). Veins, discoloration, spots, and/or dark lines correspond to the organ and/or part of the body with the disease or malfunction.

Eyes and Eyebrows

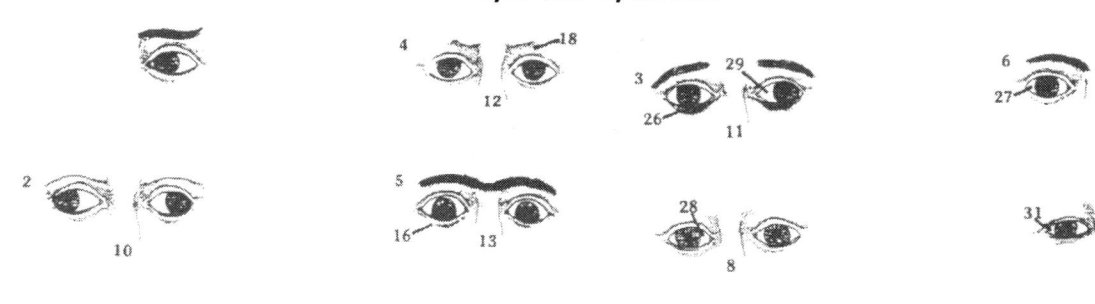

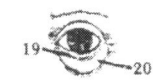

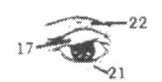

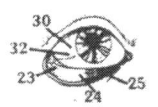

Condition	Indication
1. Inward Slant Brow	Poor protein metabolism
2. Losing Brow	Degenerative disease
3. Downward Curve Brows	Vegetarian, Fruitarian, Alkalinity
4. Eyebrows Little or None	Degenerative disease
5. Eyebrows Joined Brows	Acidic, good immune system
6. Eyebrows Thick Brows	Good immune system, acidic
7. Narrow Eye, Close to Nose	Aggressive, active, sympathetic stress
8. Large Eye, Far from Nose	Passive, gentle, parasympathetic stress
9. Cross-Eyed	Contraction, tension, high blood pressure, acidosis
10. Wall-Eyed	Passive, alkalosis, nerve damage, degenerative disease
11. One Straight, One out	Poor carbohydrate metabolism
12. White on Bottom	Degeneration, fatigue, lower organ weakness, acidic
13. White on Top	Calcification of liver
14. Bloodshot Eyes	Liquids, drugs, sugars, concentrated sweeteners
15. Blue or Red under or Around Eyes	Kidney disease, increase carbon dioxide in blood

16. Purple under Eyes
    a) Small Area
    b) Large Area
	Adrenal disease
	    a. Excess sodium chloride
	    b. Excess drugs, concentrated sweeteners

17. Styes	Poor protein metabolism
18. Hard Swelling over Eye or White Spotting	Processed and cooked fats & oils
19. Hard Red or White Bags Under Eyes	Kidney stones
20. Soft Bags or Swelling Around Eyes	Weak kidneys, kidney stones, kidney and heart stress
21. Discolored Spotting Under Eyes	Kidney stones
22. Discolored Spotting Over Eyes	Gall stones
23. Pink Sclera	Poor circulation
24. Pale Sclera	Anemia
25. Red Sclera	Inflammation or infection of circulatory system degenerative disease
26. Dark Brown Under Eyes	Contracted kidney, female sexual organ problems
27. Blue Sclera	Intestinal parasites, kidney disease
28. Soft Yellow Spot on Sclera	Liver congestion
29. Hard Yellow Spot on Sclera	Worms, Parasites
30. Yellow Bumps At end of Capillary	Cysts in corresponding area
31. Yellow Sclera	Liver problem, yellow jaundice
32. Grey Spot at end of Capillary	Clot in corresponding area
Protruding Eyes	Thyroid disease, expanded brain, heart and kidney stress
Horizontal Or Vertical Expansion of Eye	Spinal nerve, midbrain and lower brain problems

Condition	Indication
Constant Movement or Slow Reaction	Damaged nervous system
Large Pupil	Brain damage, Eating Disorder
White Ring around Iris or White Moon at Top	Nerve and brain problems, nerve stress, excess sodium
Yellow Discharge in Corner	Problems with chloride, and with protein metabolism
Few Lower Lashes	Sexual organ problems or deterioration, lower organ stress
Few Upper Lashes	Nerve problems, upper organ stress
Sharp Upward Slant of Lashes	Sex organ problems
Itchy Eyes	Lung disorder
Blinking More Than 4 Times per Minute	Weak nervous system, poor carbohydrate metabolism, kidney and heart stress

Pupil Size Distortion and Pupil Asymmetry

Healthy pupils should react to light in exactly the same way, even when only one eye is stimulated with a light. They should be centered.

Extreme Dilation (Mydriasis)
This indicates severe nervous-system stressors such as emotions, epilepsy, advanced anemia, tuberculosis, psychoses, and manias.

Wildly Fluctuating Pupils
When pupils dilate and contract under steady light it indicates cerebral congestion, nervous degeneration, weak adrenals, and/or worms (parasites).

One Dilated/One Contracted Pupil (or Mydriasis/ Miosis)
When one pupil is bigger than the other, it indicates nervous system disease (diphtheria, meningitis, and syphilis).

Pupil Discoloration and Textures
Gray: Cataracts, usually caused by arteriosclerosis or diabetes
Green: Glaucoma

Pupil Size

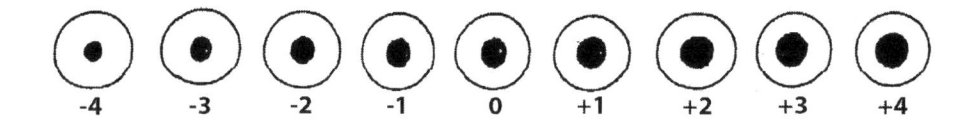

-4 -3 -2 -1 0 +1 +2 +3 +4

Pupil Size Small -1 to -4
Parasympathetic Stress, Weak Thyroid function

Pupil Size Large +1 to +4
Sympathetic Stress, weak Medulla of the adrenal gland

When light is shined on the eye and immediately the light is removed, the pupil cannot maintain constriction; the pupil will change to one of the sizes above. The cilliary muscle of the eye contracts only in response to nerve stimulation (no endocrine or local stimuli).

The neuro-transmitter acetylcholine (parasympathetic) causes the cilliary muscle to contract. Nerve polarization occurs in response to increased Sodium and decreases Potassium. Diseases can cause excess Sodium and/or deficient Potassium which can over stimulate the nerve resulting in decreased ability of the iris to respond to light (stimuli); the pupil will be unable to control its ability to keep its small size.

Eyes by the Numbers

Identify the number or numbers that the veins in the Sclera appear. Look at the Numbers Chart for this indicates the problem organ and system.

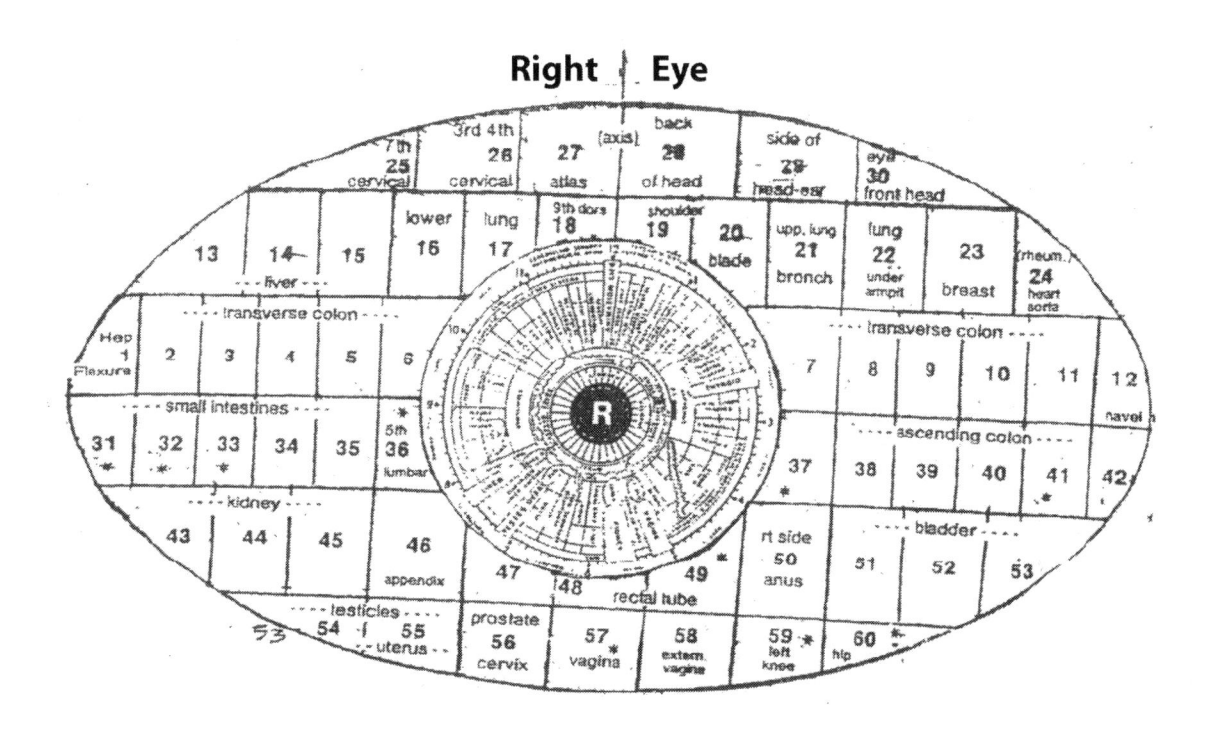

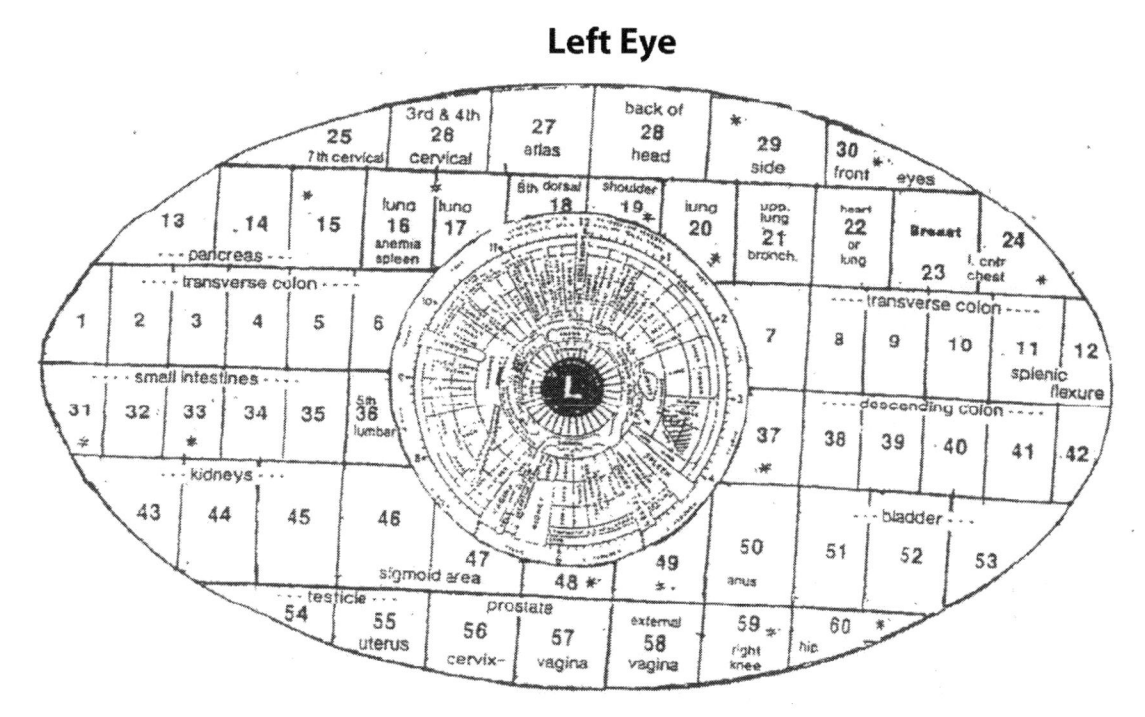

Right Eye

7th cervical 25	3rd 4th cervical 26	atlas 27	(axis) back of head 28	side of head-ear 29	eye front head 30			
13	14 liver	15	lower lung 16	17	9th dors 18	shoulder blade 19	20	upp. lung bronch 21	under armpit 22	breast 23	rheum. heart aorta 24
Hep Flexure 1	2	3 transverse colon 4	5	6			7	8 transverse colon 9	10	11	navel 12
31	32 small intestines 33	34	35	5th lumbar 36			37	38 ascending colon 39	40	41	42
43	44 kidney 45	46		47	48 rectal tube	49 anus	rt side 50	51 bladder 52	53
53	54 testicles uterus	55	prostate 56 cervix	57 vagina	58 extern. vagina	59 left knee	60 hip

Left Eye

7th cervical 25	3rd & 4th cervical 26	atlas 27	back of head 28	side 29	front eyes 30			
13	14 pancreas	15	lung 16 anemia spleen	lung 17	5th dorsal 18	shoulder 19	lung 20	upp. lung bronch 21	heart or lung 22	Breast 23	l. cntr chest 24
1	2	3 transverse colon 4	5	6			7	8 transverse colon 9	10	11	splenic flexure 12
31	32 small intestines 33	34	35	5th lumbar 36			37	38 descending colon 39	40	41	42
43	44 kidneys 45	46		47 sigmoid area	48	49	50 anus	51 bladder 52	53
	54 testicle uterus	55	prostate 56 cervix	57 vagina	external 58 vagina	59 right knee	60 hip

111

Left Eye Numbers

12	Transverse Colon C1 at navel – 12 at splenic Flex
15	Pancreas – 8th Dorsal out-
16-17	Spleen/Lower part of lung (When saliva 7.4 or higher – Spleen, below 7.4 – lower lung). When pH below 7.4 & salt is high, person should have HBP! 7.4 and above and high salt, may not register HBP because hemoglobin low.
18	8th Dorsal
19	Left shoulder – joint problems
20	Left shoulder blade – bursitis
21	Upper lung – bronchial/asthmatic problems
22	Left center chest – Angina problems 22-24
23	Breast male/female
24	Under the armpit – Angina stress
25	7th cervical
26	3rd and 4th cervical
27	Atlas
28	Back of Head Axis
29	Ear – hearing problem
30	Eye & Forehead – Strain or deterioration
31	Splenic Flexure – Small intestines to about 2" below transverse colon
32-33	Small intestines – testicles/prostate men & women Ovaries
34-35	Small intestines –men & women
36	5th lumbar
37-42	Descending colon – 37 top of Splenic Flexure counting down to 38, 39, 40, 41
43-45	Kidney
46-47	Sigmoid – where colon joins to rectal tube
48	Top of rectal tube
49	Left center rectal tube
50	Anus –protrusion possibility
51-53	Bladder
54-55	Uterus – female, Testicles Prostate– male
56	Cervix
57	Back part vagina –Can have yeast infection
58	External part of vagina –can have irritation
59	Right knee & below – calf, ankle
60	Right leg shorter than left Right & left leg at#60 – Arthritis Right and Left leg can be involved 19, 20, 59 & 60

Right Eye Numbers

1-12	Transverse Colon from Hepatic Flexure to the Navel
13-15	Liver – back hurts – 9 & 10 dorsal out of alignment
16-17	Lower lung –right lobe
18	9th Dorsal
19	Shoulder in joint
20	Shoulder, back of, in shoulder blade
21	Upper lung – bronchial area
22	Lung under armpit
22-24	Young children – scar tissue caused by Rheumatic heart or infection around heart called Pericarditis
23	Breast – women and fleshy part of men
24	Aorta Artery – where urea puts pressure near center of chest
24	Left eye – setting alone heart murmur
25	9th Cervical – a plus involves 6th & 7th and 1st and 2nd Dorsal
26	3rd and 4th Cervical, if plus add 5th Cervical
27	Atlas –possible, Atlas & Axis problems
28	Back of head
29	Ear – Hearing problem
30	Eye and forehead – strain/sinus
31-35	Hepatic Flexure, Small Intestines to Approx. 2" below Transverse Colon
35	Right along side of spine
31-32	Small intestines Men and Women
33	Ovaries
34-35	Small intestine men and women
36	5th Lumbar (R&L) can indicate kidney problems
36	Right or left eyes 4th lumbar out of alignment
36	Both eyes –lumbar region out of alignment
37-42	Ascending colon (37 at Hepatic Flex, counting down to 38, 39, 40)
41	Illeocecal valve
42	Cecum
43-45	Kidney –dehydration– kidney function decreasing
43-	Kidneys inflamed – Atlas, 5th lumbar, 7th cervical can be out of alignment to compensate – Right or Left
46-47	Appendix or appendix area scar
48	Top right of rectal tube
49	Center right side of rectal tube
50	Right side of anus
51-53	Bladder
54-55	Uterus – female, testicles, prostate – male
56	Cervix, prostate
57	Back part of vagina, can indicate yeast infection
58	External part of vagina can indicate irritation
59	Represents left knee, ankle and calf
60	Hip – left leg shorter than right

Eye Sclera

Blood vessels in the whites point to the organ and/or part of the body that is malfunctioning or diseased. Different inconsistencies in the iris appear as lines, shapes, or colors that point to an organ or body part. Inconsistency can be lighter or darker or blackish and may need a magnifier to be seen.

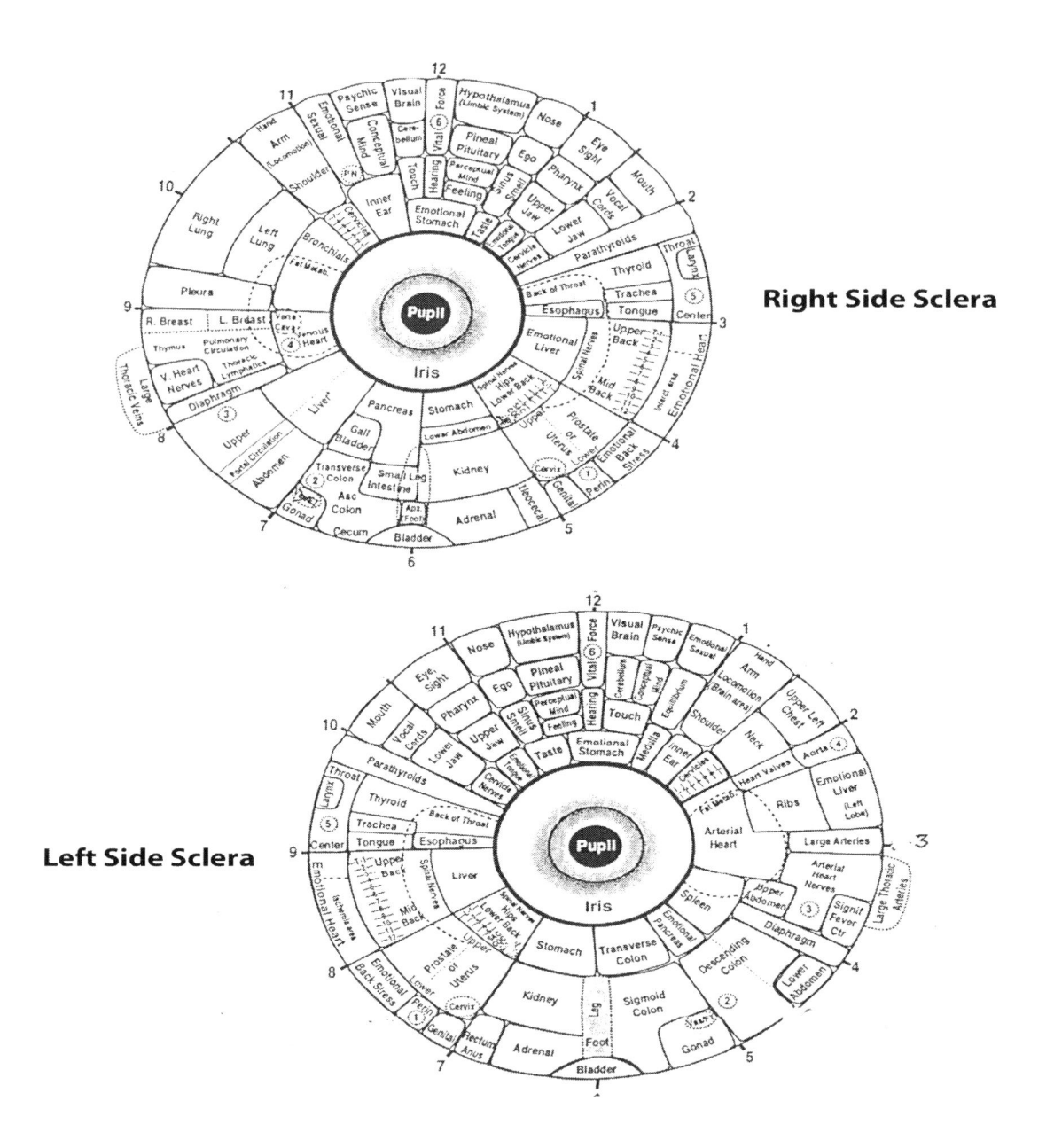

Right Side Sclera

Left Side Sclera

Iris

Different inconsistencies in the Iris appear as lines, shapes, or colors that point to an organ or body part. Inconsistencies can be lighter, darker or blackish and may need a magnifier to be seen.

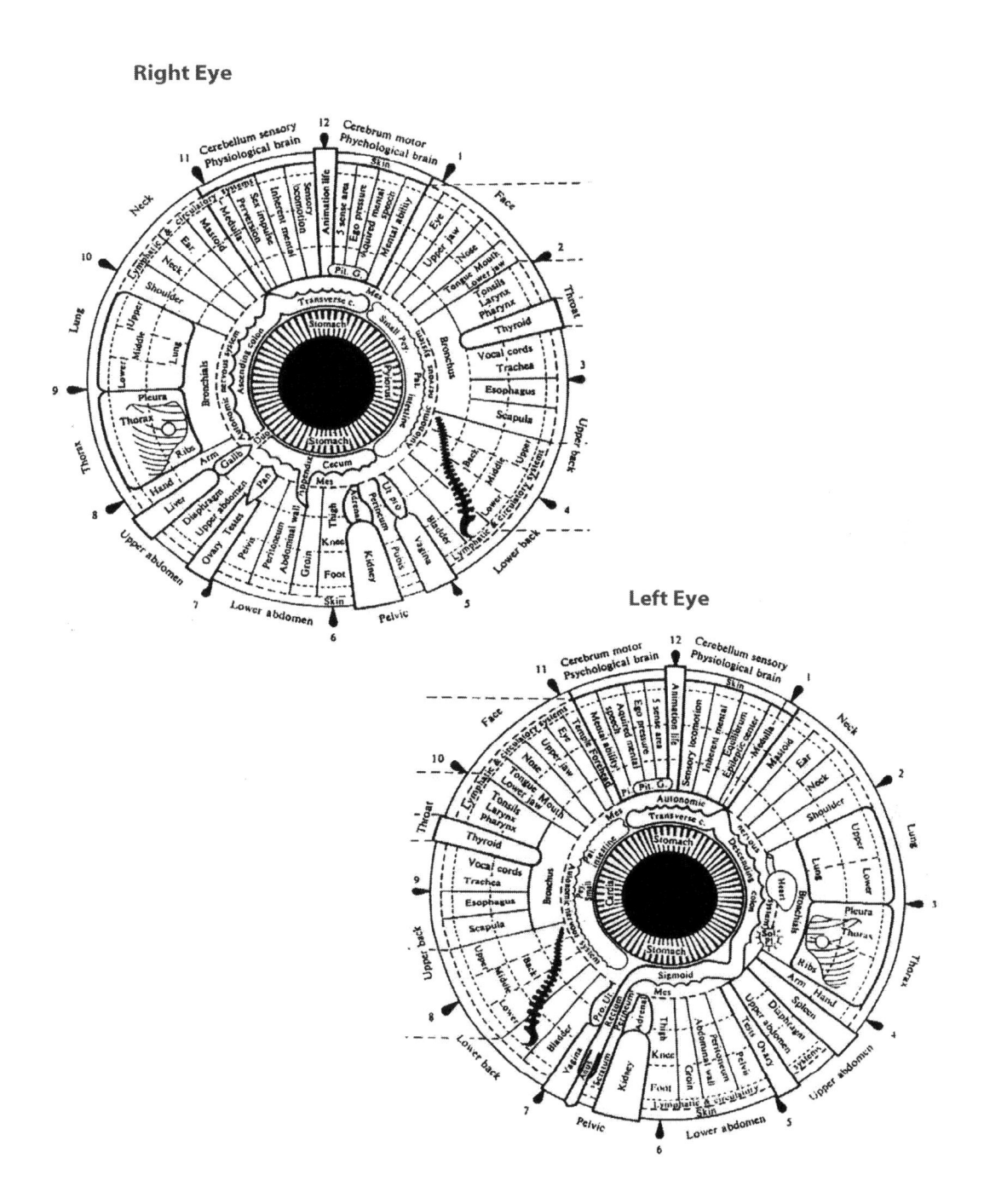

Right Eye

Left Eye

115

Vein Types in Sclera

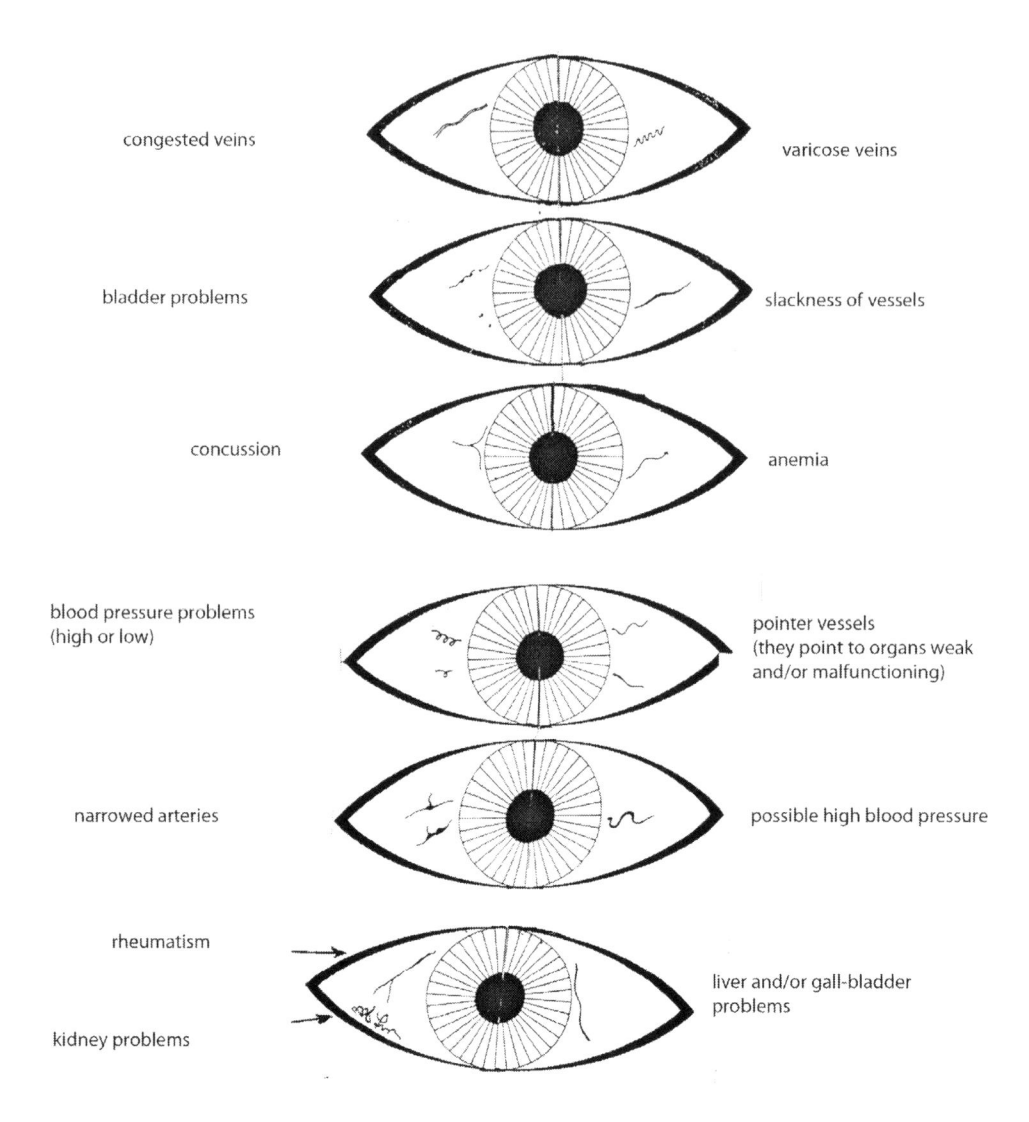

congested veins	varicose veins
bladder problems	slackness of vessels
concussion	anemia
blood pressure problems (high or low)	pointer vessels (they point to organs weak and/or malfunctioning)
narrowed arteries	possible high blood pressure
rheumatism	liver and/or gall-bladder problems
kidney problems	

Vessels on the White of the Eye

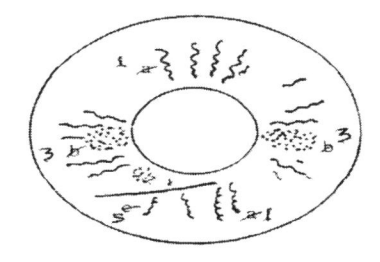

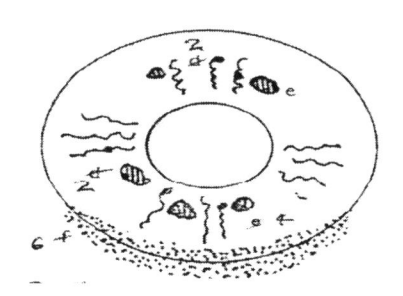

1 – Expanded blood capillaries   2 – Red spots – blood clots
3 – White mucus patches   4 – Dark spots
5 – Straight long red line   6 – Mucus under the eyeball

- **Straight, long red line** indicates problems with blood vessels or tissues and muscles.
- **Red spots** indicate blood clots and/or circulatory problems in the organs, glands or muscles in the related section of the body
- **Transparent or pale white color** indicates fat and mucus clogged, cysts, tumor growths, hormonal and lymphatic problems and, health degeneration leading to cancerous state.
- **Red color** indicates circulatory and respiratory problems. Epileptic disorders, nerve damage, and menstruation problems.
- **Yellow color** often seen in the peripheral parts of the whites indicates an accumulation of fat, congestion, liver, gallbladder and digestive problems
- **Grey or dark color** in the middle and inner section indicates deterioration of the functions of the organs and glands, digestive, respiratory and lymphatic problems
- **Cloudy white color** with grey tone tissue and/or organs are becoming too stiff to function properly
- **Mucus** at the lower part of the white, below the eyeball, is an indication of mucus and fat accumulation in the lower part of the body, fat in and around the intestines, ovaries, uterus, Fallopian tubes, and prostate glands.
- **Dark spots** indicate calcification, stones, fat deposits, cysts, tumors, and/or cancer
- **White mucus** patches indicate fat accumulation, developing cysts, tumors and/or cancer.

Vein Shapes Indicate Illness

- Accident
- Anemia
- Bladder Problems
- Clot
- High or Low Blood Pressure
- Concussion/Congestion
- Congested Veins
- Infection
- Kidney Disease
- Liver, GallBladder Problems
- Low Grade Fever
- Narrowed Arteries
- Nerve Stress
- Poor Circulation

- Pregnancy
- Pending Heart Attack
- Relaxing Stress
- Rheumatism
- Scar Tissue
- Severe Condition
- Stress
- Surgery
- Condition Worsening
- Varicose Veins
- Poor Tissue Degenerating
- Whiplash

Sclera

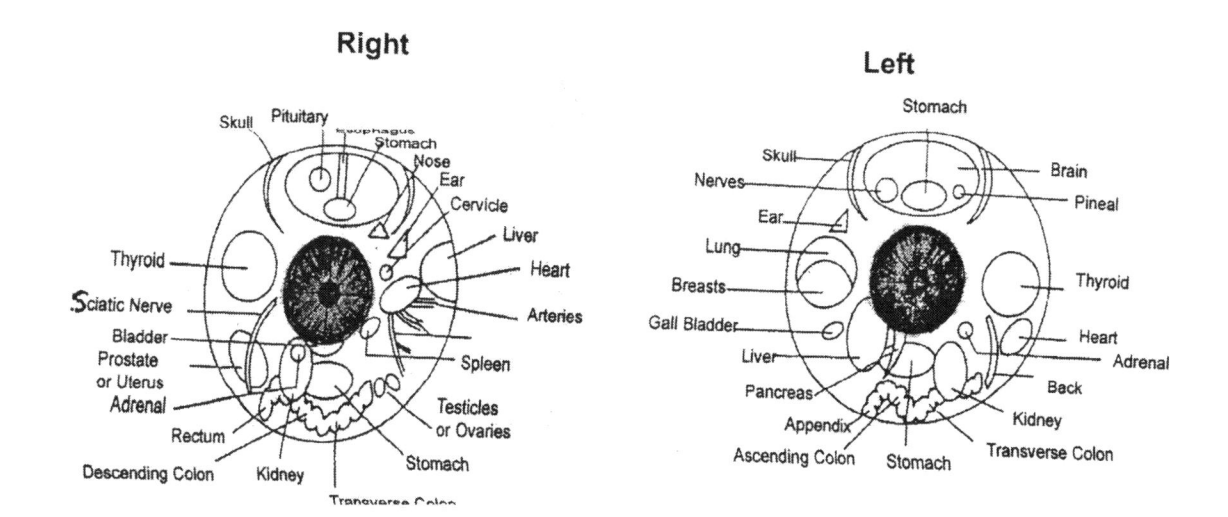

Right

Labels: Skull, Pituitary, Esophagus, Stomach, Nose, Ear, Cervicle, Liver, Heart, Arteries, Spleen, Testicles or Ovaries, Stomach, Transverse Colon, Kidney, Descending Colon, Rectum, Adrenal, Prostate or Uterus, Bladder, Sciatic Nerve, Thyroid

Left

Labels: Stomach, Skull, Brain, Nerves, Pineal, Ear, Lung, Thyroid, Breasts, Gall Bladder, Heart, Liver, Adrenal, Pancreas, Back, Appendix, Kidney, Ascending Colon, Stomach, Transverse Colon

Pupil

The condition of the pupil indicates functions of the Autonomic Nerves (Sympathetic/Parasympathetic). The pupil opens and closes according to the degree of brightness in the environment. The brighter the light, the smaller the pupil becomes; in the dark, the pupil gets larger to allow in more light. *A pupil larger than average* indicates degeneration of the automatic nerves (parasympathetic functions). Extreme dilation of the pupil arises at death. A large pupil indicates physical and mental degeneration. Fear, nervousness, anxiety, emotional and mental disorders can enlarge the pupils.

White, mucus: cloud covering the pupil indicates cataracts.
Pupil smaller: than average indicates healthy, good spiritual, physical and mental functions.

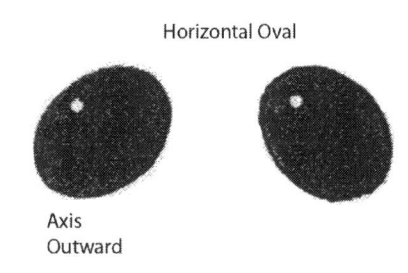

Horizontal Oval

Axis Outward

Inward Axis Oval Pupil – right pupil-indicates paralysis of the limbs, and/or painful muscular spasms.
Outward Axis Oval Pupil – left pupil-indicates muscular pain, pituitary and thyroid and/or nervous system problems
Flat Tops – A flattened upper pupil of the left eye can indicate central-nervous-system disorders (melancholia, depression, psychosis, manias, paranoia). The flatter it is, the more advanced the disturbance. In the right eye, a flattened upper pupil indicates hysteria.
Flat Bottoms – In both eyes, flat bottoms in both eyes indicate severe muscle and/or lower organ weakness. It can indicate flat feet.

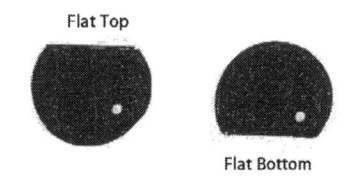

Flat Top

Flat Bottom

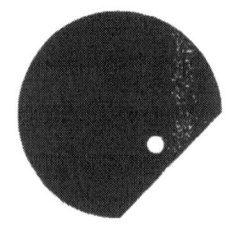

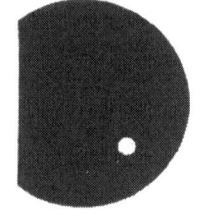

Angled Flat Side   Flat Side

Vertical Oval –Is seen when organs and organ systems are shutting down. It indicates near death, if it occurs in both pupils simultaneously. If it is only in one pupil, there is more time left. It is considered a sign of possible sudden apoplexy.
Horizontal Oval –Indicates emotional and/or psychological problems can have suicidal tendencies. Asthma or respiratory paralysis tendencies.
Flat Sides – Flat sides occurring toward the nose indicate disorders of the spine (displaced vertebra and heart problems). When flat sides occur toward the ears, it indicates respiratory weakness.
Angled Flat Sides – Toward mid-forehead indicates digestive and liver problems. It can indicate eye problems, periods of temporary blindness, emotional and psychological problems, episodes of apprehension, mania, and paranoia. Toward the temple of the left eye, indicates hormonal imbalance. Toward the temple of the right eye, indicates liver congestion.

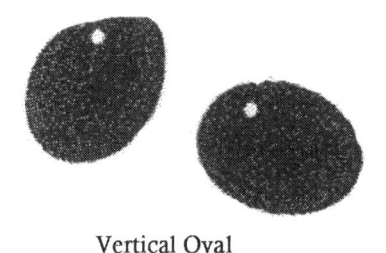

Vertical Oval

Iris Indicates Disease

IRIS HEALTH STATE	ACUTE Disease	SUB-ACUTE Disease
Good / Poor / Fair	Mild / Poor / Fair	Mild / Poor / Fair

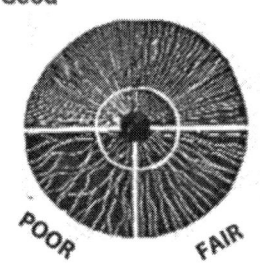

ACUTE Disease 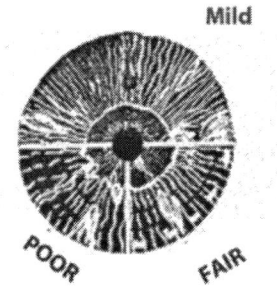 — SYMPTOMS: Pain, Inflammation, Irritable

SUB-ACUTE Disease — SYMPTOMS: Low metabolism, Weak condition, absorbing toxins. Slight pain, malfunction, metabolism

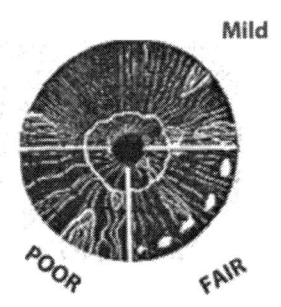

CHRONIC DISEASE
Mild / Poor / Severe

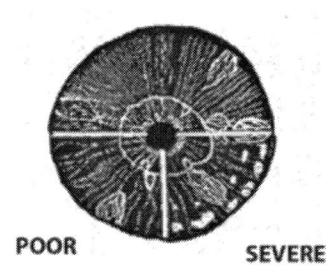

SYMPTOMS:
Weak immunity,
Waste Accumulation in cells,
Lack energy

DEGENERATIVE DISEASE
Mild / Poor / Severe

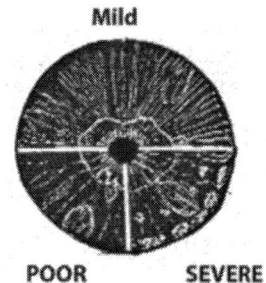

SYMPTOMS:
Cells deteriorating,
Poor Circulation,
No cleansing reaction

Iris

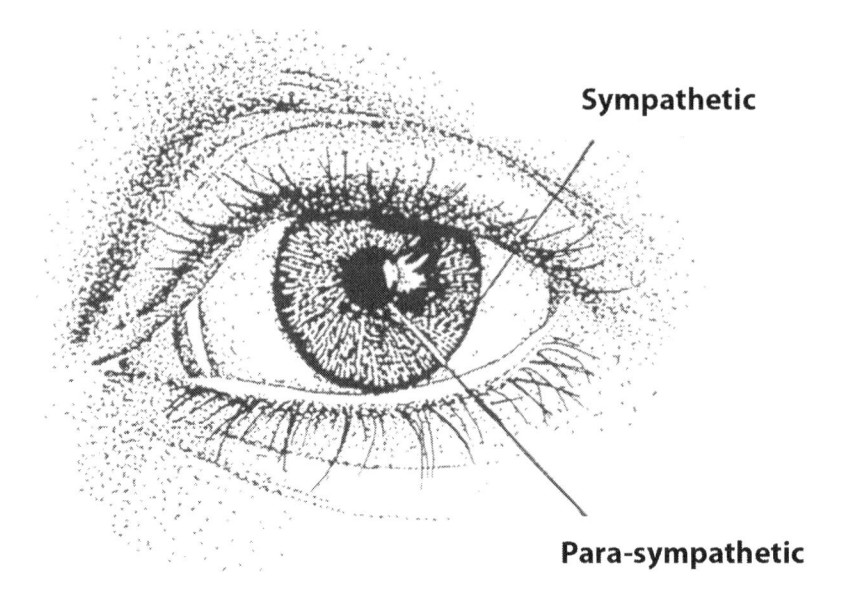

Sympathetic

Para-sympathetic

Whites Conditions

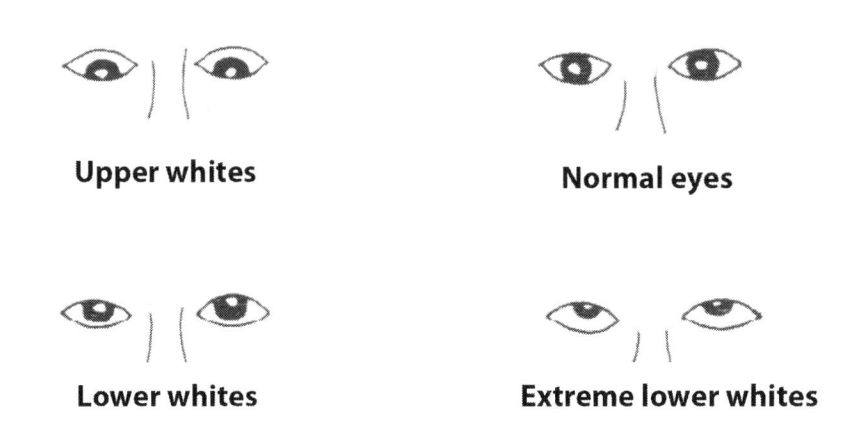

Upper whites

Normal eyes

Lower whites

Extreme lower whites

Upper Whites
Contracted eyeballs, which are normal in infants. In young children and adults can indicate abnormal emotions, mentality and behavior, aggressiveness, violence, and uncontrolled emotions.

Lower Whites
Indicates the physical, emotional, mental state is degenerating and becoming slower and weaker. With either upper or lower whites prone to accidents. In order to diagnose the lower whites, ask the person to look up at a 45-degree angle. If whites are showing beneath the iris the person has lower whites.

Inside (underside) the Eyelid

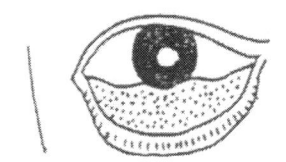

The pink area inside the lower eyelids: this area indicates the circulatory condition.
Light pink color with a smooth surface: indicates a healthy circulatory system.
Red color with expanded capillaries: indicates high blood pressure, excretory, circulatory, and nervous problems.
A whitish color: indicates an anemic condition, and dehydration foods (salt, coffee, mineral water, baked goods, soda, white sugar, white flour) consumption.
A reddish-yellow color: indicates heart, circulatory, liver, spleen, pancreas problems, expanded blood capillaries, reproductive, digestive, and circulatory problem.

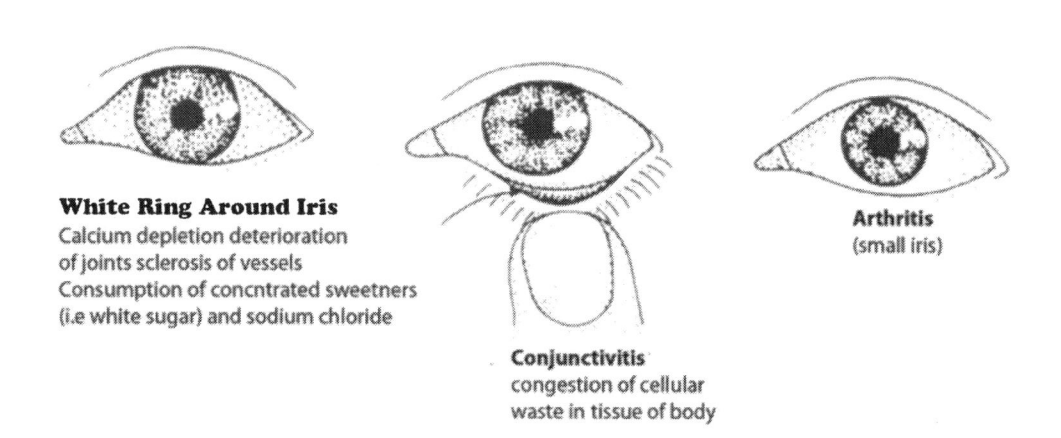

White Ring Around Iris
Calcium depletion deterioration
of joints sclerosis of vessels
Consumption of concntrated sweetners
(i.e white sugar) and sodium chloride

Conjunctivitis
congestion of cellular
waste in tissue of body

Arthritis
(small iris)

Eye Blinking

The average speed of eye blinking is four times per minute, or once every fifteen seconds. Blinking is a sign of Female Principle. A baby does not blink at all. A healthy person's eye can go without blinking for many minutes. A person who blinks more than four times per minute is in poor health. If blinking is frequent it indicates nervous disorders, fear, timidity, irritability, and over sensitivity.
The inside of the eyelids: The skin inside the upper and lower eyelids is pink with a smooth surface.
Small dot-like pimples: Indicates liver and kidney stress, and protein molecule lacrimal clogging tissue.
A white color: deoxygenated blood, anemia, poor circulation and low hemoglobin.
A reddish-yellow color: Indicates expanded blood capillaries accumulation of fat, mucus, heart, kidneys, and glandular problems.

Eye Floater

Floaters inside the eyeball's gel-like fluid (vitreous) are pieces of skin that detach from the retina. The vitreous can become concentrated and thick which pulls pieces of skin from the retina. Eating processed foods, diabetes, concentrated, processed sugars, sodium chloride, alcohol, and drugs can cause slightly thick vitreous that pulls tissue loose inside the eye. The floaters eventually settle at the bottom of the eyeball and out of vision. If the floater is seen with flashes of light it could be a sign of retina detachment.

Arcus Senilis

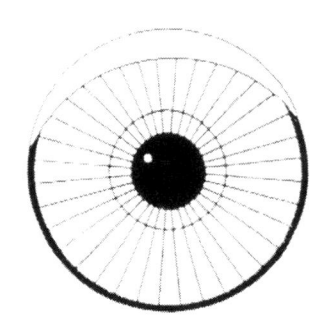

An arch (arcus) opaque film similar to a half circle referred to as a mineral ring on the upper half of the iris indicates bodily system deterioration.

Arcus Senilis can indicate arteriosclerosis, malnutrition of the nervous system and brain, and/or as well as kidney and heart stress.

Eye Nerve Signal

The eye is an out growth of the brain. The light that enters the eye strikes the Rods and Cones, which stimulate the eye's Retina nerve that connects directly to the brain. The eye has over 90 million Rods that refract only Black and White colors from the light. The eye can send 9Megabits per second to the brain. The female's X-chromosome gene carries the Cone's (4.5 million) Red, Blue, and Green color. The male's Y Chromosomes carries the Black and White rod's gene. This results in a high amount of men with a faulty version of color. Consequently, men are the most colored blind (10%) of the Sexes.

The eye can blink 10 times per minute. In the 1/3 second of time it takes to blink there is a moment of blindness. This results in several minutes of blindness per hour. Added to this, the eyes changing from one image to another causes the new image to be blurry and out of focus until the new image is adjusted into focus. It takes 1/10 of a second for the eyes to re-focus blurry time by substituting it with a created image, imagine image, or a false image. The Rods and Cones nerve ONLY transports signals. The brain reads the signal and interprets it into information. In other words, you see with your brain as well as hear, feel, smell, touch and taste with your brain.

The speed of the nerve signal and the speed of the brain substituted created false image is very difficult to separate. The Myelinated nerves are able to travel 330 feet per second (100m/sec) or 200 miles per hour (260 kph). Un-Myelinated nerve (are not covered with fat) signals travel 3.3 feet per second (1m/sec). Therefore, the brain can make separating the real image from the false image impossible.

Eyelash Types

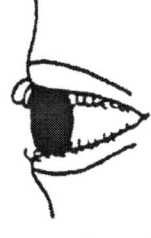

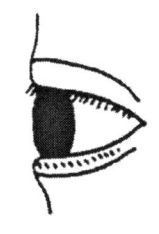

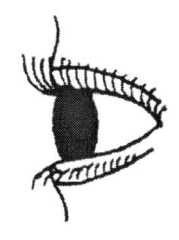

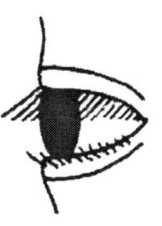

Curving Inward **Shorter Eyelashes** **Curving Outward** **Long Eyelashes**

Eyelashes that curve outward: indicates nervous sensitivity, degeneration of reproductive functions.

Shorter eyelashes: indicates acidic blood caused by salty food, roasted and/or baked flour, cooked meat and less intake of whole grain and raw vegetables.

Eyelashes that curve inward: indicates over consumption of large quantities of salt (sodium chloride), meat, eggs, fish, poultry, excess processed grains and cooked vegetables. Deterioration of the reproductive functions, menstrual cramps or lack of menstruation caused by acidic contraction of the ovaries.

Color Around the Eyes

The colors around the eyes change when the spiritual, emotional, mental, and physical health changes. It can fluctuate daily with the health state.

Clear, clean, natural skin color: indicates balanced harmonious, emotional, mental, and spiritual functions.

Dark color: Indicates an acidic toxic condition, weak kidneys, adrenal glands exhaustion and weak hormones. This can be caused by consumption of junk food, salt (sodium chloride), and concentrated sweeteners.

Eye Exercise and Massage

Eye Exercise

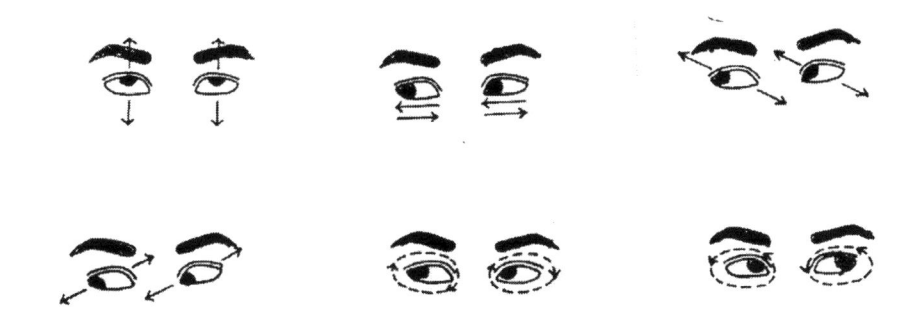

Eye exercise strengthens the eyes, acts as disease prevention and enhances the function of the liver (right eye) and pancreas (left eye). Slowness in eye movement can indicate alkalinity, patience, methodical thinking, under stimulation and the Female Principle. Fastness in eye movement can indicate acidity, impatience, quickness in the thinking, overstimulation (nervousness) and the Male Principle.

Viewing television, computer monitors and screens as well as inadequate time in the sun, and/or outdoors in a natural setting (forest, park etc.) can cause poor circulation in the eye and eye muscle weakness. Eye exercise and stimulation of eye acupressure points can enhance eye circulation and muscle tone. Stimulation should be done in sets of repetition or in your own creative way.

1. Begin by keeping the head straight, than look up toward the ceiling and then down at the floor. Repeat this motion several times. Move the eyes slowly up and down.
2. Next, look to either side of the head. Make the eyes look at the corners of the eyelids toward the ears.
3. Then look up and down into the opposite corners of the eyes.
4. Then rotate the eyes in a clockwise direction, then in a counterclockwise direction. When done slowly it takes up to ten minutes.
5. Always follow these eye movements with a rubbing of the hands together until they get warm and then press the palms onto the eyes to bring heat and energy into them.

Eye Stimulation Massage

Press and/or rub the points indicated to stimulate eye health.

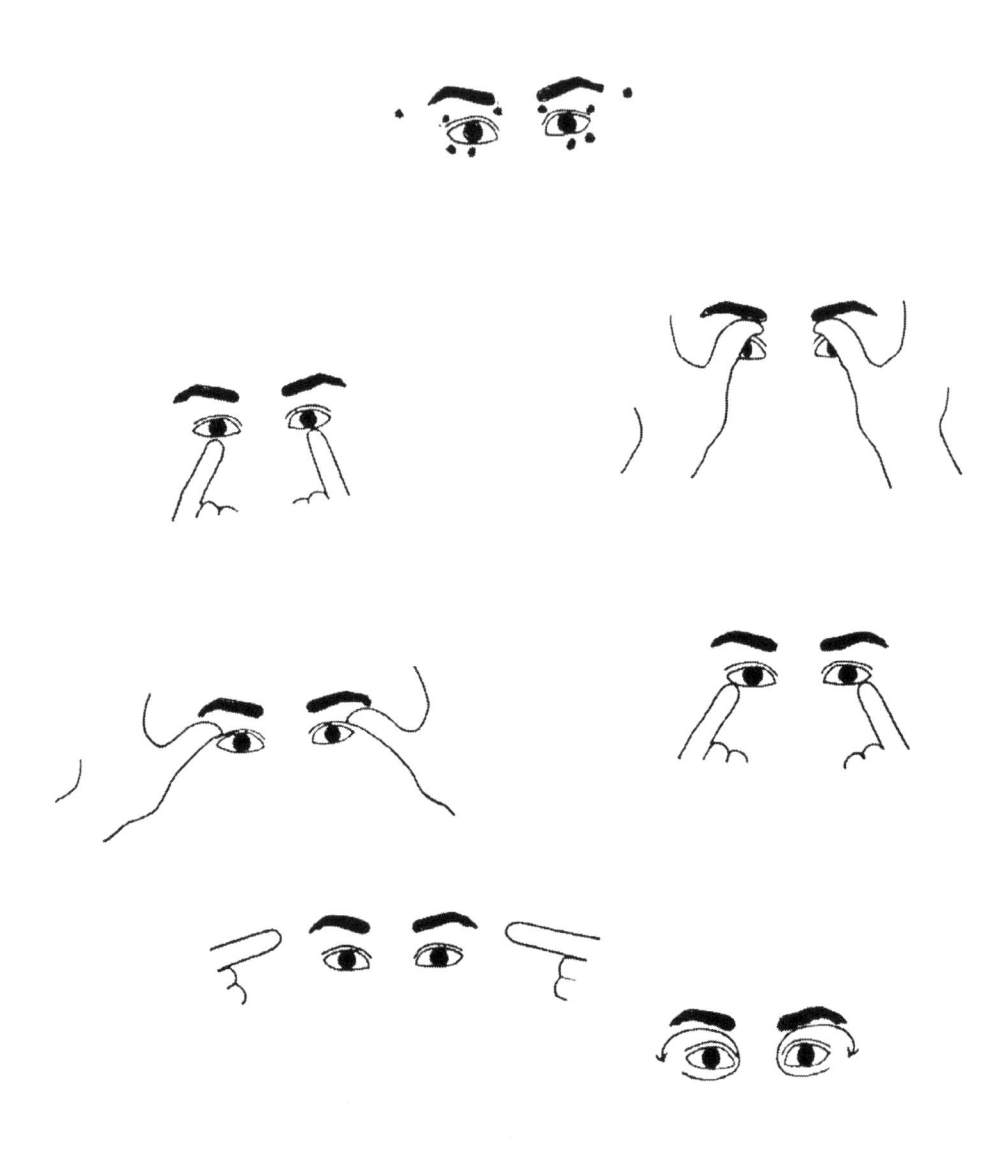

Eye Exercise Chart Guide

Muscles that are attached to the eyeball can become weak, resulting in farsighted (associated with stress) or nearsighted visions. These muscles contract or expand the lenses in order to adjust the vision for objects that are close up or far away. The six muscles change the shape of the eyeball. Four muscles flatten the width of the eyeball lengthwise making eye muscles strong which maintains and increases good vision. You will no longer need eyeglasses or contacts or surgery.

Exercise the eye muscles by putting your nose approximately ½ inch from the square in the center of the Eye Exercise Chart.

Exercise
1. Start the exercise by looking at the top of the upper most upside down triangle and look in a counter clockwise direction at each Triangle. Do this three times. Close your eyes very hard for approximately three seconds then open them.
2. Look at the outermost upside down triangle (Female/Uterus) at the top. Then, look at each outermost triangle in a clockwise direction. Do this three times. Close your eyes very hard for approximately three seconds. Then open them.
3. Follow the above for the middle and inner triangle.
4. Repeat steps 1, 2, and 3 in a counter clockwise direction.
5. Start at the top right hand corner (broken lines) and let your eyes follow the broken line diagonally down to the left corner base (----↙). Do this three times.
6. Start at the left base and follow the broken diagonal line up the top right corner. Do 1 repetition (do it three times). Then, close your eyes very hard.
7. Start at the top left corner and follow the exercise procedure of number 5. In other words reverse number 5.
8. Start at the lower right corner and look up then look down, to the top left. Follow number 6.

You can be creative with the exercise (use variations, mix them up). You can listen to music, sing, deep breathe, or cover an eye and do one eye at a time, then do both eyes.

Eye Exercise Chart

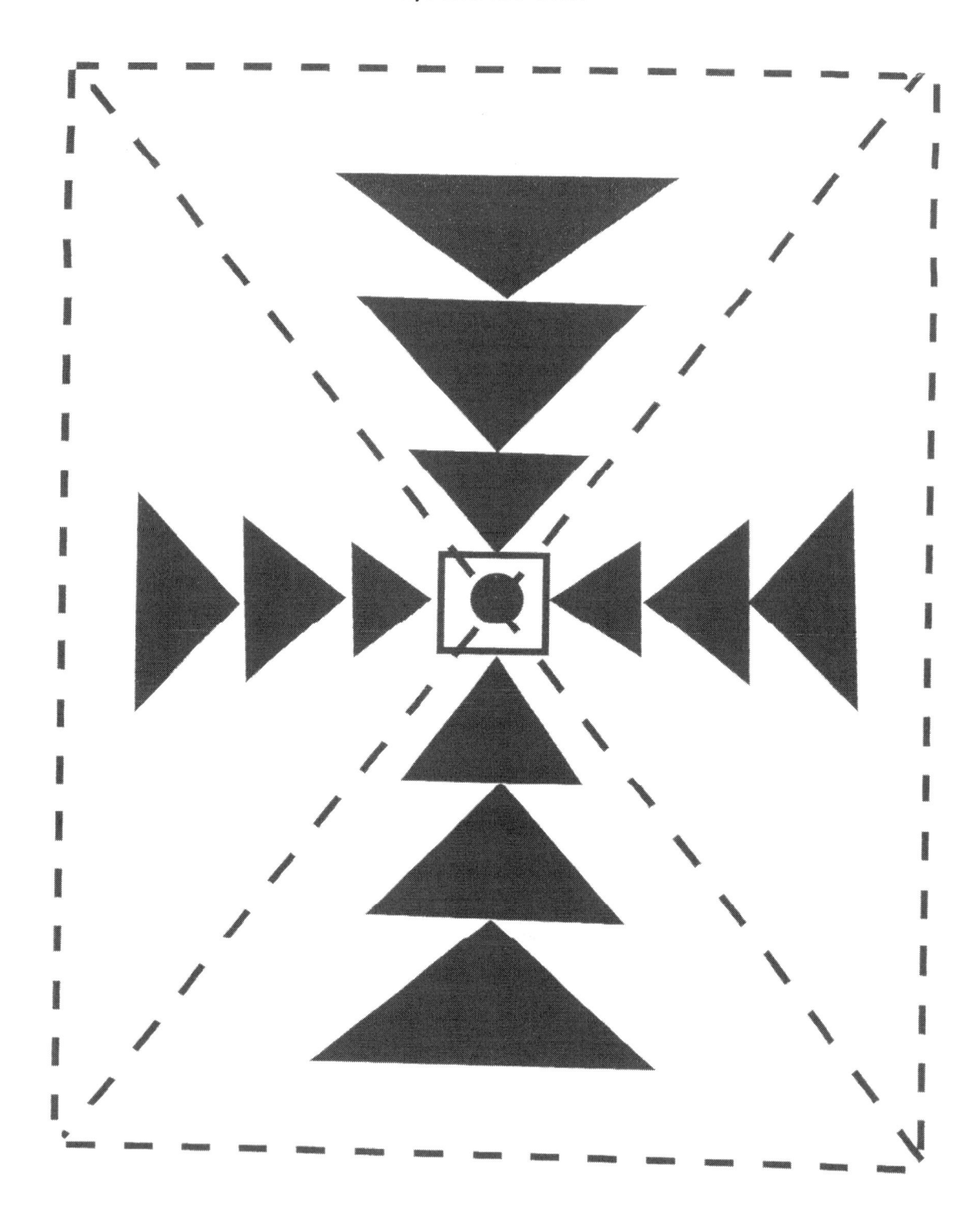

Hair

Hair Chart

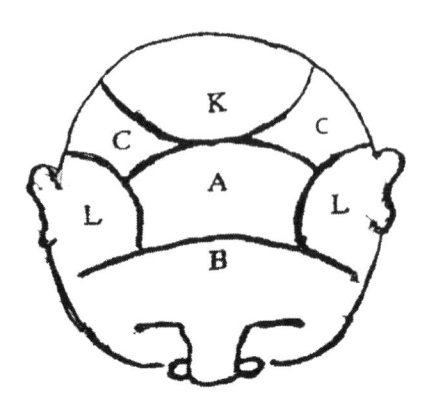

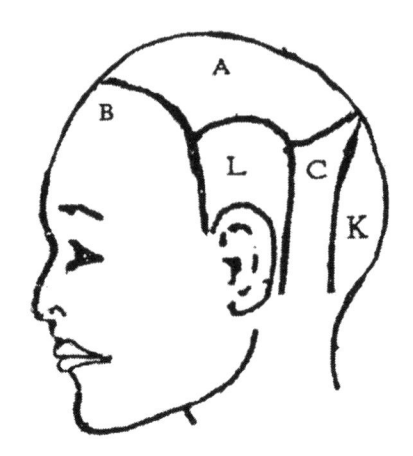

B—Front
Excretory system, Kidney, Bladder, Sex Organs
L—Side
Lungs, Large Intestine, Respiratory System
A—Top
Blood, Circulatory System, Small Intestine, Heart
C—Back
Digestive System, Stomach, Pancreas, Spleen
K—Back (hairline)
Liver, Gallbladder

Hair Spiral and Hearing

The Female Principle dominates the reception of sound if the hair spiral is on the right side of the head. A spiral on the left indicates the Male Principle is dominant. There is a tendency to slightly favor the ear or tilt the head on the side of the spiral. The ear that dominates hearing is the one closer to the center of the spiral. This helps sounds to be centered inside the head. Hearing is better through the sector parallel to the axis of the spiral.

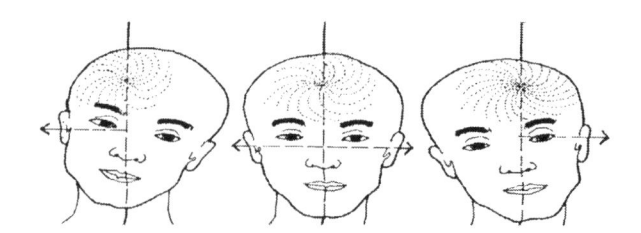

Ear

Ear Acupuncture Points

Acupressure can be applied to the points with the fingertip and/or the tip of a wooden matchstick. A point with inconsistency in the skin, texture, color, dryness, soreness, darkness, lightness, rash, bump, temperature change can indicate a disease or a problem with that specific organ or body part.

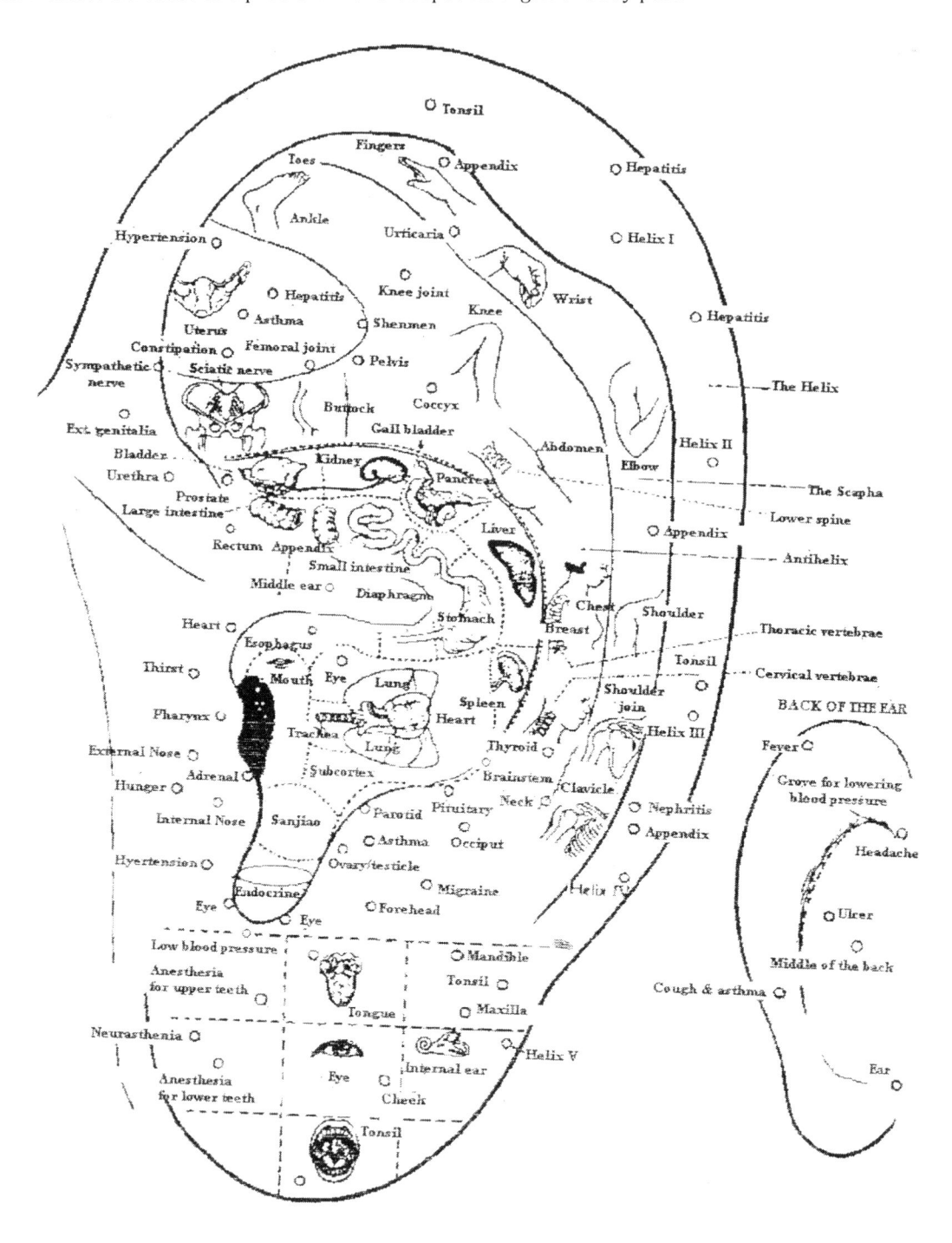

Helix Points may be used to reduce Sympathetic stress, acidity, inflammation, fever, swelling. **Sanjiao** is used for circulatory, glandular, and hormonal problems.

Ear Points

Acupressure points are used for many illnesses. Using prolonged finger pressure helps to stimulate the ear points. Hold each point for a minute. The points which are most sensitive to pressure should be held for several minutes or until the soreness decreases.

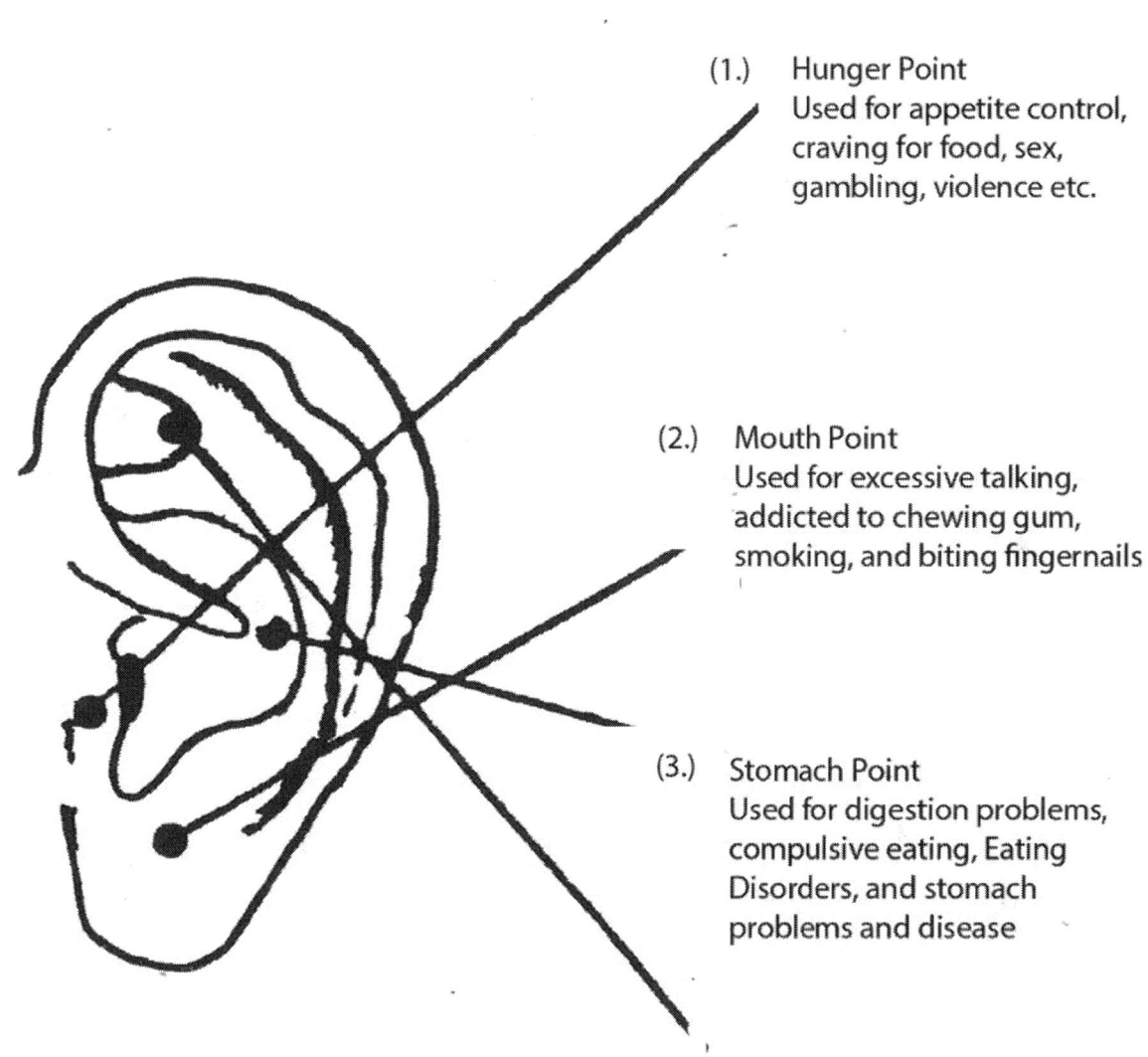

(1.) **Hunger Point**
Used for appetite control, craving for food, sex, gambling, violence etc.

(2.) **Mouth Point**
Used for excessive talking, addicted to chewing gum, smoking, and biting fingernails

(3.) **Stomach Point**
Used for digestion problems, compulsive eating, Eating Disorders, and stomach problems and disease

(4.) **Immunity** Increase the effectiveness of parasypathetic system, Female Principle, and Sympathetic system Male Princple. This point is used for emotional problems (anger, nervousness, mood swings, stress, anxiety, etc) and can help balance thoughts and improve thinking.

Ear and Body

The outer layer corresponds to the circulatory and excretory system. Spleen and lymphatic problems are indicated if there is a reddish color. If the earlobe is clearly separated from the head, it indicates a good reproductive system, a healthy nervous system and a balanced emotional thinking process. A purplish color indicates circulatory problems and low oxygen content of the blood. The upper area of the ear (earlobe), if it tends to be enlarged it indicates a potential for Hypo- or Hyper- glycemia.

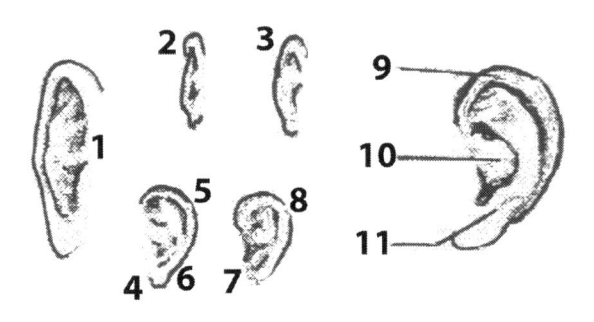

Area of Ears	Indication
1. Protrusion of Middle	Good immunity
2. Uneven	Imbalance function of Male and Female Principles, health is unstable
3. Sticking Out	Weak immunity, narrow viewpoint, weak health tendencies
4. Detached Lobes	Good glandular function (adrenals etc.),
5. Periphery slightly dark	Digestion and spleen problems
6. Creased Lobes	Hearing problems
7. Slight amount of Lobe attached	Poor vitality and weak nature, weak glands, acidic tendency
8. Ears slightly dark	Kidney problems, acidic tendency
9. Outer Ridge	Circulatory system
10. Middle	Digestive system
11. Inner Ridge	Nervous system
Small ears	Limited perspective, stays fixed and rigid emotions, ideas, and health view points
Wiggling	Excess protein foods tends to be acidic
Vertical Slant	Food choices, unhealthy
High on Head	Proud, egocentric, dualistic, rigid about health
Excess Wax	Liver problems, overconsumption of processed fats
Delicate Ear	Kidney and reproductive organs weak, malfunction

Ear Chart

Inconsistencies such as discoloration, rash, bumps, sores, scratches, texture, dryness, oiliness, sensitivity, hair growth, variation in skin temperature in an area can indicate malfunctioning, stress or disease with an organ, body section and/or system.

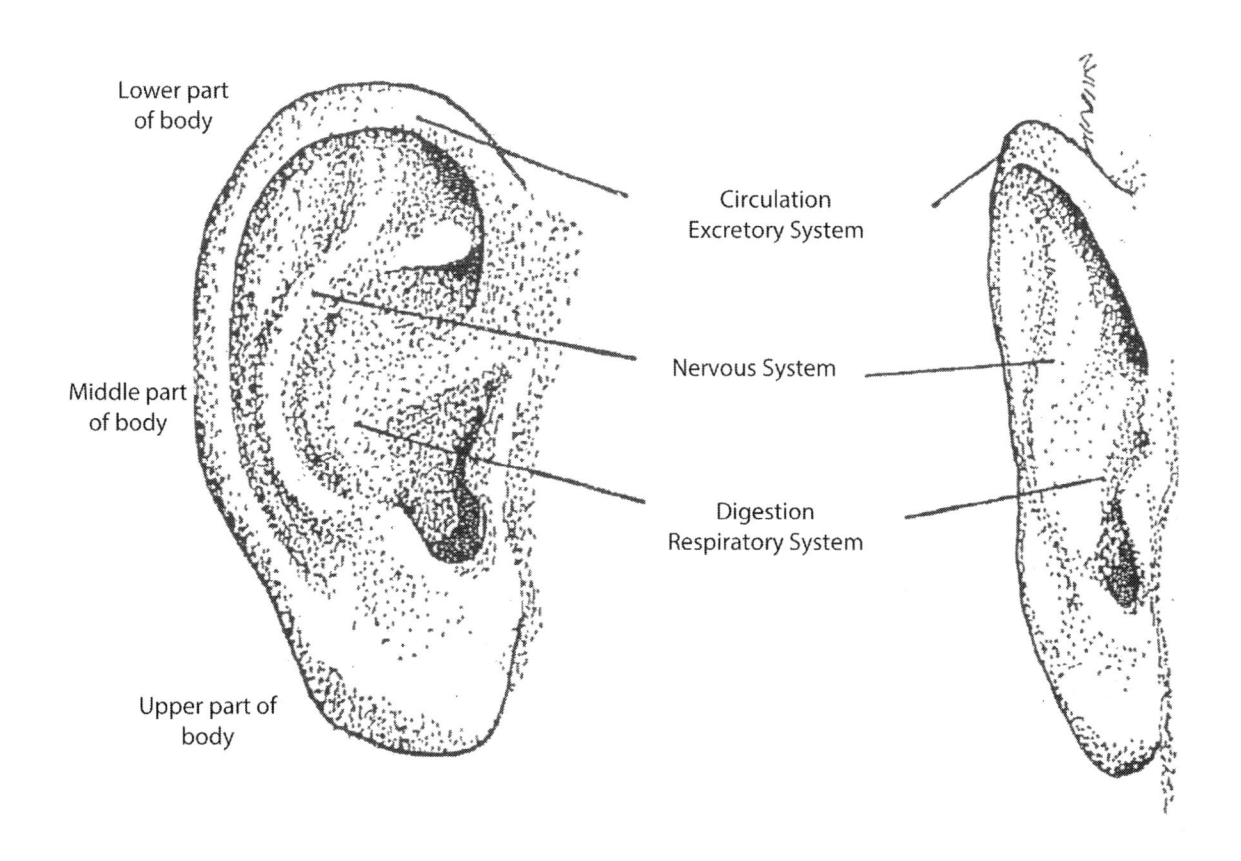

Lower part of body

Circulation
Excretory System

Middle part of body

Nervous System

Digestion
Respiratory System

Upper part of body

137

Ear Position and Shape

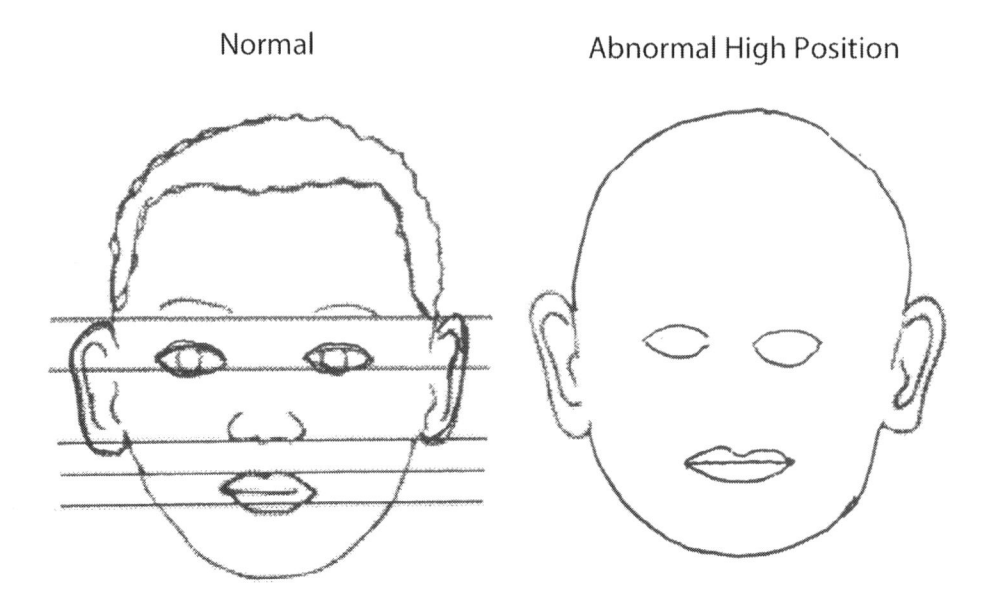

Normal   Abnormal High Position

Normally the ears begin at eye level, indicating good immunity and health. Earlobes should extend down to nose level. The lower part of the ear should slightly attach to the head around nose level. A small earlobe, or no earlobe, can indicate undernourishment, an inadequate diet, nervous, mental, and emotional problems. Slightly pointed ears can indicate overconsumption of protein, aggressiveness, emotional rigidity and narrowed mindedness. A large middle region of the ear in relationship to the upper and lower portions can indicate balanced emotions, thoughts, and good immunity. Ears positioned high can indicate a tendency to be acidic and a predisposition for aggressiveness, attitudinal problems and unbalanced thinking and emotions.

Ear Angles

Small ears can indicate a tendency to eat a diet of processed foods, meat, poultry, and eggs. A person with small ears has a tendency to focus on the present and have a lack of planning for the future; they need to put things in a wholistic conceptual perspective. Thick ears indicate balanced mental and emotional processes and holistic tendencies. Thin ears can indicate a tendency to eat unbalance meals, be critical, prejudice, and lack emotional balance. Ears lying flat close to the head have a tendency for a good metabolism, and wholistic lifestyle. Ears slightly separate from the head; within about a 30 degrees angle of the head, tend to be more mental than physical. Ears that stick outward beyond a 30-degree angle tend to be acidic, emotional and mental narrow, negative suspicions, skeptical of others, and/or abuse chemicals.

Normal
Ears lie flat against the head

Abnormal
Ear angle is more than 30 degrees away from the head

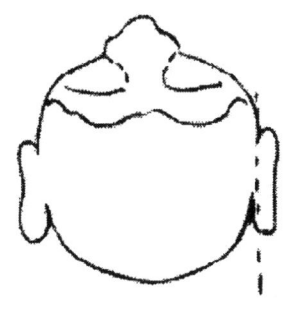

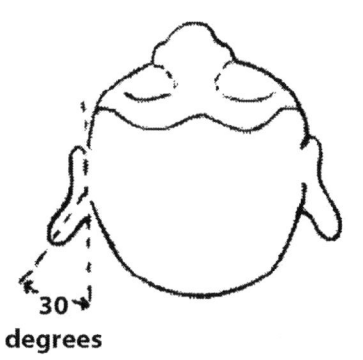

30 degrees

Sounds

People tend to use non-word phonetic sounds in between their words, sentences, before or after saying a statement, when trying to think of asking or answering a question, when picking up an item, when getting ready to tell a lie, before uttering a word, during laughter, when reacting to pain or sexual intercourse, and conversations. People tend to use one non-word sound more than another. The sounds they repeat more than another con indicate the health status. These non-word utterances can indicate problems with a part of the body related to the sound. The sounds can be used for healing by taking a deep breathe, exhale and then make the sound.

Emotional Center

Effects	Sound
Balances the entire body	A - E - I - O – U (make sound of letter, don't say letter name)
Lungs, sinuses, skull	HUM – HUM –HUM
Ears, auditory tube (Eustachian) to emotional brain	N - N - N
Nasal passages, sinuses (headaches)	MA – MA – MA
Jaw (tension headaches and migraines)	YA - YOU - YAI
Stomach (indigestion, acid indigestion, gastric reflux, food craving)	HUH - HUH - HUH

Cheeks

Cheeks

The skin of the cheeks indicates the state of health or a disease.

- **Firm clear skin**: good digestion and respiratory system
- **Tight thin skin**: the tissue of the two systems (digestive and respiratory) are high in acid, impacted with waste, the of thinning the systems skin
- **Brownish purplish:** deoxygenation (low oxygen) of the digestive and respiratory systems. The speed of circulation and breathing may be increased in order to get enough oxygen. This can over stimulate the sympathetic nervous system resulting in nervousness, oversensitivity and/or hypertension
- **Slightly dark:** mucus congestion and fat accumulation within the tissue of the digestive and or respiratory systems and/or the formation of cyst and tumors.
- **Darker:** intestinal, kidney, and excretory problems
- **Skin eruptions**: (pimples, bumps) mucus congestion and fat accumulation, stress on the lungs, reproductive organs and/or intestines, possible cyst in and around the ovaries or prostate, weak functioning of the digestive and/or respiratory systems.
- **Swollen wrinkles:** mucus or fat impaction of the digestive tract
- **Slight greenish brown skin**: the deterioration of the respiratory system, intestinal bleeding and/or blood thick with waste
- **Blue/Brown skin:** hardening of the gallbladder, degeneration of the liver's metabolic function
- **Pale brown:** bacteria infection, anemia, weakening of the lungs
- **Hair indicates:** hormone imbalance, the two systems are weak, deterioration of reproductive system

Teeth

Teeth

Inconsistency in color (mineral deficiency), shape, slight and deep vertical ridges, light or dark spots, misalignment, slightly too short or too long, shifts in the thickness and thinness, and spaces between teeth can indicate problems with the organ related to the tooth.

Direction of growth: Front teeth growth outward indicates that while the teeth were growing there was a diet of raw vegetables, fruits, excess concentrated sweeteners, and undiluted fruit juices. Teeth growing inward indicate that junk foods were eaten; including processed dairy, meat, white flour products, sodium chloride (salt) and cooked food and oils. Teeth that are usually straight and there is no overbite or under-bite indicate a balanced diet and lifestyle.

Spaces between the teeth: This related to Pituitary stress, which causes a shift of teeth and, widen of jawbone. People with this tend to be mindful of their thinking and attitude.

Size of the teeth: Large teeth indicate stable minerals and a balanced diet, while smaller teeth indicate that the diet was nutritionally poor while teeth where growing.

Abnormal tooth surface: Vertical ridges on the tooth surface are caused by a diet of concentrated sweeteners (white sugar), bleached white flour, sodium chloride (salt), junk foods, and a lack of vegetable protein and uncooked fat. Teeth with small, pinhole-like dots result from a lack of mineral or calcium, vegetable protein, raw fats, fresh vegetables, and an excess of sodium chloride (salt) and cooked minerals. Serrated edges on the front teeth often result from the same cause, and weak protease enzymes.

The number of teeth: Children usually have 20 teeth. Adults have 32 teeth; eight incisors, four canines, eight premolars, and twelve molars. A under nutrition diet results in the third molars (wisdom teeth), growth problems which may cause deformed molars, gum problems and pain while growing.

Tongue Exercise and Gum Massage

This exercise may be done after meals, upon waking, and at other appropriate times.

1. Roll your tongue around your mouth and across your gums and teeth. Use your tongue as you would a toothbrush.
2. As you roll your tongue around your mouth, saliva will be secreted by the salivary glands. Do not swallow it, but allow it to collect until you have a mouthful of saliva.
3. Swish the saliva around as if you were using a mouthwash. Wash the entire inside of your mouth including the gums and in between the teeth.
4. Swallow the saliva until your mouth is clear. As you swallow it, feel its energy as it descends to your stomach.

Gum Pressure Points

The organ placement on the lips has the same placement points on the gums. The gums can be pressed with the fingers to stimulate the meridians that supply energy to the mouth, teeth, and gums. Feel free to do this exercise any time of the day or after meals. Press these pressure points firmly with a rubbing movement to energize areas.

Teeth Deformities

Straight Growth

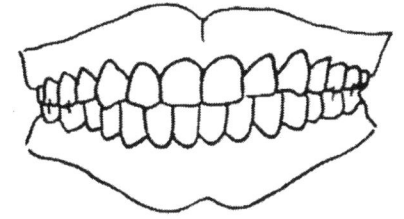

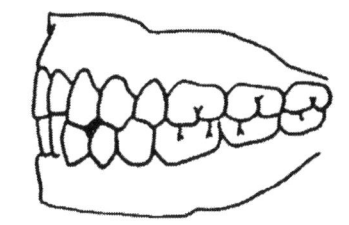

Outward Growth

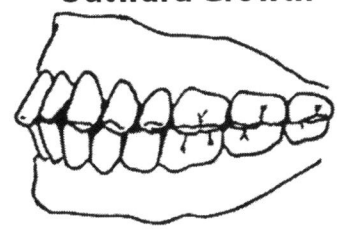

Inward Growth

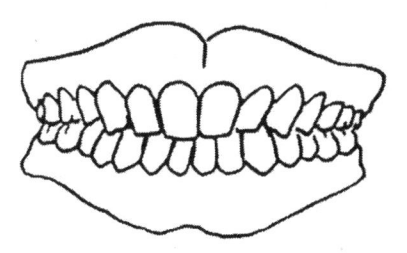

Vertical Ridges

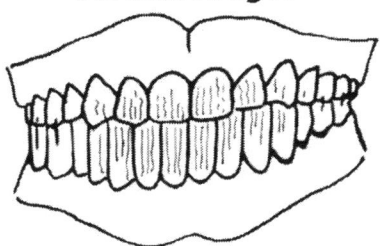

Small, pinhole-like dots

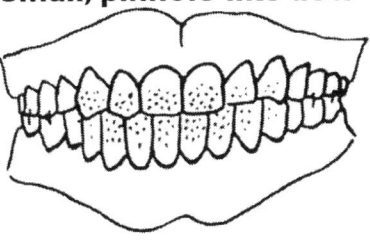

Spaces Between

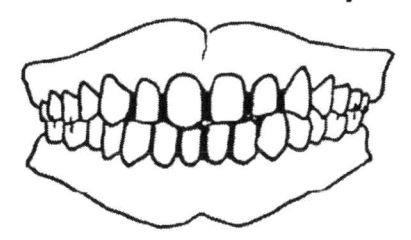

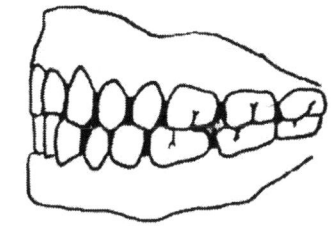

Serrated Edges

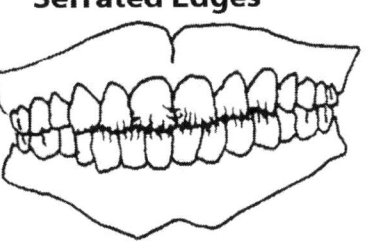

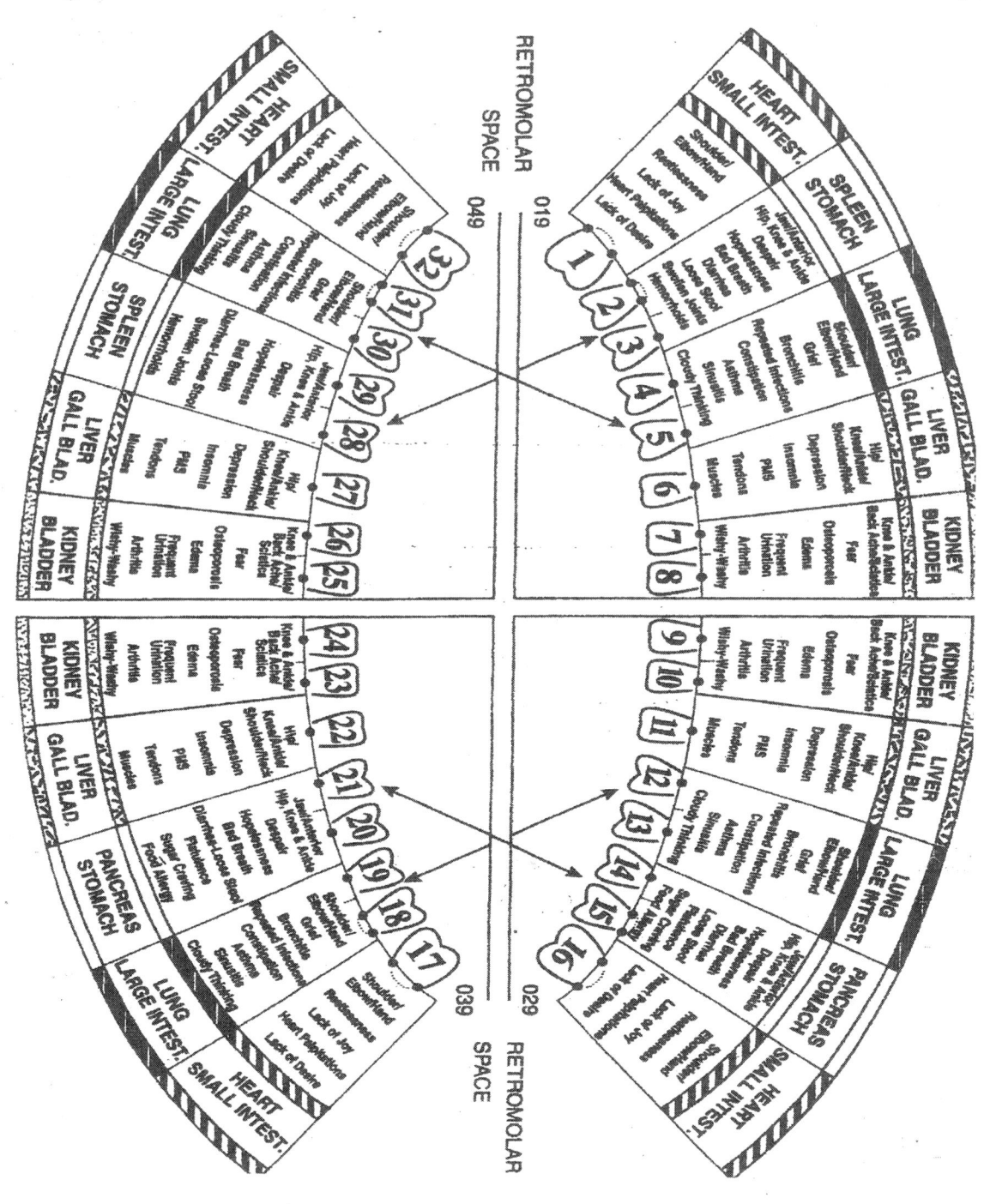

Each tooth is associated with glands, organs, and the anatomical structure on the same meridian. The electrical flow of action (acid) and the reaction (alkalinity) conductivity can be altered and decreased to glands, organs, bones, muscles, emotions, and thoughts when blocked by dental implants, cavities, infected teeth, dental fillings, crowns, root canals, bleaching, drilling, fluoride, and tooth paste glycerin which blocks re-enamalization (healing). Electro Acupuncture according to Voll (EAV) measurements indicates decrease electrical flow to teeth that have had dental work and or cavities. Cavitat (acoustic seismology) indicates dental tooth drilling, which is similar to Fracking, which causes microscopic cracks in the jawbone, degenerates, overheats, and damages the tooth's blood vessels and nerves.

Unnatural Tooth Gaps Exam

Adults have thirty-two teeth. This includes your four wisdom teeth that may be under the gum. Starting with the tooth farthest back in your lower right jaw, count your teeth. You will need a dental mirror to count because touching the teeth to count them is not reliable. If you have fewer than twenty-eight teeth, then examine the gaps where teeth are missing. Where a tooth is missing, check the corresponding tooth in the other jaw to see if it is growing into a space left by the missing tooth. Then keep your jaws closed and separate your lips with your fingers; look at the tooth opposite the empty space to see if it extends up or down farther than the teeth on either side of it. If any of the teeth are bginning to move or grow into a space where a tooth is missing this indicates a dental problem.

Adult Teeth **Children's Primary Teeth**

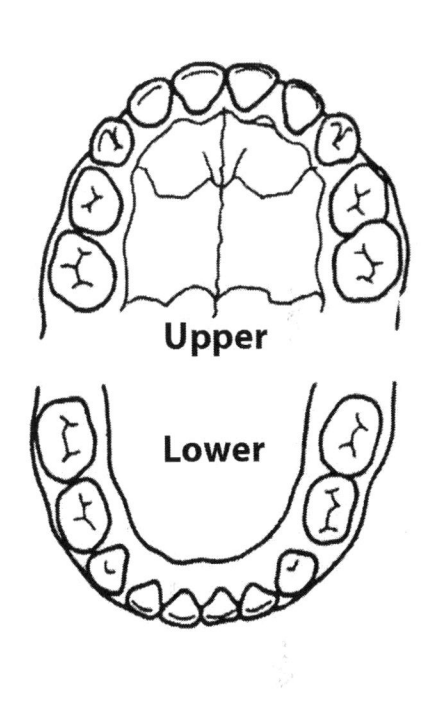

(Dentist numbering system)

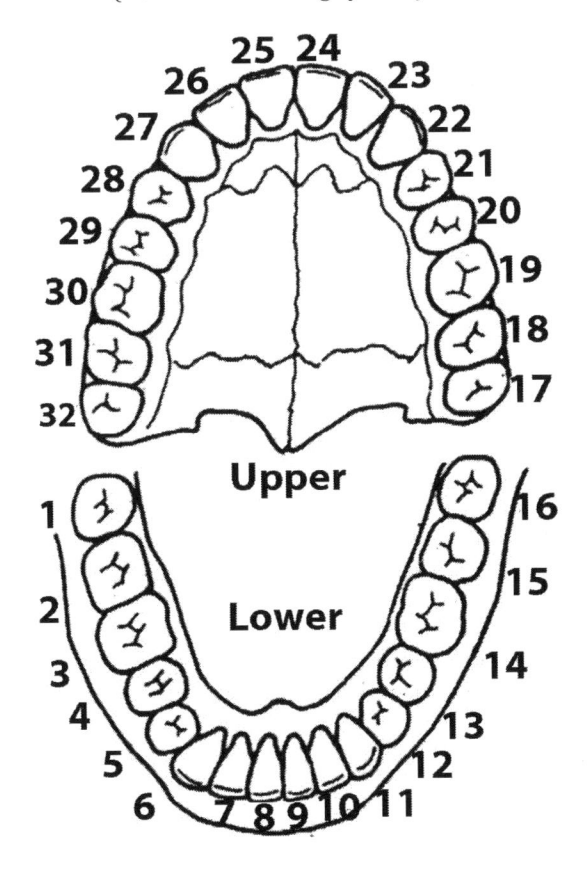

Children's Primary Teeth and Growth

The average dates when teeth appear vary from child to child.

Primary Teeth	Months
Central Incisors	6 – 8
Lateral Incisors	9 - 11
Eye Teeth	18 – 20
First Molars	14 – 17
Second Molars	24 - 26

Adult Teeth and Growth

Adult Teeth	Approximate Age	Tooth Number
Central Incisors	7 to 8	24
Lateral Incisors	8 to 9	23
Canines	12 to 14	22
First Premolars	10 to 12	21
Second Premolars	10 to 12	20
First Molar	6 to 7	19
Second Molar	12 to 16	18
Third Molar (Wisdom Tooth)	17 to 21	17

Tongue

Tongue Diagnosis

Any inconsistency in the skin of the tongue or papilla (buds) on the tongue as well as cracks, vertical and horizontal lines or wrinkles or a change in color, texture, bumps, and over sensitivity can indicate a problem with the organ related to that area. A change in color, dark taste buds, enlarged taste buds, white-coated areas, redness, paleness indicate problems to organs or functional disorders to the tongues related organ.

Tongue and Organs

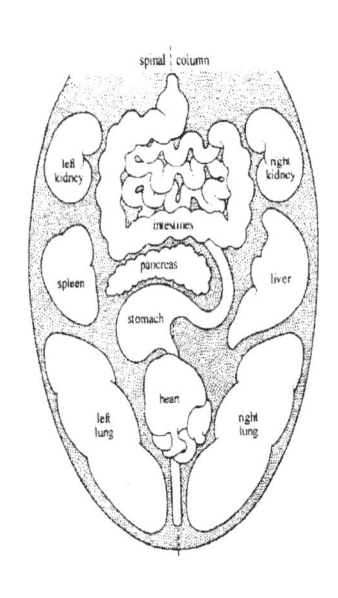

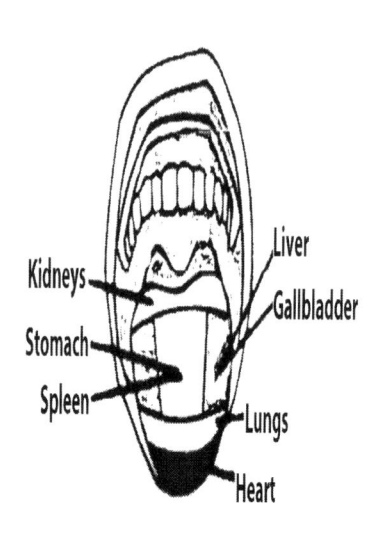

Tongue Description	Indication
Cleft tongue	Heart disorder
Dry tongue	Stomach disorder
Warts and growths	Protein congestion, see corresponding organ
Wart on tip	Stressed, overactive heart, kidneys deteriorating
Soft tongue	Digestive system congested with cellular waste
Hardness	Mucous waste congestion
Fur	Stomach disorder

Tongue Description	Indication
Pale	Digestive system, malfunctioning
Yellow	Acute stomach disorder, liver and gallbladder disease
Green	Liver and Kidney problems
Blue	Kidney and bladder problems
Violet	Liver and pericardium disorder, oxygen starvation, drugs
Grey/Black	Heart and kidney problems
Trembling	Nervous and brain disorder
Black at root	Kidney disorder, possible cancer
Purple tongue and/or gums	Uterus and bladder disorder
Slimy	Spleen problems
Foul breath	Intestines and stomach constipated with manure
Watery voice	Excessive liquid, kidney disorder

Description of Tongues

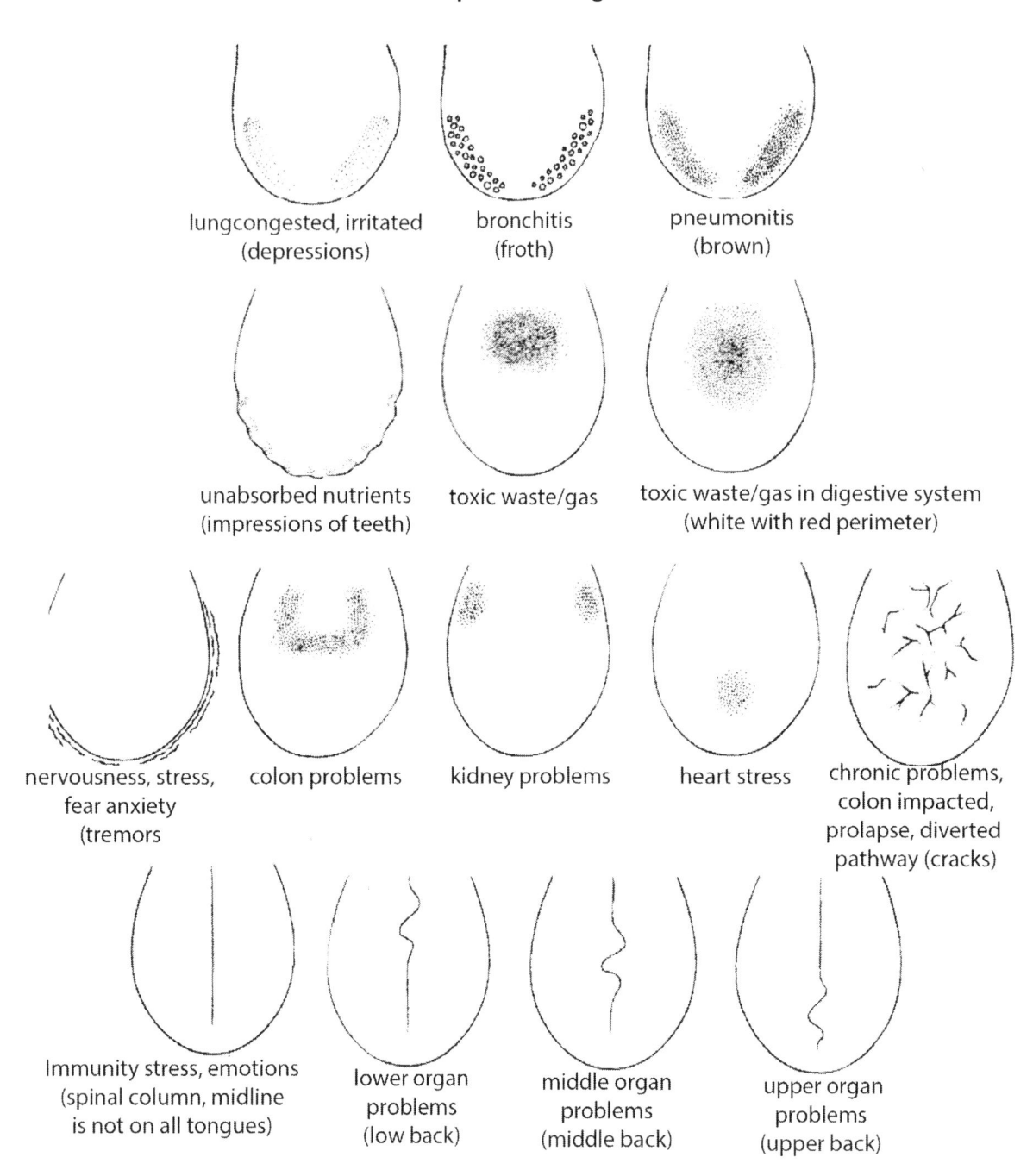

- lung congested, irritated (depressions)
- bronchitis (froth)
- pneumonitis (brown)
- unabsorbed nutrients (impressions of teeth)
- toxic waste/gas
- toxic waste/gas in digestive system (white with red perimeter)
- nervousness, stress, fear anxiety (tremors
- colon problems
- kidney problems
- heart stress
- chronic problems, colon impacted, prolapse, diverted pathway (cracks)
- Immunity stress, emotions (spinal column, midline is not on all tongues)
- lower organ problems (low back)
- middle organ problems (middle back)
- upper organ problems (upper back)

Tongue Shapes

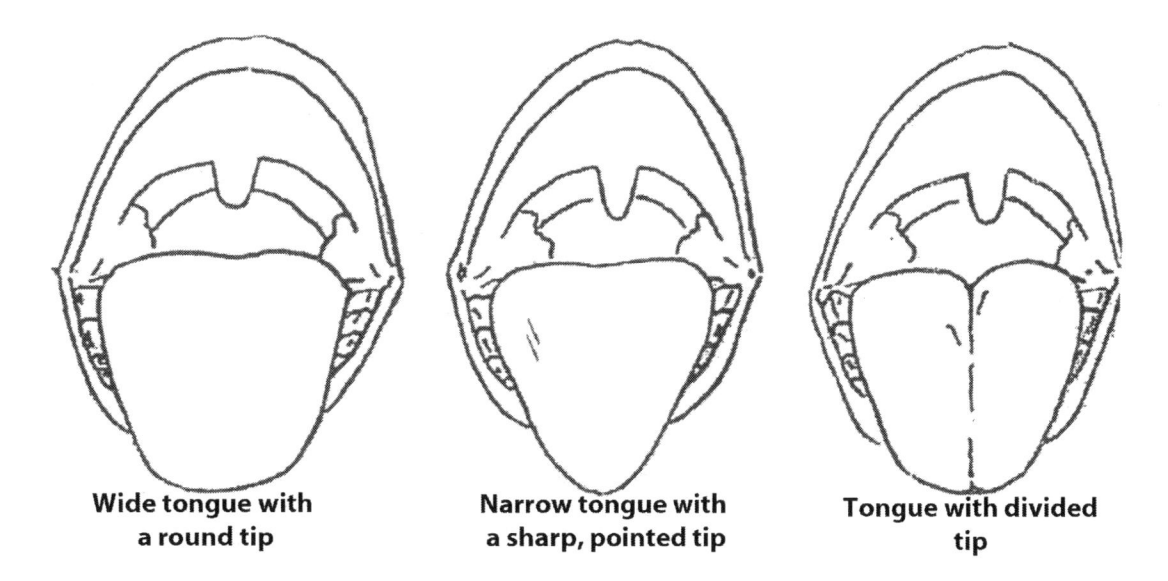

Wide tongue with a round tip

Narrow tongue with a sharp, pointed tip

Tongue with divided tip

- ❖ **Wide tongue with a round tip:** Indicates alkalinity tendency. The physiological and psychological conditions are generally harmonious, gentle and understanding.
- ❖ **Narrow tongue with a sharp, pointed tip:** Weak protease enzymes. Tends to be physically rigid and tight, and mentally aggressive and have rigid opinions and emotions.
- ❖ **Tongue with divided tip:** Nourishment unstable, and has a tendency to be indecisive and emotionally changeable.
- ❖ **Flat tongue:** Tends to have good metabolism. Tendency to be in a harmonious environment.
- ❖ **Thick tongue:** Tends to have weak lipase and protease enzyme, and shows a more active and aggressive character.

Tongue Motion

Parasympathetic	Stress	Sympathetic
Complete absence of vitality	**Mild**	Slight Motion
No motion	**Acute**	Moderate Motion
Very little motion or slow	**Chronic**	Fast Motion (Tremor)

Disease And Taste

Disease and Taste

An excessive taste (craving) for one type of food can indicate a problem with an organ. There are five primary tastes (sweet, sour, pungent, bitter, and salty). Pungent is not actually a taste. Pungent is the sensation (Touch) of hot/burning feeling when food touches the tongue. There is also the Glutamate (protein) and Savory (pleasure, enjoyable). Taste buds are on and under the tongue, in the roof of the mouth (Palatine), in the throat, lungs, and nasal passage.

Organ	Taste	Symptoms
Pancreas and Spleen	Sweet	Wet mouth, Ulcers, Greasy foods, indigestion, heaviness of body, low body temperature to extremities
Liver	Sour	Cataract, Weakness, Overheating, Insomnia, Pain-right side, nausea, like it cold
Lungs, Large Intestine	Pungent	Mucous, Congestion, Loose Stools, Cracked Lips, Cramps, Never thirsty, Hemorrhoids
Heart, Small Intestine	Bitter	Swelling of nose and hands, Emotions unstable, Shortness of breath, Perspire, Respiratory disease (bitter expands/ opens lungs)
Kidney, Sex Organs	Salt	Hair Loss, Dandruff, Arthritis, Dry Mouth, Weak Ankles, Painful Swollen Legs, Sex Organ Deterioration, tends to eat hot spicy foods

Fingers And Fingernails

Curvature of fingers

Curve toward the Middle Finger: indicates Male Principle tendency. Curve away from the Middle Finger: Female Principle tendency. When the fingers are stretched, they should be straight and balanced. Fingers that curve inward or outward, indicates certain organs and functions in the body are overactive or underactive.

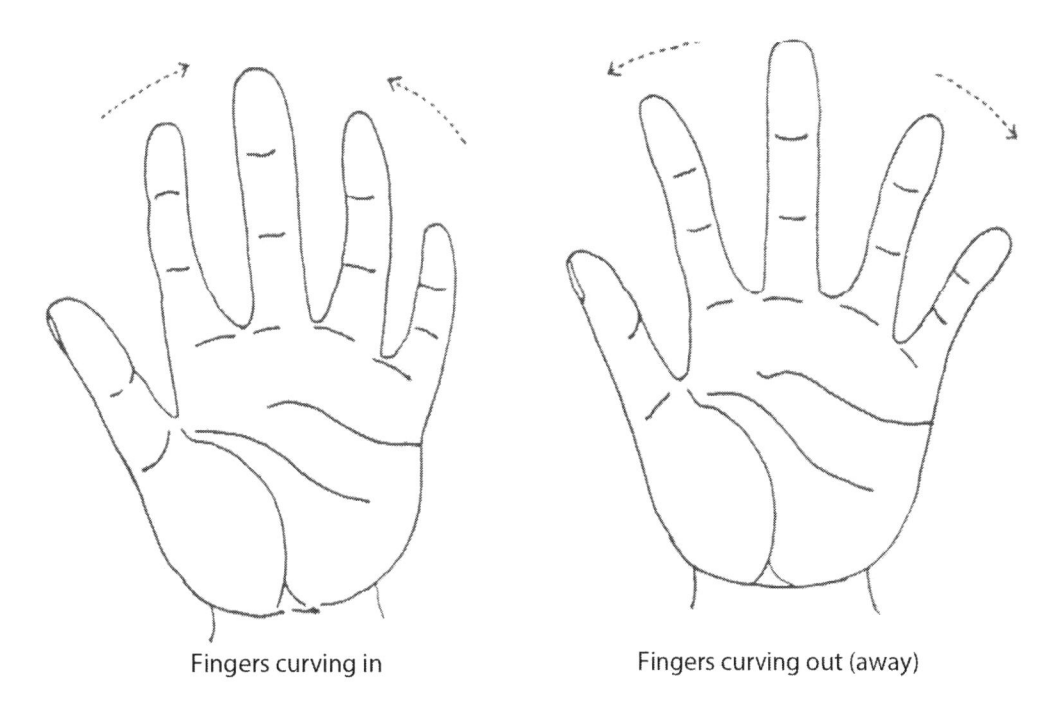

Fingers curving in   Fingers curving out (away)

Fingers and Organs

Fingers	Organs and Functions
Thumb	Lungs, respiratory system
Index finger	Large intestine and its functions
Middle finger	Three Melanin Clusters, (chakras) heart, the circulatory, and reproductive systems
Ring finger	Three Melanin Cluster (chakras) and the metabolism, heart, intestines, stomach
Little finger	Heart and small intestine

Finger Placement

The way the fingers are set in the hand indicates a personality type. If a finger is set higher than the others, it has high influence on the personality.

Fingers Set on a Line: Fingers that are evenly set on the palm, indicates stability, a positive attitude self-confidence, and can follow treatments for disease.

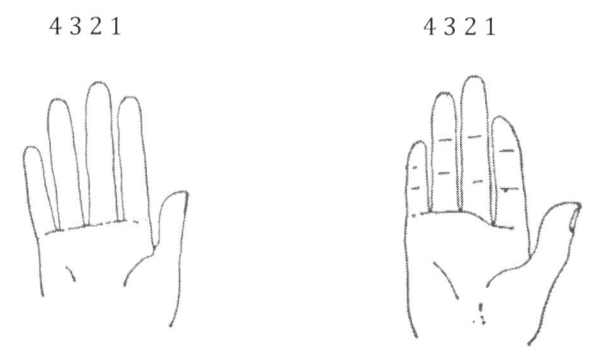

Low Set First Finger: The First (Jupiter) finger sets lower on the hand indicates lack of self-confidence and a need to be encouraged. May tend to get neurotic or nervous. Needs nurturing to stay healthy. Tends to let emotional stress cause them to become ill.

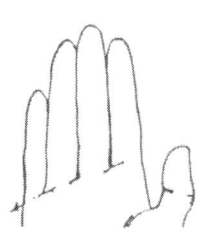

Low Set Fourth Finger: Little finger set low in the hand can indicate problems with balancing the emotional personality. They have difficulty eating a balance diet. Tends to lack tact and social grace, which can cause negative reactions. If the thumb were straight, it would indicate an outspoken individual.

Fingertip Conditions

- **Cracked, split**: Problems with the circulatory, and excretory functions. Degeneration of the reproductive system. Sexual weakness, which manifest itself as a loss of desire.

- **Pale, fatty skin:** The digestive and lymphatic system problems. The kidneys and liver may be forming cysts or tumors. Tendency to accumulate fat and mucus in the lungs.

- **Red or purple:** The respiratory and circulatory systems are malfunctioning. There is a tendency to have nervousness, irritability, depression, mood swings, and hypersensitivity.

- **Hard, flaky skin:** Tendency to have hardening of the arteries and muscles. Mental and physical rigidity.

- **Soft, peeling skin**: Heart and circulatory systems are stressed. Kidneys and excretory functions are declining. Tendency to be easily agitated, irritated, and oversensitive.

Nail Diagnosis

Inconsistency in shape, texture, or color of the nail can indicate a health problem.

- Pale color, anemia is indicated.
- Yellow indicates a liver weakness.
- Blue indicates lung and heart weakness.
- Blue Lunar crescent at the base of the nail indicates liver problems.
- Red Lunar is a sign of cardiac failure.

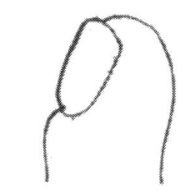

Weak heart and lungs (clubbed nail)

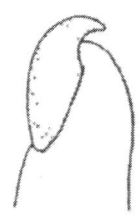

Chronic cough (hook-like)

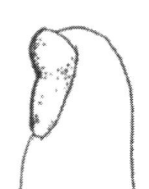

Chronic fever, long standing disease, degenerative disease (transverse groove)

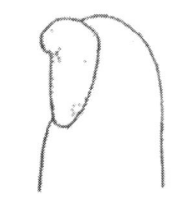

Chronic lung infection (bump at the end of nail)

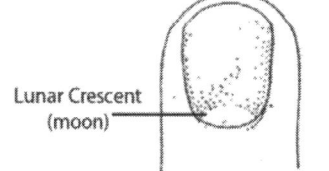

Lunar Crescent (moon)

Calcium or Zinc deficiency (white spots)

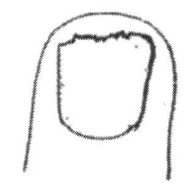

Hormone imbalance nervousness (brittle)

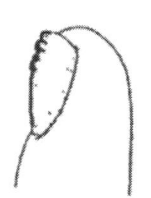

Malnutrition (stepped nail)

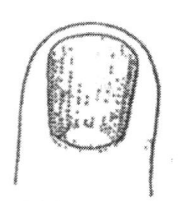

Malabsorption (longitudinal striations)

Fingernail Diagnosis

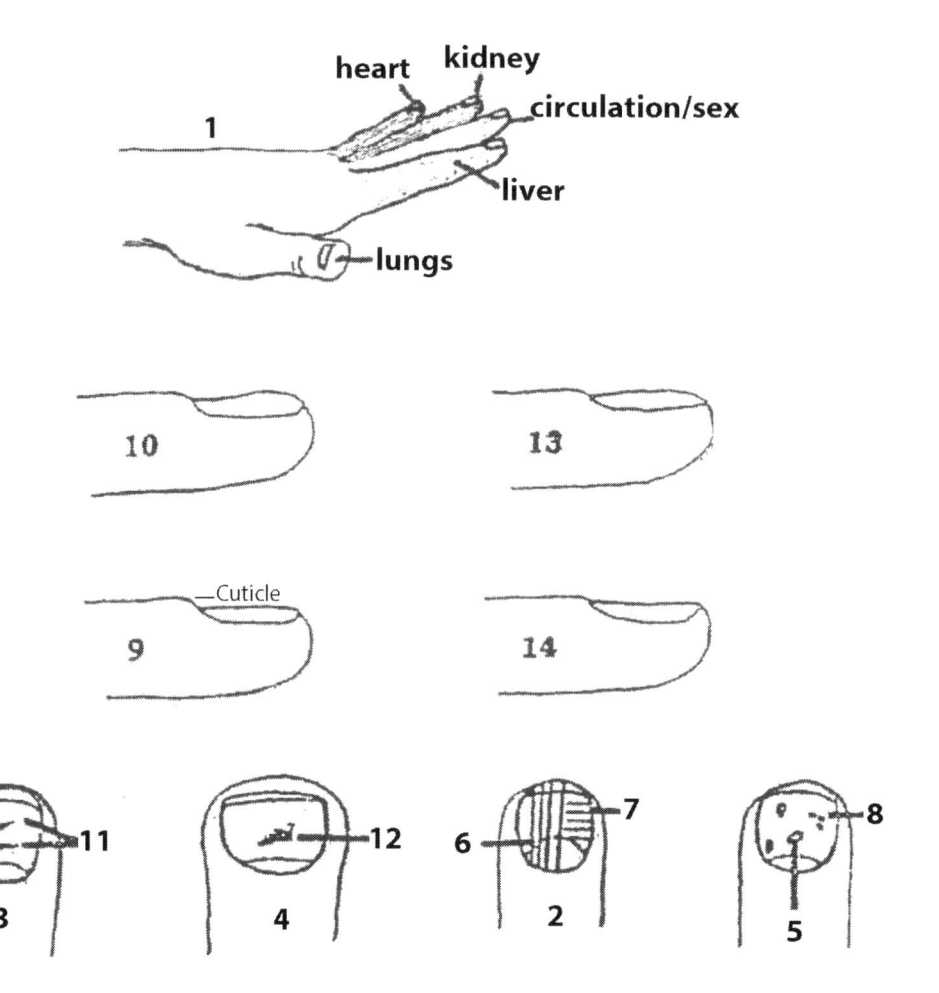

Nail Description	Interpretation
1. Fingers become pale when they are stretched tense and then relaxed	Anemia
2. Large Moons (Lunar crescent)	Excess protein, weak digestive protease enzyme
3. Small or No Moons	Good Immunity
4. Short & Square Nails	Strong immunity
5. White Spots	Zinc or Mineral deficiency, concentrated sweeteners
6. Verticle Lines	Possible bacteria or worms in intestines
7. Horizontal Lines	Unstable diet or major environment change
8. Small Red Dots	Pin worms
9. Thick or Inflamed Cuticle	Excess protein, protease problems

160

10. Concave Nail	Intestinal parasites
11. Diagonal Indentation, Wide at Bottom	Round worms
12. Diagonal Indentation, Wide at Top	Tape worm
13. Bulging Nail	Strong corresponding organ
14. Flat Nail	Weakness in corresponding organ
Narrow Nails	Weak immunity
Cracked Nails	Sexual organ deterioration, hormonal problems
Biting Nails	Worms, nervousness
Bulging Nail Becoming Flat	Metabolic disorder

Shape and Size

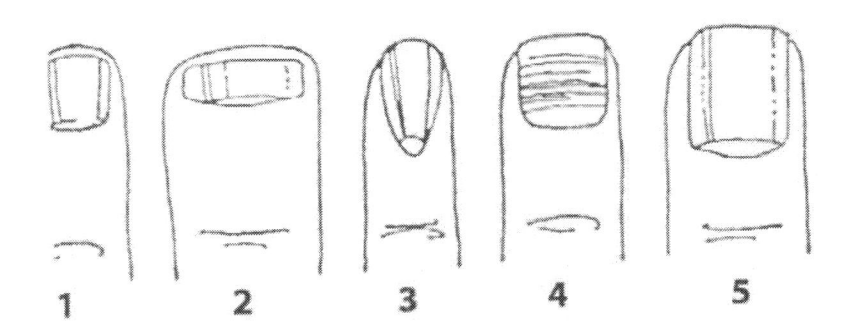

Use the moon of the nail bed when you judge the size of the nail.

1. Short nails: Critical

2. Short and broad nails: Sensitive and Aggressive; can negatively misinterpret others words and/or emotions, and can react with abusive words and/or violence.

3. Filbert shape nails: Tends to have nervous energy. They put everything they have into a healing task. When it's finished, they collapse from physical and/or emotional exhaustion.

4. Ribbed nails: Traumatic shock.

5. Long and broad nails: An open and frank type approach to disease and wellness.

Finger Analysis

Top Knot: Indicates an orderly person (sequential) and mentalistic (Thinker). Complex disease and treatments seem simple and simple disease and healing modalities can seem confusing.

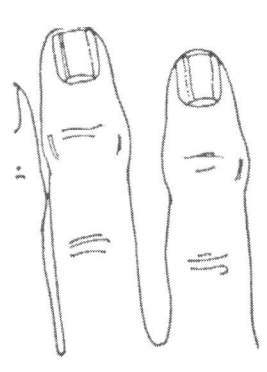

Lower Knot: They can feel uncomfortable when behavior, words and/or emotions lack order (sequence). A knot on the lower joint indicates a practical approach to wellness.

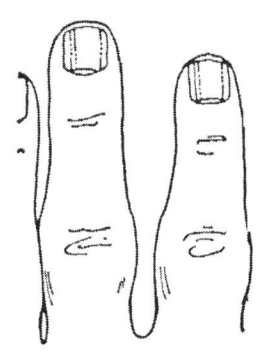

Smooth: Fingers that have smooth joints indicate an intuitive mind. They grasp healing ideas, concepts and assignments quickly. Short, smooth fingered people may get themselves into difficulties. They tend to be spontaneous and act without full information about a disease or health treatment disorderly and chaotic situations.

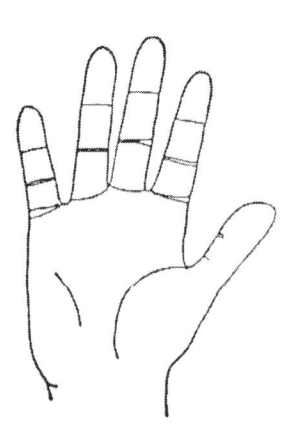

Long Smooth Fingers: Long, smooth fingers indicate creativity. Long fingers give them the intuitive ability and patience to follow intuitive treatments.

Knotted: Fingers with knots on both joints belong to the philosophic type. They tend to be skeptical about disease and wellness. Health problems are solved with attention to details.

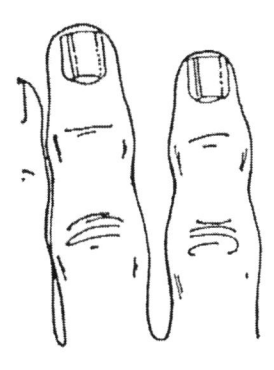

Fingers and Measurement

In the ancient past the fingers were used as a standard for measurement. The width of your four fingers is equal to the width of the Palm of your hand.

4 Fingers width = 1 Palm

4 Palms = 1 Foot

6 Palms = 1 Cubit

4 Cubits (24 Palms) = Your Height

Fingernail Form

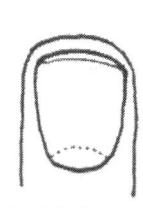

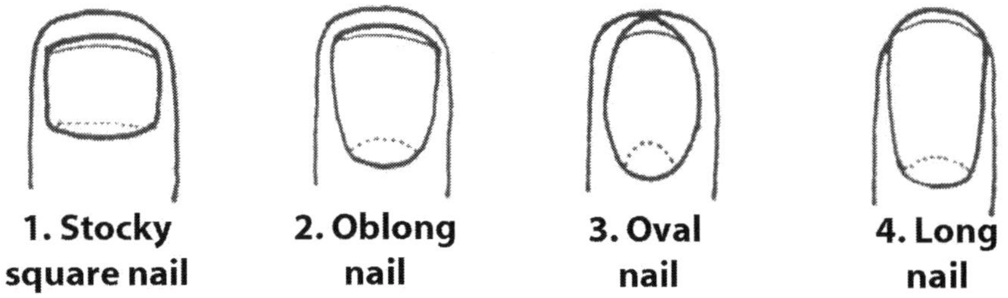

1. **Stocky square nail**
2. **Oblong nail**
3. **Oval nail**
4. **Long nail**

1. **Stocky, square nails:** Indicates tendency to be physically active and mentally inflexible.
2. **Oblong nails:** Indicates a spiritually harmonious person with episodes of rigidity.
3. **Oval nails:** Indicates an emotionally sensitive person with a high level of rationalization.
4. **Long nail:** Indicates digestive, respiratory, and physical weakness. A tendency to be emotional and oversensitive.

Hardness and thickness: Harder and thicker nail indicate physical and mental vitality.

Softer and thinner nails: Indicate a more passive weak person.

Fingertip Forms

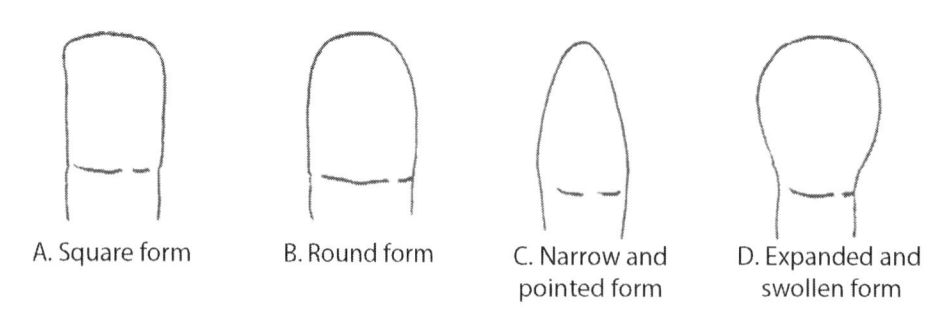

A. Square form   B. Round form   C. Narrow and pointed form   D. Expanded and swollen form

A. **Square fingertips**: Indicates determined, theoretical, aggressive, and physically active individual.
B. **Round fingertips**: The parents had a good and healthy lifestyle. This is an energetic, positive personality, sympathetic, active and a good disposition.
C. **Narrow, pointed fingertips**: Tendency to be physically weak, and the emotional ability to be manipulated and to manipulate.
D. **Expanded, swollen fingertips**: An aggressive, self-centered, discriminating person with tendencies to have offensive episodes.

Nail Color

Pinkish red nails: Good circulation and nutrition.

Reddish-purple nails: Circulatory, digestive, and excretory system have problems. There is a tendency for insomnia, constipation, diarrhea, fatigue, depression, mood swings, and psychosomatic problems.

Dark red: Excessive fatty acids, cholesterol, and/or minerals in the blood, heart, circulatory, kidneys, excretory, liver, gallbladder, and spleen stress. Hardening of the arteries and muscles. Inflexibility of the emotions and thoughts can be a disease consequence.

Whitish nails: Poor circulation and low hemoglobin. The accumulation of fat and mucus in and around the heart, liver, pancreas, prostate, and ovaries can be in progress. Leukemia and other types of cancer.

Twelve Types of Fingernails and the Zodiac

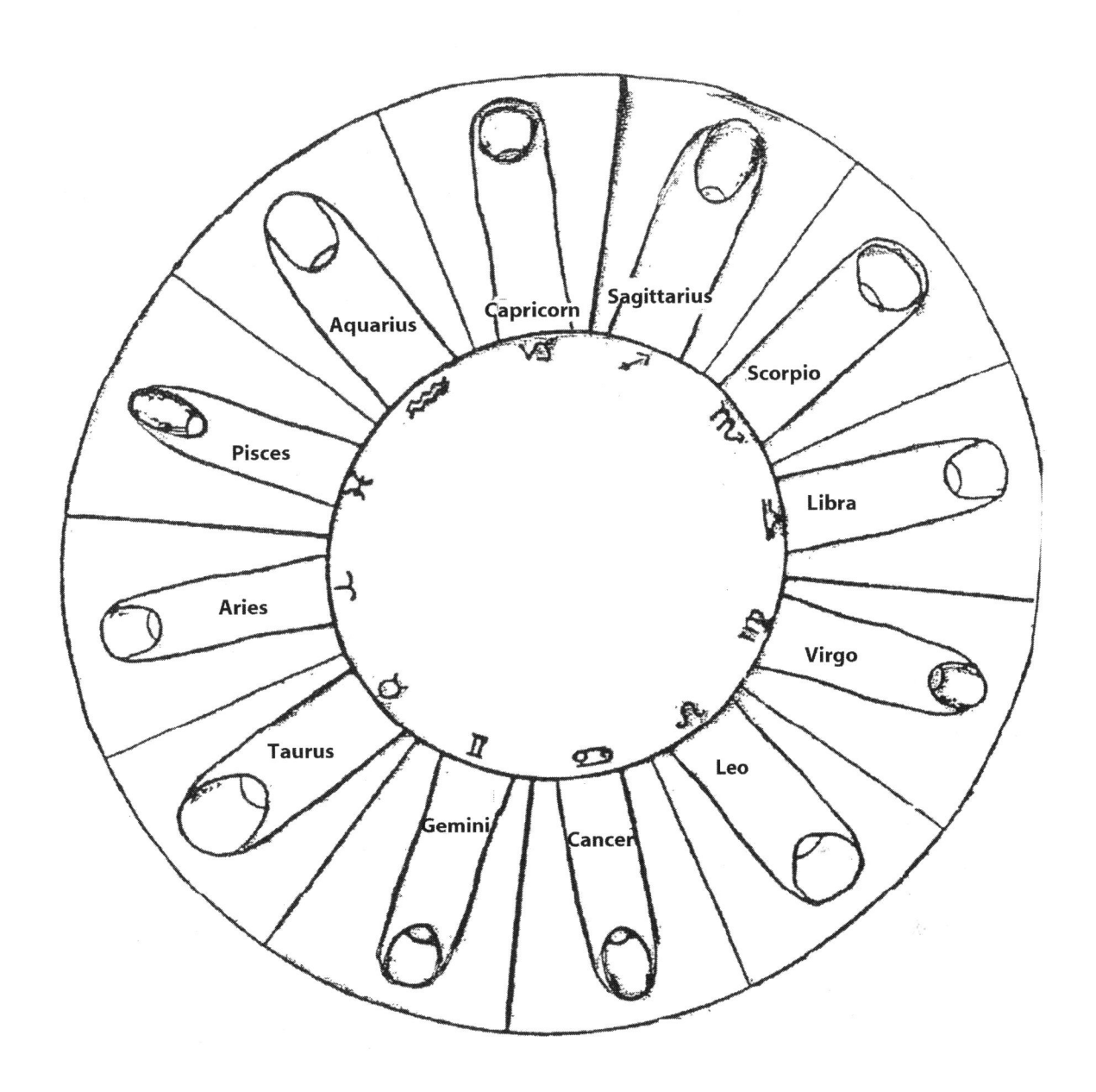

See Zodiac and Body Chart on next page

Zodiac and Body

Zodiac	Tends to have problems with
Aries	Eyes, cerebrum
Taurus	Neck, cerebrum, lower back
Leo	Heart, thymus
Libra	Kidney, adrenal
Cancer	Breast, veins, arteries
Virgo	Intestine, liver, pancreas
Sagittarius	Sciatic nerve, thigh
Scorpio	Genitals, gonads
Aquarius	Lower leg, colon, bladder
Pisces	Feet, circulation
Capricorn	Knee, teeth, bones
Gemini	Arms, fallopian tubes

Finger Shapes

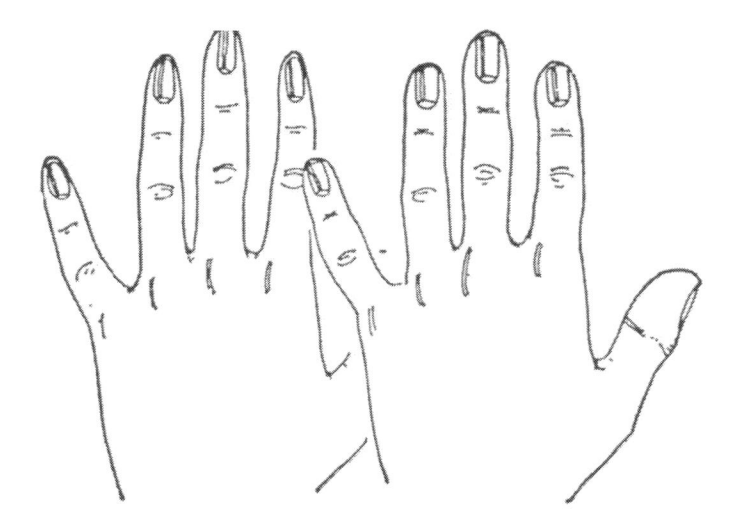

Square Fingers: They are practical and earthy. Healing modality must have a practical application. A natural for business. Excellent for the artistically talented.

Conic Fingers: Tend to be receptive to treatment. Rounded tips are associated with truly feminine women and artistically receptive men.

Pointed Fingers: Tends to like creative healing modalities. A spiritual approach to healing suits them. The practical approach to wellness is of little interest. Intuition is highly developed and they act on it. The term "scatter brained" is often applied to them.

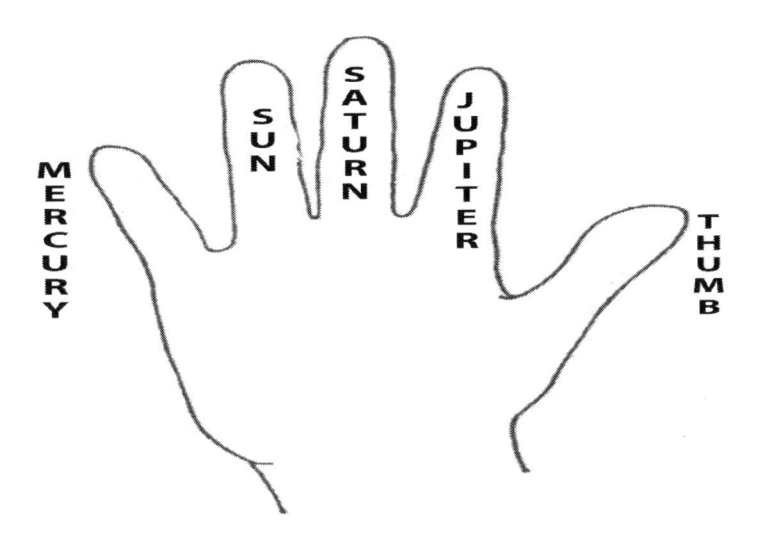

Planets and Fingers

If there is inconsistency in a finger's skin texture, dryness, oily, moisture, temperature, discoloration etc., the corresponding planet can indicate a health condition. SEE Face Types (Planets) and Health Problems

Finger Shapes

Spatulate Fingers: Tends to be active. They must always be doing a useful healing activity. Their wellness thoughts tend to be random, and go from one non-related idea to another non-related healing activity or idea. Their emotions guide their ability to be well.

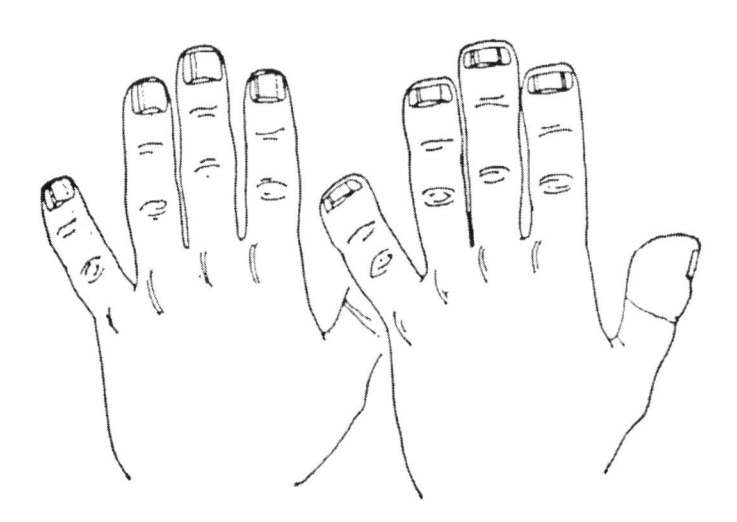

Mixed Typed: A combination of several different finger types. They are versatile. In order to obtain an accurate diagnosis examine each finger individually.

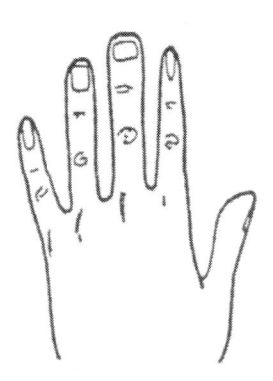

Fingers

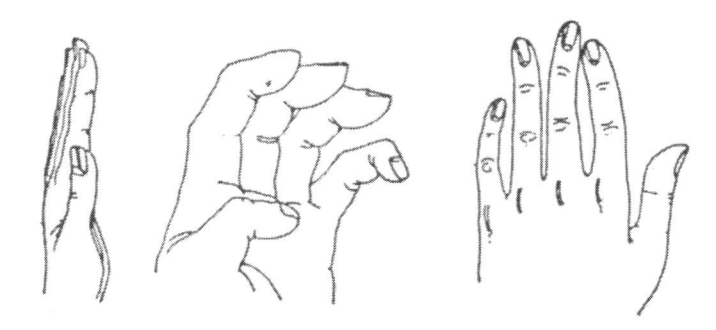

Straight Stiff Fingers: If a finger or fingers are stiff it can indicate a rigid (stiff) mind or the organ related to the corresponding finger is congested with waste. The related organ has lost it flexibility (alkalinity).

Long Fingers: Indicate a rational thinker and conservative person. They can be skeptical and suspicious about a new disease or healing ideas, changes and disease treatment protocol. Can have a tendency to hold onto their ideas. It can indicate the corresponding organ is overactive in response to a disease or toxins. Their diseases can be of long duration.

Inward Curve: Fingers that curve toward the palm indicates striving to achieve wellness objectives despite emotional or financial obstacles. It indicates that the corresponding organ is stressed and/or malfunctioning as a reaction to a disease or toxins.

Twisted Fingers: This indicates that the emotions and thoughts are dysfunctional. The organ related to this finger is exhausted in its attempts to achieve wellness and it is weak.

Finger Spaces

Narrow Spaces: Earthy stable and not easy to change from disease to wellness. They do not take risk on unfounded, exotic or untested healing programs. They hold on to old time folklore healing systems. If you are married to this type, better have another source of income that's yours alone or else you will live cheaply and do not expect them to spend money on various treatment professionals.

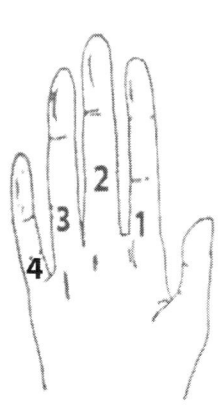

Wide Spaces: Sickness flows in and out of them easily. With very wide spaces between the fingers, will easily try alternative remedies. They are knowledgeable about holistic remedies and enjoy talking about them, but will not apply that awareness to themselves.

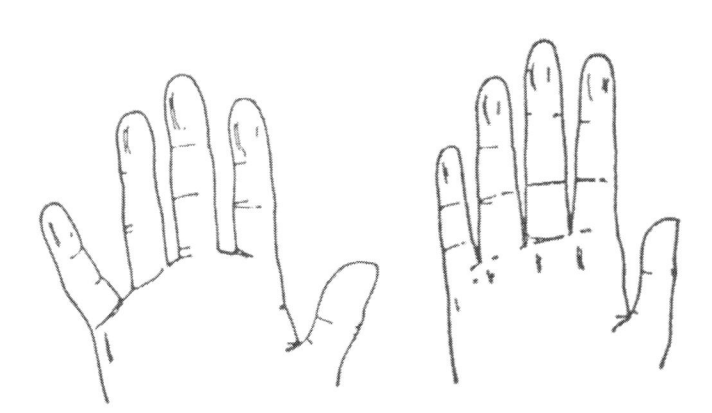

Color of the Center of the Palm

The center of the palm is slightly indented. Palm centers that do not have clear color, feel rigid and tight or have slight pain indicate physical, emotional, mental, spiritual, digestive and/or circulatory difficulties. A change of color in this area indicates disorders in the body as follows:

Palm Center Colors

Color	Systems
Red	Circulatory
Purple	Respiratory and Reproductive
Dark	Excretory
Yellow	Liver and Gallbladder functions

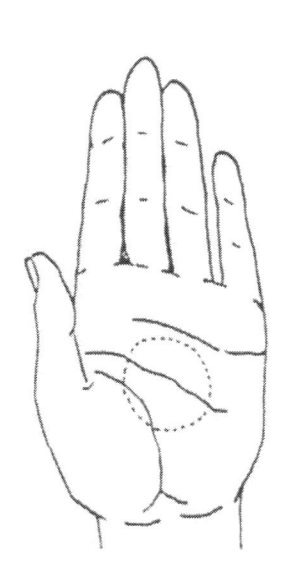

Points at the Base of the Palm

Base of the Palm Swollen: Press along the bony, fleshy region at the base of the palm, if swollen occurs at the wrist joint immediately under the palm, the following disorder can be indicated;

Point 1 –(base of the thumb) indicates lungs, respiratory functions, and large intestine problems.

Point 2 –(center of the hand) indicates circulatory, and reproductive difficulties.

Point 3 –(base of the little finger), indicates heart and circulatory system, small intestine, and digestive tract problems.

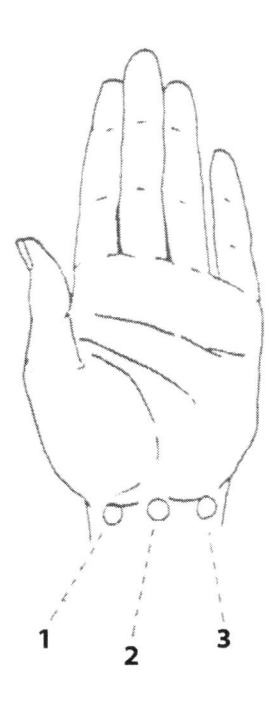

Finger Regions

Fingers be divided into three regions according to the areas indicated:

A. **Base Area:** Digestive and respiratory functions.
B. **Middle Area:** Nervous System functions.
C. **Tip region:** Circulatory and excretory functions.

Fingernails are constructed from the elimination of excessive elements in the form of minerals and protein. Incidentally the root of the hair inside the skin is alive while the visible nail is dead. This is built in the same manner. Nails and hair indicate waste by products that reflect the health during the period of growth.

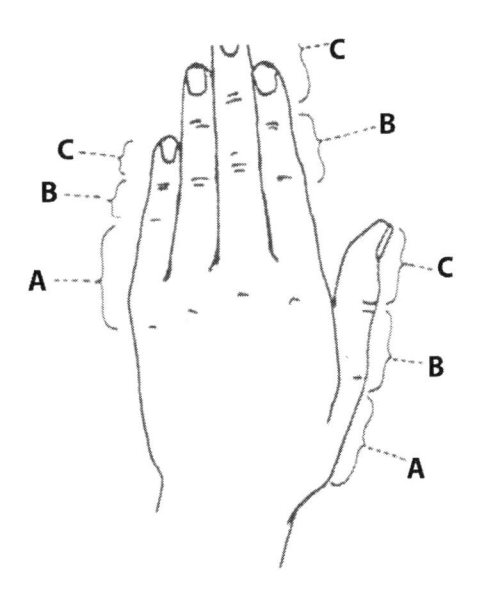

Space Between Fingers

Spaces between the fingers: When the fingers are held closed and viewed from the back of the hand, and no space is showing, it is an indication of good health. When spaces show between the fingers, it is caused by nutritional deficiencies, especially imbalance among carbohydrates, proteins, fats, and minerals. This can reflect imbalances in the body, spirit, emotions, physical, and thoughts. The space between closed fingers indicates the easy flow of emotions, thoughts, and the easy change from disease to wellness.

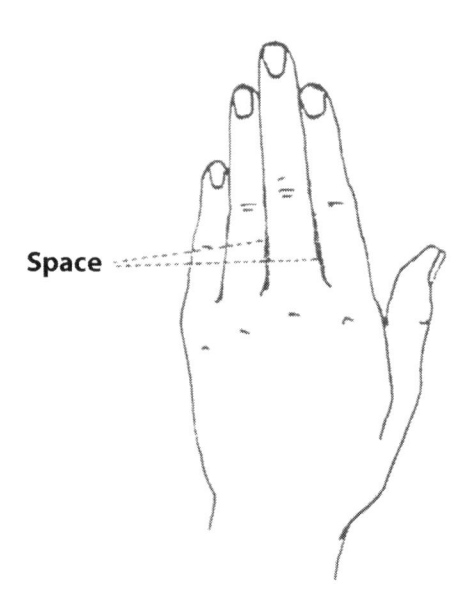

Space

Webbed Fingers

When the fingers are spread, webs appear between them at their roots. If the webs are large, it indicates acidity, chemicals, drugs and medications. When the webs are small, the diet of the mother during her pregnancy was balanced. Embryos that are nourished with junk food tend to have large webs that are sometimes surgically removed.

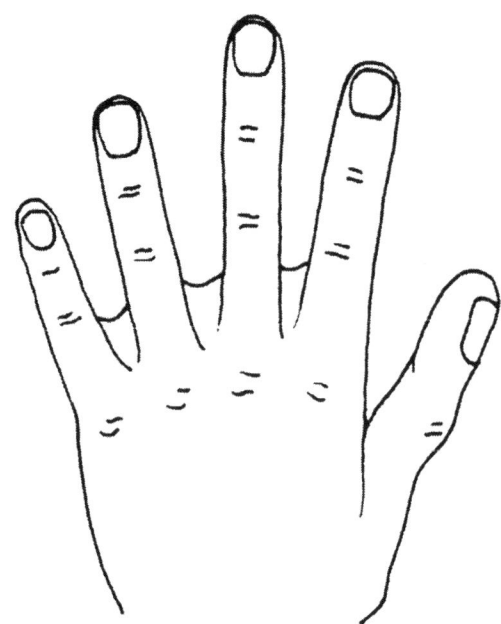

Long and Short Finger

Long Fingers: Indicates a personality that is skeptical about healing modalities, but once they have the facts, they master the treatment protocol in a slow and steady manner. They are cautious by nature, and want to have an outline of the healing process in order to start. They require step-by-step remedy instructions and favor a sequential process.

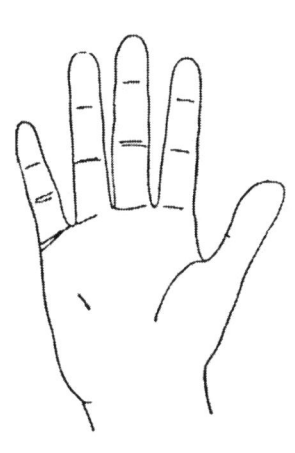

Short Fingers: Indicate a need for a treatment plan. They are emotionally impulsive and tend to shift from one healing method to another. They require little information to figure out the disease or healing process. They can be emotional eaters and moods can be a factor in choice of remedies as well as food.

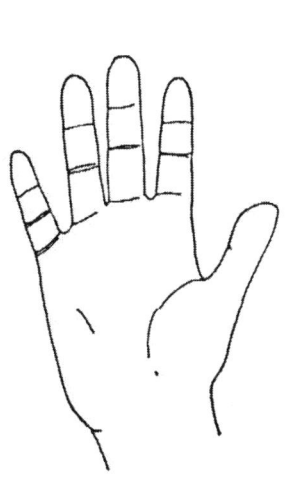

The Wrist

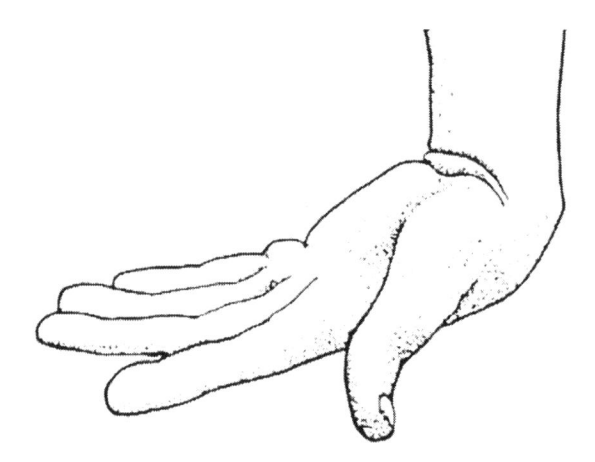

The wrist of a healthy person is flexible enough to bend backwards at a 135-degree angle without any pain or discomfort. If the angle is of less degree it can indicate hardening of the joints, muscles, and/or arteries, and the process of degeneration of tissue, organs, and bones.

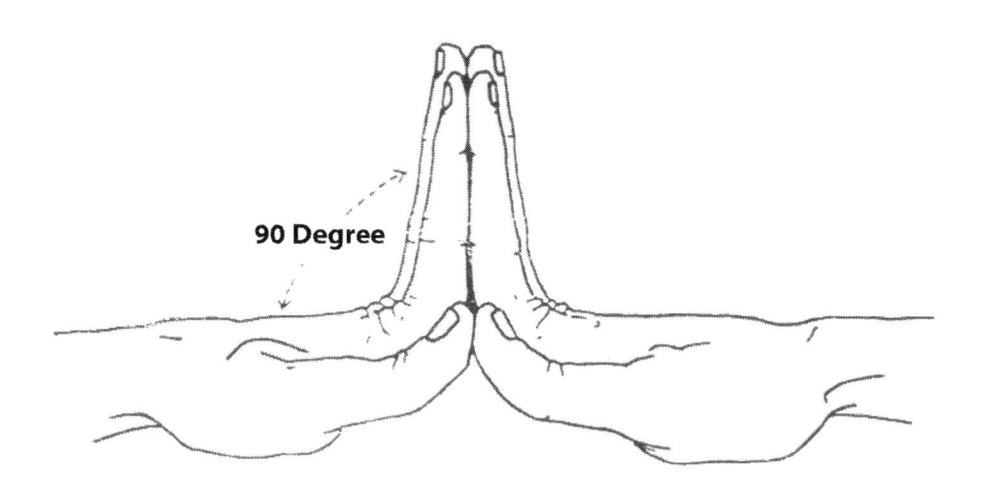

Hold the palm of the hands horizontal, put the fingers together, and then bend the fingers 90 degree. When this cannot be performed it indicates inflexibility, hardening of the arteries, nerve problems, and rheumatism. Make a fist and push with your finger between the knuckles. If your finger cannot make an indentation between the knuckles, there is hardening of the arteries, and kidney problems. Hold the fingers out straight and see whether they are straight or curved. Straight is normal. If they are curved check to see which acupuncture meridian is on the finger and/or organ is related to the finger. Curving away from the thumb is the Female Principle, and towards the thumb is the Male Principle.

Fingers And Planets

1st –Jupiter Finger Indicates: pride, ambition, administrative ability, threat, direct attack, reciprocity, spiritual, sequential, assertive, can rationally understand disease and treatments, emotions can cause disease.

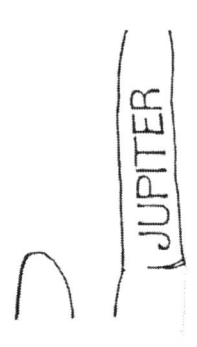

Stiff: Difficulty in changing disease-causing lifestyles. Lacks flexibility

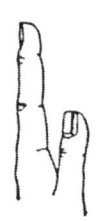

Knotted: Difficulty in changing disease-causing lifestyle. Lacks flexibility

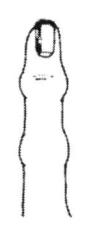

Thick second joint: May neglect health in pursuit of pleasures, asserts self to achievement of material success.

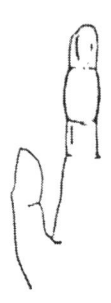

Thick Third Joint: Over eats, eats for emotional reasons.

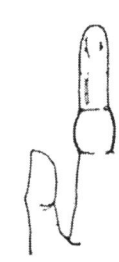

Thin: Can be very strict with diet and appetite control. Tends to be slightly built. Good self control.

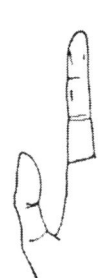

Thick: Loves comfort. Sensual appetite. May medicate emotional problems with snacks and junk foods. Enjoys leisure time eating.

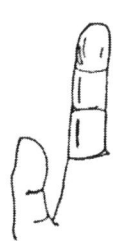

Short Third Joint: Indigence, lack of push. Needs encouragement and nurturing to achieve wellness. Can be apathetic, lacks aggressiveness

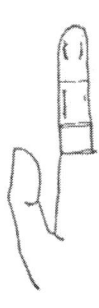

Thin Third Joint: Has self-control and can develop a healthy lifestyle. Tends to be balanced in approach to diet. No extravagance in eating or lifestyle.

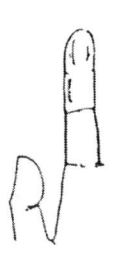

Long Third Joint: Does not find it easy to change but when changes tend to follows treatment regiment. Earthy, and has a desire for recognition.

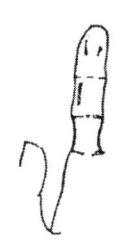

Flexible: Can adapt to illness and wellness, Emotionally flexible, good social skills.

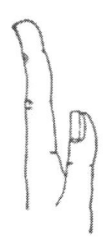

2nd - Finger Saturn

Saturn Finger Indicates: Enjoys learning about health. Tends to be a loner, questions health ideas and researches holistic treatments before action upon them.

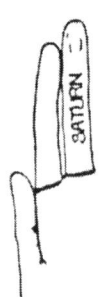

Long: Emotionally try's different health modalities, can have sad moods; distrust their healing ability. Seeks alternative medical ideas, enjoys philosophy and intellectual matters.

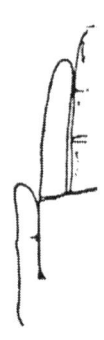

Conic: Tends to gradually become positive about achieving wellness.

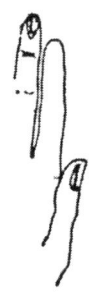

Thick and Short: Enjoys sharing and participating in health groups, co-ops etc. Tends to be an extrovert, socializer, does not frivolously plans activities.

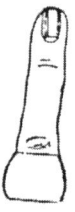

Thick and Long: Tend to have a strong desire to be knowledgeable about health. Can be avarice, and self-centeredness.

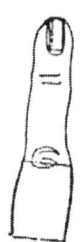

Thin Third Joint: Likes to know the reason why disease exist. Will try many different types of healing systems.

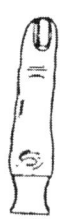

Long Third Joint: In attempts to be healthy their negative emotions can defeat wellness.

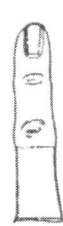

Thin Second Joint: Needs a scientific explanation of remedies to accept health protocols. Enjoys science and tends to be realistic.

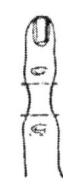

Pointed: Tends to disregard disease treatments and does not follow a healthy lifestyle. Tends to neglect responsibility for health. Good ability to process medical science.

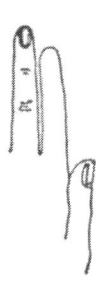

Short: Sporadic health habits. Has difficulty with sequential healing methods. Emotions cause instability and disease. Does not accept the seriousness of illness.

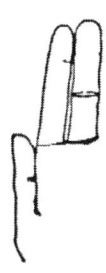

Short Third Joint: Tends to rationalize about health instead of using common sense. Gets too involved in rational thinking while overlooking reality of illness.

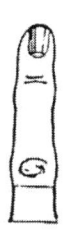

Long Second Joint: Understands health matters. Good ability with mathematics and scientific rationalizations for diseases and alternative medicine.

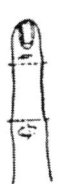

Short Second Joint: Tends to lack application of healing protocols and knowledge of holistic health. Overlooks practical solutions to health problems. Thoughts can cause unawareness of health.

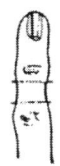

Thick Second Joint: Tends to like herb usage and will practically use them. Has a realistic and practical approach to getting well.

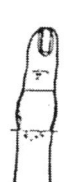

3rd Finger (Sun)

Sun Finger Indicates: Need for emotional attention, and nurturing self for wellness.

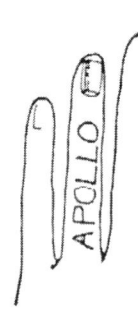

Short: Emotional avoidance of facing reality of disease and wellness protocol.

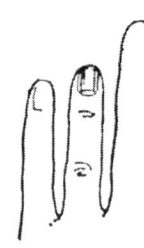

Thick First Joint: Sensual feeling approach. Has total emotional involvement in obtaining wellness. Has a need for touch and attention to emotions to get well.

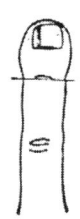

Knotted: Needs step-by-step sequential approach outline to achieve wellness. Emotionally desires to overcome disease.

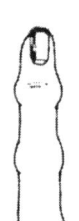

Stiff: Limited emotional vocabulary can cause illness.

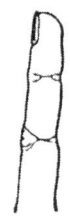

Smooth: Emotionally spontaneous instead of using a sequential approach to healing.

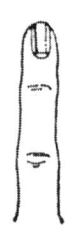

Long: Needs nurturing and emotional attention, to obtain wellness.

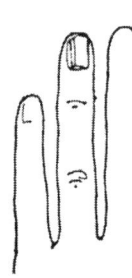

Long First Joint: Emotions tend to rule health choices. Relies upon how they feel about disease to solve illness.

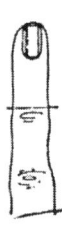

Thick: Needs emotional attention in order to get well.

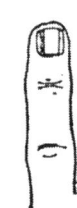

Conic: Usually needs emotional appreciation and nurturing to seek out healers and/or accept healing protocol.

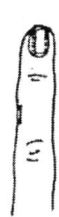

Thin: Takes an intellectual approach to emotions, which can cause emotional problems and disease.

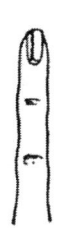

4th - Finger (Mercury)

Mercury Finger Indicates: Good social skills and communication ability. Uses logical approach to disease and wellness. Enjoys health literature. Organizes healing routine.

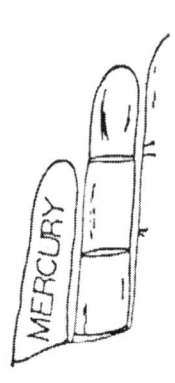

Pointed: Good skills at explaining steps toward disease. Knowledgeable about health concepts.

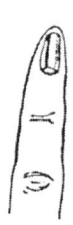

Conic: Understands the shrewd and eloquent way drug companies sell drugs. Being emotionally connected to others helps wellness.

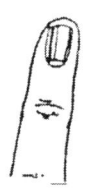

Thick Third Joint: Budgets finance so that money can be allocated for wellness.

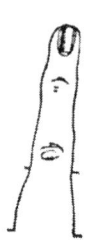

Thick Second Joint: Enjoys social interactions with others of like mind about alternative medicine.

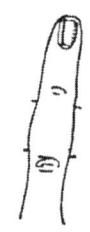

Long: Clearly understands and communicates signs and symptoms of disease. Easily understands health protocols.

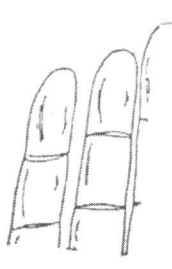

Square: Uses a sequential and logical approach to disease and wellness.

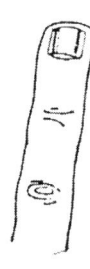

Long Third Joint: Tends to emotionally re-arrange health facts, which can cause misunderstanding of disease and wellness.

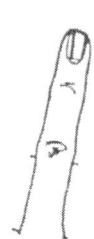

Short Second Joint: Tends to allow other financial matters to overshadow money needed for their wellness.

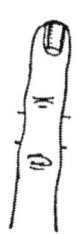

Short: Good comprehension of disease and easily arrive at healing solutions.

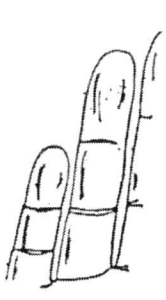

Spatulate: Good at sports, and exercise, which can contribute, to wellness or injuries.

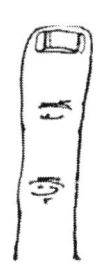

185

Fingers and Emotions

Thick First Joint on Second Finger: Intellectual understands need for health. Lacks emotional balance, and have lack of tact.

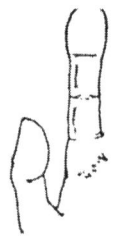

Thin First Finger: Interaction with others can be emotionally abusive which can cause them to be diseased.

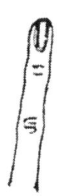

Long Second Joint on First Finger: Has a practical approach to health matters. Good ability to budget money for the cost of wellness.

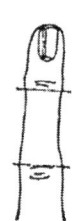

Long Third Joint on First Finger: Desires to be well and enjoys self-love to the point of overindulgence, which causes emotional illness.

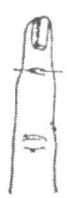

Flexible First Finger: Open to new alternative medicine ideas.

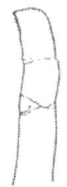

Thin First Joint Second Finger: Emotional imbalance can cause diseases such as depression.

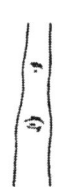

Square Second Finger: Fixed in ways, emotionally rigid and does not tolerate deviation and change in health protocol.

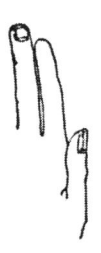

Stiff Second Finger: Tends to feel social activities will have a negative outcome causing emotional and/or physical disease.

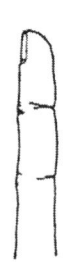

Knotted Second Finger: Enjoys emotional attention. Has a scientific aptitude and easily understands diseases and wellness.

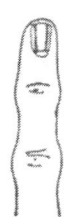

Long First Joint on Fingers: Has aptitude for sequential and rational ideas about disease and wellness.

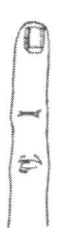

Thin First Joint on Fingers: Tends to focus more on spirituality, and philosophical rather then upon their physical health.

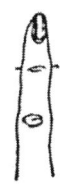

Thick Second Joint on Fingers: Tends to be realistic about disease and healing protocol use. Fails to face emotions directly.

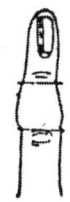

Thin Second Joint on Fingers: Mindful of emotional self and how it impacts their physical and mental well-being.

Long Second Joint on Fingers: Has an objective, non-emotional approach to emotions. Tends to rationalize and analyze, and not emotionally accept their contribution to disease.

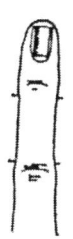

Spatulate Fingers: Behavior indicates emotional problems cause illness. Tends to feel insecure and pessimistic about becoming healthy.

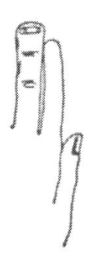

Flexible on Second Finger: Concern about other's feeling causes them to ignore their health.

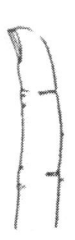

Stiff Fingers: Tends to be aware of the impact of behavior and thoughts on physical health.

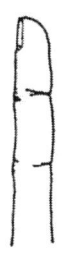

Spatulate Fingers: Constantly in search of for emotional ways to achieve wellness.

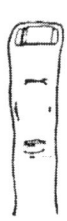

Thick Third Joint on Fingers: Tends to overlook physical health.

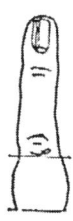

Square Fingers: Achievers wells when a detail of disease is understood.

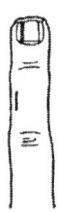

Pointed Fingers: Looks for emotional reasons, mythological reasons for disease.

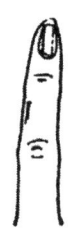

Thin Fingers: Has a lean build and a tendency to allow emotions and spirituality to cause illness.

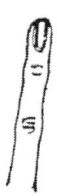

Short Fingers: Passive attitude can cause illness.

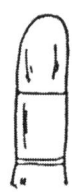

Long Fingers: Needs emotional nurturing and if does not get it becomes ill

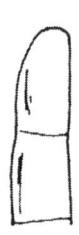

Spatulate Second Finger: Tends to search for the hidden meanings of disease.

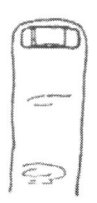

Long Second Joint on Fingers: Aggressive drive, accomplishes task, despite obstacles of having health problems.

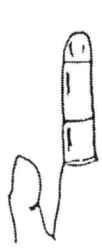

Thick Fingers: Tends to allow emotions to allow sadness and depression to cause disease.

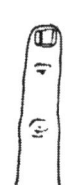

Thin First Joint on First Fingers: Can be emotionally rigid and overwhelm others with attitude that they are always right. This rigid behavior can cause illnesses.

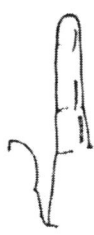

Long First Joint on Fingers: Allows feelings, spirit, and emotions to interpret disease problems.

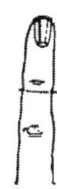

Short First Joint on Second Fingers: Seeks after success through materialism instead of seeking to overcome disease.

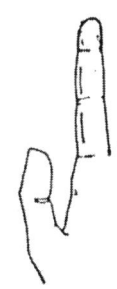

Smooth Fingers: Allows emotions to place too much importance on intuition and inspiration to solve disease problems instead of science.

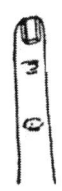

Flexible Fingers: Enjoys hidden meanings of disease. Has a high degree of tolerance does not dwell in negativity. This helps wellness

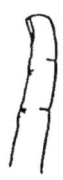

Short Second Joint on Fingers: Tends to favor paying attention to thoughts and dreams, does not devote energy to practical matters solution to health problems. Overlooks own behavior and be careless about health matters.

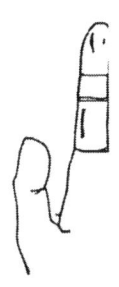

Knotted Fingers: Analytical, pays attention to health remedies. Question health ideas and our conclusion about wellness.

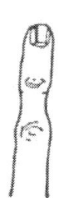

Square Fingers: Enjoys discovering the truth about and illness. Rigid beliefs and intolerant to other beliefs causes health problems can be knowledgeable about of alternative medicine.

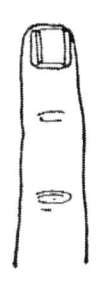

189

Palms of Hand

Hands

Inconsistency in the skin texture, dryness, oiliness, discoloration as well as tenderness to touch indicates an inconsistency with the organ and anatomical part related to the area.

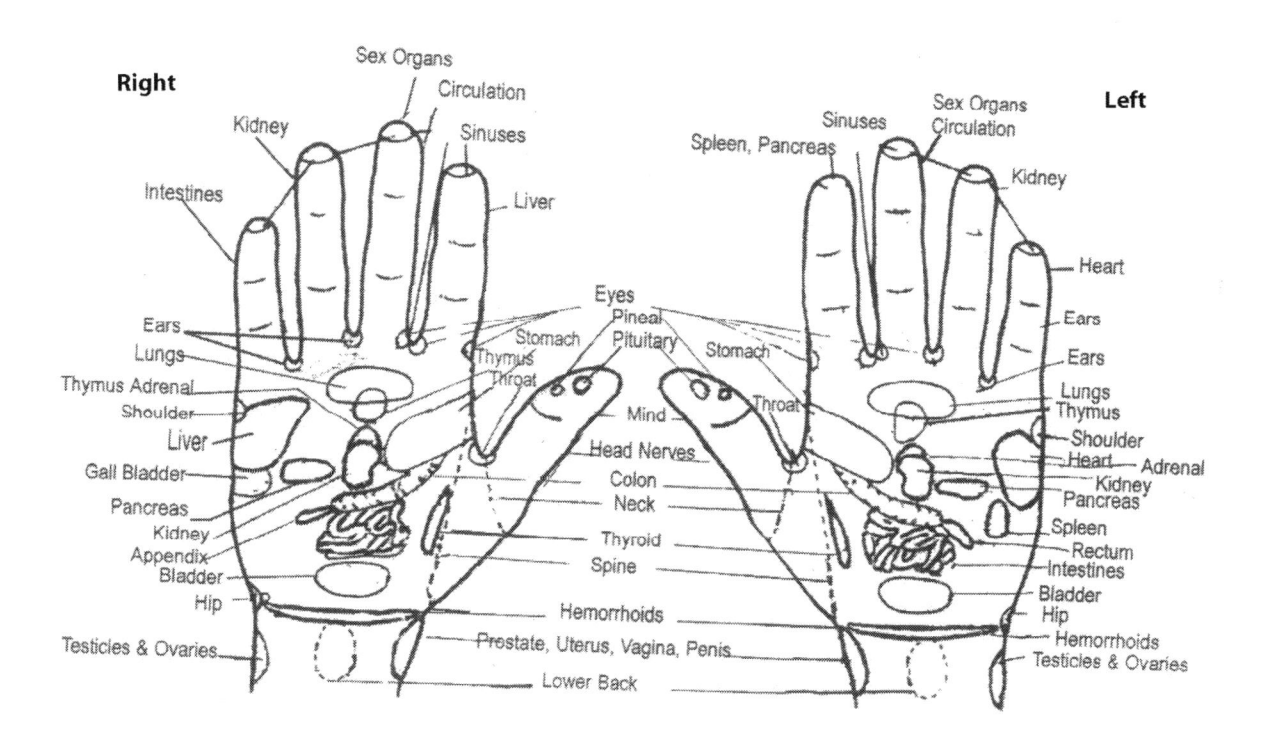

Lines in the Hand

Inconsistency in the lines of the hands such as brakes, excessive crossing wrinkles in it or over it, thinness, thickness, blotchy, paleness, redness around or on the line, splits in the line, or skin texture change on the line or around the line etc. reveal problems in the Upper, Middle, and Lower Function of the system.

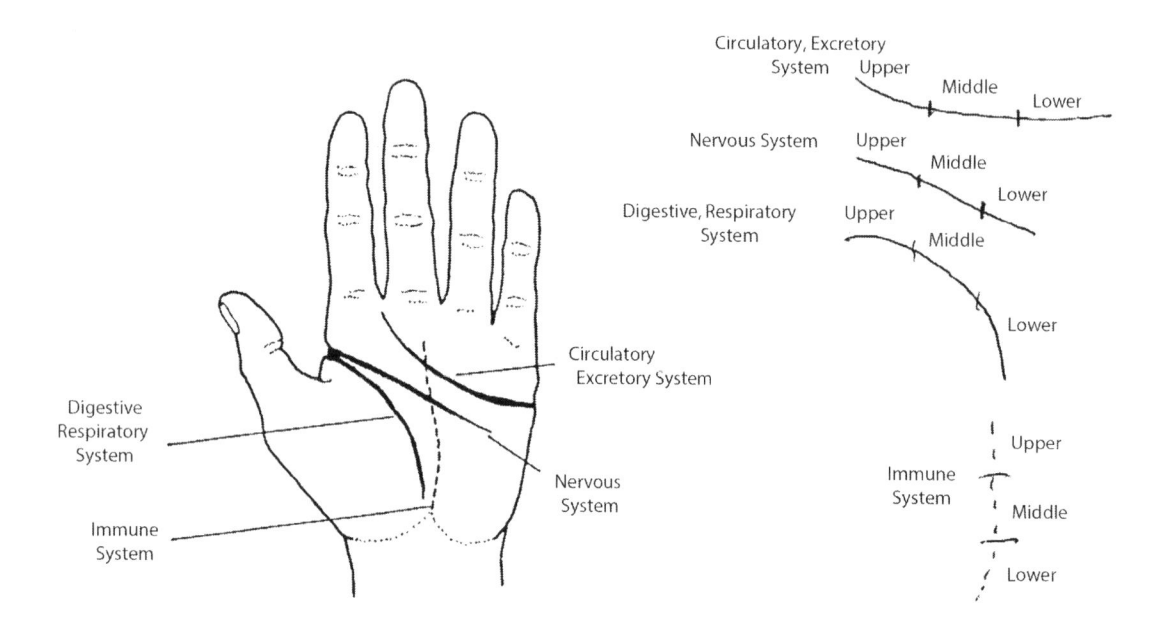

Hand (Palm) Moisture

Dryness	Disease Progression	Moistness
Slightly Dry =	**+ Sub acute**	= Slightly Moist
Dry =	**+ Acute**	= Very Moist
Very Dry =	**+ Chronic**	= Sweaty
Extremely Dry =	**+ Degenerative**	=Very Sweaty

Moisture Decreased

Problems with building and repairing of cells caused by alkalosis

Kidneys causing Alkalosis

Pancreatic Enzyme Weak

Pancreatic Insulin Problems

Sympathetic Cortex Problems

Moisture Increased

Problems with building and repairing of cells caused by acidosis

Kidneys and/or Potassium Acidosis related to excessive mineral salts and/or sodium chloride

Sympathetic Stress = increased perspiration over entire body

Parasympathetic Stress = unstable equilibrium = perspiration of hands and feet

Thyroid Stress

Inadequate Pancreatic Insulin and/or Glucagon

Inadequate Testosterone amounts

Hand Temperatures

An above or below normal temperature of the hand, veins, arteries flexibility (vasoconstriction vs. dilation), body temperature or metabolic rate problems can be indicated.

Temperature (Sympathetic)	Disease Progression	Temperature (Parasympathetic)
Cool =	**= Mild =**	= Slightly Warm
Cold =	**= Acute =**	= Warm
Very Cold =	**= Chronic =**	= Very Warm
Icy Cold =	**= Degenerative =**	= Extremely Warm

Temperature Low

Sympathetic Stress

Bodily Organs are acidic

Problems with regulating temperature

Inadequate Function

Inadequate Parathyroid Function

Testosterone Low Level

Temperature High

Parasympathetic Stress

Kidneys and/or Potassium Excess Acidosis due to excessive mineral salts, sodium chloride

Thyroid Stress

Parasympathetic causing Adrenal Cortex Stress

Pancreatic Insulin and/or Glucagon Problems

Adrenal Cortex overworked related to emotional, physical, spiritual stress

Hands

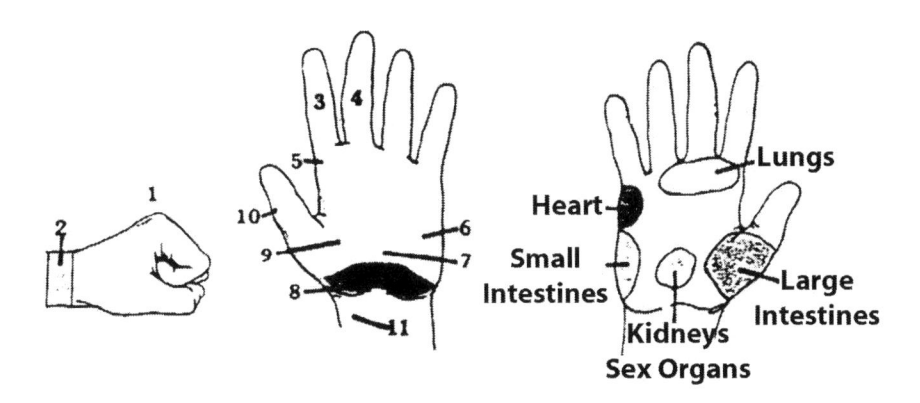

Hand Indications

Physical Condition	Symptoms
1. NO INDENTATION between KNUCKLES when FIST is made	High Blood Pressure, hardening of arteries, kidney problems
2. WRIST, ABNORMAL COLORATION	Sexual organ problems
3. FINGER CURVES towards THUMB	Energetic, healthy, over stimulated corresponding organ
4. FINGER CURVES away from THUMB	Weakness deteriorating in corresponding organ
5. BLUE LINE	Mucous, congestion in stomach
6. SPLOTCHY HAND	Blood stagnation, emotional addiction
7. PURPLE or BLUE PALM	Deoxygenated (carbon dioxide) blood
8. DARK RED HEEL of PALM	Uterus, bladder and prostate problems
9. YELLOW PALM	Pancreas, spleen, and liver problems
10. BLUE SIDE of THUMB	Digestive tract problems
11. MOVING toward WRIST, PRESS with THUMB in a STRAIGHT LINE to one inch below WRIST; IF BULGE FORMS	Excess liquids, edema, soft tissue damage
FLEXIBLE FINGERS	Organs healthy
WIDE TOP SECTION	Healthy corresponding organ
SWOLLEN FINGERS	High blood pressure, edema
LESS THAN 90 DEGREES BACKWARDS FLEXURE at WRIST on HARD SURFACE	Sexual organs degeneration
PAINFUL JOINTS	Kidney disorder

WIDE HAND and SHORT FINGERS	Aggressive, active
NARROW HAND & LONG FINGERS	Intellectual, artistic
WEBBING between fingers	Concentrated sweeteners, refine carbs, diabetic tendency
HOT HANDS	Overactive liver, acidity, sodium chloride, excess protein
COLD HANDS	Synthetic Chemicals, poor circulation
BULGING VESSELS on back of hand	Edema
WET HANDS	Liver problems
FINGERS TREMBLE	Nervous disorder, nerve damage

Fingers, Relationship to Systems, and Organs

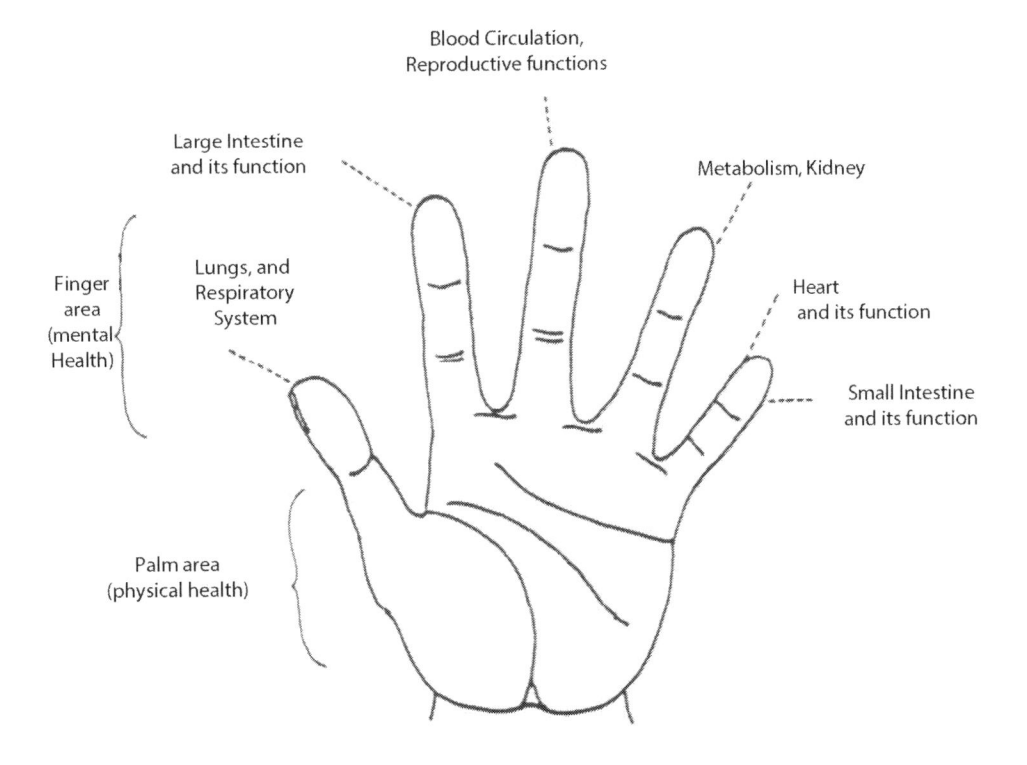

Blood Circulation, Reproductive functions

Large Intestine and its function

Metabolism, Kidney

Finger area (mental Health)

Lungs, and Respiratory System

Heart and its function

Small Intestine and its function

Palm area (physical health)

Thickness: A thick palm indicates a good immunity. A thin palm indicates imbalance nourishment, weak health, and tendency to have emotional conflicts.

Length: When the palm is longer than the fingers, the person is physically active. When the fingers are nearly the same length as the palm, or longer, the mental capacities are more active and there is a tendency to be physically weak.

Wet and Dry Palms: Wet palms indicate heart, circulatory, kidney, and excretory functions are overactive. Has a tendency for mental, and physical fatigue. Excessive sweat, unpleasant body odors indicates Liver problems; insomnia, mood swings, and unfocused thinking and memory problems. When the palms are cold there is contraction of tissues, blood vessels and capillaries, overconsumption of refined processed foods, drugs, and poor circulation. Can be physically, mentally rigidity, and inflexible. Good rationalizing ability, rigid, inflexible, narrow minded, prejudice, and an emotional conflict. In normal health the palm is slightly moist with cool temperatures.

Width of Palm: Physical strength, good health, and immunity. A narrow palm width indicates physical weakness and tendency to have weak immunity.

Mounts

The finger mount has a fleshy raise part at the base similar to the large raise part at the base of the thumb. This raise part is called a Mount. Any inconsistency in the skin of the mount, slight temperature change, dryness, oiliness, discoloration, tenderness, slightly small and/or large mount indicates health problems associated with that planet.

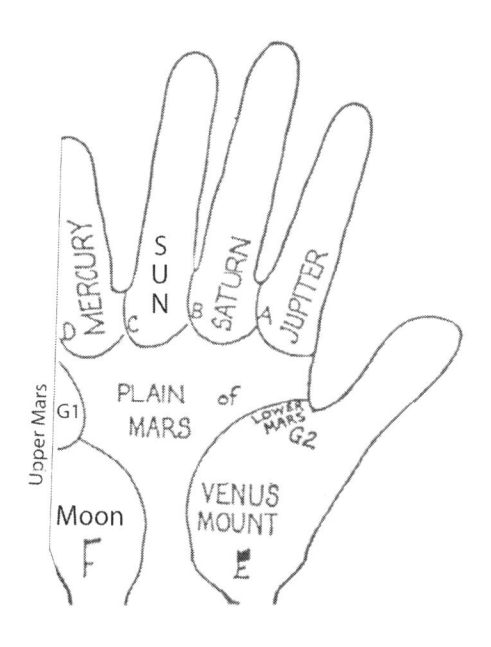

Mount	Symptoms	Type
A. Jupiter	Heart disease, artery and vein weakness	Ambitious, conceited, intellectual, open minded
B. Saturn	Mucous membrane, dehydration, edema, digestion problems	Cautious, rigidity, restrictive
C. Sun	Neuritis, respiratory problems	Artistic, expressive, self centered, generosity
D. Mercury	Thyroid, kidney, throat problems, infections	Shrewd, communicator, stress, tension
E. Venus	Arthritis, rheumatism, fractures, spinal, dental, and/or skin problems, gall stones	Sentimental, careless, harmonizer, emotional
F. Moon	Liver problems, hepatitis, pancreas disease, obesity, skin problems	Imaginative, moody, instinctive, emotional
G. Mars	Swellings, inflammation, fevers, infection, blood disease, accidents	Fighter, aggressive, conflicts, conqueror, sexual interest

Palm Line and Age

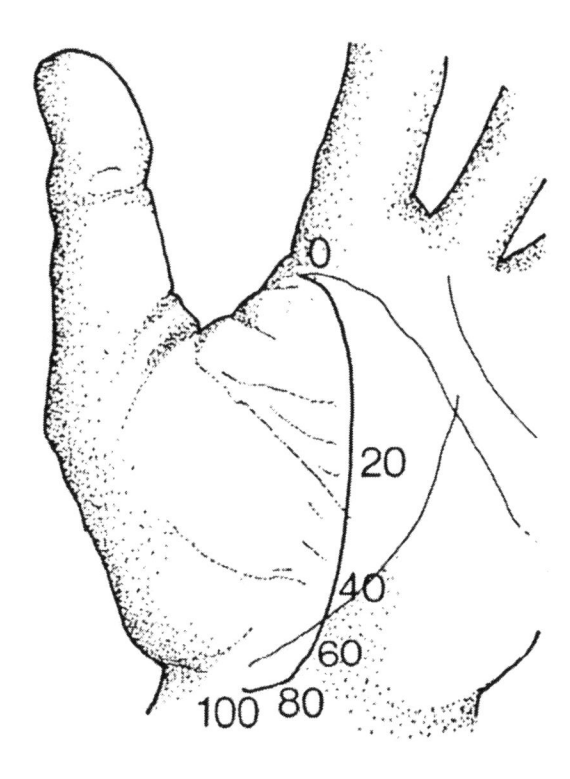

The positions of the Palm Line corresponding to the age of the person.

The palm line in the middle, it indicates the age of about twenty. The part to the junction or fork (if there is one) indicates forty-three to forty-five. This line should be clear and long, going all the way around the bottom of the hand. If it is doubled, the mind is split: around the corresponding age there will be social and mental difficulty. If the line is jagged and unclear, the digestive and respiratory systems are weak, and sickness may occur. A break in the line indicates that there will be sickness or death.

Hand Acupuncture Meridian Points

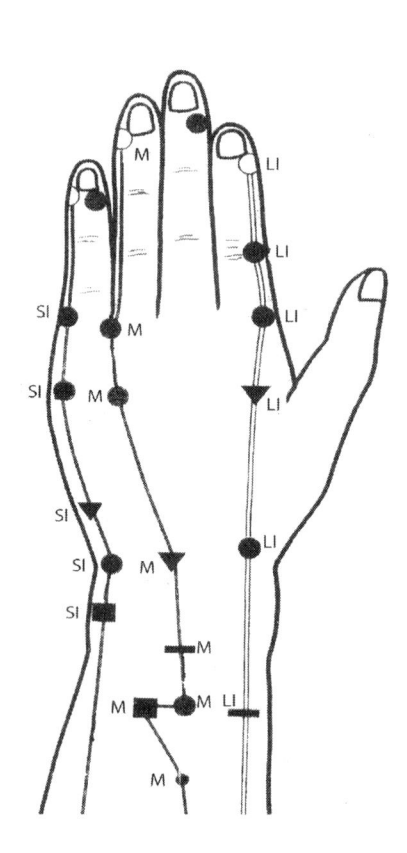

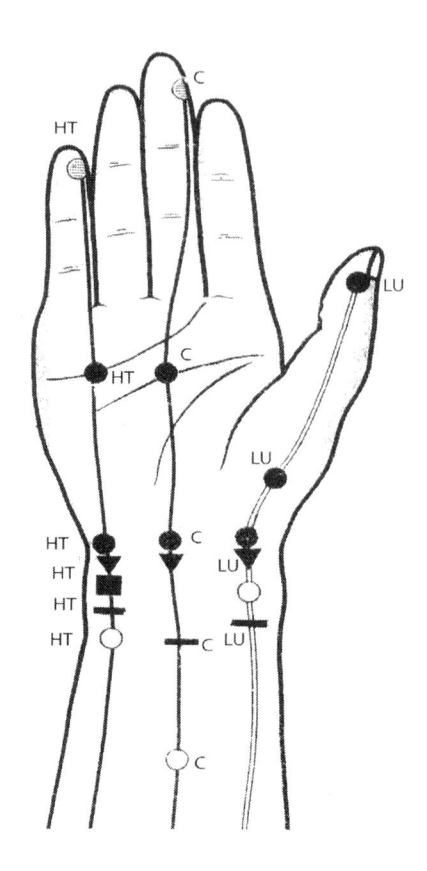

Shapes of Points Meridians	Function of Meridian
Points on Hand (solid circle)	Circulatory, Nervous, Digestive, Immune, and Excretory Systems
Source Point (triangle)	Actual origin
Accumulating Points (solid square)	Gathering of quantities of toxins can be blockages
Connecting Points (solid rectangle)	Joins and links systems together
Alarm Point (oval circle)	Warning of problems
Associate Point (solid half crescent)	Related in bodily functions

Pulse (Palpitation) Diagnosis

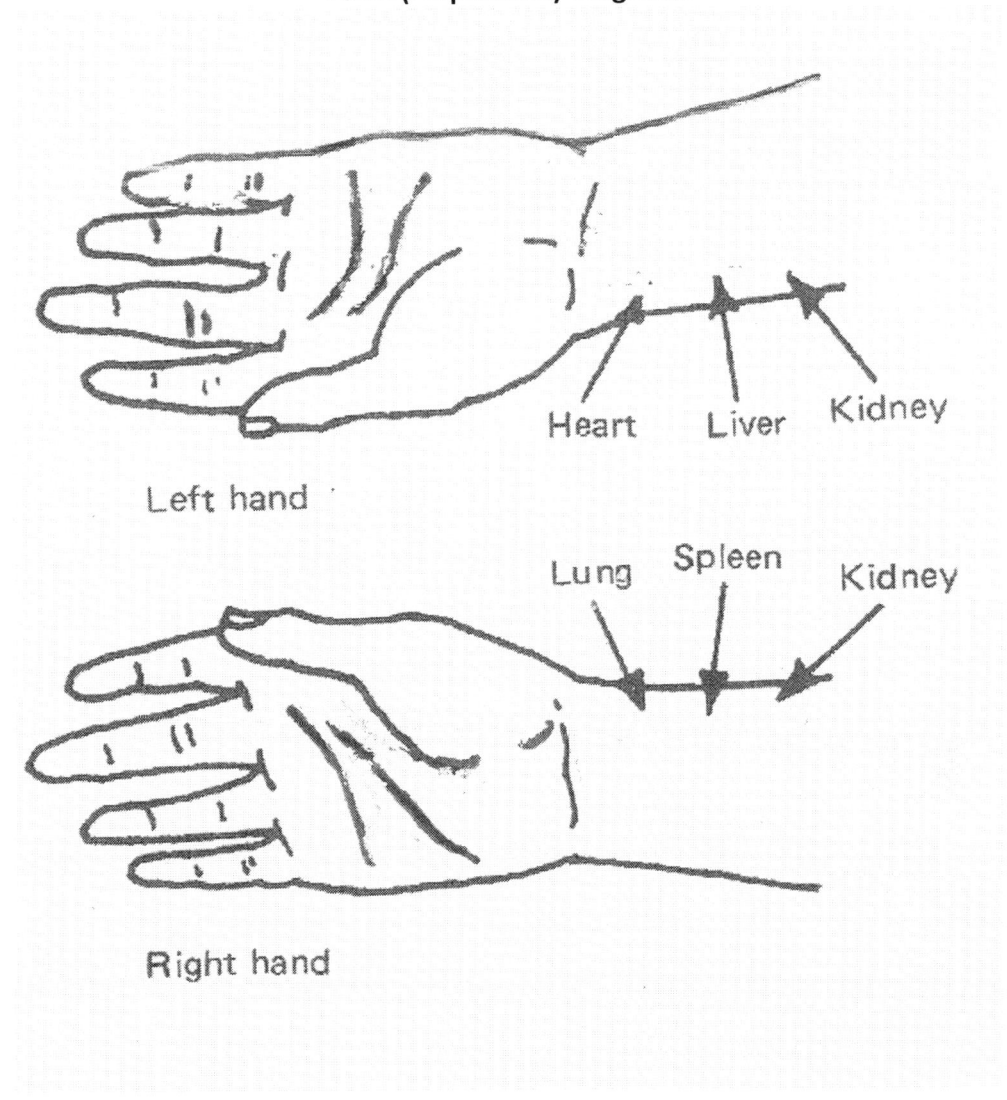

Left hand — Heart, Liver, Kidney

Right hand — Lung, Spleen, Kidney

Normal Pulse

The blood flow usually is soft and smooth in the oxygen-carrying artery. The groves inside the inner artery walls cause the blood to spin. The grooves can widen or narrow causing a slight slowing down or speeding of the spin of blood. The muscular structure of the artery and grooves create a wave-like movement of the blood. The wave should not be rough, choppy, flat, or bulge too high. The quality of the blood flow should not change easily or irregularly. The superficial, middle, and deep palpation should feel the blood clearly.

The pulsating blood flow and rhythm can be affected by:
- The ability of the kidney's Renin and liver's Heparin to thin the blood
- Arteriosclerosis and or Atherosclerosis
- Acidity and alkalinity
- Oxygen amount in the blood (capillary exchange)
- Clogged or blockage
- Electrolyte congestion
- Blood pressure
- Excretory system ability to rid blood of waste
- Emotions, diet, drugs, exercise
- Muscle weakness of arteries
- Sympathetic or Parasympathetic stress
- Nitrate problems

Pulse Divisions

The Three Pulse Points are:
- Distal which is at the wrist crease (farthest distance from elbow)
- Middle slightly medial to the radial styloid process
- Proximal (nearest to the elbow)

Three Levels of Touch (Palpating)
- Gentle Light (Superficial) Touch: Upper Organs
- Semi-Deep (Middle) Touch: Stomach, Spleen
- Deep Touch: Liver, Kidneys

Radial Pulse Location
The three positions at the wrist, along the radial artery, each Pulse Point is palpated at the superficial, middle, and deep levels.
The pulse indicates:
- Distal: Upper organs
- Middle: Middle organs
- Proximal: Lower Organs

Feel pulses (palpitation) with the pads of the fingers. Do not use fingertips. Hand must be relaxed- neither tense of limp. The hand and fingers should be in the pulse-taking position.

Exercise: Make the hand muscles flex (contracted) and tense as much as possible. Then relax and let the hand droop. Gradually without too much effort allow your hand to lift the fingers. This is the ideal condition of the hand for pulse taking, relaxed, and flexible. Place the third (middle) finger pad on the radial artery slightly medial to the styloid process. The index finger placed in the distal position at the wrist crease and the ring finger in proximal position. Usually with a small individual, the fingers will have to be squeezed close together. In a large individual the fingers may need to be spread open. Use equal pressure with three fingers to feel the radial artery pulse. Release the pressure on the middle finger slightly to compensate for the styloid process. The pressure of the radial artery on the styloid can cause an artificial pulse reading when the same amount of pressure is exerted. This can make the pulse seem to be excessive in the middle position. When you feel the radial artery and have adjusted the pressure, release the pressure equally until you can feel the pulse. This is the superficial position. Then press as deeply as possible until you stop the pulse. Release the pressure until the pulse slightly returns. This is deep position.
- Timing: The ideal time is early morning
- Position: The arm should be horizontal and not higher than level of heart
- Finger Placement: Keep the three fingers on the pulse points and lift fingers slightly to feel different levels.
- Breathing: Your breathing should be normal in order to be more receptive.

The person's pulse being diagnosed is correlated with the pulse reader's Breathing Cycle in order to determine whether the pulse is slow or rapid.
- Normal pulse: 4-5 beats per breath of the pulse reader.
- Three beats or less: Slow Pulse
- More than five beats: Rapid Pulse

The pulse can be counted using a watch according to following table:

Pulse Table

Age	Rate
1-4	90 or above
4-10	84
10-16	78/80
16-35	76
35-50	72/70
50+	68

Factors that influence a Pulse Reading

- Weather: Pulse is deeper in the winter, more superficial in summer (thinner blood).
- Gender: Men's pulses are slightly stronger, and the left pulse is slightly stronger. In women the right pulse is slightly stronger.
- Occupation: Sedentary workers have a mild pulse. Those doing heavy physical work should have a stronger pulse.
- Ideally the person must wait 1 hour after eating because the stomach pulse will read very high, and other organ reading will be decreased.
- Medications, stimulants, caffeine, nicotine, as well as drugs can affect the pulse.
- Read the pulse 15 minutes after urination, drinking liquids, or having a bowel movement
- Pulse diagnosing should take place in a calm quiet place.

Pulse and Disease

Disease	Pulse Description
Abdomen/ Stomach/ Intestine Problems	Curly type movement, weak, rapid
Abscess	Rapid, slippery, crooked
Acidic	Slippery, slow, large, shaky
Addison	Fast, weak
Anemia	Weak, faint, rapid
Angina Pectoris	High tension
Anxiety	Low tension, slow, weak
Asthma	Hollow, full with all fingers, Superficial, slippery
Boils/ Skin Eruption	Slow, crooked, thick
Chickenpox	Unstable, crooked, rapid
Cholera	Jumpy, faint, irregular, weak
Colds	Weak, trembles, restless, fluctuates
Constipation	Forceful, crooked, strong
Diabetes	Thread, thin, knotty, fluctuates between quick and slow beats
Diarrhea	Jumpy, weak, Superficial: quick, Deep: weak, slippery, small
Edema	Thin, weak, can be large, crooked with slowness, can suddenly stop and start
Exhaustion	Extreme scatter
Eye Problems	Hard, crooked, slippery, moves slowly
Epilepsy	Slowly moves up and down, weak, Superficial: slow delayed, Deep: quick, small
Gouty Arthritis	Moves slowly, thick, intermittent
Headaches	Seems unstable, weak, jumpy
Hemorrhoids	Moves slowly, short
Indigestion	Beats slowly, hard, crooked
Liver Problems	Thread, faint, Superficial: small, thread, large
Nephritis	Full and quick, rapid
Obesity	Steady, mild, plump
Rheumatism	Weak, rapid, thin
Sciatica	Crooked, slow, thick
Sinus Problems	Very slippery, crooked, downward motion
STD	Thin, slow, slippery, knotty
Stroke	High tension, slow
Thyroid Problems	Hyperthyroid: rapid, hypothyroid: slow
Ulcer	Restless, shaky type motion
Worms	Almost undetectable

Pulse and Organ Problems

Organ Problem	Palpitation Pulse Indicators
Heart	Vigorous beats, long duration
Lungs	Strong and long beats
Stomach	Long, strong
Liver	Sinking, long, strong, tension moves with fullness
Spleen	Upper Organs: Long strong
	Lower Organs: Soft, scattered

Disease Pulse Readings

A few descriptions of Pulse Readings are:
- Slowed down or Relaxed- A normal pulse is relaxed. An abnormal pulse is loose, slack, and tends to get slow (about 60BPM). The beats come and go slowly, feels thick, and the rate is like normal but becomes slow at the end of a beat.
- Choppy, Hesitant- Relaxed, slow, difficult, fine, and can stop and loose a beat but then recover. It is not smoothly flowing.
- Excess, Full, Forceful, large, hard pulse, and feels full at all 3 levels.
- Slippery, Rolling- Smoothly flowing beats come and goes fluently and smoothly will also feels slippery and slick.
- Surging, Flooding- Wide and similar to a wave, floating pulse starts strong and ends weak "Coming onto the shore with force and retreating without force"
- Leathery, Feels like a Drum skin, Hard- Large (wide) with an empty center; feels like a string that is hollow and felt with light pressure. Floating, large, and hard and resistant to pressure.
- Hollow- Pressure causes it to get weaker and will disappear. Reappears when pressure is floating, soft, large body, but empty in the center. Forceless—large and weak. Digestion problems, inadequate blood-flow.
- Soft or Soggy- Floating, fine, soft and flexible. Felt with light pressure and not with heavy pressure. "Floating, thread and soft" similar to a string in water. Blood flow obstructed or blocked, spleen problems.
- Scattered- floating, large (feels wide) and without root: with light pressure becomes irregular, scattered and chaotic: with heavy pressure cannot feel pulse.
- Forceless, Empty, Deficient- A term used for various types of forceless pulses. Pulse can feel like it is floating, large, slow, empty, deficient, soft, forceless pulse image.
- Deep- Located near the bone and felt with heavy pressure, and can be felt with lighter pressure.
- Firm, Confined- Hard, not changeable, large, and long. Felt with heavy pressure.
- Weak- Soft like a thread and fine.
- Slow- Below 60 BPM or less than 4 beats per breathe of the pulse read.
- Tight, Tensehas strength, feels like stretched and twisted rope.
- Faint, Minute, Indistinct- Very fine, soft, weak, barely palpable. It can be felt and then sometimes it is lost. Very thread and soft.
- Thready, Thin- Feels like soft thread, weak, without strength but not moved by pressure.
- Regularly Intermittent- Relaxed and weak, pauses at regular intermittent intervals. Intervals can be strikingly to long.
- Rapid- Above 90 BPM, or more than 5 beats per breath.
- Rapid-Irregular, Skipping, Abrupt irregularly interrupted.
- Moving, Throbbing, Stirring- Forceful, slippery, rapid, strong, and throbbing abruptly.

Feet

Feet

Inconsistency in the skin of the foot such as slight warm or cold areas, deep vertical or horizontal wrinkles, thickness, or thinness of skin, sensitivity, soreness, changes in texture, dryness, paleness, redness, dark or light spots, bumps etc. in areas indicates organ problems. Foul odor of the foot can indicate liver problems. Fungus infection (Athlete's foot) can indicate consumption of processed concentrated sweeteners, fungus (mushroom) and fermented foods (i.e. vinegar) as well as weak immunity (Antibiotics Kill Fungus).

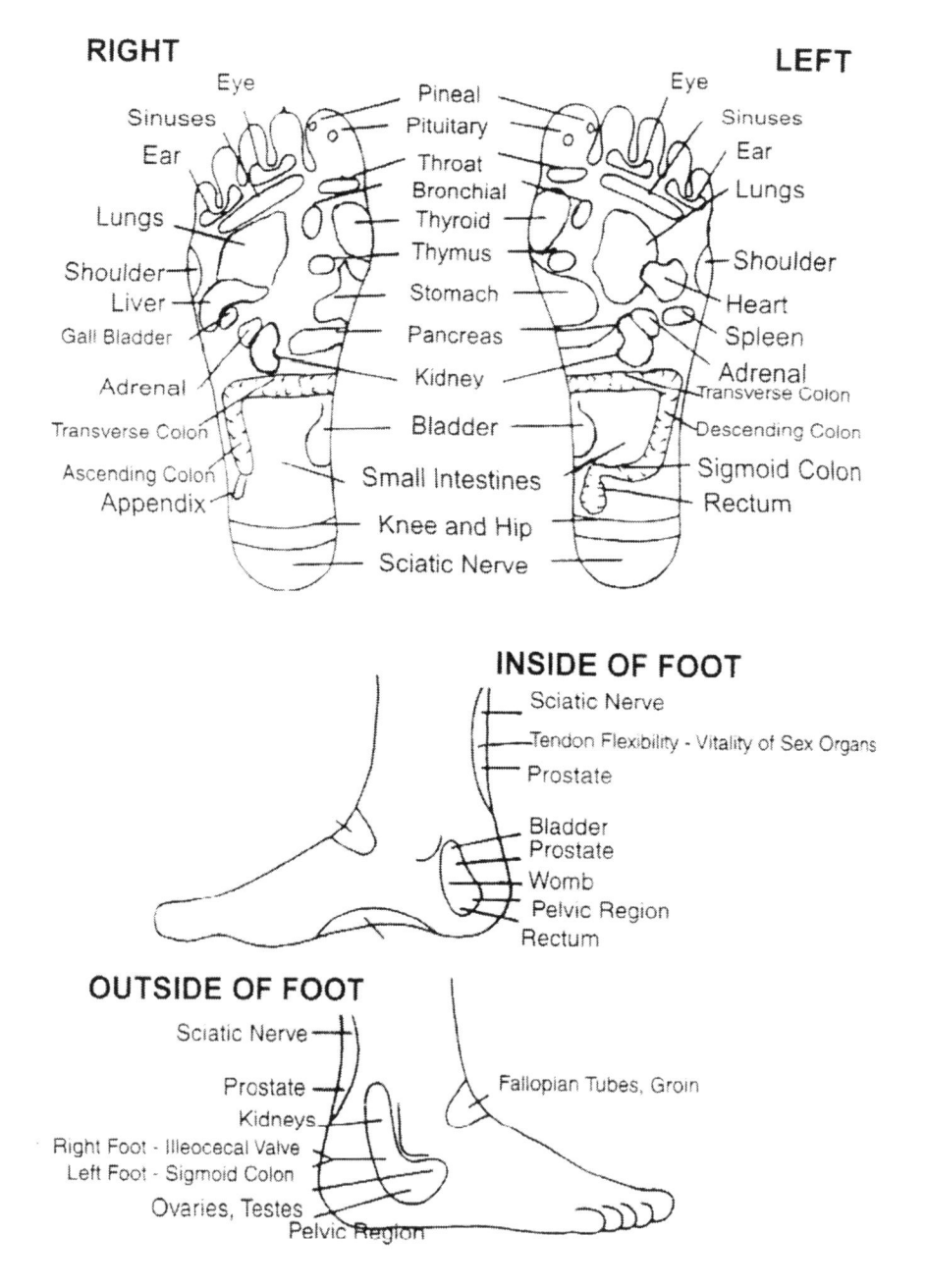

Feet, Toes, and Ankle Correlation

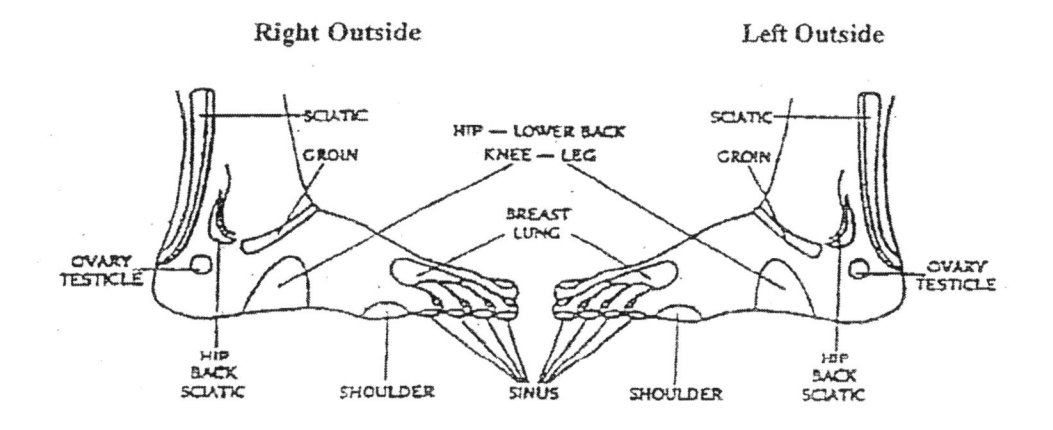

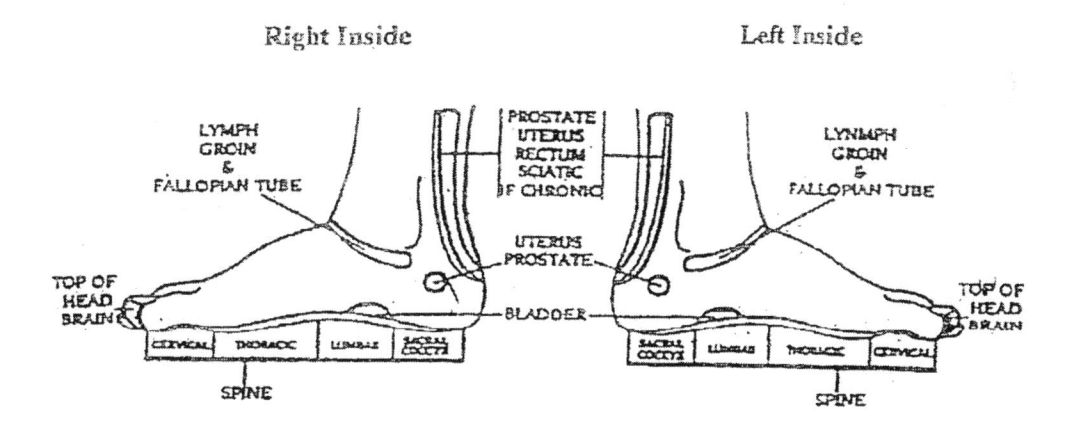

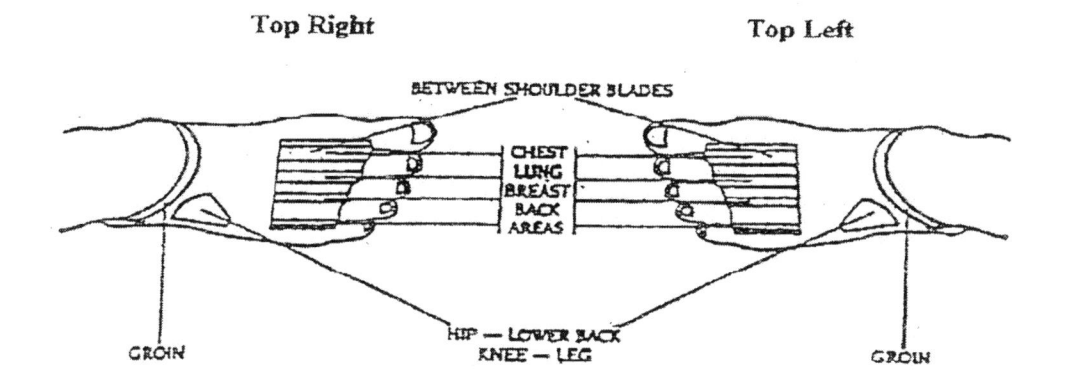

Feet, Glands, Lower Blood Pressure

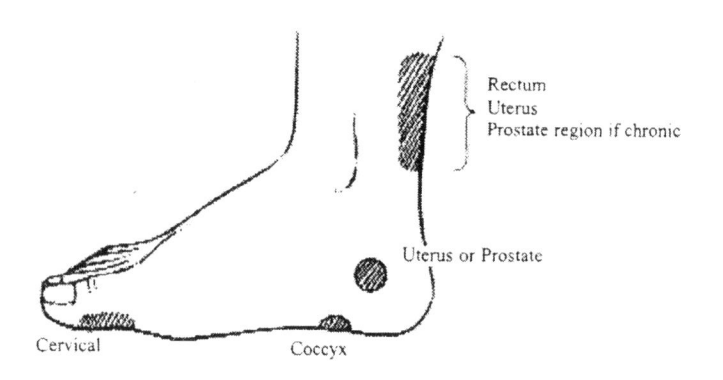

Rectum
Uterus
Prostate region if chronic

Uterus or Prostate

Cervical Coccyx

Right Food, lateral view.

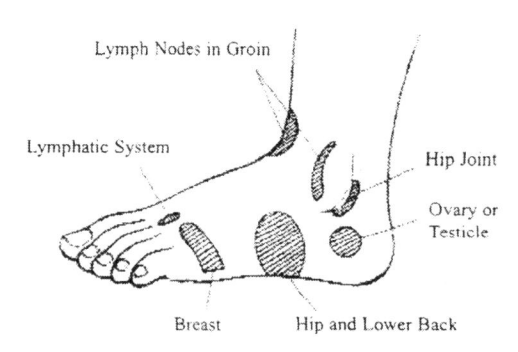

Lymph Nodes in Groin
Lymphatic System
Hip Joint
Ovary or Testicle
Breast
Hip and Lower Back

Left Foot.

LOWER BLOOD PRESSURE

To lower high blood pressure, acupressure to center of the sole of the foot.

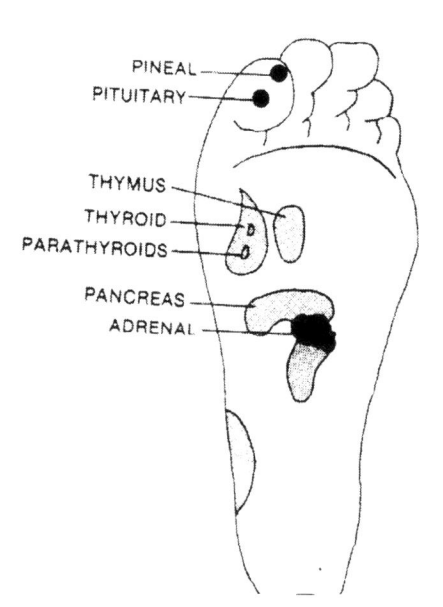

Glands

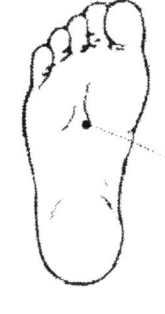

PINEAL
PITUITARY
THYMUS
THYROID
PARATHYROIDS
PANCREAS
ADRENAL

Feet Indications

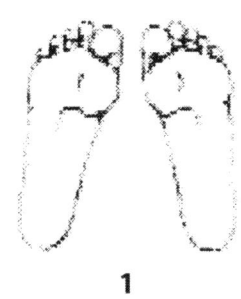

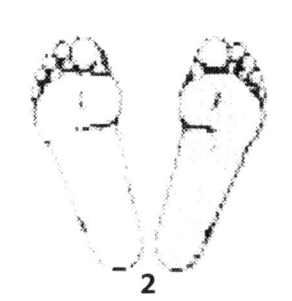

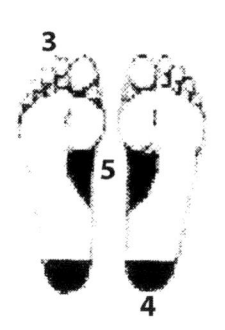

Feet	Symptom
1. Pigeon Toed	Compensating
2. Outward Angle	Expansion, weakness
3. Straight	Balance
4. Heel Pains	Heart problems
5. Fallen Arches	Nervous system problems
Athletes Foot	Kidney disorder, cellular waste
Bad Smell	Liver problem, waste congestion
Cracked Feet	Spleen, pancreas and digestion problems
Cracked Nails	Liver problems, worms
Shrunken Toe	Undeveloped organ
Pain in Toe	Corresponding organ problems

Foot Pressure Points

A change in the skin color, bumps, peeling, dryness, slight coldness or warmth and/or texture change indicates disease or a malfunction of the corresponding organ and/or part of the body.

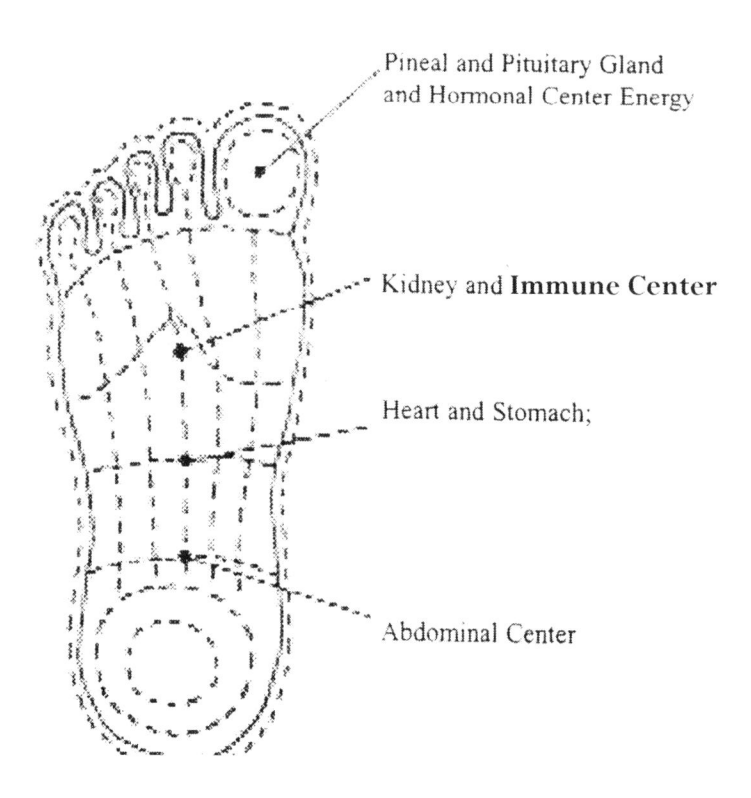

- Pineal and Pituitary Gland and Hormonal Center Energy
- Kidney and **Immune Center**
- Heart and Stomach;
- Abdominal Center

Two Diagnosis Points on the Foot

Two points formed by the junctions of bones extending up from the toes can be used for a diagnosis of the internal organs: (1) the indented point in the small valley formed by the junction of the bones extending up from the first and second toes: and (2) from the fourth and fifth toes. If pain is felt when point (1) is pressed, it indicates problems in the stomach and liver, and physical and mental fatigue. If pain is felt when point (2) is pressed, it indicates a tendency toward mineral deficiencies and inadequate metabolism causing fatigue and sleepiness. It can indicate the formation of cyst and stones in the gallbladder.

Foot Diagnosis Points (1, 2)

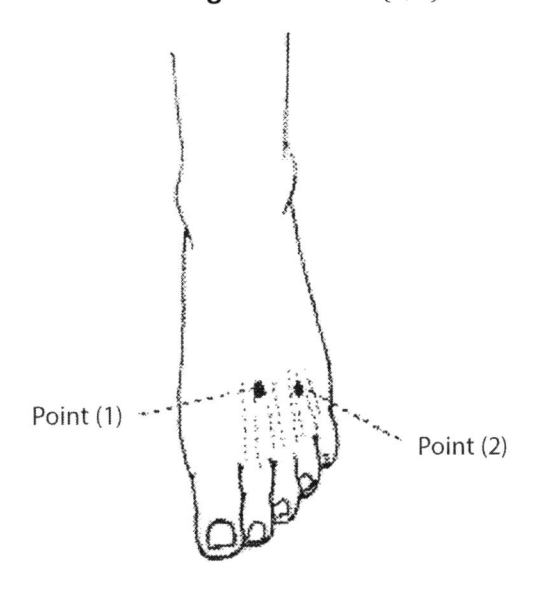

Point (1)   Point (2)

Length of Toes

From the first toe to the fifth toe, the length of the toes gradually decreases. The second and/or third toes are longer than the first two toes. It indicates stomach disorders such as gastritis, ulcers, cancer, and digestive tract stress. A second and third toe longer than the first toe indicates weakness of the stomach.

Curving Toes

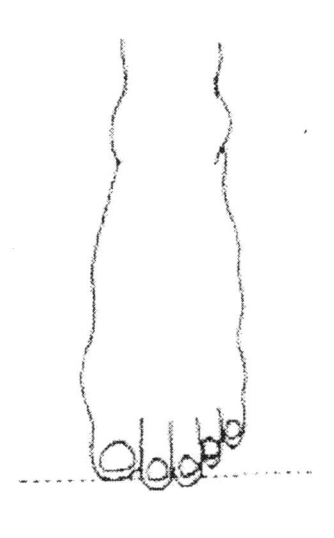

1   2   3 4 5

If the First Toe (Great Toe) curves toward the second toe, it indicates that the spleen, pancreas and lymphatic system are being stressed and the liver is underactive and needs glandular support from the spleen and pancreas. If the Fifth Toe is curved towards the fourth toe, it indicates that the kidney, bladder, excretory systems, gallbladder, lung, and respiratory system are stressed to a point of fatigue and under-activity. The wearing of pointed shoes or high heels or shoes too small causes deformed feet.

Callouses

Callouses indicate that excessive fat, mucous, acid, protein, and waste has caused a nutritional imbalance. This imbalance caused malfunctions in organs. If a callous is on the fourth toe, then the liver's gallbladder is deteriorating. If a callous is on the sole of the foot (on the knuckle center) it indicates kidneys stress caused by eliminating cellular waste.

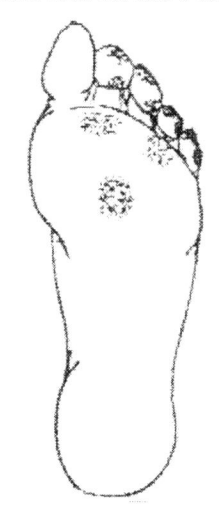

Callouses on the Feet

Callous at the tips of the toes: is an indication that the corresponding organs have an imbalance in the metabolism of minerals, proteins, fats, carbohydrates, or vitamins. This also indicates acidosis, and an eating disorder, which has stressed organs.

First (large) toe curving inward

Fifth (small) toe curving inward

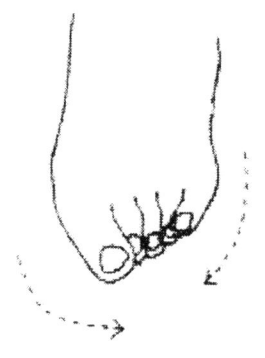

All toes curving inward

Toes- Organ Correlation

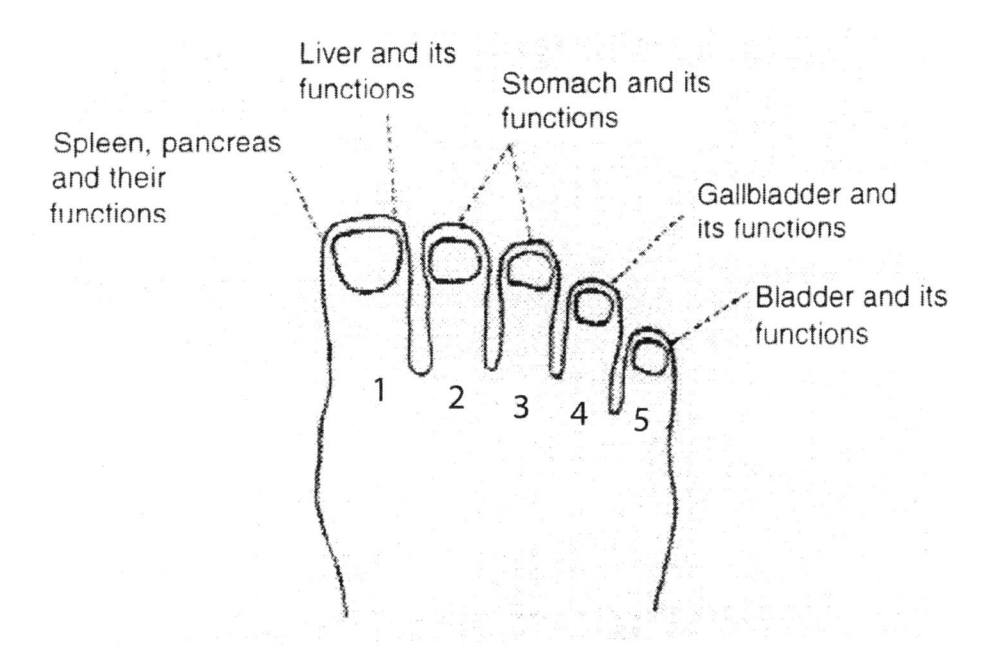

Diagram showing top of foot with toes numbered 1-5 and organ correlations:
- Toe 1: Spleen, pancreas and their functions
- Toe 2: Liver and its functions
- Toe 3: Stomach and its functions
- Toe 4: Gallbladder and its functions
- Toe 5: Bladder and its functions

The toes and toenails indicate organs and their functions. The first toe and its nail are related to the spleen, and pancreas. The outer area is related to the liver, especially at the inner area. The second and third toes and their nails indicate the stomach. The second toe indicates the stomach and digestive organ. The third toe indicates the stomach and duodenum. The fourth toe and its nail indicate to the gallbladder. The fifth toe and its nail are related to the bladder.

Toe Nail Color

The toenails are normally harder than the fingernails. The condition of the toenail varies according to the health status. The normal pink color of the toenails is slightly darker than the pink fingernails. The surface of the toenails should be smooth, indicating good health and nutritional balance. Darker colors of the toenails including dark blue and dark purple indicate imbalance nourishment. Pale white color and rugged surface often appear on the fourth and fifth nails. Indicates liver, gallbladder, kidneys, and excretory system problems.

Toes and Body Functions

On the bottom of the foot, the area at the base of each toe corresponds to an organ and glands ability to function. The condition of the foot indicates disease conditions. If there is soreness, tenderness, dryness, moisture, hard or soft skin, rashes, bumps, discoloration, cracking, pain, peeling, coldness, or excess warmth in an area: it is related to the corresponding organ or system. In this way, you can diagnose the inner body and systems.

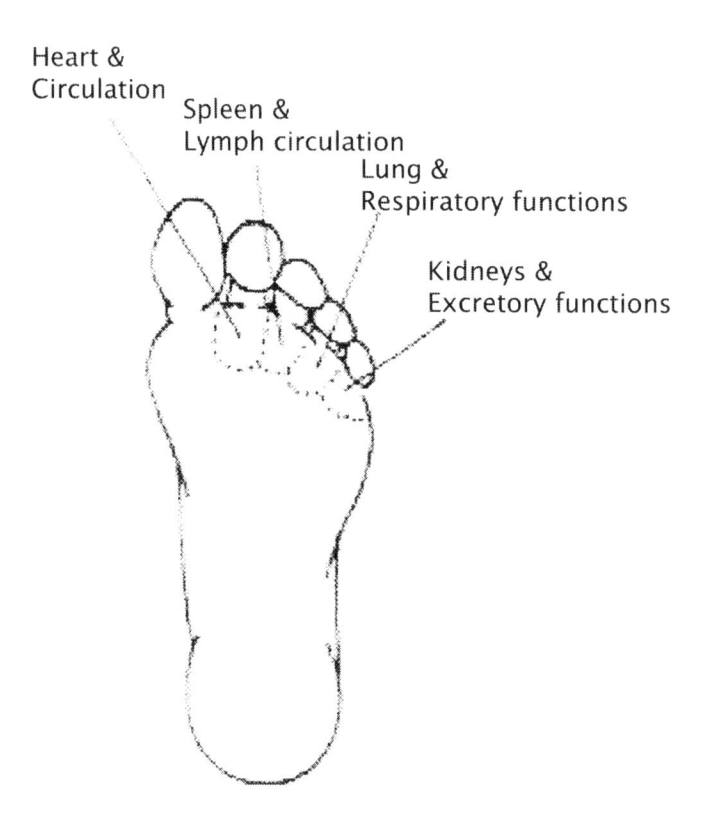

- ❖ Area under the second toe: heart and circulation.
- ❖ Area under the third toe: spleen and lymph circulation.
- ❖ Area under the fourth toe: lungs and respiration.
- ❖ Area under the fifth toe: kidneys and excretory system.

Foot Colors and Disease

Skin darker than usual, purplish green, or bluish brown coloration indicates a problem or disease with the organ related to that area.

A. Stomach

B. Spleen, pancreas, and lymph gland, can indicate Hodgkin's disease.
C. Gallbladder.
D. Bladder, uterus, ovaries, and prostate.

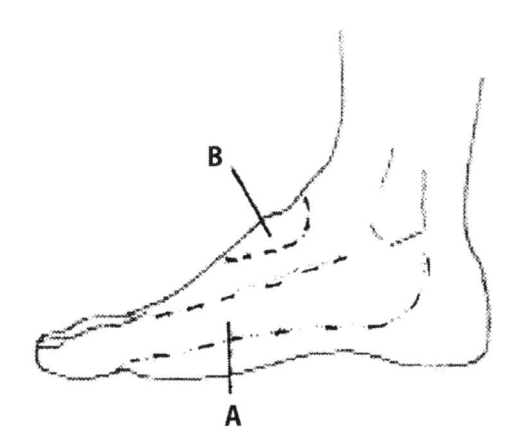

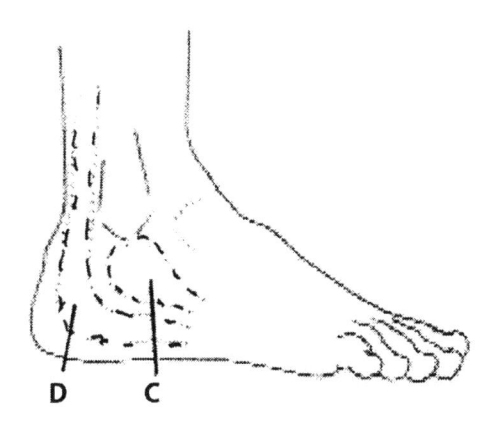

Acupuncture Meridian Points on Lower Leg and Foot

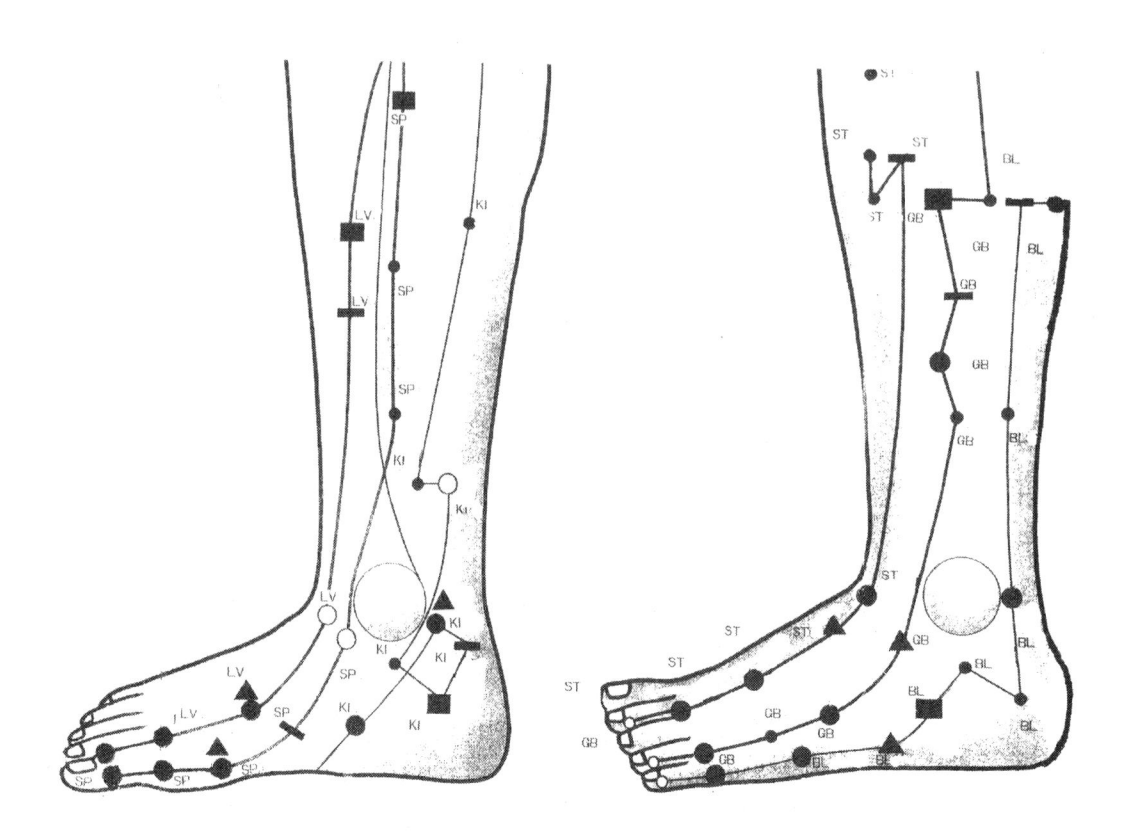

Shapes of Points on Meridians	Function of Meridian
Points on Hand (solid circle)	Circulatory, Nervous, Digestive, Immune, and Excretory Systems
Source Point (triangle)	Actual origin
Accumulating Points (solid square)	Gathering of quantities of toxins can be blockages
Connecting Points (solid rectangle)	Joins and links systems together
Alarm Point (oval circle)	Warning of problems
Associate Point (solid half crescent)	Related in bodily functions

Body's Effect on Shoes and Feet

Diagnoses Using Shoes

Inconsistency in the wear of the sole of the shoe is caused by unequal distribution of weight related to a misaligned spine. A misaligned spine causes nerve messages of organs to be altered. This alters the organs ability to function properly, which alters the health.

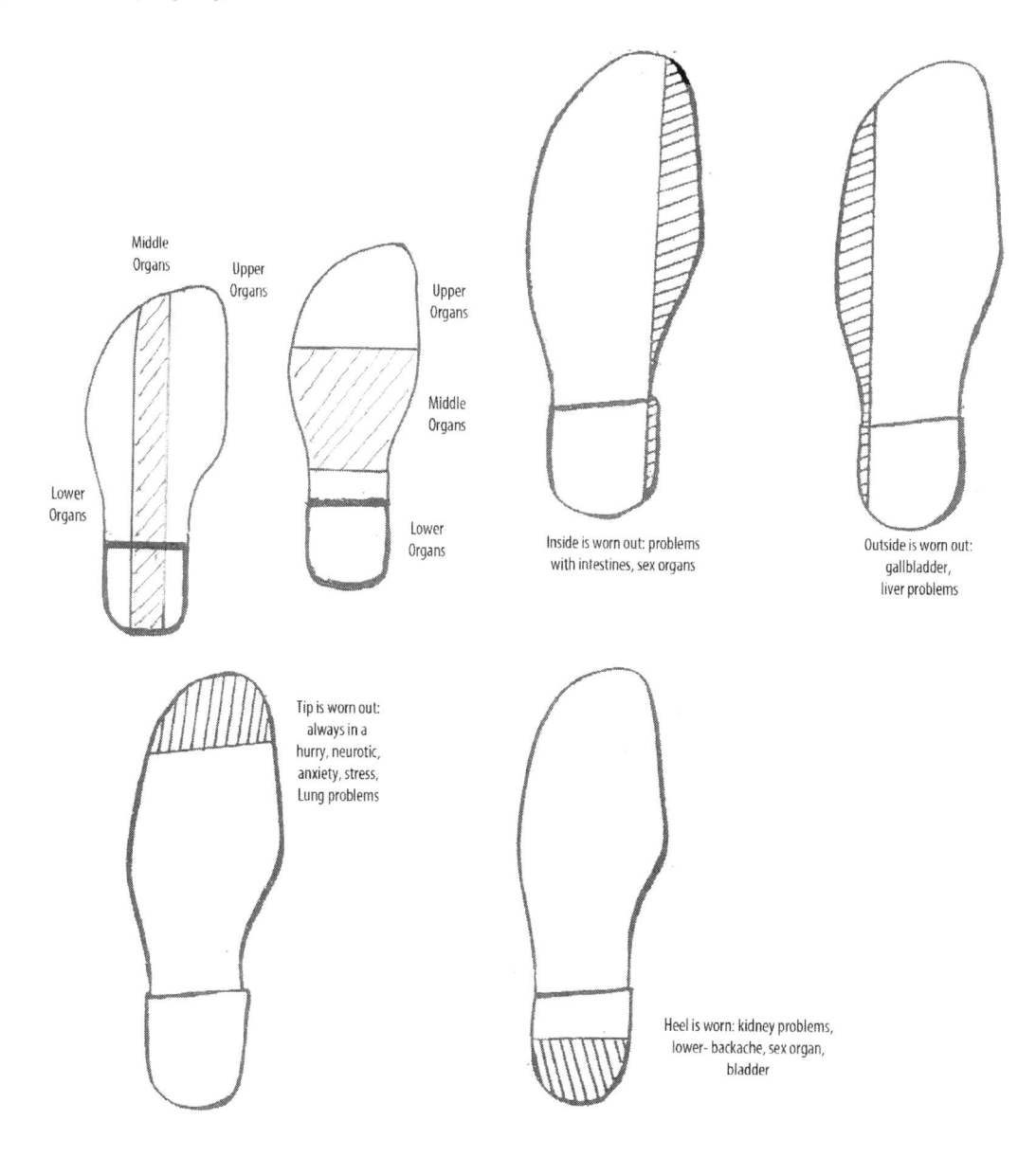

Middle Organs / Upper Organs / Lower Organs

Upper Organs / Middle Organs / Lower Organs

Inside is worn out: problems with intestines, sex organs

Outside is worn out: gallbladder, liver problems

Tip is worn out: always in a hurry, neurotic, anxiety, stress, Lung problems

Heel is worn: kidney problems, lower- backache, sex organ, bladder

Position of Feet

When lying on the back (supine) the feet will form angles.

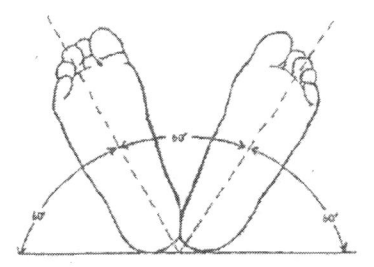

Normal position: the ideal position of the feet; hip sockets, legs and the shoulders are balanced.

The left foot is turned out more than 60 degrees; Left hip socket is loose, left leg is shorter, and more weight is put on the left foot.

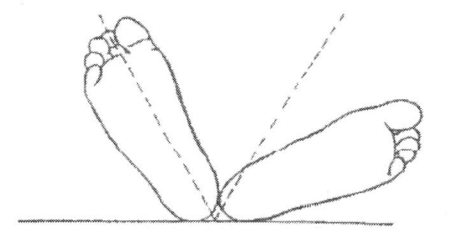

The right leg is turned out more than 60 degrees. Right hip socket is loose, right leg is shorter, and more weight is put on the right foot.

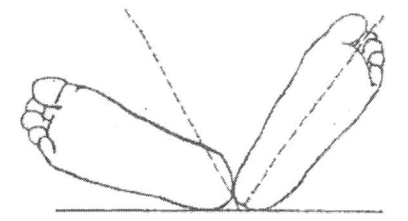

When both feet are turned out more than 60 degrees, both hip sockets are misaligned.

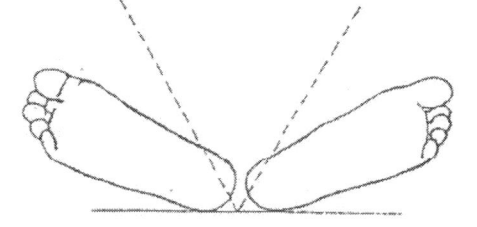

Angle of Feet

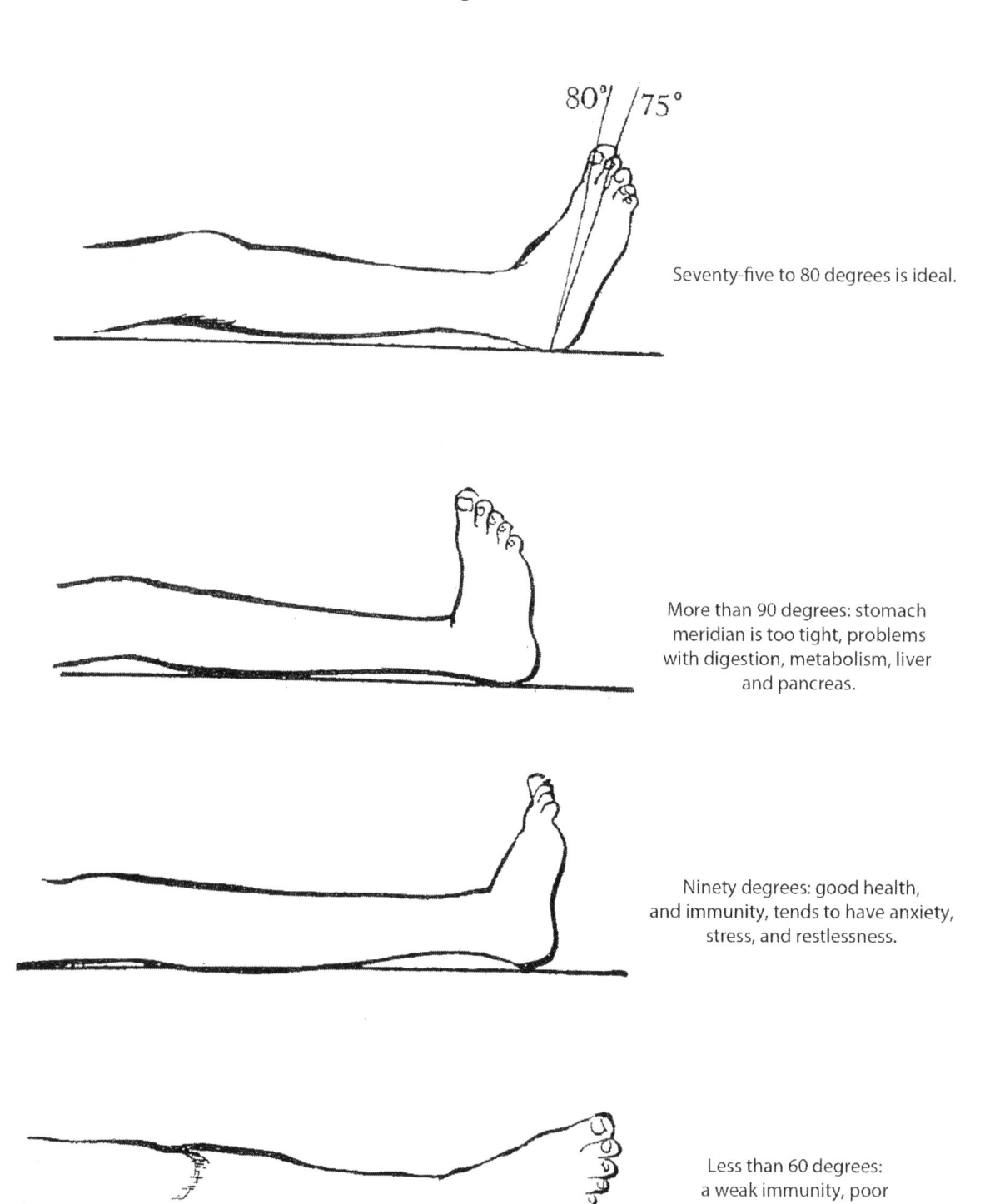

Seventy-five to 80 degrees is ideal.

More than 90 degrees: stomach meridian is too tight, problems with digestion, metabolism, liver and pancreas.

Ninety degrees: good health, and immunity, tends to have anxiety, stress, and restlessness.

Less than 60 degrees: a weak immunity, poor health, chronic sickness.

Acupuncture

Acupressure Finger Position

Acupressure is the application of 2 to 3 pounds of pressure to points on the body related to organs, organ systems, and anatomical structure. If the pressure reveals soreness, tenderness, pain, and/or discomfort it indicates a problem. Inconsistencies of the skin on a point as well as Muscle Testing on a point can identify problems. At points where there is little or no muscular tension, apply firm but gentle pressure. Use the pad of the finger rather than the tip. At points, which feel tense, use just enough pressure to feel the tension, so that you feel the hardness of the muscle at your fingertips. Gradually rub the point for reaction. At points of muscular tension gradually apply pressure until you feel the tension.

Correct Finger Pressure Position

Incorrect Finger Pressure Position

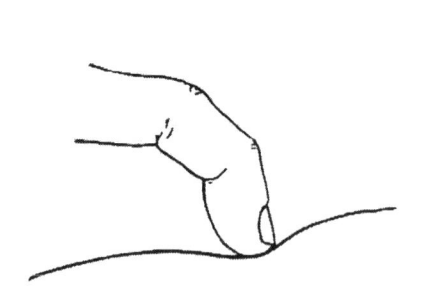

Organ Energy Points

Inconsistency in skin or if acupressure is applied and there is sensitivity to your touch that indicates a problem with that organ. If the skin on a point is inconsistent in color, texture, rash, bumps, dryness, oiliness, change in hair texture or color etc. it indicate a health problem related to the organ on that point.

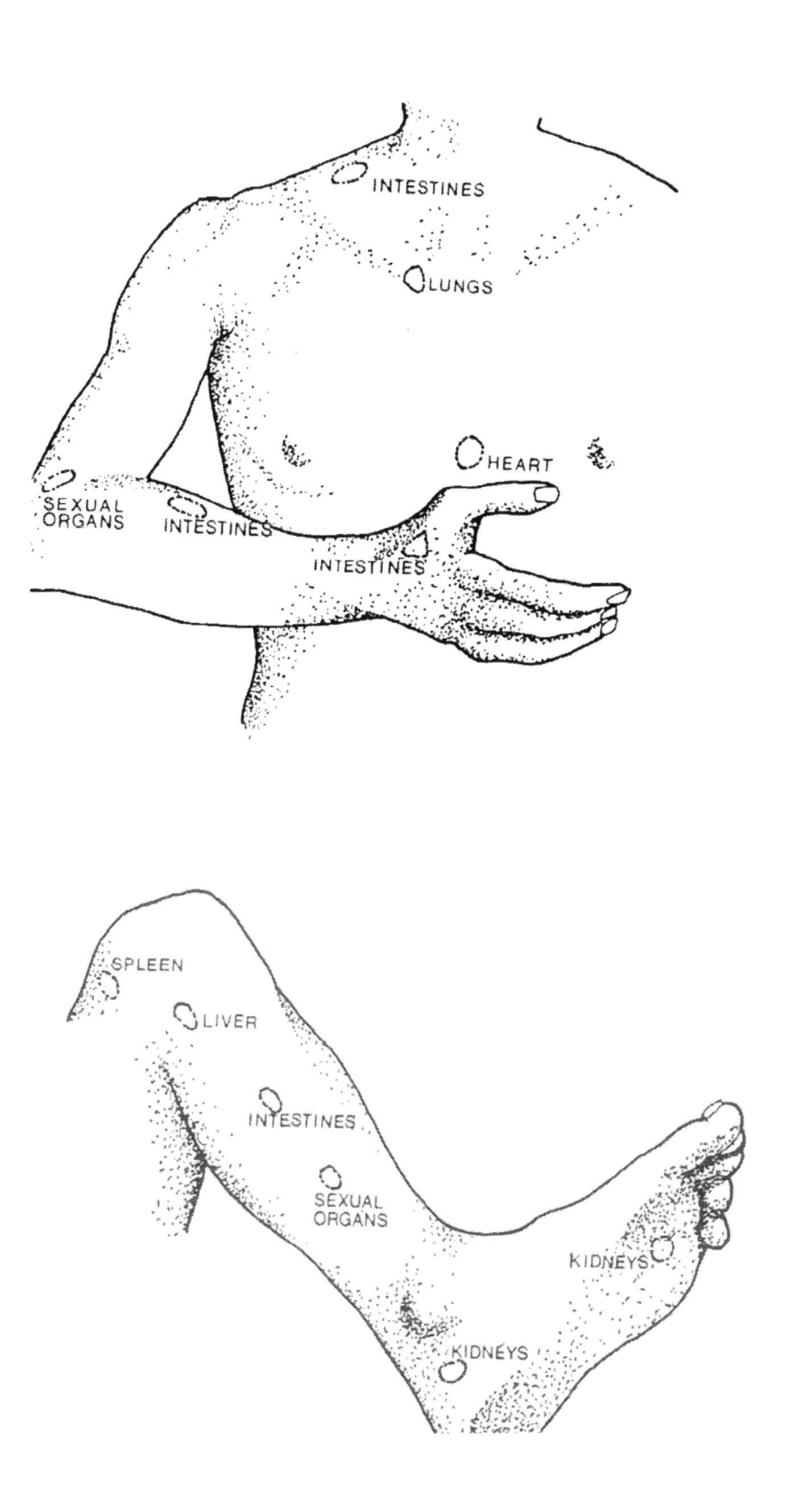

Amino Acid Points

An *inconsistency* in skin or if acupressure is applied and there is sensitivity to touch or pain it indicates an inconsistency in absorption, metabolism of an amino acid, or a deficiency in that amino acid.

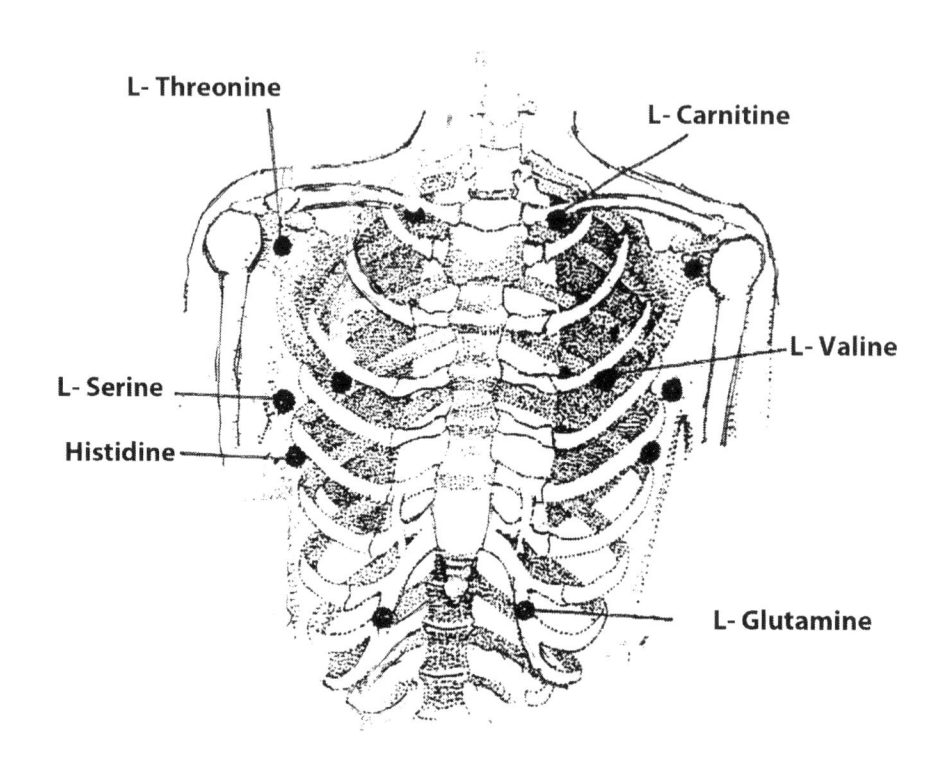

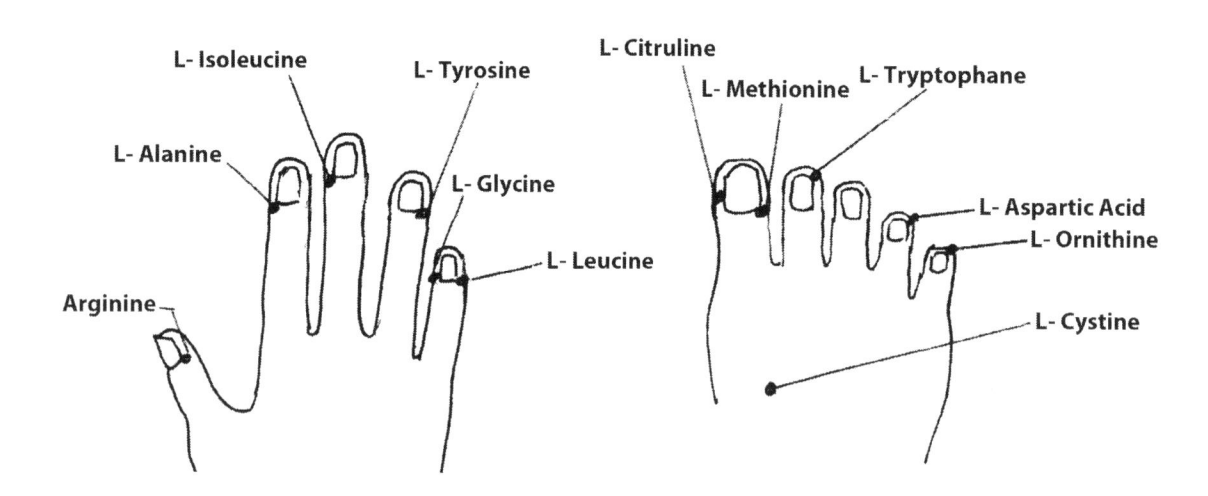

Acupressure/Acupuncture Points on the Body

An inconsistency in the skin or if acupressure to the part causes pain or is sensitive to touch it indicates an inconsistency of the function of the organ.

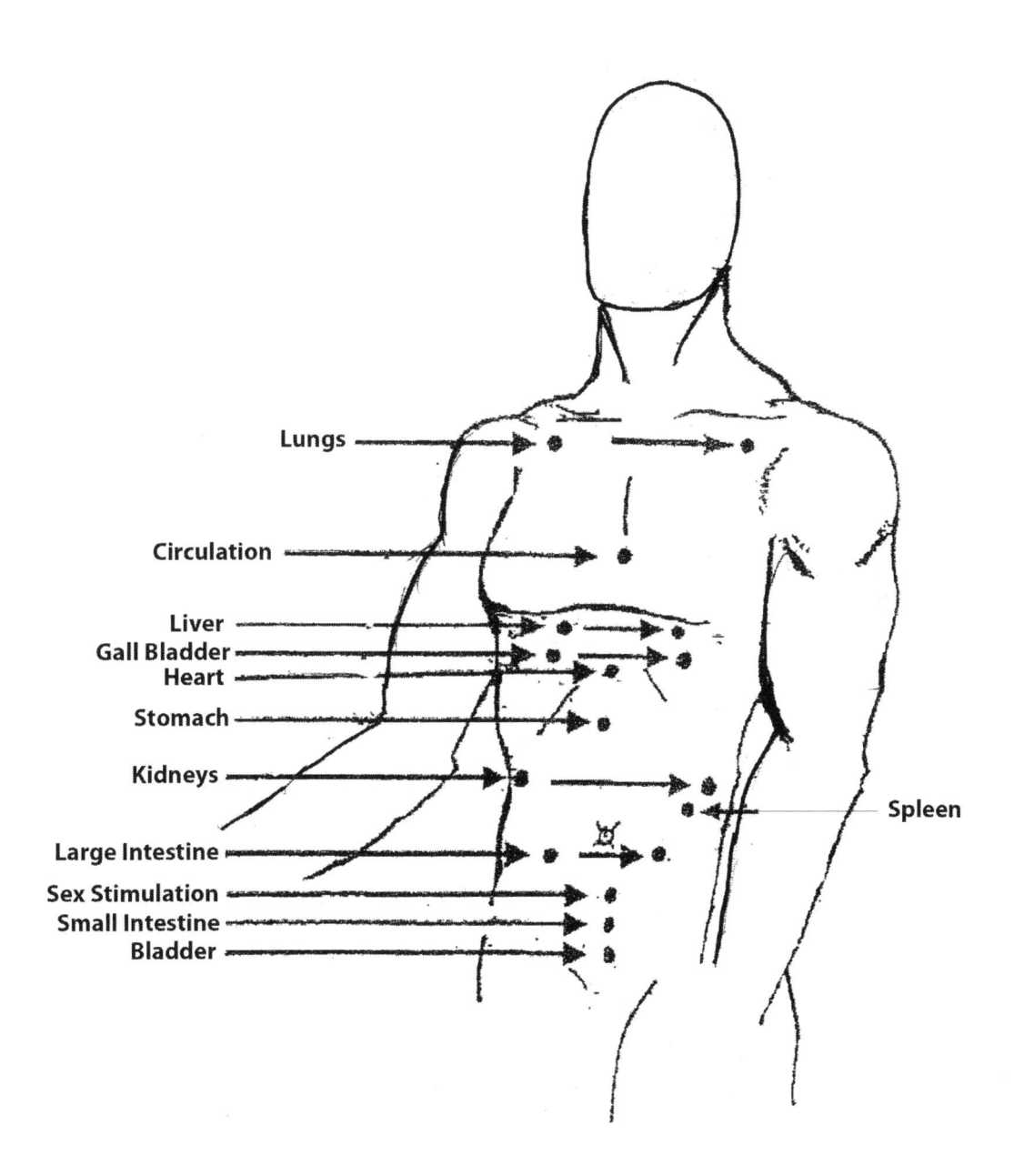

- Lungs
- Circulation
- Liver
- Gall Bladder
- Heart
- Stomach
- Kidneys
- Large Intestine
- Sex Stimulation
- Small Intestine
- Bladder
- Spleen

Acupuncture/ Acupressure Meridian on Body

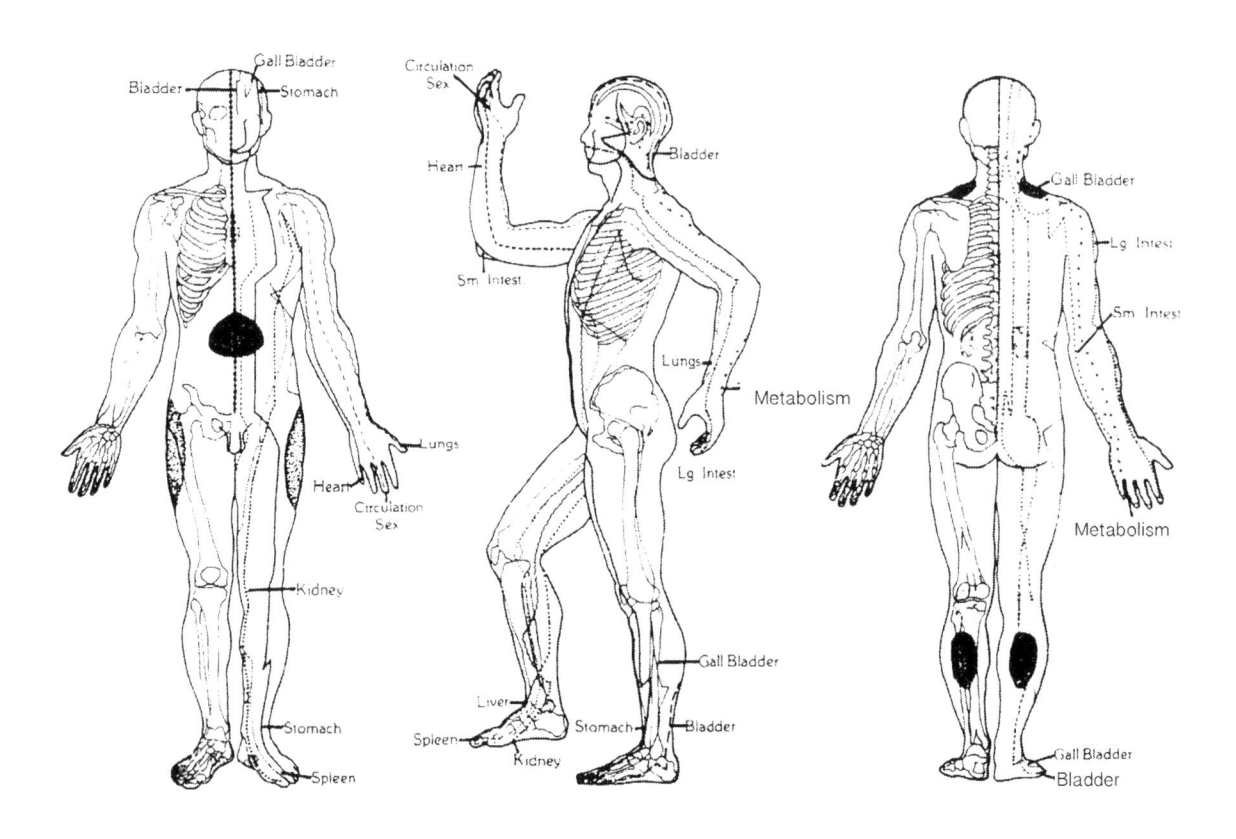

The Meridian broken lines correspond to organs and functions. If there is discoloration, bumps, rashes, dryness, oiliness, excessive hair growth (appears longer than surrounding hairs), lack of hair (appears shorter than surrounding hairs), change of texture of skin or hair, a series of scars, marks or bruises, soreness and/or oversensitivity to touch on a Meridian can indicate problems with corresponding organ and/or function.

Points on Body Chart

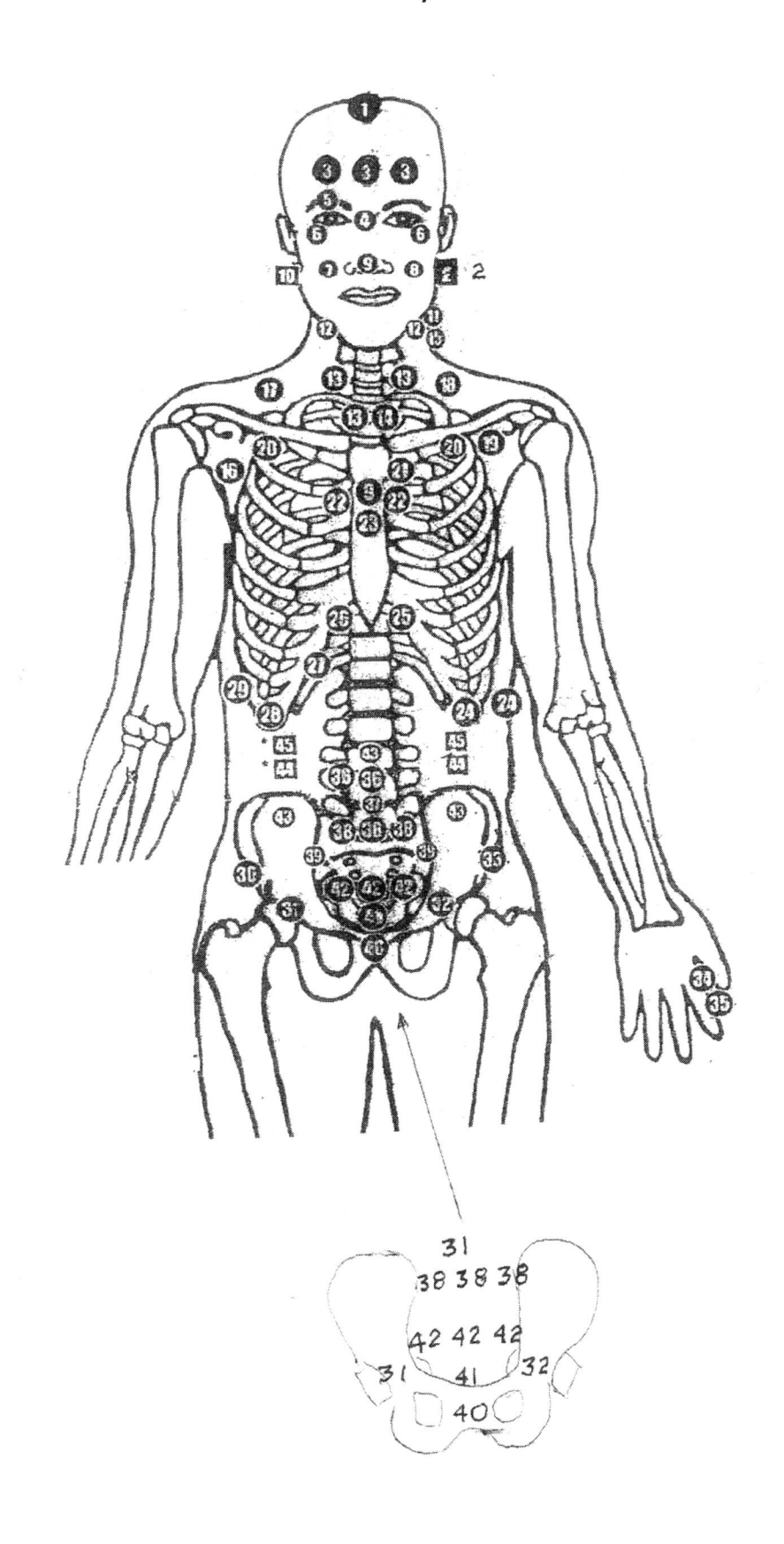

227

Points on Body

Skin inconsistency, acupressure that causes slight pain or discomfort, and muscle testing that causes weak response indicates problems with the nutrient that corresponds with that point.

Head and Neck	Torso	Pelvis
1. Blood Pressure	16. Vitamin E	31. Iron
2. Protein	17. Vitamin F	32. Vitamin D
3. Stress	18. Calcium	33. Copper and Phosphorus
4. Pineal Gland	19. Vitamin C	34. Parasites
5. Vitamin A	20. Lungs	35. Yeast
6. Allergy	21. Bioflavonoids	36. Pancreatic Digestion
7. Potassium	22. Cardiovascular	37. Virus
8. Sodium	23. Allergies Systemic	38. Magnesium and Manganese
9. Allergy	24. Pancreas	39. Vitamin B
10. RNA/ DNA	25. HCl (Hydrochloric Acid)	40. Lead
11. Lymph	26. Enzymatic	41. Bladder
12. Parotid	27. Acidophilus	42. Male/Female Organs
13. Thyroid	28. Bile Salts	43. Colon
14. Iodine	29. Liver	44. Kidney
15. Trace Minerals	30. Zinc	45. Adrenals
		46. Arthritic or Rheumatic Pain

Organ Zones on Body

- The more central part of the body indicates the function of the internal organs.
- The peripheral area of the back indicates the central part of the front of the body, digestive tract, and the organs in the middle part of the back.
- The middle back area indicates the function of the stomach, pancreas, kidneys, and the duodenum.
- The lower back (thoracic) indicates the function of the lower lungs, liver, gallbladder, spleen, and the diaphragm.
- The sacral and buttock area indicates the function of the uterus, ovaries, prostate, testicles, rectum, and bladder.
- The area directly above the waist indicates the functions of the transverse colon, and upper small intestines.
- The waist area correlates to the lower small intestine, ascending colon, descending colon, and their functions.

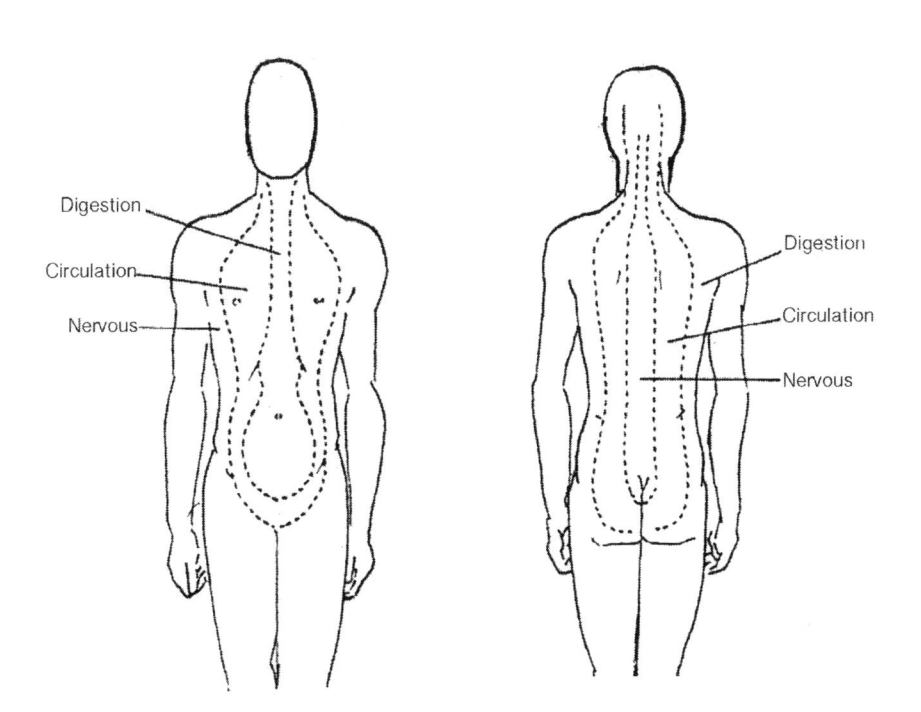

Melanin Energy Lines and The Pulses

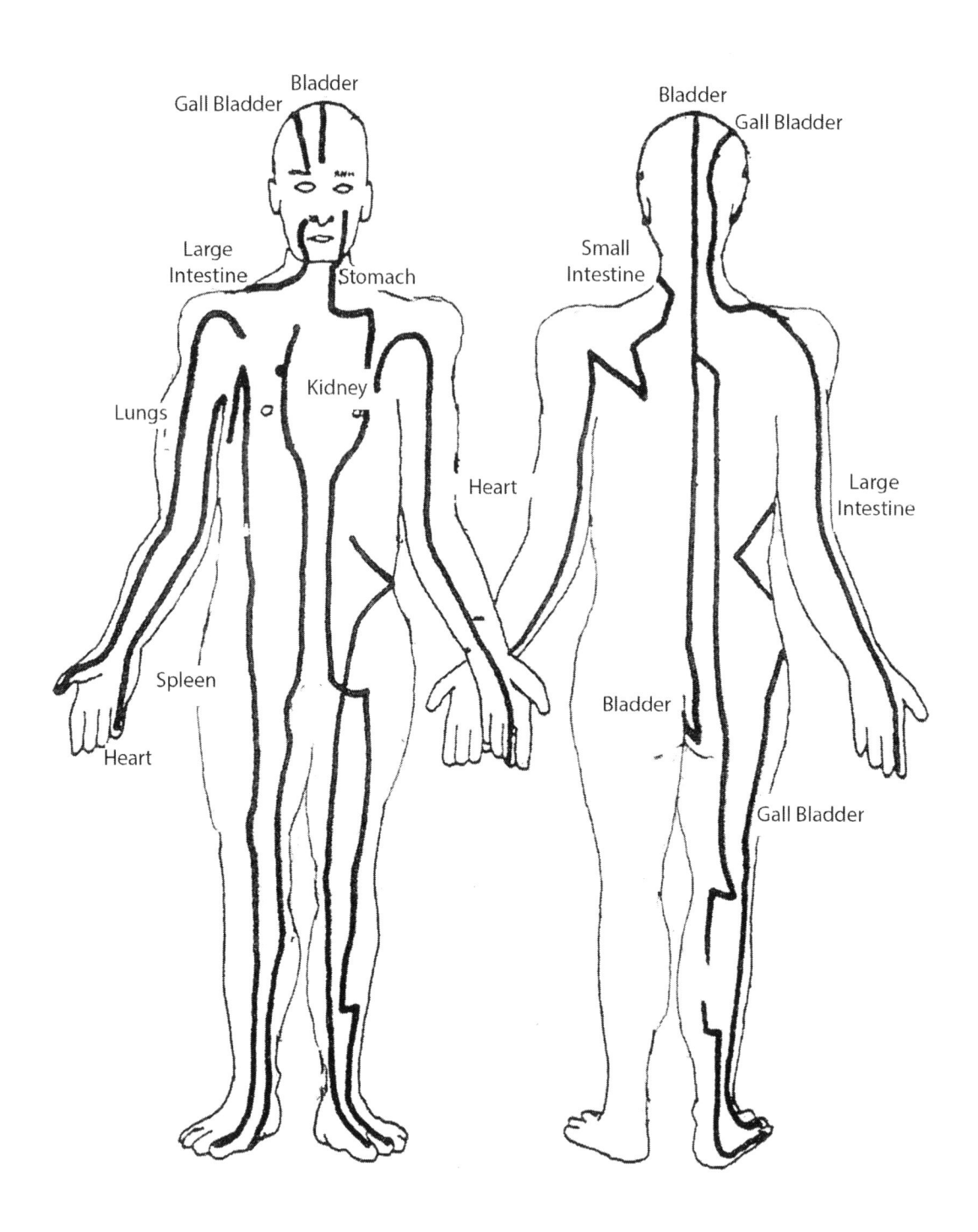

Acupuncture Points

If pressed and there is discomfort or pain, skin irritation such as rashes on area, discoloration, or bumps on points it can indicate a disease. Muscle Test, if there is a weak response it indicates problems with that organ.

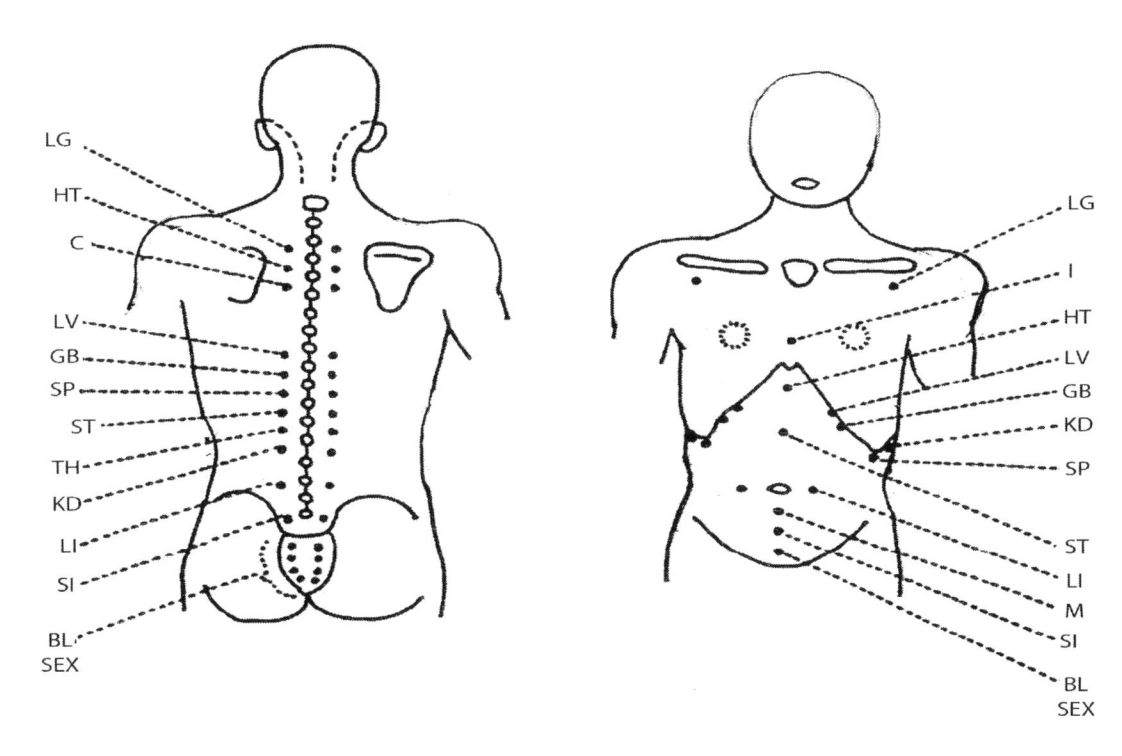

LG	Lungs
HT	Heart
C	Circulation
LV	Liver
GB	Gallbladder
SP	Spleen and Pancreas
S	Stomach
M	Metabolism and Heart Energy
KD	Kidneys
LI	Large Intestine
SI	Small Intestine
BL-SEX	Bladder and Sexual functions
TH	Thyroid
I	Immunity

231

Acupuncture (acupressure) Points

Apply acupressure/ acupuncture to a specific point if there is soreness, oversensitivity, discoloration, and a bump or rash on the point or an unpleasant feeling reaction in the organ itself it indicates a health problem related to that organ. Muscle Test can be used, if weak response there is problems with that organ.

Anterior Chest Region

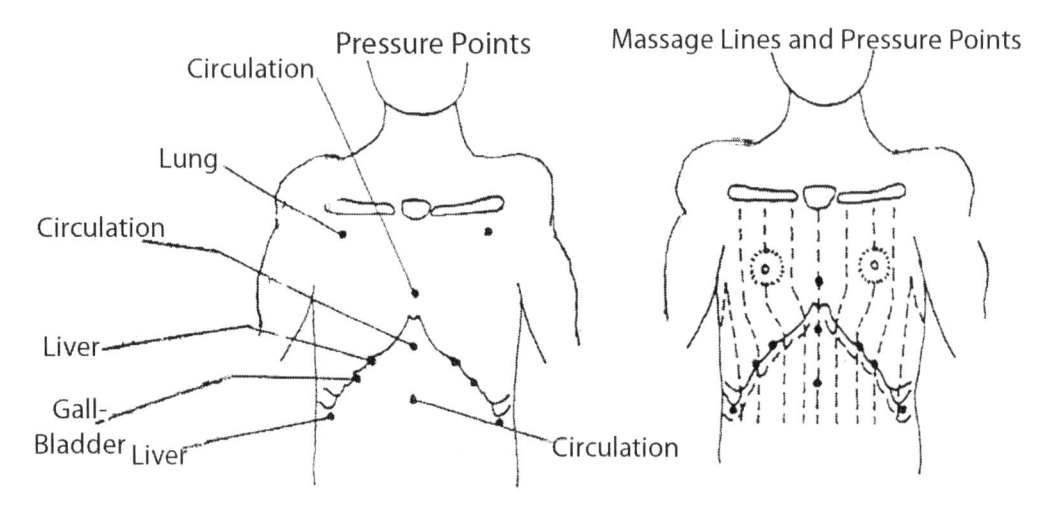

Meridians on Front and Side of Torso

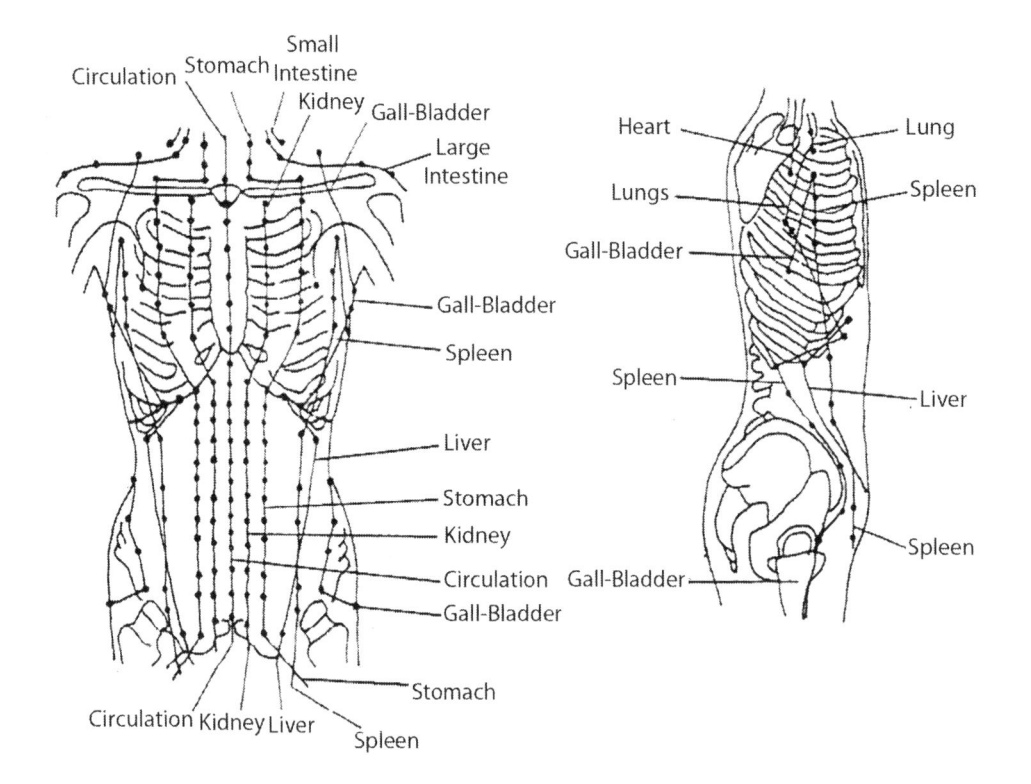

Abdominal Section

If the skin on these points has inconsistencies such as discoloration, roughness, dryness, rashes, bumps, soreness, oversensitivity, excessive heat or cold, hair is shorter or longer than surrounding hair or a change of texture of hair it can indicate disease or malfunction of related organ. Muscle Testing can be used; if there is a weak response there is a problem with that organ.

Incoming and Outgoing Energy Points

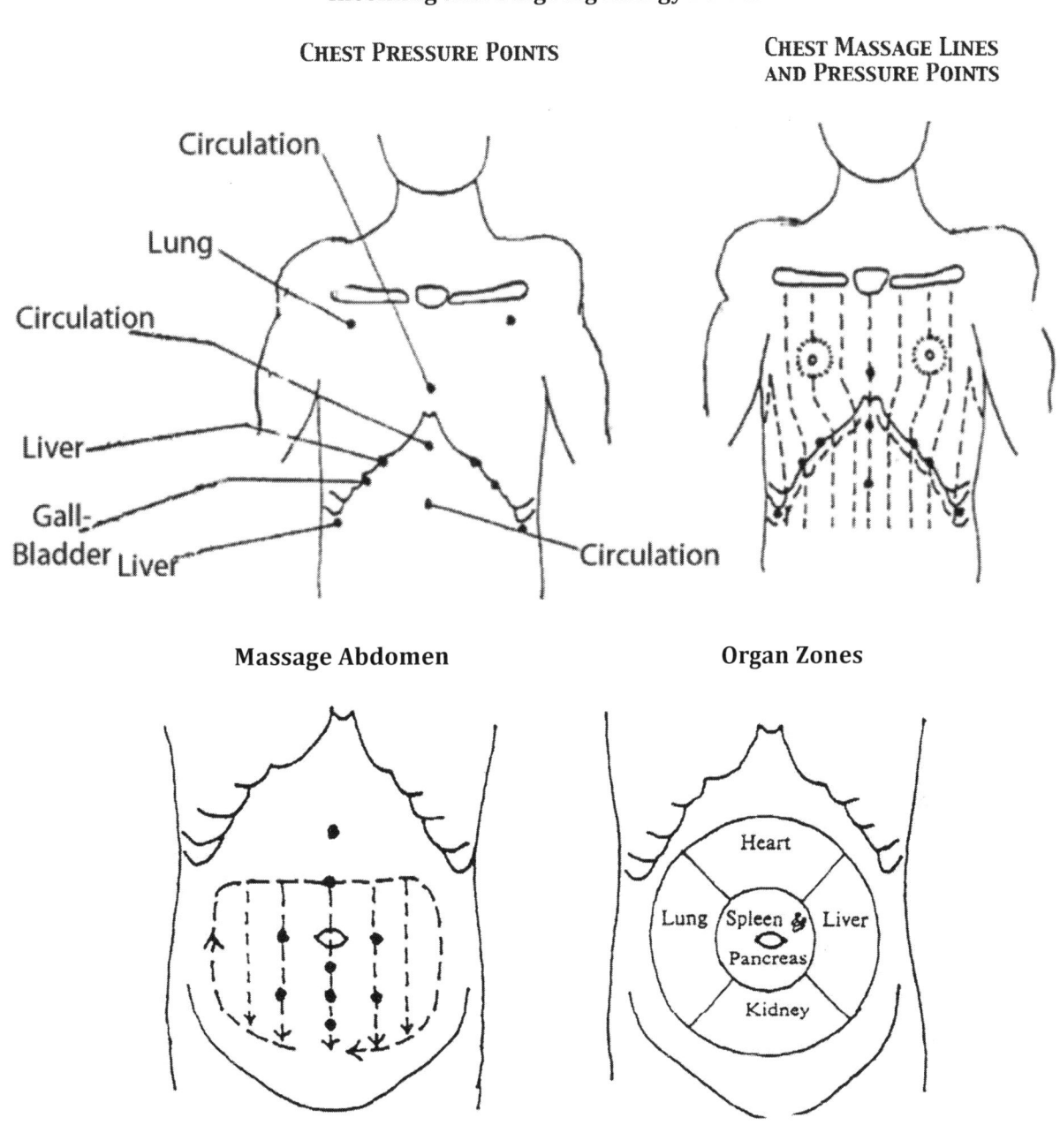

CHEST PRESSURE POINTS

- Circulation
- Lung
- Circulation
- Liver
- Gall-Bladder
- Liver
- Circulation

CHEST MASSAGE LINES AND PRESSURE POINTS

Massage Abdomen

Massage in direction of arrow for treatment.

Organ Zones

- Heart
- Lung
- Spleen & Pancreas
- Liver
- Kidney

Apply acupressure to zones diagnose by looking and/or touching and noting inconsistencies.

233

Organ Areas

An inconsistency in the skin and/or hair texture, color, temperature, or sensitivity changes in the areas indicate disease and/or malfunction of related organs.

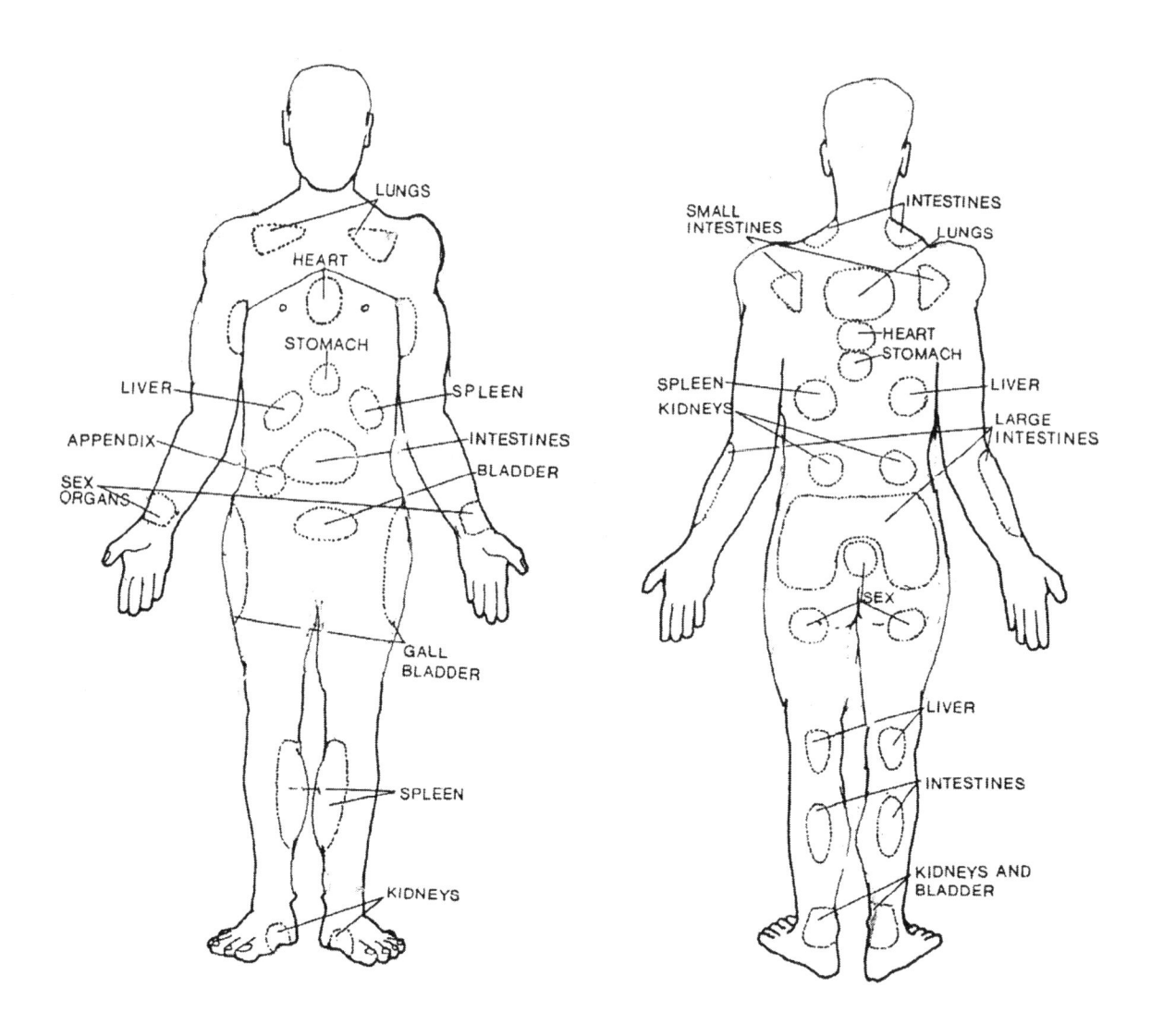

Disease and Body Areas

If there is longer hair in one area, sensitivity to touch, discoloration, bumps, texture change, oily or dry skin, increase or decrease in temperature, rashes in the area it indicates these diseases.

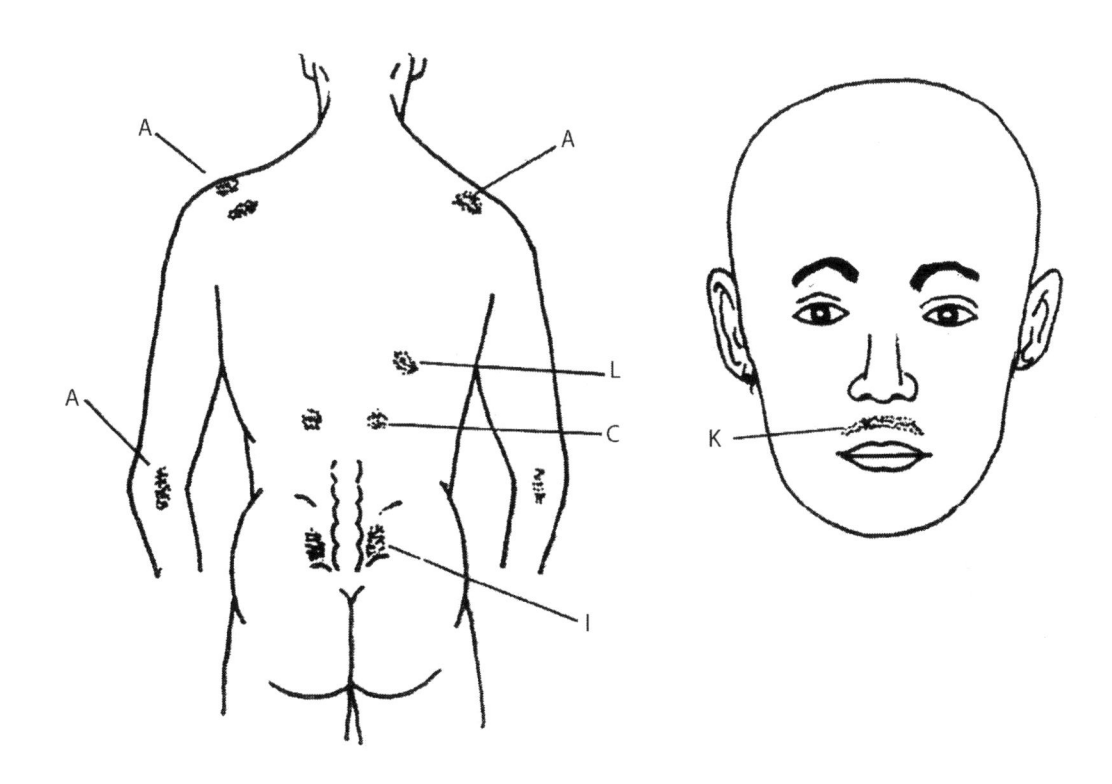

A-Arm arthritis and/or rheumatism

L- Liver disorders

C- Colds Influenza, and/or inner ear infections

I- Intestinal disorders

K- Kidney disorders and/or Athletes foot

Disease and Leg Hair

If the hair in the areas is longer, exceptionally coarse or fine, or change in color and/or texture it can indicate a disease.

- A- Leg arthritis
- B- Leg rheumatism

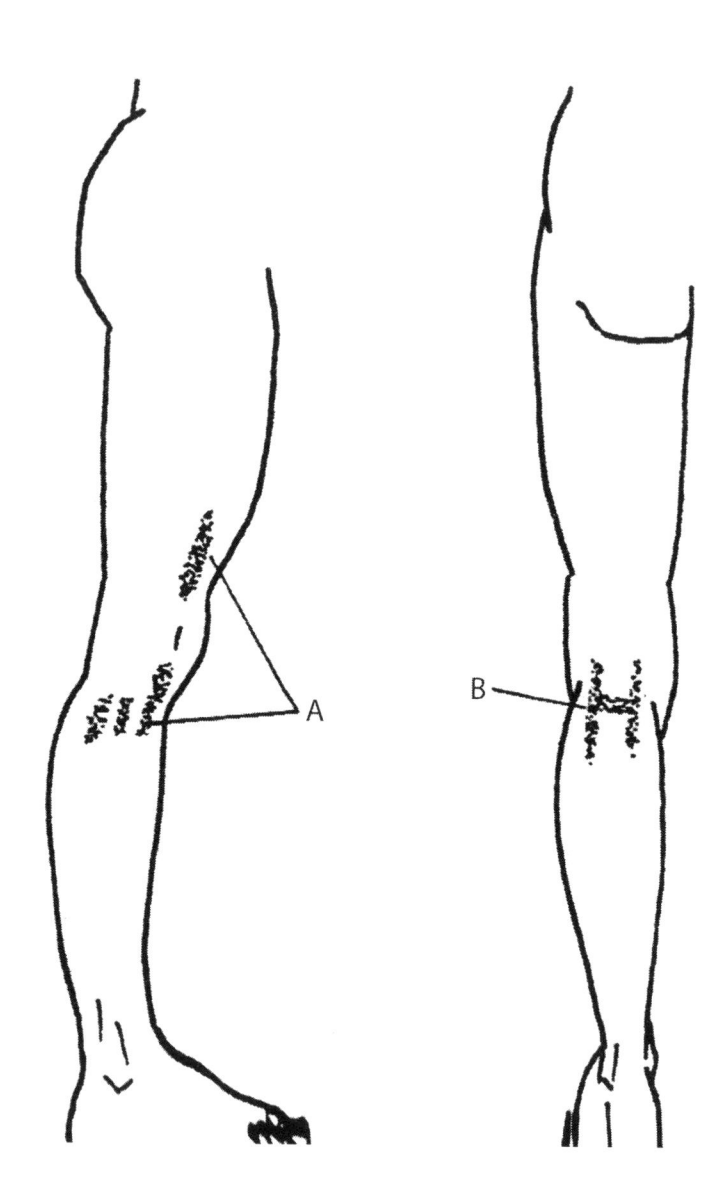

Handwriting Diagnosis

An individual's cursive handwriting is a type of literary DNA and fingerprint. It reveals the inner subconscious subliminal personality, which is peculiar to that individual. There are many methods used to understand the personalized information contained in individuals handwriting. Only a few techniques are used in this diagnosis. The letter or words that are inconsistent in shape, lack proper symmetry, deformed and/or irregular in the lower, middle, and/or Upper Area indicates problem.

How to Do a Writing Diagnosis

Looking at people's handwriting is good for practice and developing efficiency. However, a formal diagnosis is ideal. When diagnosing handwriting the paper used should be unlined, use the same weight and size paper for each diagnosis. A black ink ballpoint or a very sharp pencil should be used. For a diagnosis the person should write about a recent event, observation, handwrite a text message, write about a social or news event or write a letter to themselves. The diagnosis sample should be sign and dated. Place tracing paper over the writing diagnosis sample or make notations on separate piece of paper or on the diagnosis sample.

1. Underline letters, words, or phrases that are not normal
2. Circle letters and words that are unusual
3. Underline Lower, Middle, and/or Upper, areas that deviate from normal
4. Indicates baseline, deviations, slants, size to small and/or too large, spacing, connecting strokes, stroke pressure, shapes, loops, adornments
5. Note emotional and health issues

Letter Size

The normal height of letters is ⅛ inch (3ml). Writing with normal size letters indicates the ability to be practical and the ability modify the lifestyle in order to achieve wellness. Smaller than normal letters indicates that the person likes to obtain information about healing modalities. They can be introverted and independently pursue remedies (see Female Principle). Larger than normal indicates that the person needs emotional attention and nurturing to gain wellness is not achieved immediately (see Male Principle).

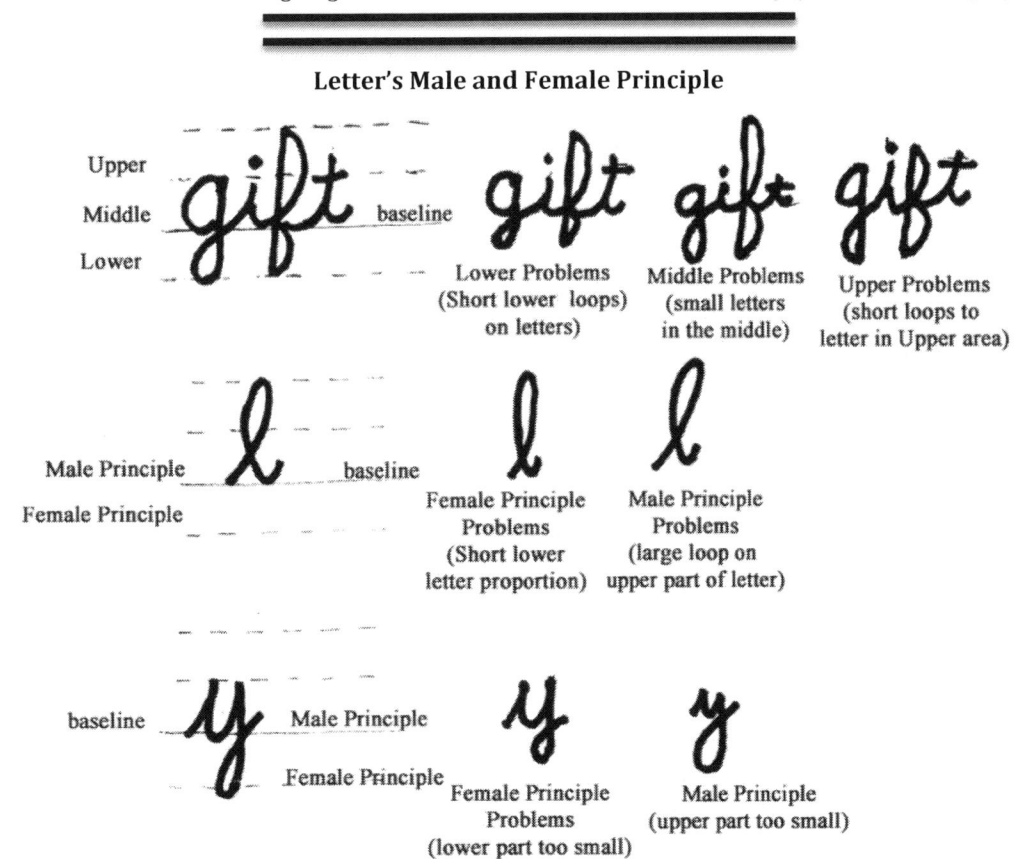

Letter's Male and Female Principle

The letter of letters that is in consistent, lack proper symmetry and proportionality and are deformed and/or Upper area indicates a health problem in that area. Choose the area with the highest amounts of abnormal letter shapes as the focus of health concerns.

Letter Strokes Male/Female Principle

Downward letter strokes are Male Upward letter strokes are Female. Strokes moving to your left are Male. Strokes moving to the Right are Female. Each single stroke can be divided into 3 sections. The starting point of the stroke is related to the Lower Organs. The mid-section of a stroke is related to the Middle Organs. The ending section of a stroke is related to the Upper Organs. See the Holistic Chart for more information.

Letters and Emotions

Attention Deficit- letter strokes have reduced pressure upward strokes and rightward strokes
Anger/Frustration- letters in lower area angular, long, and full
Aloof/ Anti-social- Middle area loopy and large, uses angles
Anxiety/Uncertainty- fragments of letters or broken parts of letters can be at the baseline
Behavior full of Drama- very decorative artistic signature
Believes in their own illusions/ fantasies- Upper area very looped
Clever- writes in a string thready manner, uses many angles, curly coils
Cover Ups Dysfunctions- letters are blurry and unclear
Cunning- complicated adornments, loops and arches on letters
Compulsive- periods of words too far behind or too far forward of the letter
Detached/Aloof- large spaces between letters, lines and/or words
Does not like being told what to do/ Rebellious- strokes to letters not in normal written direction, counterstrokes
Deceitful- written words seem too neat, typed in appearance or can be to clear or too complex in shape
Easily Manipulated- uneven pressure on pen (normally upward strokes have light pressure, downward strokes slightly heavy pressure)
Emotionally Influenced- very light pen stroke pressure
Fakes outward personality and behavior- writes slowly
Fakes niceness- rigid baseline conformity as if drawn by a ruler (normally words written on baseline have slightly wavy flow)
Guilt Feelings- many circular adornments, loops, and arches around and/or over letters and words or at the end of letters/words
Hides Feelings/Thoughts- heavy stroke pressure, ovals usually full or no open space inside ovals, artistic decoration on the tail end of letters and loops, letters backward and/or upside down
Hypocrite/ Mental Problems- very angular letters with artistic type decorations in the form of loops, curly coils, decorative ending tails on letters
High hopes/ Ideals/Ambition- very tall upper are letters
Ideas impractical/ Illusionary- short letters in lower area, tall in upper area
Immature- excessive roundness to letters
Indirect- letters difficult to understand, not legible
Misses the point of life/ Ideas/Conversation- first letter is clear followed by letters omitted or unclear
Manipulator- some thready letters with uneven letter sizes
Mood Swings- letters in consistent in slants, spacing, and/or size. Can be erratic.
Non-commitment- does not write the whole word or letter, omits small parts of letters, letters awkwardly written
Narrow-minded- letters or words crowded and cramped together
Opportunist/Takes advantage- unsteady or snake-like on baseline
Poor will power- no horizontal line on the letter "T", absent or weak horizontal line
Resentful- unsteady pen pressure on letter strokes, letters with angles
Secretive- circular-like adornments, loops, line arches over letters, words, or letters of words close together, thready, curly ovals
Sudden Fluctuation in Moods/ Expression- pressure used for writing letters sporadic and erratic
Thinks they are important- tall capital letters
Truthful- consistent uniform letters, middle area of letters usually same size: tends to avoid decorative letters, slant and spacing of letters consistent
Untruthful- letters inconsistent in slant, spacing and size erratic writing, gaps and main letters omitted or unclear and thready string-like
Unsatisfied- Middle area letters not consistent or very flat

Unpredictable/ Ambiguous- letters within words clear at the beginning of the stroke and ending of stroke, thready string-like strokes and letters

Vain / Conceited- circle "i" dots, decorative letters with flourishes, large loops

SEX ORGANS

Female Genitals (Side View)

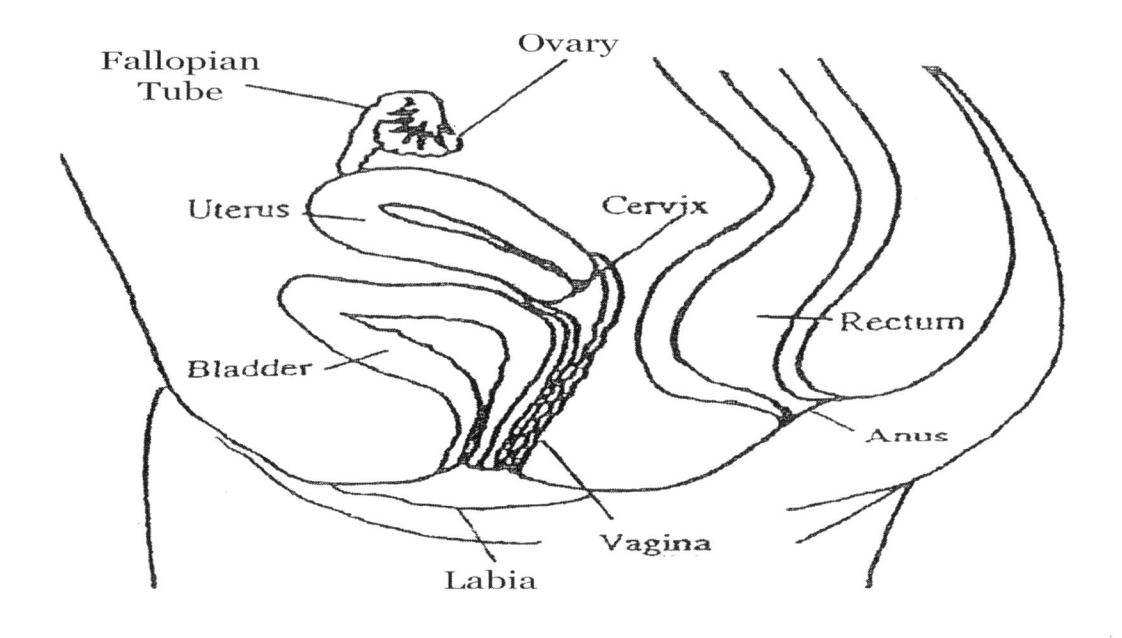

Male Genitals (Side View)

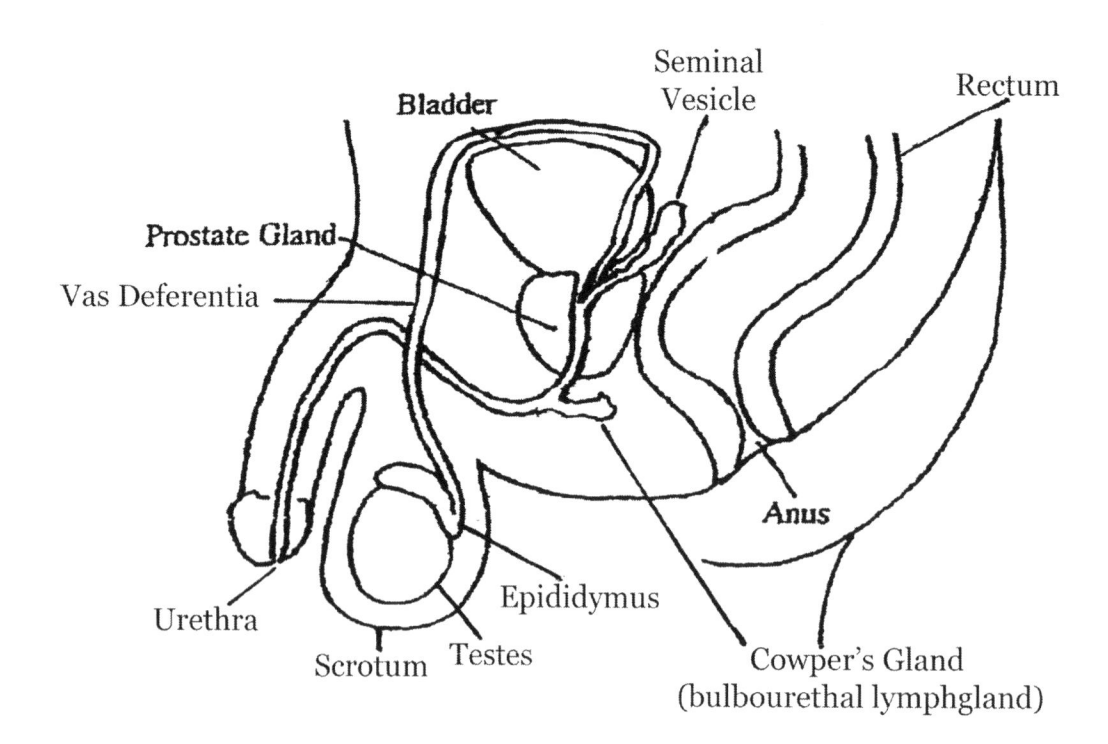

Female Sex Organs

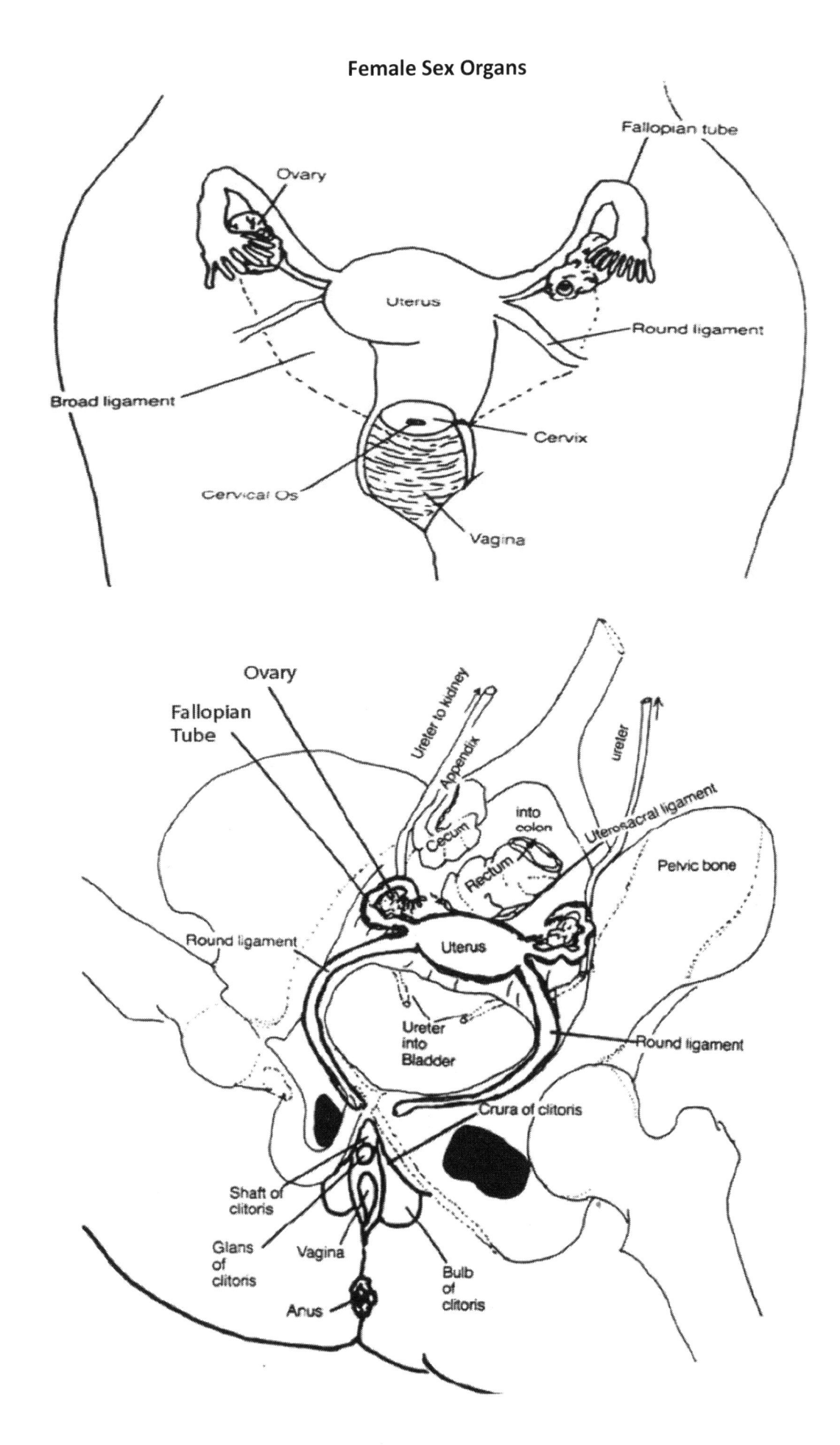

Male Sex Organs

The sperm that fertilizes the female egg are manufactured in the testicles. The testicles are in a small sac called the scrotum. The scrotum hangs outside the body cavity behind the penis. The temperature of the sperm is regulated by the up and down movement of the testicles inside the scrotum. From the testicles tubules the sperm moves into the convoluted Epididymis (tube folds over itself, almost 20 feet or 6.1 meters long), which curves over the back and top of each testicle. In the Epididymis the sperm incubates and matures in about 3 months. When sperm is ready to be ejaculated it travels through the Vas Deferentia (singular: vas deferens).

The Vasa Deferentia are the two slender muscular ducts (tubes) which sperm use to travel out of the testicles and up into the main body cavity.

The Vas Deferntia ducts circle around the bladder, they enlarge slightly to form the Ampulla, and then narrow into the Ejaculatory Ducts that goes into the center of the prostate. The prostate is a muscle and gland about the size of a walnut. It weighs about 20 grams and secretes a thin opalescent alkaline fluid. It is located at the neck of the bladder and wraps around the Urethra. The Urethra is a tube which urine passes out. The Ampulla is below the pouch like Seminal Vesicle. Seminal Vesicles secrete fluid that goes into the Ejaculatory Duct. Semen is a mixture of prostate fluid, bulbourethal (two pea size Cowper's gland) lubricating fluid, which nourishes and mixes with sperm from the Ampullar portion of the Vas Deferens.

The semen as well as urine passes out through the tube called the urethra. The tube ends at the head of the penis. The penis is sponge-like tissue. This sponge-like tissue becomes engorged with blood and trapped, causing the penis to become erect. In response to sexual arousal the ejaculatory ducts empty into the urethra. The prostate gland fluids, 1 to 5% sperm cells and neurotransmitters, endorphins, hormones, immunosuppressant, cortisol, oxytocin, Thyrotropin Releasing Hormone, melatonin, serotonin, FSH (follicle stimulating hormone), prolactin and LH (luteinizing hormone) called seminal plasma. This and other fluids are ejaculated out the urethra by muscular contractions. A circular muscle around the neck of bladder closes. This prevents urine from passing into the urethra and semen from backing up into the bladder. The penis shape has been analyzed with the logico-deductive technique called reverse engineering. The head of the penis is a bulging mushroom crown bulbous glan, which is wider than the shaft. The bulbous glan head seems to push another's male's sperm (ejaculated earlier) out of the vagina-semen displacement. The thrusting of the penis into the vagina during sexual intercourse draws another male's sperm away from the uterus. Another male's sperm can survive 50 minutes to 4 hours in the female's reproductive tract and can fertilize the egg. The male currently having sex within 4 hours of another male would not remove his own ejaculated sperm because after ejaculation the erection deflates to flaccid and leaves his sperm. Other male animal's do not have a mushroom shaped head to the penis such a apes, monkeys, horses, cats, dogs, and whales etc. Male cats have about 150 sharp backward pointing spines on their penis. This causes pain to the female cat and she hollers in pain. The irritation of the female cat's vagina by the penis spines causes the vagina to come slightly inflamed and swell which blocks another cat's sperm from entering the uterus. In previous eras of time fast-ejaculating (Premature) males could mate within 4 hours with several females in one sex episode during the human mating season. Women in this modern era do not breastfeed and use birth control and their use of condoms causes women to demand longer sexual episodes. Therefore, the Premature Ejaculators are now considered Maladaptive sexual failures, or suffers Erectile Dysfunctions.

Sexual Response

I. Sympathetic Nerves (Predominately Right Nostril Breathing) Above Waist Activity
    1. Active: Lungs, Thyroid Gland ("Ah" sounds)
       Inactive: Large Intestine (Heavy breathing)
    2. Active: Heart, Thymus Gland
       Inactive: Small Intestine (Lips and Labia swell, erect clitoris and nipples)
    3. Active: Pancreas (Energy release, "O" sounds)
       Inactive: Stomach
    4. Active: Adrenals (Muscle contractions, "A" sounds)
       Inactive: Kidney
       (Wet vagina, Cowper gland wets penis)

II. Parasympathetic Nerves (Predominately Left Nostril Breathing) Below Waist Activity
    5. Pubis (Genital) and Cranial Bones Expand
       Active: Pituitary
       Inactive: Excretory System
    6. Active: Liver
       Inactive: Gallbladder
    7. Increase of Blood to Muscles (Prostate, Uterus, Vagina) Decrease to the other Internal Organs
    8. Body Muscles Relax (reach threshold)
    9. Active: Pineal Gland

The state of health, sympathetic or parasympathetic stress, disease, emotional injury and diet has a direct effect on the sex glands and organs, and the sex response. When an organ has a problem or hormonal imbalances, it can cause a person to avoid a step in the sex response. Sex Hormone imbalance can be caused by physical stress, excessive exercise, over working and inadequate nutrition. Sex stimulants can cause an acidic state, sympathetic stress, and hormone imbalance. There is a social tendency to focus only on Part 1 of the Sympathetic Nerves phase of sex and ignore Part 2. The high level of male and female masturbation adds to the focus on Part 1 of sex. All these factors weaken the ability to experience Part 2 and to allow the sensation to be holistic. Disease organs can get weaker if they are drained of nutrients caused by excessive sex stimulation (i.e.=, sex songs, talk about sex, sex in movies, pornographic visuals and audios, or sexual intercourse). Consequently, Regenerative Sex non-climaxing, non-ejaculatory sex needs to be used to promote healing.

Rhythm Theory

Age x .2 = Frequency of ejaculation in days.
For example a person 40 years old would need 8 days between ejaculation (40 x .2 = 8). This would allow nutrients to be replenished, and sperm to mature. If less days between ejaculations then increase amounts of supplements are needed.

Metabolic Sexual Intercourse Factors
Increase Fatty Acid activity (dysaerobic) in males.
Increase sterols (anaerobic) in females.
Changes are made on the organism level, pH, pulse, temperature, blood pressure, hormones, vitamins, enzyme and mineral levels.
Females, in general, have a higher percentage of positive lipids than males.
Females are anaerobic; males are dysaerobic.

Sexual Response Time

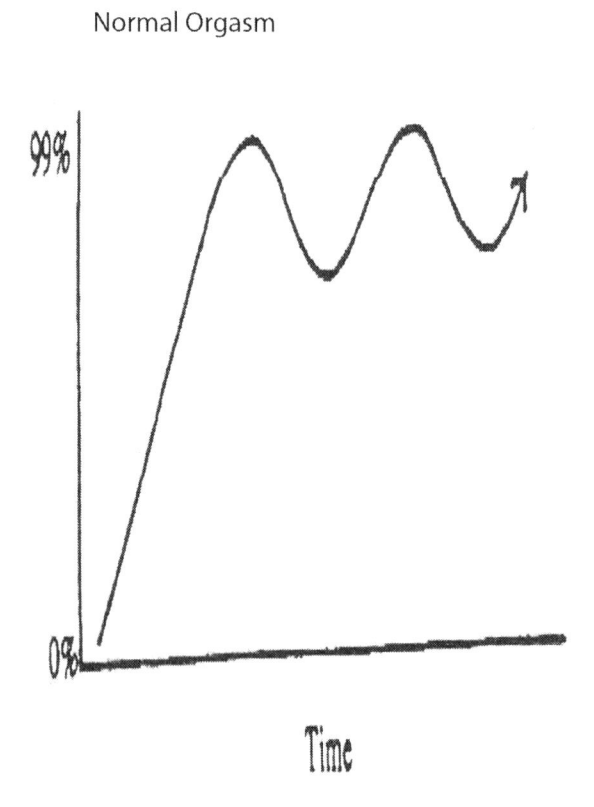

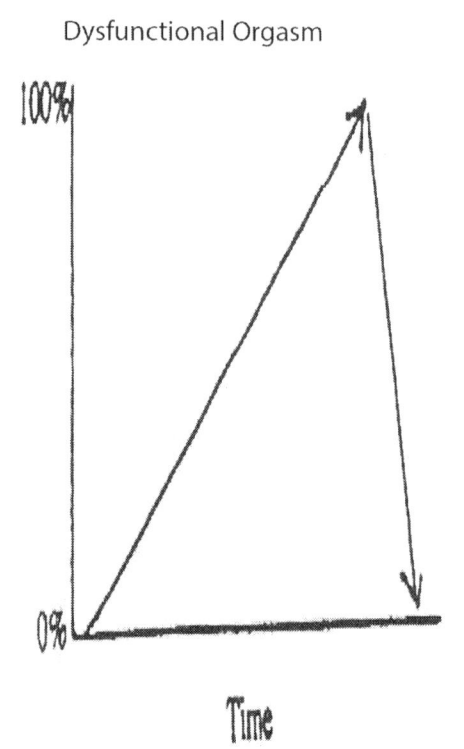

Normal Orgasm

Dysfunctional Orgasm

Dysfunctional Orgasm
It is usually caused by sympathetic stress, acidity, hormonal imbalance, and/or sex organ problems.

Intercourse Position

These positions are considered ideal for sperm delivery into the uterus.

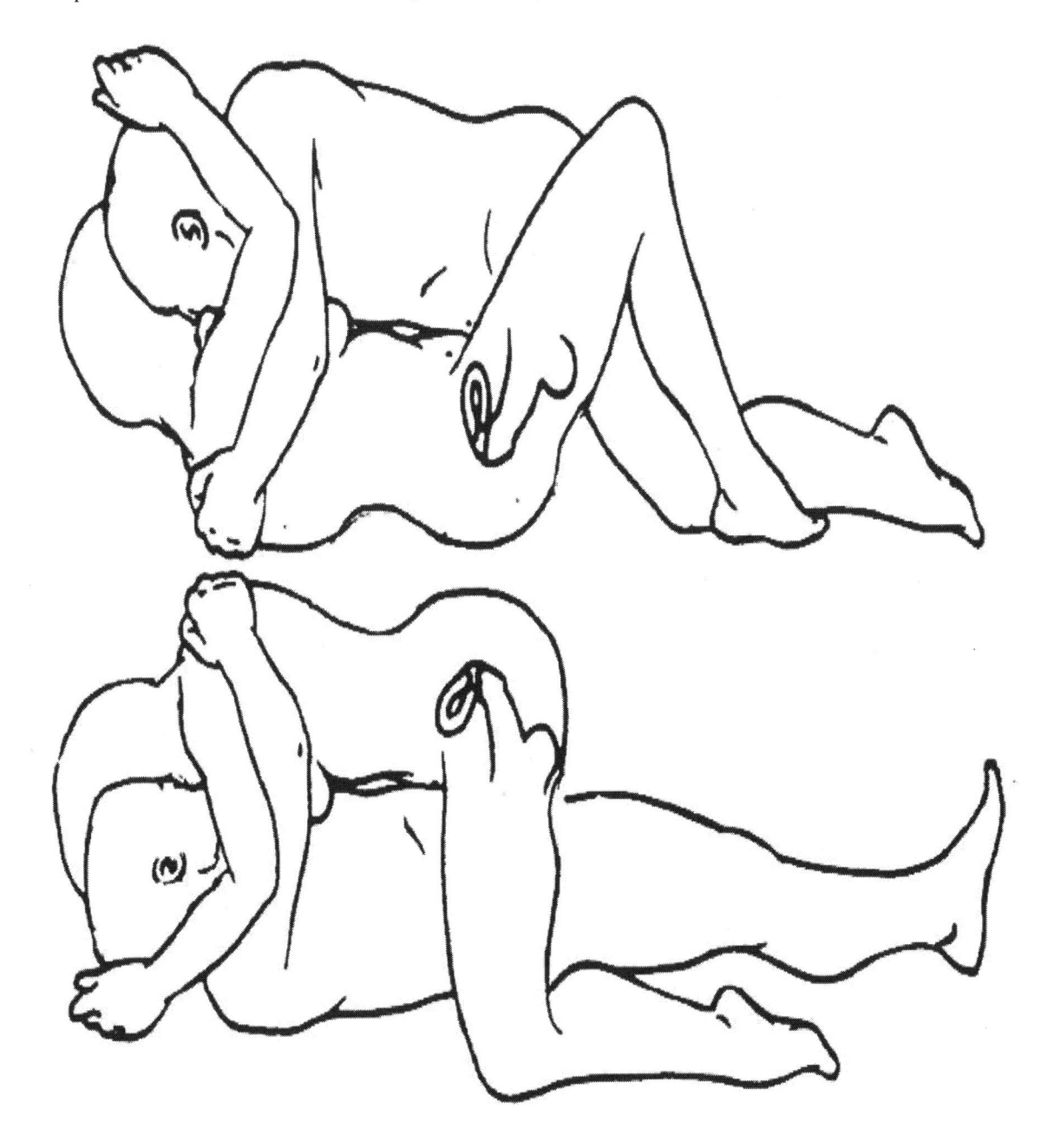

Types of Sexual Intercourse Positions

A variety of sexual positions should be used to avoid energy nutrient draining and quick ejaculation climaxes. The variety of positions sustains sex pleasure and helps achieve Holdbacks. Sexual activity can be prolonged when you use positions you do not like and/or a variety of positions are used.

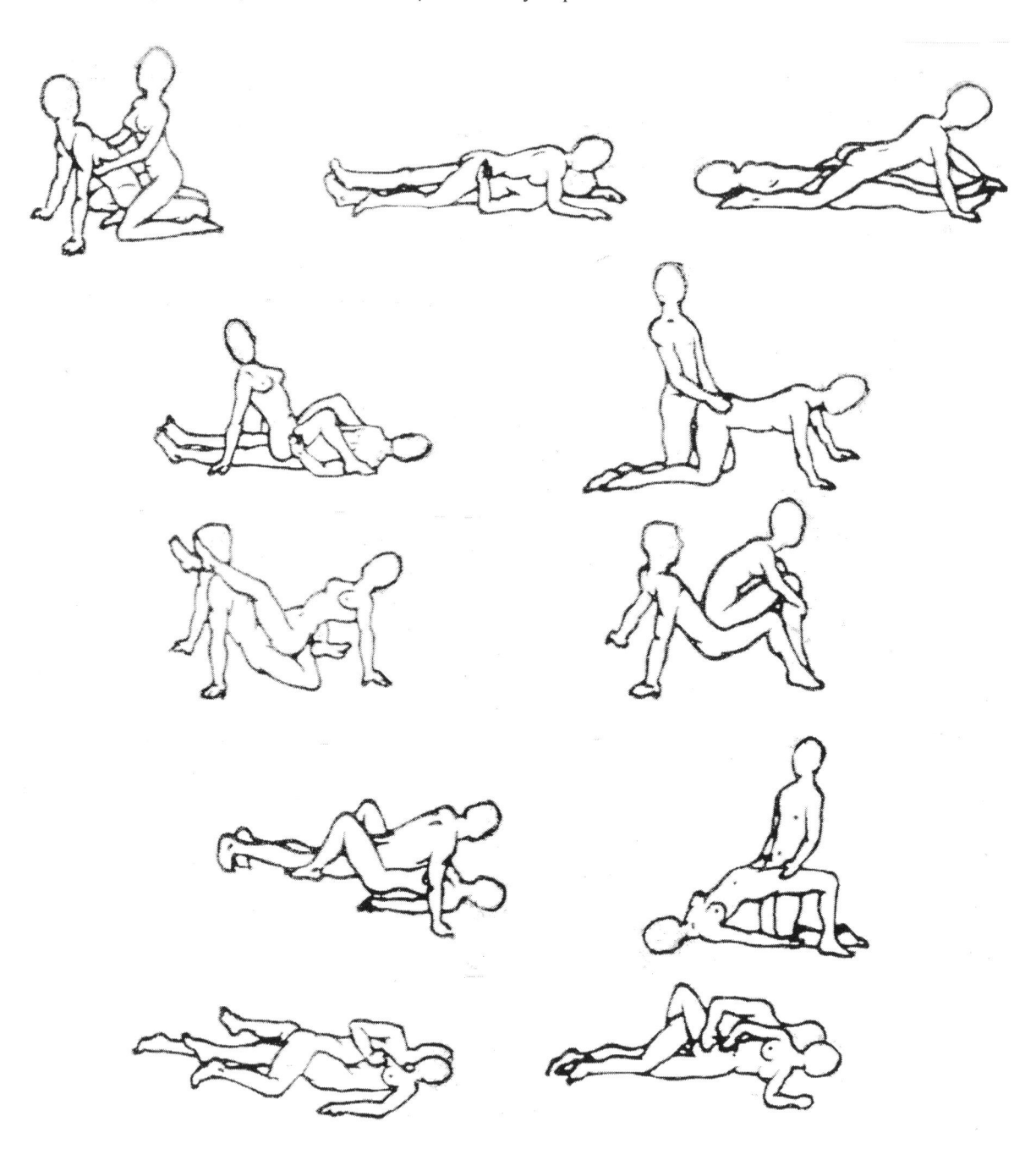

Sex Response

- Lips of vagina
  - Labia Majora, opens, flattens (erect and flattens)
  - Labia Minora, extends (erect like)
- Urethra (tissue around base gets erect)
- Clitoris get Erect
- Cervix (neck of uterus) gets erect and engorged with fluid
- Penis gets erect
- Hair on back gets erect (male and female)
- The upper part of labia, base of urethra, upper part of cervix become very pleasing when stimulated (erogenous)
- Breast Swell
- Dark area around nipples get darker and larger
- Vaginal Shaft gets longer (erect like)
- Vagina moves upward, small cup is formed to hold sperm at opening of uterus
- The thrusting action of penis rubbing against the vagina muscles causes the uterus to slightly swing back and forward. This tends to slightly stretch the ligaments that suspend the uterus. After sex the uterus ligaments rebound shorten to there inactive state causing orgasmic sensation to sustain
- Frenulum (on underside of the penis) triggers perineum, prostate and urethra to pulsate and contract. Frenulum in females is where the labia attaches to clitoris.
- Skin gets highly sensitive
- Orgasm sensation spread into the labia, vagina, clitoris, uterus, sex organs, and hip areas.
- Skin of labia darkens indicating orgasmic level
- Orgasm
  - Foreskin darkens
  - Lips of vagina darken
- Climax Plateau
  - Clitoris shortens, lifts, too sensitive to touch
  - Vagina contracts
  - Larger lips (Majora) swell
- Anus sphincter muscle closes
- After play
  - Close hugging and caressing
- After Orgasm
  - 30 minutes to 1 hour to return back to normal
  - The female's uterus ligaments, muscles of the vagina erectile tissue of the clitoris, cervix, labia's, and uterus vibrate as it returns to the normal state. This action tends to sustain the orgasm pleasure.
  - Area around nipples get small, nipples stay big

Sex Organs and Your Body

- Nose close to eyes = Long vagina shaft / Long penis
- Nose far from eyes = Short vagina shaft / Short penis
- Narrow cheeks and jaw = Small sex organs
- Deep lines at mouth = Strong sex feelings
- Few lashes on lower eyelid = Mild sex feelings
- Few hairs and / or small amount of hair around sex organs = Sexual control
- Wet mouth while talking = Easily aroused
- Tongue = Associated with clitoris / penis

The distance from the heel of a person's hand to the tip of the fourth finger is the approximate length of that person's erect penis / or erect vagina.

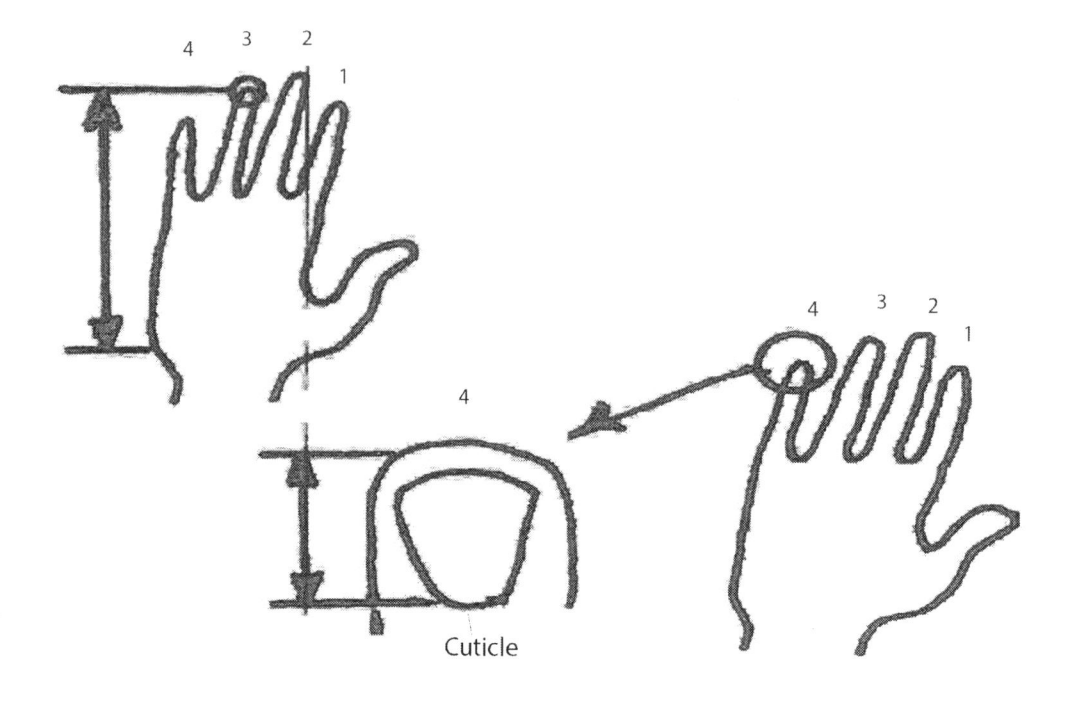

On the female's hand the distance from the cuticle of the small fourth finger to the fingertip is the approximate length of that female's erect clitoris.

Female Hormones and Glands

The female's hormones and glands are interconnected. The glands and hormones act and react to each other. A gland that is weak or stressed causes the gland above it or below it to COMPENSTATE. For example, a weak Pituitary gland secretes a decreased amount of Follicle Stimulating Hormone (FSH) and Lutein Hormone (LH), which cause a low sperm count and sperm that does not have enough movement (motility). A weaken Pituitary decreased FSH and LH can cause infertility in women. The Hypothalamus, Pituitary, and Adrenal Gland (HPA) circuit acts and reacts to physical, emotional, and behavioral changes. The Hypothalamus stalk is connected to the Pituitary that is located beneath it. When the Hypothalamus reacts to stress it signals that the Pituitary, then the Pituitary signals the Adrenals to secrete Adrenaline/Epinephrine (Fight/Flight). This chain reaction causes the sex hormones to decrease its reproductive hormones (Estrogen, Progesterone). After the stress episode is over the Morphine-like oxytocin is needed to relax the body.

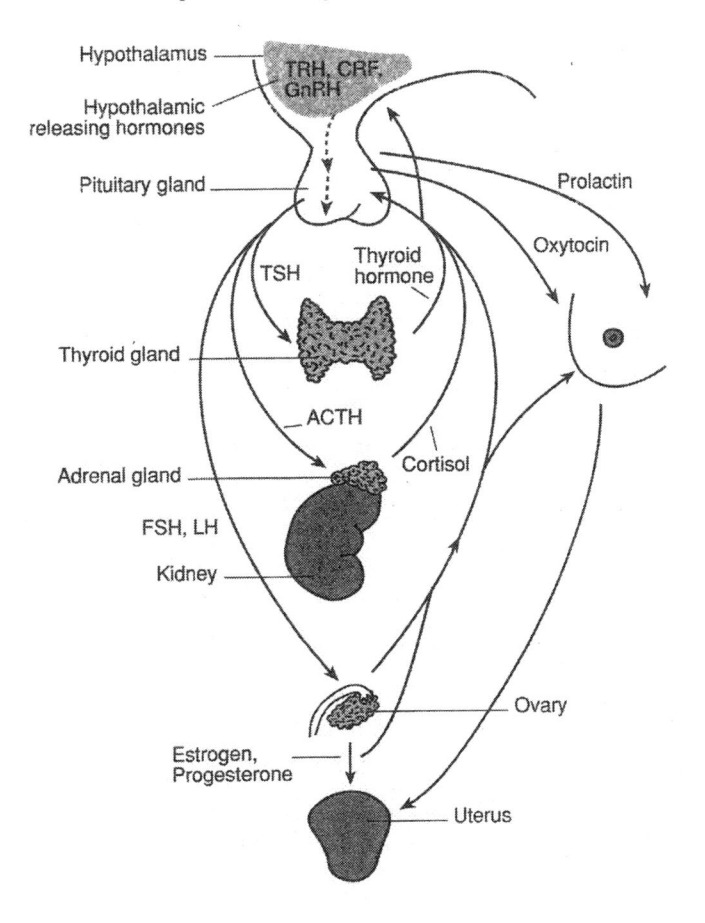

TRH- Thyroid Releasing Hormone
CRF- Corticotrophin Releasing Hormone
GnRH- Gonadotropin Releasing Hormone
TSH- Thyroid Stimulating Hormone
ACTH- Adrenocorticotrophic Hormone
FSH- Follicle Stimulating Hormone
LH- Luteinizing Hormone

Fibroid Tumor

The Eyes Iris in the lower portion can appear a partial, slight, or large teardrop slightly darkens shape. This can indicate pregnancy or an enlarged prostate or a fibroid tumor. If the female is pregnant the teardrop in the left eye indicates a girl, while the right eye indicates a boy.

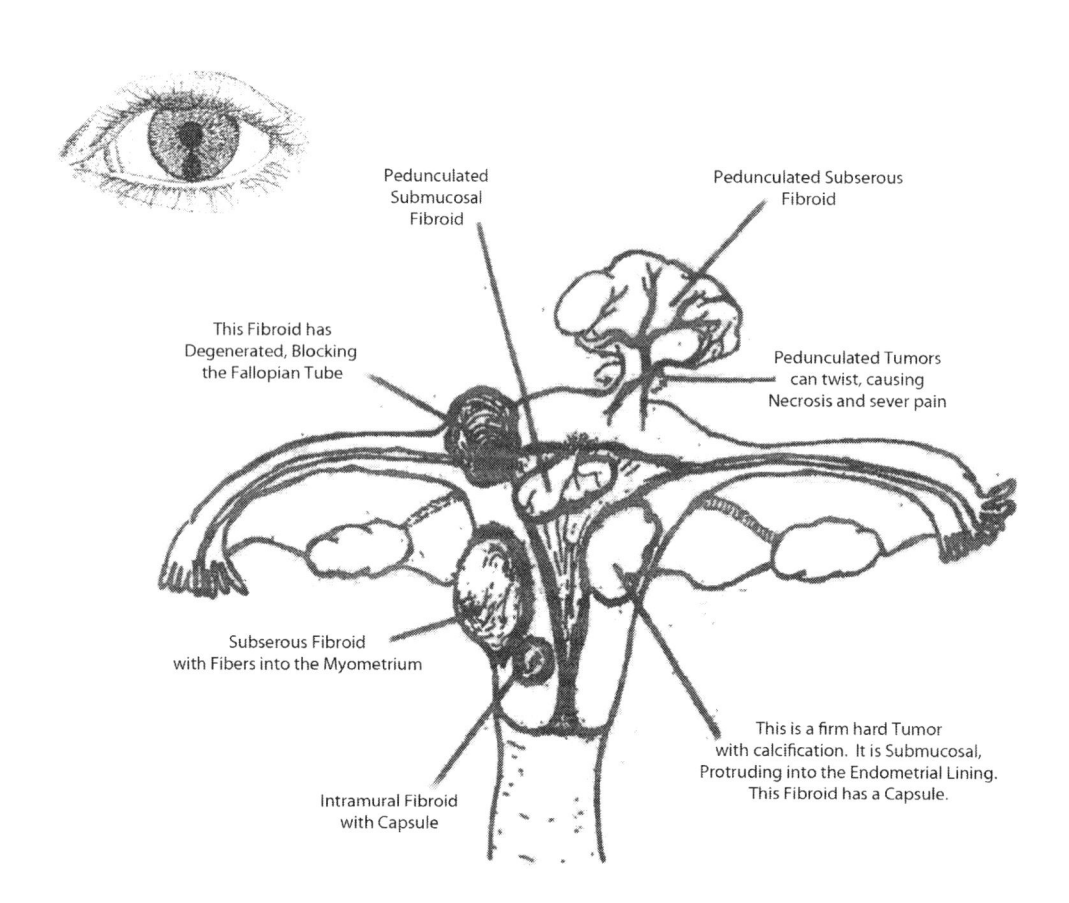

- Pedunculated Submucosal Fibroid
- Pedunculated Subserous Fibroid
- This Fibroid has Degenerated, Blocking the Fallopian Tube
- Pedunculated Tumors can twist, causing Necrosis and sever pain
- Subserous Fibroid with Fibers into the Myometrium
- This is a firm hard Tumor with calcification. It is Submucosal, Protruding into the Endometrial Lining. This Fibroid has a Capsule.
- Intramural Fibroid with Capsule

Female Warning Signs for Cancer

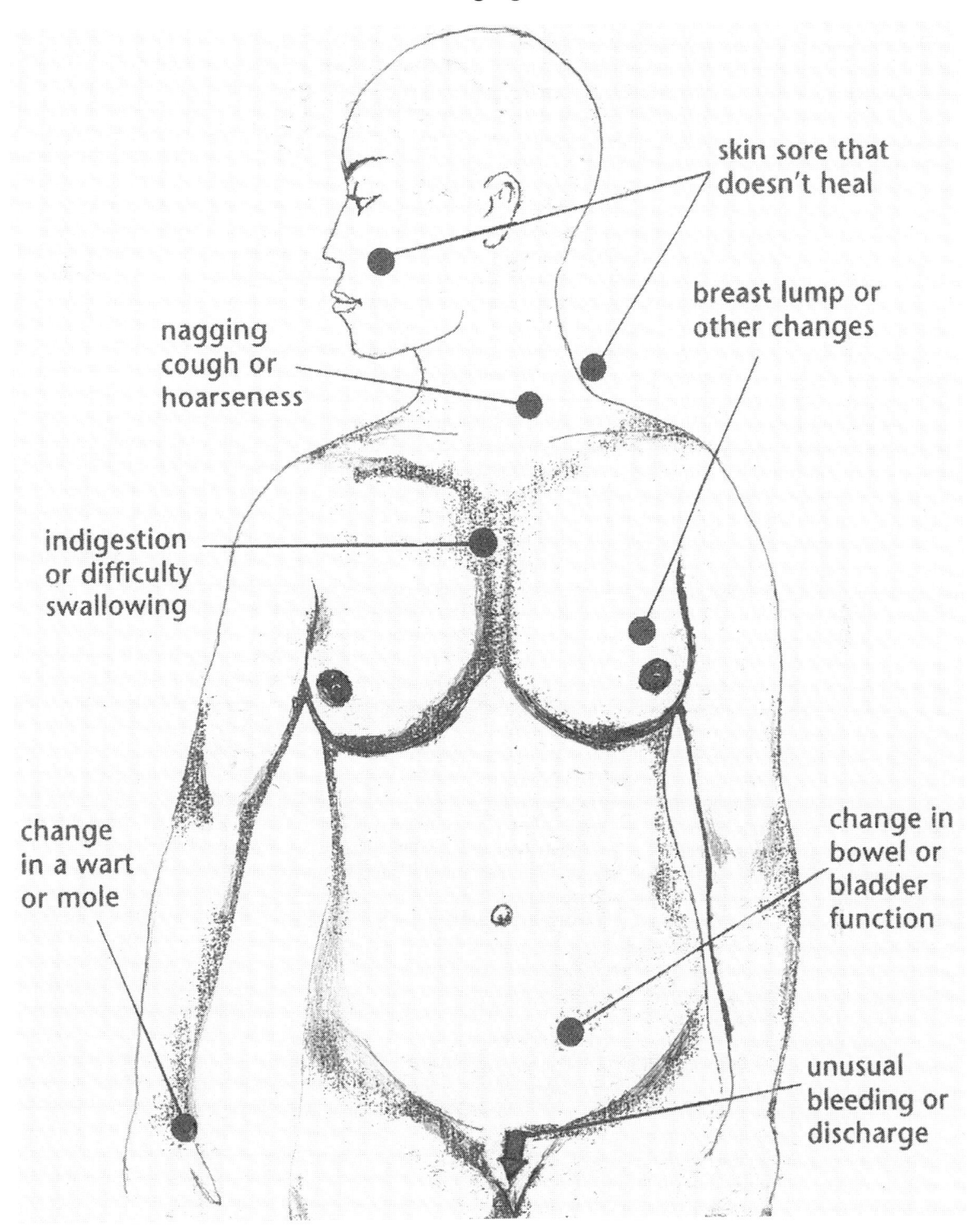

- skin sore that doesn't heal
- breast lump or other changes
- nagging cough or hoarseness
- indigestion or difficulty swallowing
- change in a wart or mole
- change in bowel or bladder function
- unusual bleeding or discharge

Enlarge Prostate

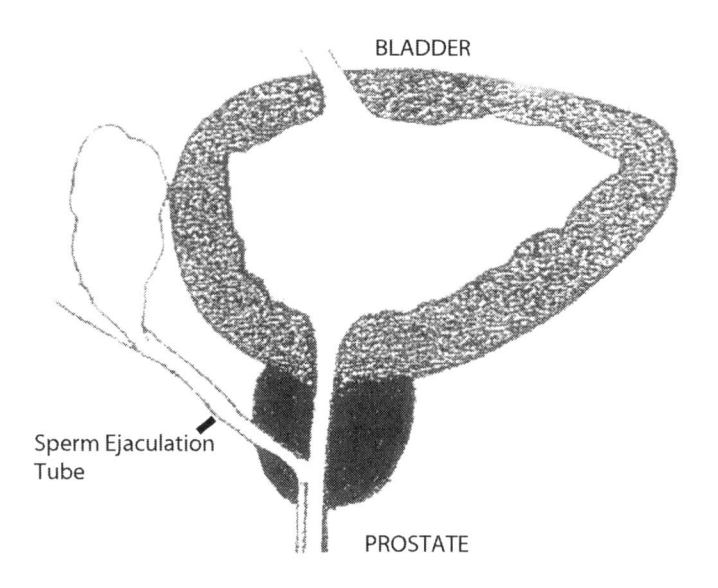

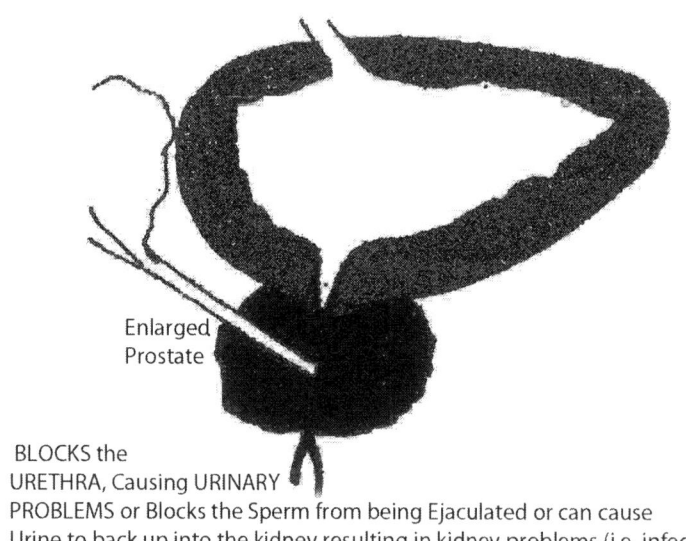

BLADDER

Sperm Ejaculation Tube

PROSTATE

Enlarged Prostate

BLOCKS the URETHRA, Causing URINARY PROBLEMS or Blocks the Sperm from being Ejaculated or can cause Urine to back up into the kidney resulting in kidney problems (i.e. infection).

Female Sexual Process (6 Erections)

Sexual process starts hormonally and then the uterus, vagina, labia, and clitoris move from inactive to active. The sexual arousal is emotional and physical. The hormone oxytocin (morphine-like hormone) causes the desire to bond. The larger lips (labia) on the outside get erect and clasp the penis. The inner lips (labia) get flat and erect widening the opening of the vagina. The erectile tissue around the urethra get erect and bulge down into the vagina creating an erogenous area, the vagina gets erect and longer. The neck of the uterus (cervix) gets erect and the uterus tilts forward, and the clitoris gets erect. The neck of the uterus and vagina fills with fluid and lubrication to the uterus and vagina increases. The muscles of the vagina start to contract and relax which stimulates the penis.

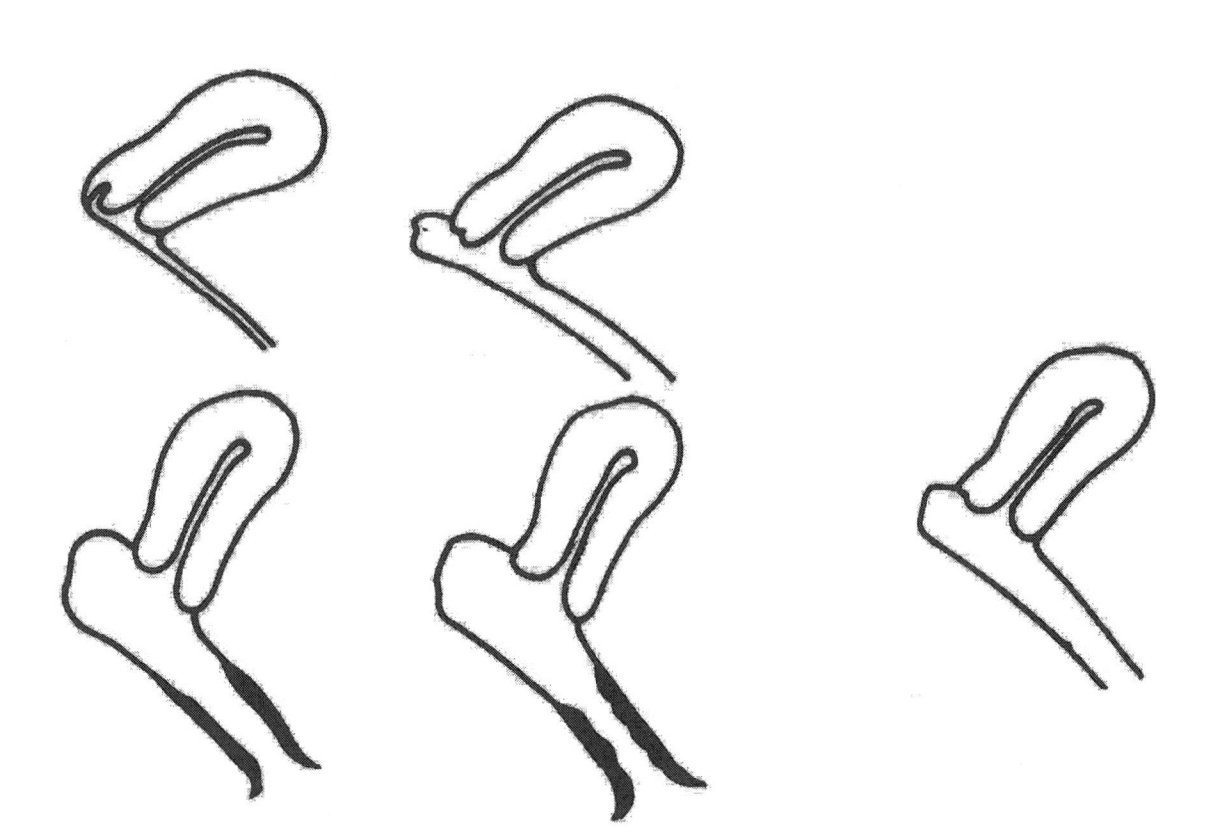

Uterus and Vagina

Vagina Organ Zones

If one area stimulated is more non-pleasing or pleasing than another area or the skin is inconsistent, and feels uncomfortable this can indicate problems with the organ in the vagina organ zone.

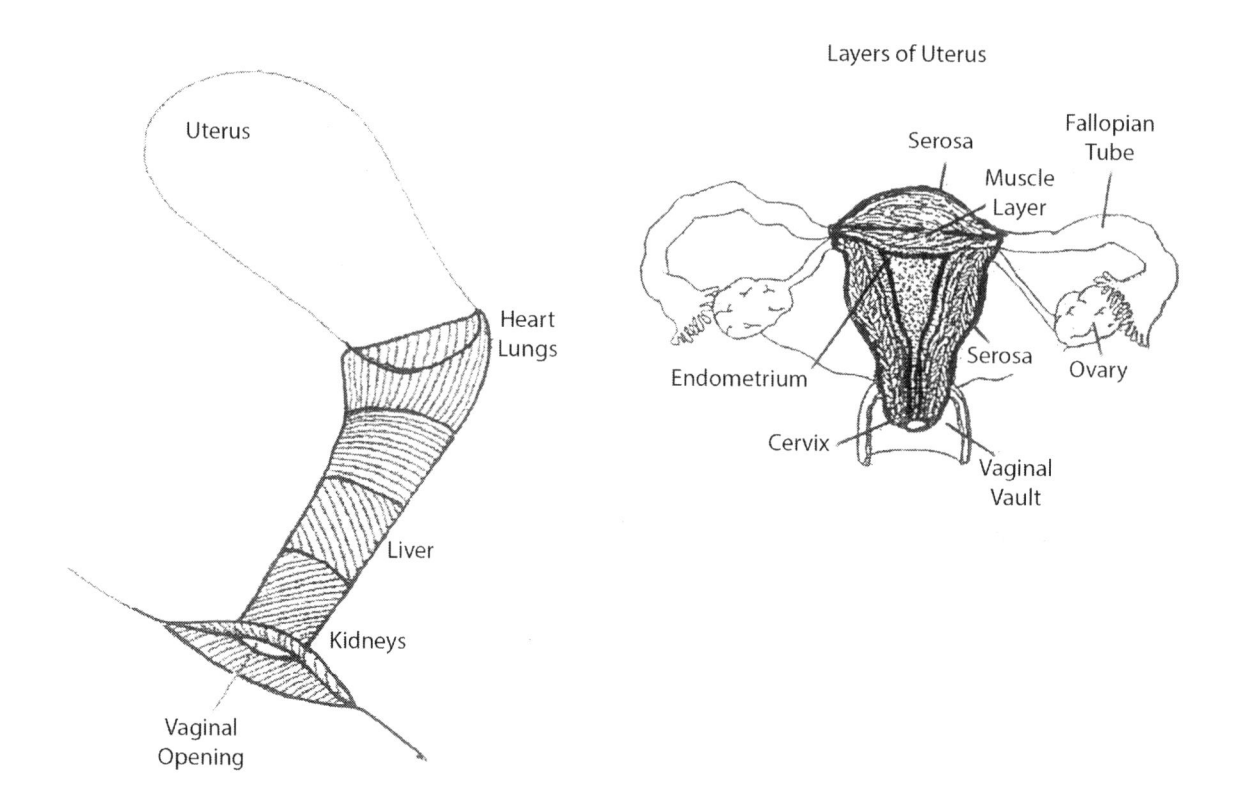

Zodiac Vagina and Acupressure Points

Each woman has nerves in and around the vagina that cluster more in one area (Acupressure Meridian) than another. The numbers surrounding the vagina are similar to the houses of the Zodiac. If the nerve cluster area (House of the Zodiac) has skin that is inconsistent, irritable, uncomfortable, or too sensitive it indicates a problem with the organ associated with that house. The hair surrounding the vagina can be inconsistent (grey in area, long, thin, thick, and short) it indicates a health problem in the Zodiac sign.

The nerve clusters are different in each woman resulting in different sexual pleasurable areas. This creates a physical and emotional sexual personality similar to the Zodiac sign that has the nerve cluster.

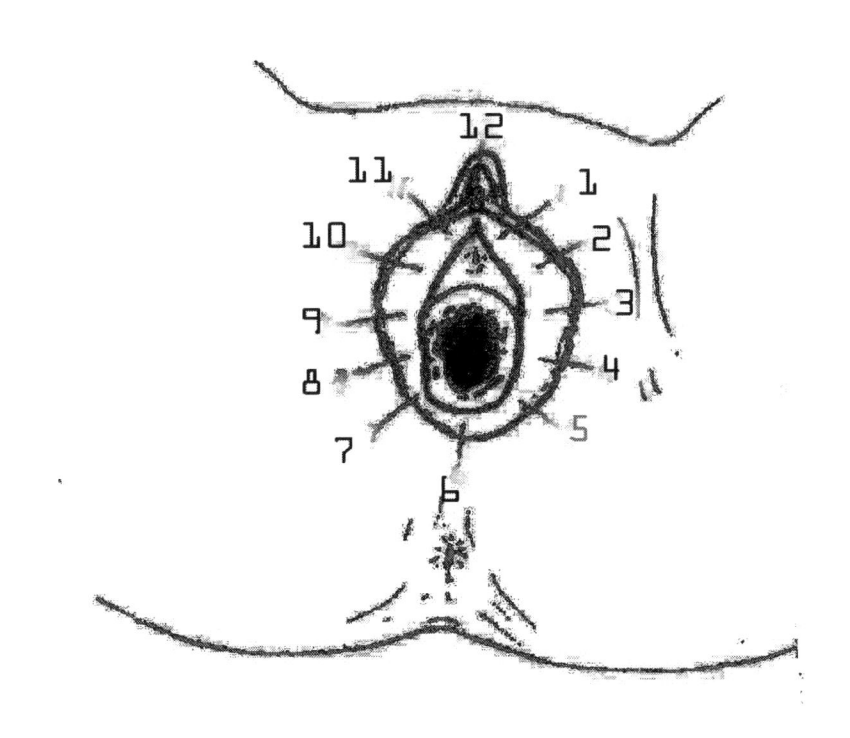

Breast Shape

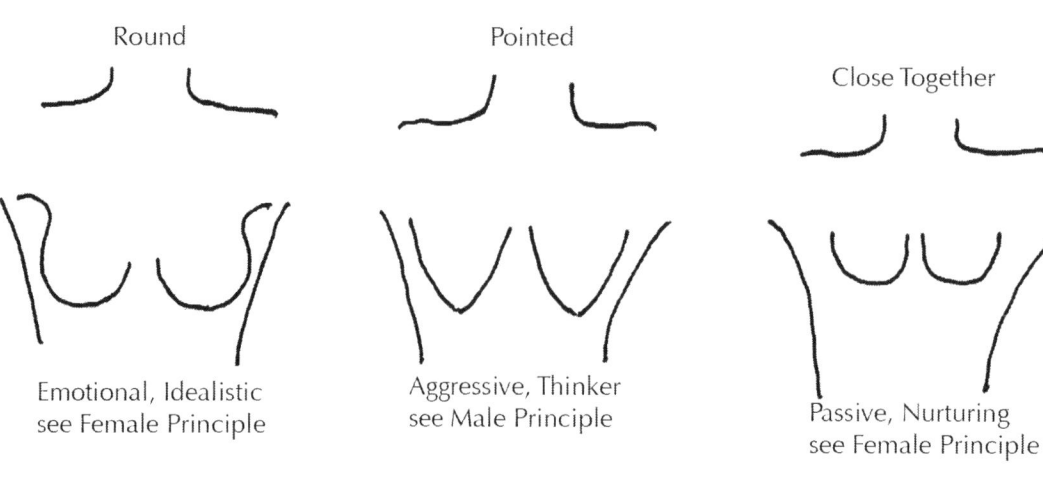

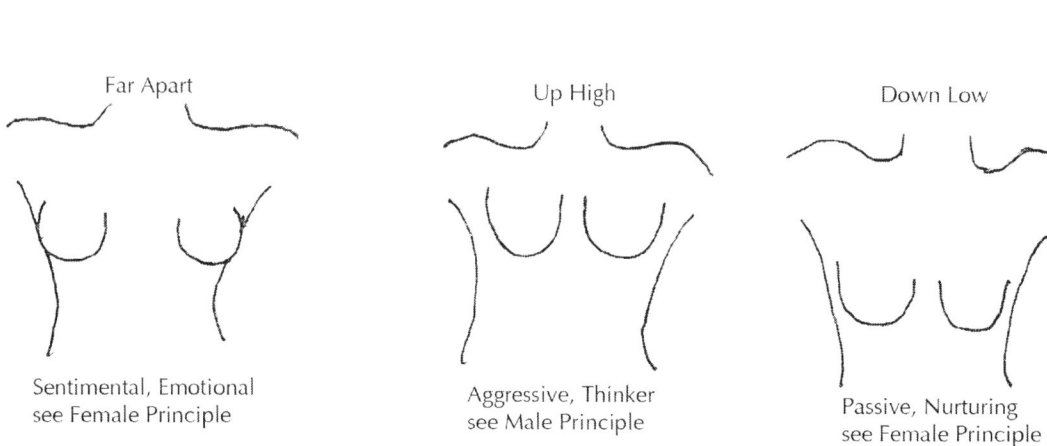

Round
Emotional, Idealistic
see Female Principle

Pointed
Aggressive, Thinker
see Male Principle

Close Together
Passive, Nurturing
see Female Principle

Far Apart
Sentimental, Emotional
see Female Principle

Up High
Aggressive, Thinker
see Male Principle

Down Low
Passive, Nurturing
see Female Principle

Breast Areola

Areola circular dark area around the nipple corresponds to the Zodiac Houses. The entire breast also corresponds to the Zodiac. Any inconsistency of the skin, light or dark area, long hair in an area, or noncircular shape in an area of hair growth on the areola can indicates problems with an organ or part of the body. Breast lumps in a house can indicate the cause of the lump.

Zodiac Sign	Related Body Part
1. Aires	Head, face, cerebrum, eyes, nose, pituitary
2. Taurus	Neck, throat, cerebellum, mouth, thyroid, vocal cords
3. Gemini	Arms, shoulders, lungs, fallopian tubes
4. Cancer	Stomach, breast, arteries, diaphragm, uterus, veins
5. Leo	Cardiac region, spleen, heart
6. Virgo	Small intestine, pancreas, lower abdomen
8. Scorpio	Small of back, adrenals, kidneys, bladder
9. Sagittarius	Pelvis, reproductive organs, gonads, colon, rectum
10. Capricorn	Knees, bones, gallbladder, teeth, cartilage
11. Aquarius	Calves, ankles, bladder, retina of eyes, parathyroid
12. Pisces	Feet, circulation, lymphatic system

Breast Exam While Standing

Perform breast self-examination by feeling the breast with the hand flat and the fingers flatten together. Do not pinch bits of tissue between the thumb and forefinger. Do the examination during a bath or a shower when the hands glide over the wet soapy skin. Move your hand over every part of the breast and feel for hard knots, lumps or thickening. Use the right hand to examine the left breast. Feel the entire area from the middle of your chest to central part of the breast to the middle of the side of your body and the armpits. Become familiar with your breast. Identify one or two particular milk glands and then identify them again on another exam. This makes it easier to recognize a change in the anatomy of the breast.

Areola   Zodiac House Circle

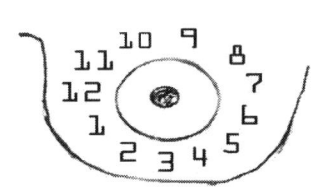

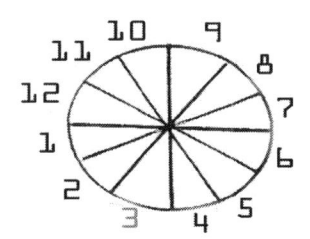

Breast

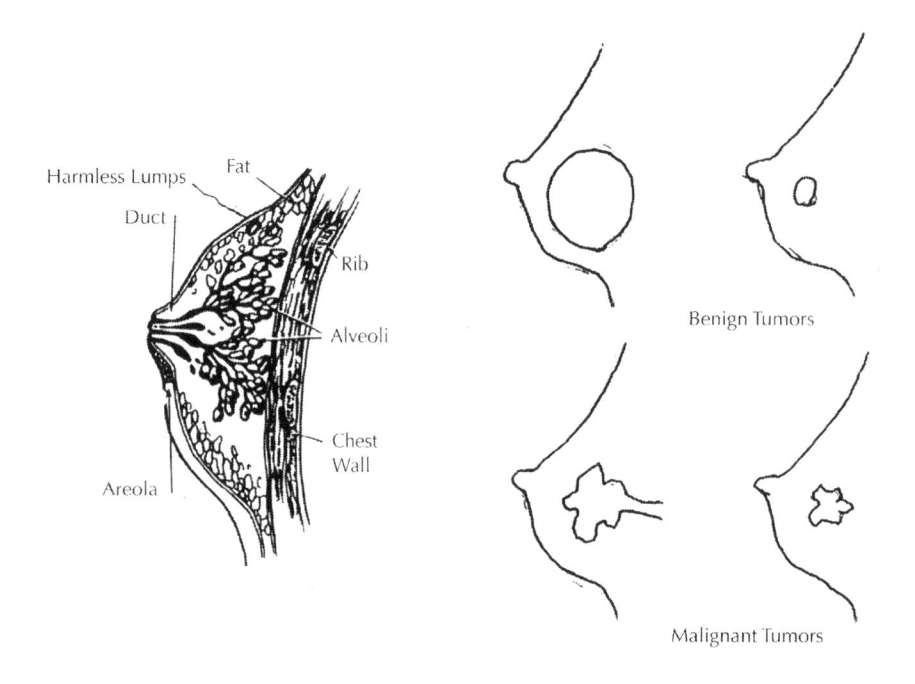

Penis / Organ relationship

If one area is more pleasing when stimulated than another area, or if the skin is inconsistent (color, texture, dry, etc.) this can indicate problems with that organ in that area.

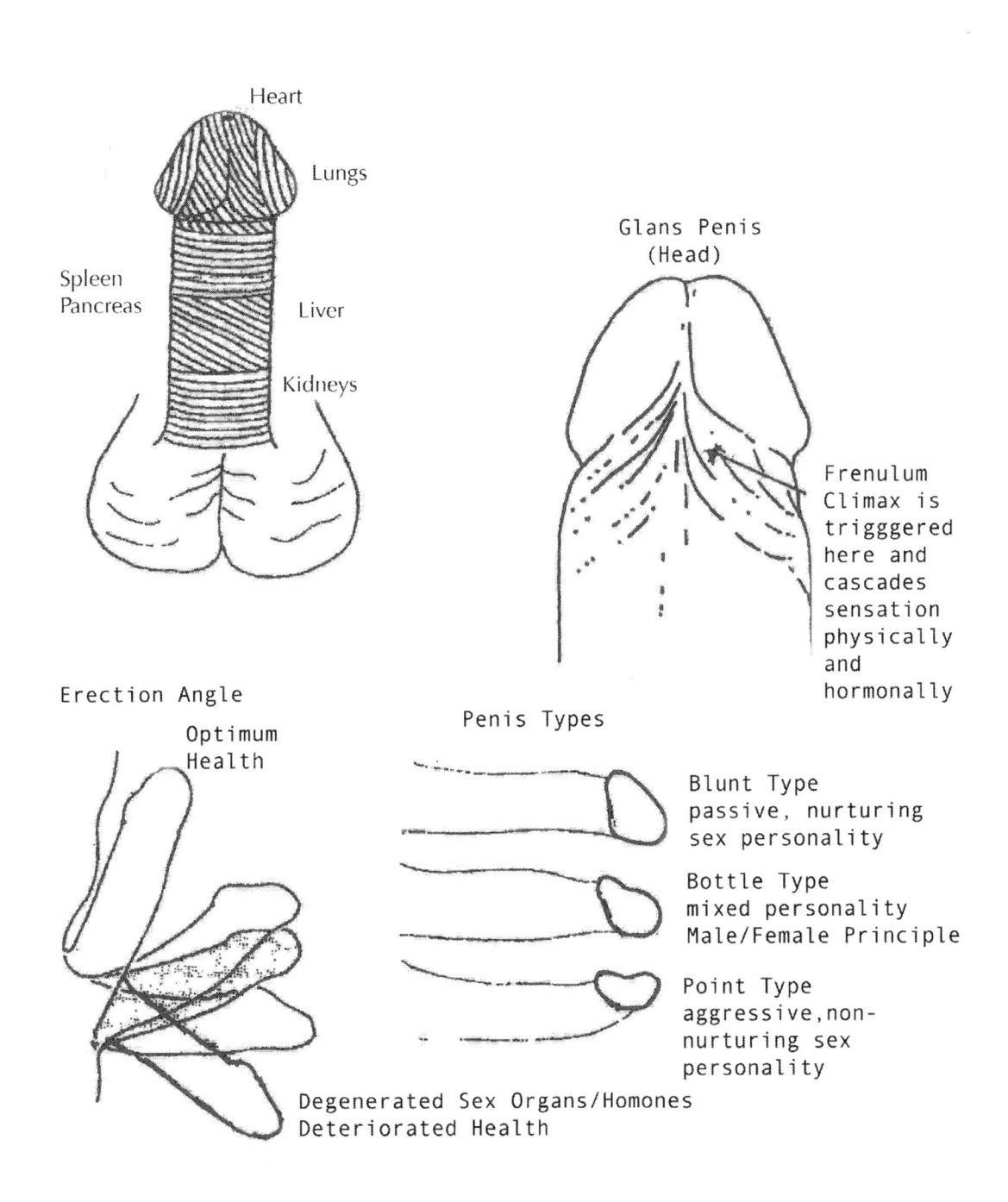

Heart
Lungs
Spleen Pancreas
Liver
Kidneys

Glans Penis (Head)

Frenulum Climax is trigggered here and cascades sensation physically and hormonally

Erection Angle
Optimum Health

Penis Types

Blunt Type
passive, nurturing sex personality

Bottle Type
mixed personality
Male/Female Principle

Point Type
aggressive, non-nurturing sex personality

Degenerated Sex Organs/Homones
Deteriorated Health

Penis and Testicles Sexual Process

1. Excitement Levels:
    Sex stimulates the Frenulum, which triggers an automatic reflex; this sends blood flowing into the spongy tissue of the penis. The spongy mass swells and presses against the sheath of the skin. This causes the penis to become stiff and sticks out at an angle from the body pointing upward. Muscular contraction pulls the testes closer into the body. This stage can be maintained for long periods or can sporadically decrease or increase without orgasm, several times.

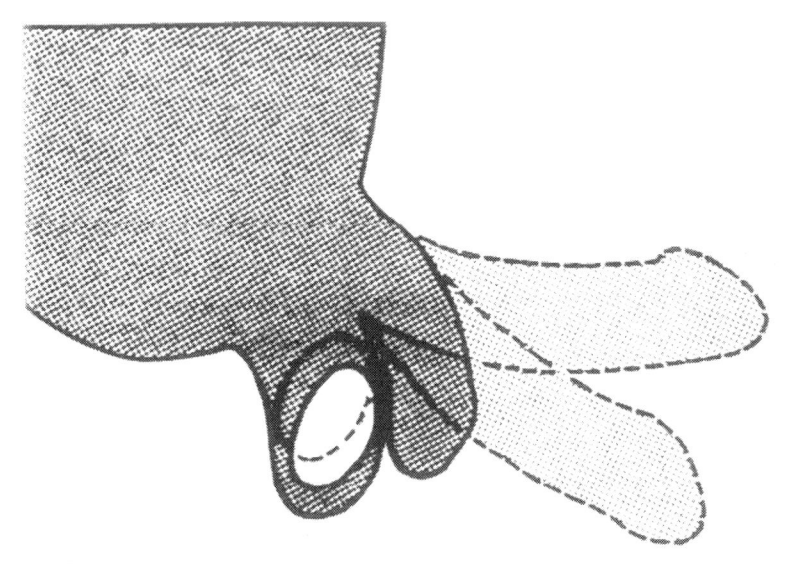

2. Plateau Level
    The testes are drawn closer to the body. The penis increases slightly in diameter, near the tip, and the opening in the tip becomes more slit- like. The tip itself may change color, to a deeper purple.

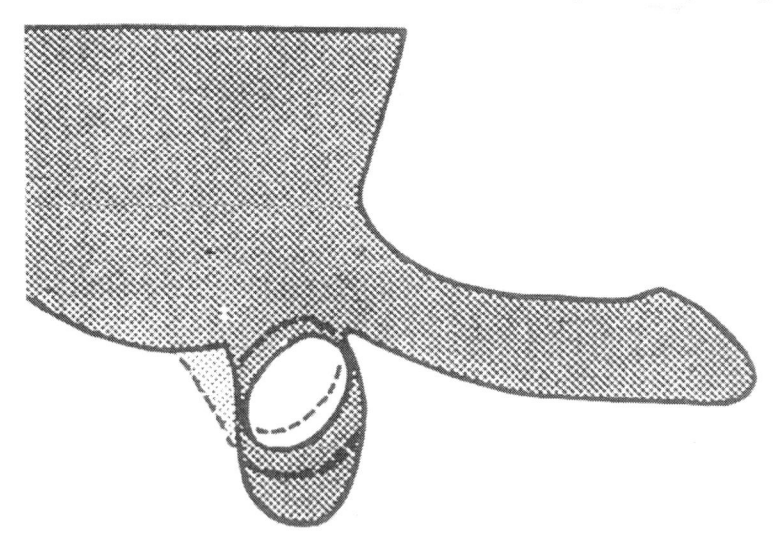

3. Resolution
   Often there is first a very rapid reduction in penis size to about 50% larger than its normal state; followed by a slower reduction back to normal. Each of the stages can be prolonged (if the penis remains inserted in the female genitals).

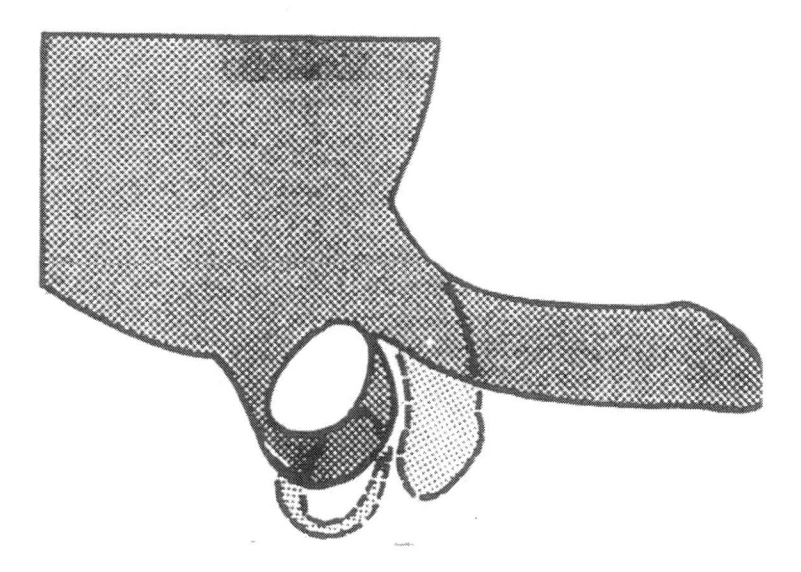

4. The muscles around the urethra give a number of rapid involuntary contractions. This causes semen to be ejaculated out of the penis with force. There are usually three or four major bursts of semen, one every 0-8 seconds, followed by weaker, more irregular, muscular contractions.

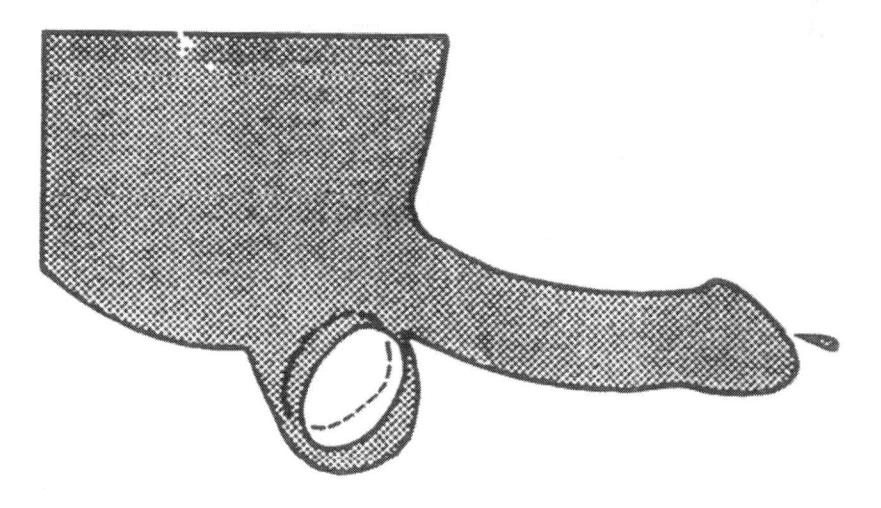

Reduce Sexual Arousal

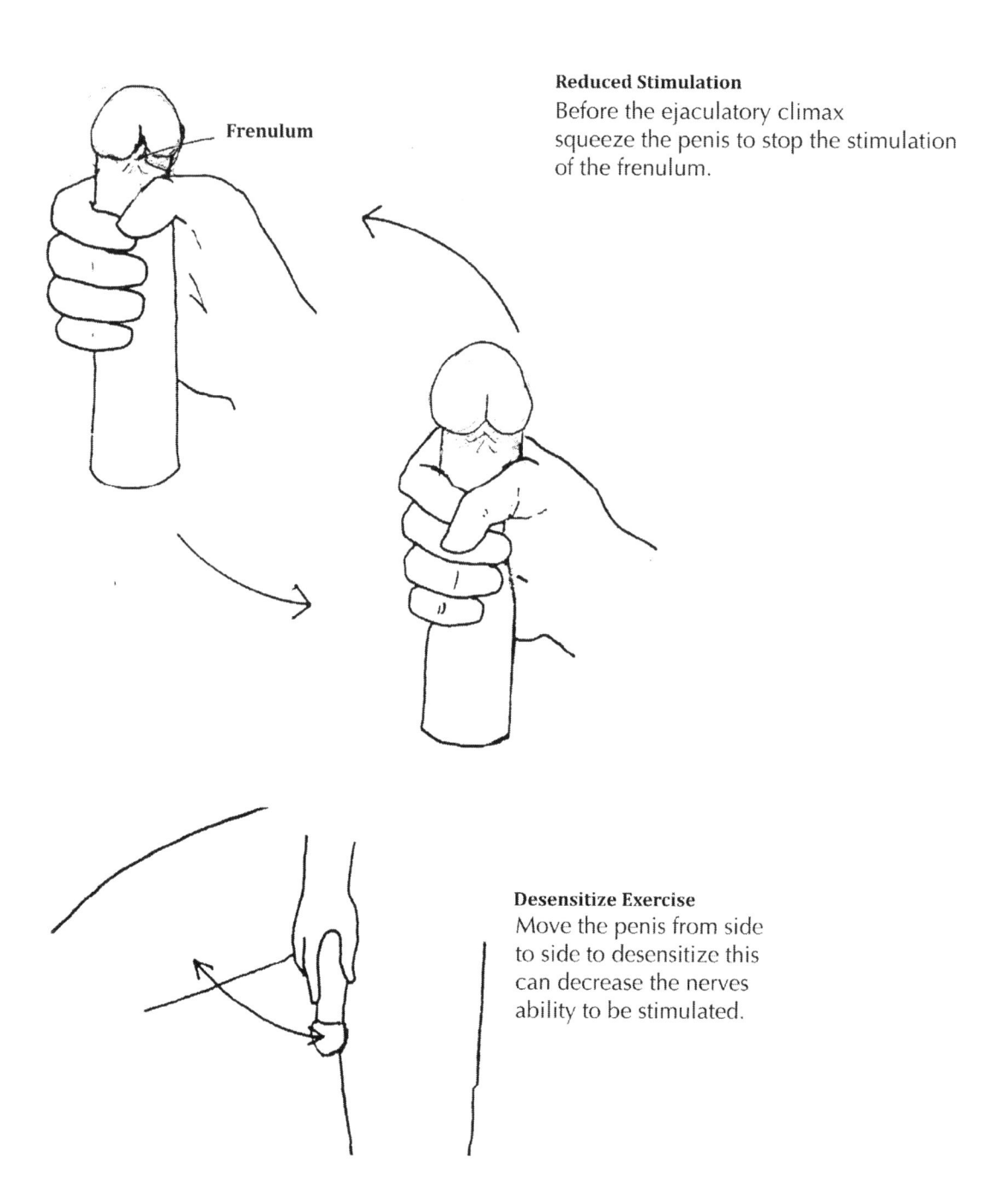

Frenulum

Reduced Stimulation
Before the ejaculatory climax squeeze the penis to stop the stimulation of the frenulum.

Desensitize Exercise
Move the penis from side to side to desensitize this can decrease the nerves ability to be stimulated.

Inguinal Hernia

Inguinal hernias are a soft mass of a bulging of the intestines through the inguinal within or just above the scrotum. A hernia is part of an organ or a part of tissue that has protruded through another tissue (of the inguinal). Usually, an inguinal hernia is caused by a portion of a bowel (intestines) that has slipped into the inguinal canal.

Approximately a month before birth, the testicles of the male fetus are located in the abdomen. The testicles descend into the scrotum. This occurs before or shortly after birth. Once it creates an opening and the testicles descend, the passage close. When the inguinal canals do not close completely. This creates weak tissue in the abdominal wall. Straining the muscles from lifting items, sexual intercourse, constipation, coughing can tear the abdominal wall tissue. This increases abdominal pressure causing the canal to tear and reopen resulting in a hernia. The bowels can get twisted in the hernia, pinch the blood supply and deteriorate the bowels and/or get them inflamed or swollen. The hands can be used to push back hernia through the inguinal, or standing on the toes and bouncing forcefully on the heels can lower the hernia.

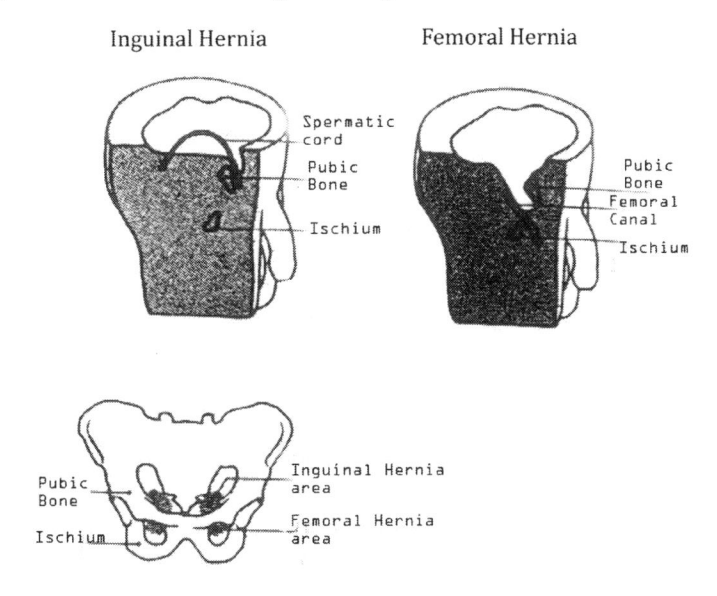

Test For Prostate

Test the prostate gland by palpating; insert your lubricated glove with index finger into the rectum. On the anterior (front) rectum wall (skin) slightly pass the anorectal (ring) then palpate the prostate. The gland should feel smooth, rubbery and is the size of a walnut.

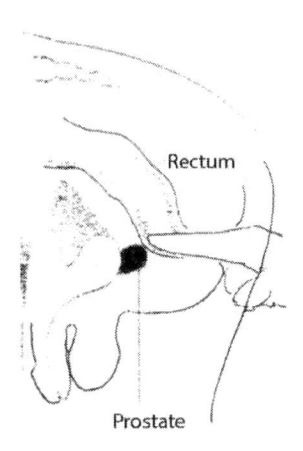

Sexual Energy Center (Acupuncture Meridian Point)

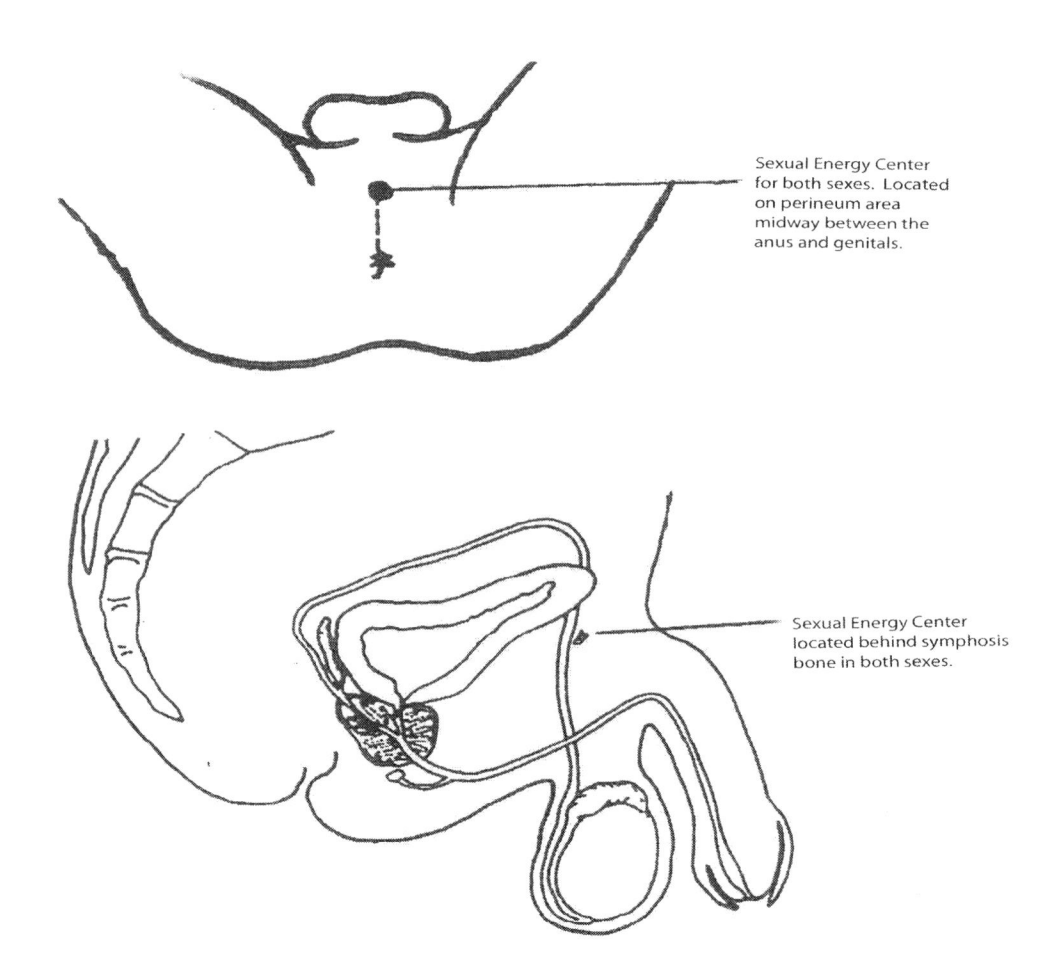

Sexual Energy Center for both sexes. Located on perineum area midway between the anus and genitals.

Sexual Energy Center located behind symphosis bone in both sexes.

Two Mineral Imbalances Which Can Weaken Sex Organs
- Sodium to potassium ratio of less than 6= emotional inhibitions.
- Sodium to potassium ratio of more than 6 = emotional aggressiveness.
  FEAR = Low sodium (inadequate sexual assertiveness)
  High potassium (excess sexual defensiveness)

Sexual Regeneration Orgasm

The reproductive system is weakening because of inadequate nutrition, and the lack of utilizing Sexual Regeneration (Part 2 of sex) to reach orgasm. Sex that is primarily focused on achieving orgasm and ejaculation causes the decline of the sex organs.

Sexual regeneration is using injaculation (Holdback the ejaculation) to achieve orgasm. The angle of the erect penis can indicate deterioration. The erection angle is the angle made by the penis and the torso.

Erection Angle (fingers represent penis angle)
The erection angle is the angle made by the penis and the torso.

Teens (about 45 degrees)

20's (about 60 degrees)

30's (about 90 degrees)

40's (about 105 degrees)

50's (about 135 degrees)

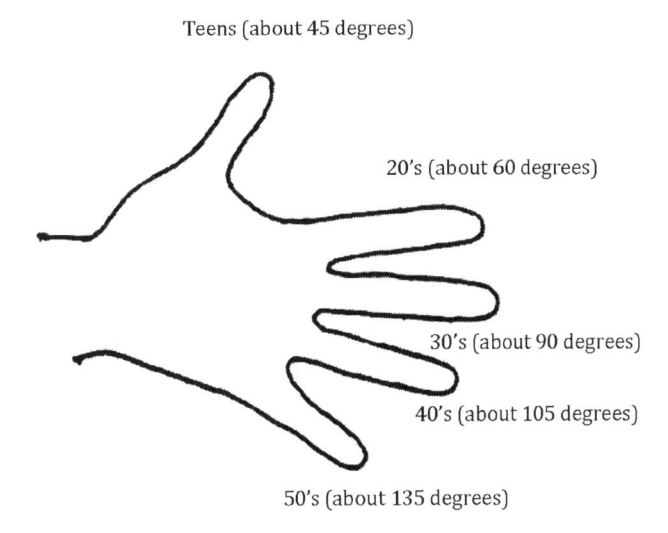

Young babies and boys (teens) sex organs are vital and have not deteriorated. Their erection angle can be 45 degrees. Men with weak or deteriorated sex hormones and organs angle can be 90 degrees to 135 degrees. They tend to have long hairs in the nose or ears. Women with weaken or deteriorated sex hormones and organs tend to have excessive or long hair around the mouth. Sex is a hormonal and nutritional activity. And, a decrease in either is indicated by the sexual degeneration.

Orgasm Chart

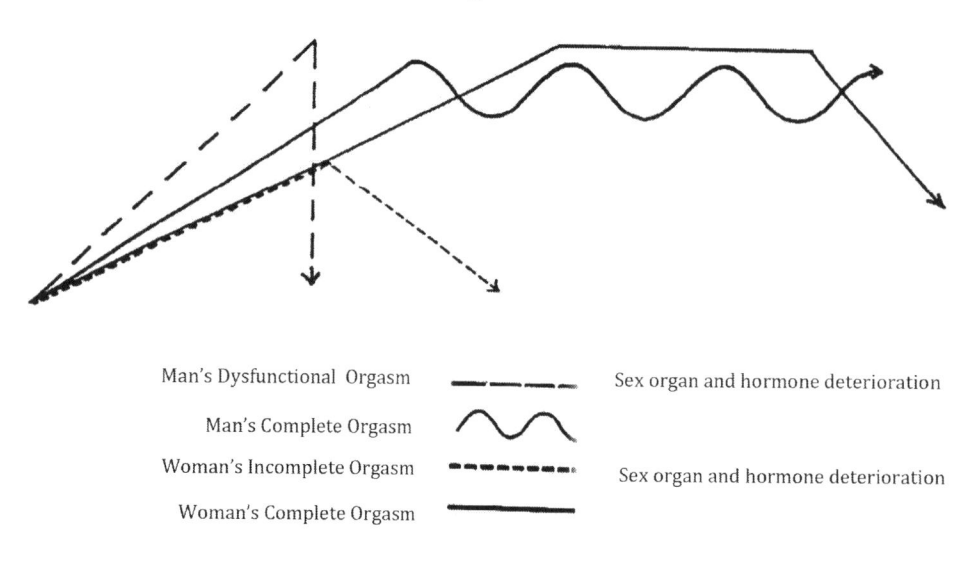

Man's Dysfunctional Orgasm — — — —   Sex organ and hormone deterioration
Man's Complete Orgasm ∿∿
Woman's Incomplete Orgasm ▪▪▪▪▪▪▪   Sex organ and hormone deterioration
Woman's Complete Orgasm ─────

Broken lines represents the woman's orgasm using Holdbacks

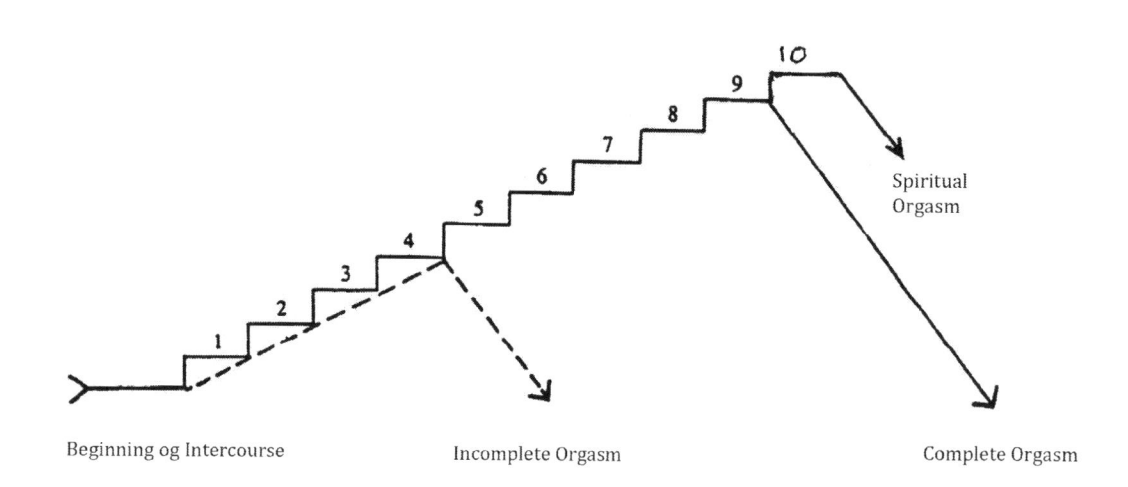

Beginning og Intercourse   Incomplete Orgasm   Complete Orgasm

Spiritual Orgasm

Sex Holdback Method

Holdback   **Benefits to the Body**

1. Strengthens and nourishes the body.
2. Strengthens the eyes and ears.
3. Strengthens the immune system, and lymphatic.
4. Strengthens and nourishes the internal organs.
5. Improves the circulatory and nervous system.
6. Nourishes bones and joints.
7. Develops a strong aura.
8. Heals all kinds of sickness.
9. The man and woman nourishes spirit and the Pineal Gland is stimulated.

The Holdback is achieved by not allowing the orgasmic feeling to reach a climax (women) and no climax causing ejaculation (men). Just before the sensation of climax or ejaculation is reached the sex activity must stop and the penis has to be removed from the vagina. During the pause of sexual activity a Prayer, Positive Affirmation, Poem, Song, or Talking can take place to allow time for the sexual excitement to calm down. This pause allows the Holdback sexual excitement to lessen and is needed before the sex act starts again. Each time there is a pause during sex that stops a climax and ejaculation is called a Holdback. Holdbacks are done in succession from 1 to 9. It may take some time before you can do more than 2 or more Holdbacks. You may want to start with 2 Holdbacks and work your way up to a succession of 12. Using various sexual positions that are different or that do not cause too much excitement sustains the duration of sex and reduces over stimulation, which can cause a climax and ejaculation. The objective of the Holdback is to allow the climax and ejaculation sensation to stay in the body. Visualize or think about or pretend the orgasmic sensation goes from the genitals up the spine to the brain and back down to genitals. The orgasmic sensation should go from the genitals to the brain during each pause in the sex activity (Holdback). This orgasmic energy is believed to strengthen and nourishes the body, mind, spirit, and is called Sexual Regeneration.

Sex Organs and Your Body

- ✓ Small mouth = Small vagina / penis
- ✓ Long fingers = Long shaft of vagina, long penis
- ✓ Big lips = Large lips (labia) to vagina
- ✓ Bulging eyes = Small penis / vagina
- ✓ Deep set eyes = Long penis / long shaft to vagina
- ✓ Thick eyelids = Short shaft vagina / penis
- ✓ Thin eyelids = Long shaft vagina / penis
- ✓ Thick wide lips = Thick penis (girth)/ thick lips on vagina

Sexual Hormonal Rhythm Method

Take the temperature in the morning before getting out of bed, and before going to the toilet. There are Ovulation Microscopes (ovuscope) that are the size of a cigarette lighter and Ovulation Watches are available as well as Ovulation Computer Programs. The circle shows the pattern of temperature during the menstrual cycle. Low temperatures are at the outside, high at the center. There is a rise in temperature before ovulation. Ovulation devices and computer programs make tracking ovulation easier than thermometer.

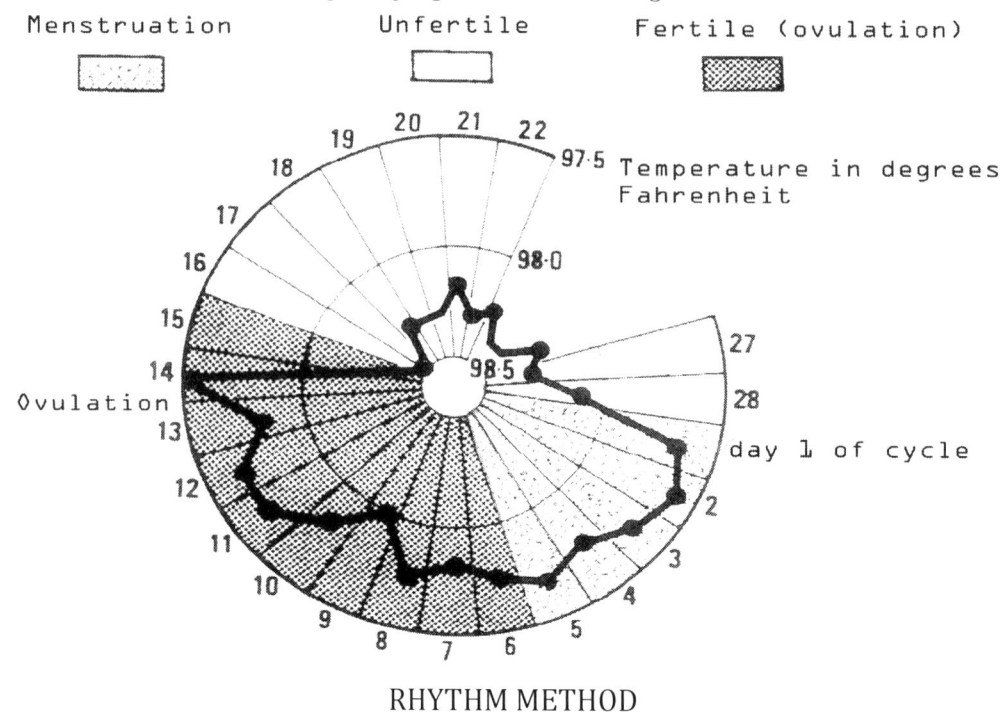

RHYTHM METHOD

Suppose a woman had menstruation regularly every 28 days. Ovulations released egg would be most likely on the 15th day of the cycle, but could happen anytime from the 13th to the 17th a period of 5 days. The egg and sperm works as a team and one egg is chosen while the other eggs decrease their nutrient demand so that one viable egg is released from the ovary. The egg is caught by the fimbria (fingers) of the fallopian tube. Inside the fallopian tube the sperm fertilizes the egg. Sperm can live up to four days in the uterus. Ideally, the sperm should be in the fallopian tube before the egg is released. Sperm teamwork is necessary, it takes many sperm to eat through the protein and sugar shell around the egg so that one sperm can get into the egg and fertilize it.

The ovary and fallopian tube each have a cycle. An ovary may release an egg each month or alternate. An ovary can release an egg then stop for two to three months while the other ovary releases its eggs. If the fallopian tube hormonal cycle with an ovary is interrupt or broken because surgery removal of the ovary, the cycle will be obeyed. The right ovary can be removed and the right fallopian tube will obey its cycle and will cross over the uterus and pick up an egg from left ovary.

The cycle is hormone and nutrient dependent. Therefore, the cycle can be altered by sympathetic stress (i.e. excessive female exercise) or poor nutrition. For example, if the manganese level is very low the hormones are altered. This can cause a female to go into hormone imbalance causing menopause. The manganese can decrease at any age (8 years old) causing temporary menopause symptoms for hours or a day. The bodily system can be healthy enough to rebound to normal hormone levels. However, the female's sex hormone production can be deteriorated or aged. This can decrease or stop the sex hormone rebound resulting in temporarily or permanent menopause. Consumption of sex hormones in processed foods and refine-cooked oils (junk food, baked, and fried foods) can cause puberty (menstruation, ovulation) to start in 8-year-old girls. Female's natural ability to store energy in the form of fats starts ovulation (must store 10 to 25% fat). The calories from stored energy are needed for pregnancy and breastfeeding. The body naturally converts carbohydrates, protein and fats, into a type of sugar and then stores the sugar in the form of fats (glycogen). Young boys that consume sex hormones in processed foods are starting to have reduce testicle size, low sperm count and ejaculating sperm at 10 years old and younger.

HEALING AND DISEASE SEX POSITIONS

Sexual Positions

These sexual positions can indicate health or emotional problems, especially if a person tends to favor a specific position more than another. This can indicate a problem with an organ or system associated with the position. These sexual positions can be used to treat various health problems.

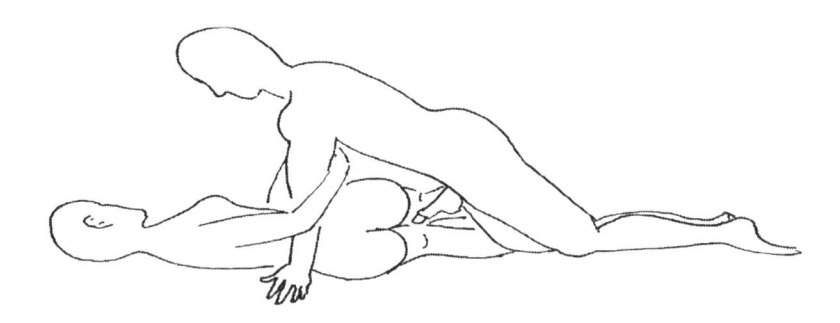

Men that suffer from impotence, erectile dysfunction, premature ejaculation, prostate disease can use this position, for sex organ related problems.

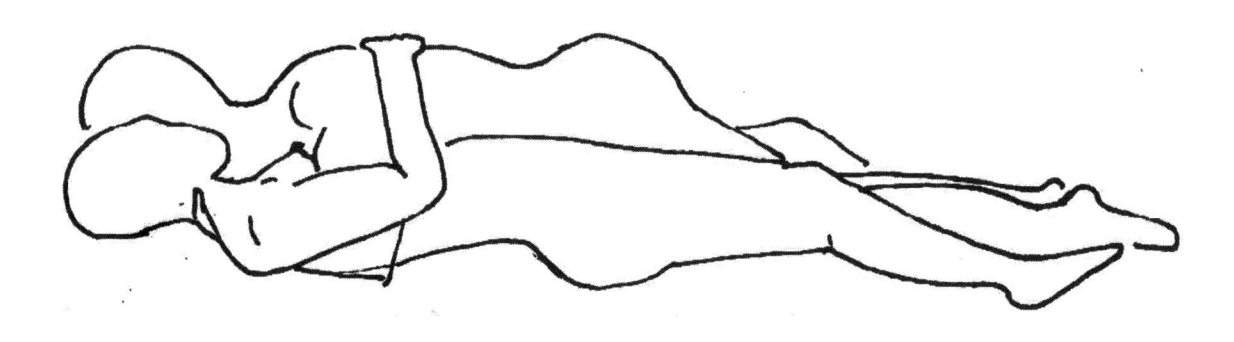

Chronic fatigue, blurred vision, acidic breathing patterns (shallow breathe), excessive perspiration, rapid heartbeat, weakness, and fainting.

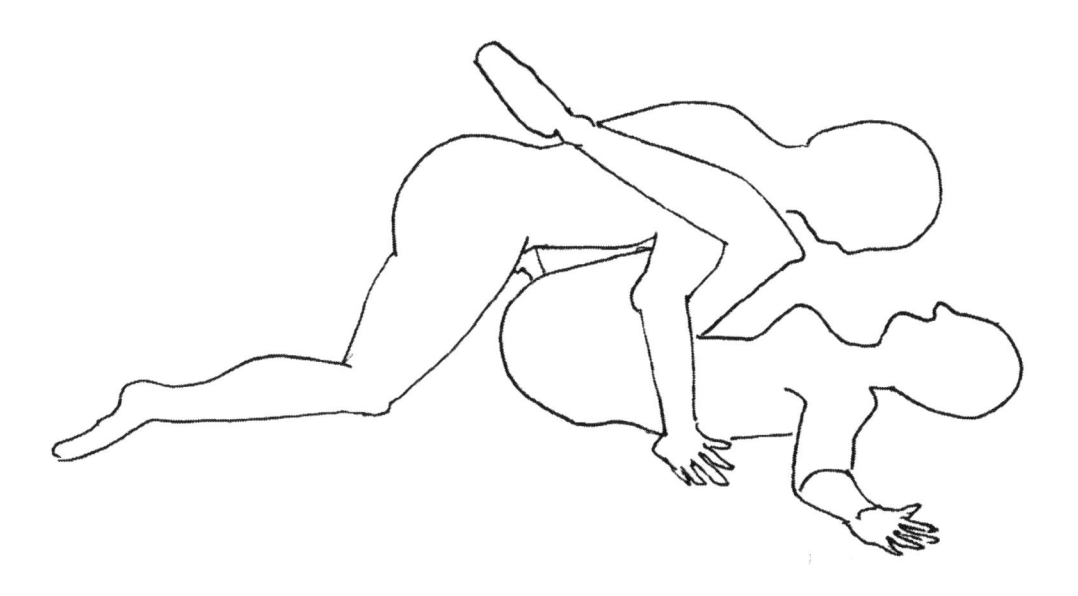

Excessive perspiration (liver problems), rapid heartbeat, weakness, and fainting, Undernourishment, anemia, dry skin, poor circulation

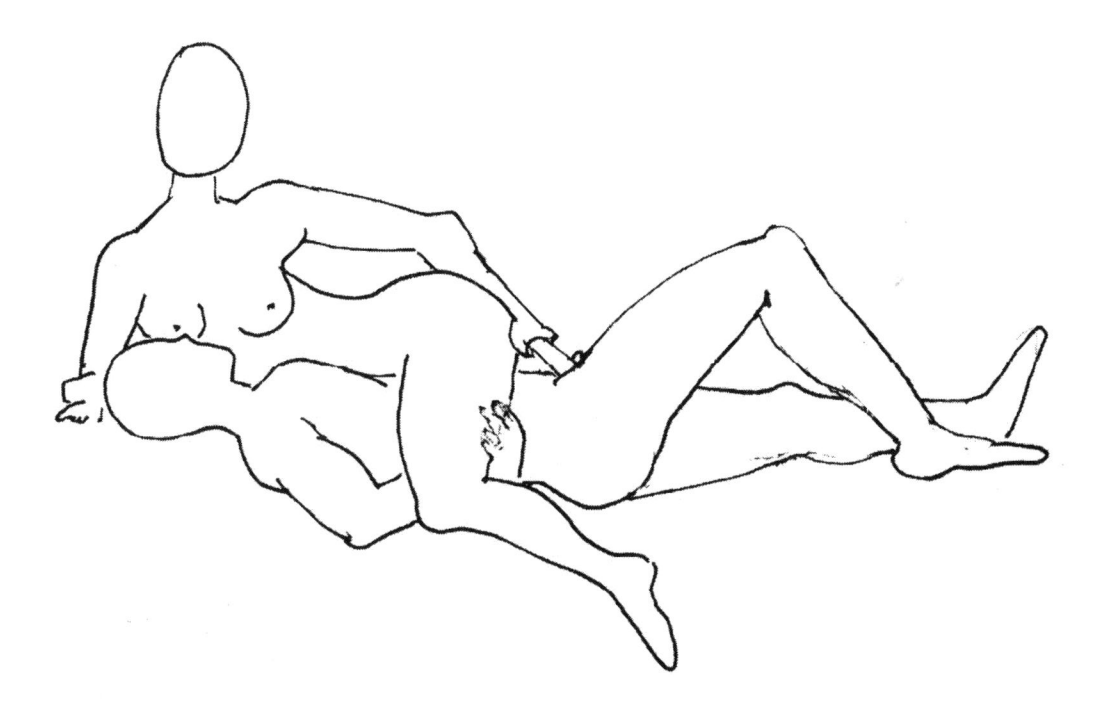

Poor circulation, cramps, headaches, abnormally heavy or light menstruation, no period, hormone imbalance, blockage of meridians menstrual problems

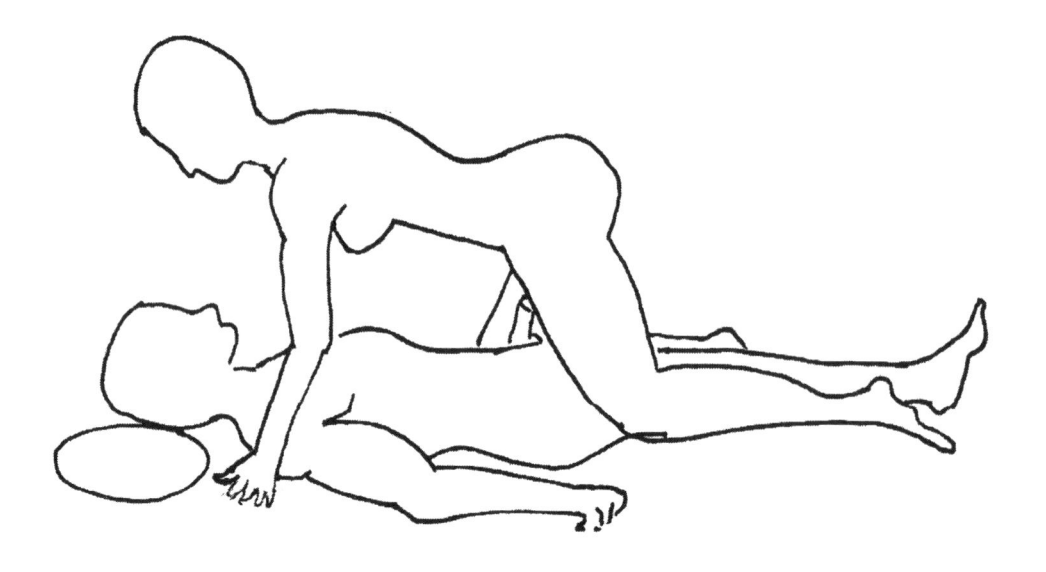

Hormone imbalance, stress and nervous system problems, menstruation problems

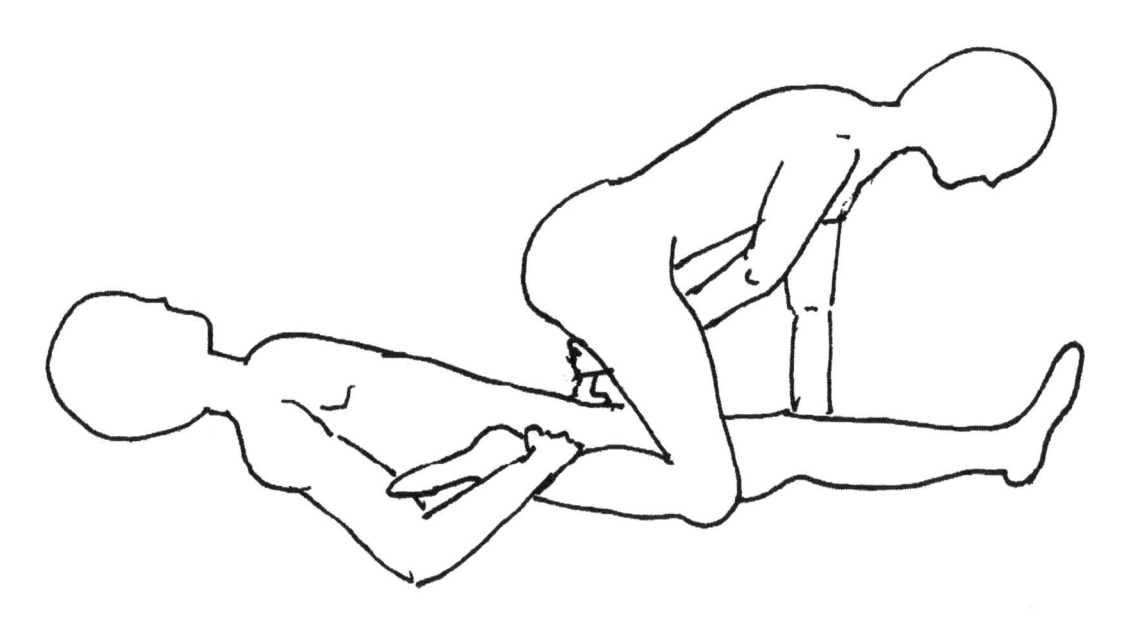

Edema reduces circulation resulting in excess electrical heat that raises body temperature not a fever

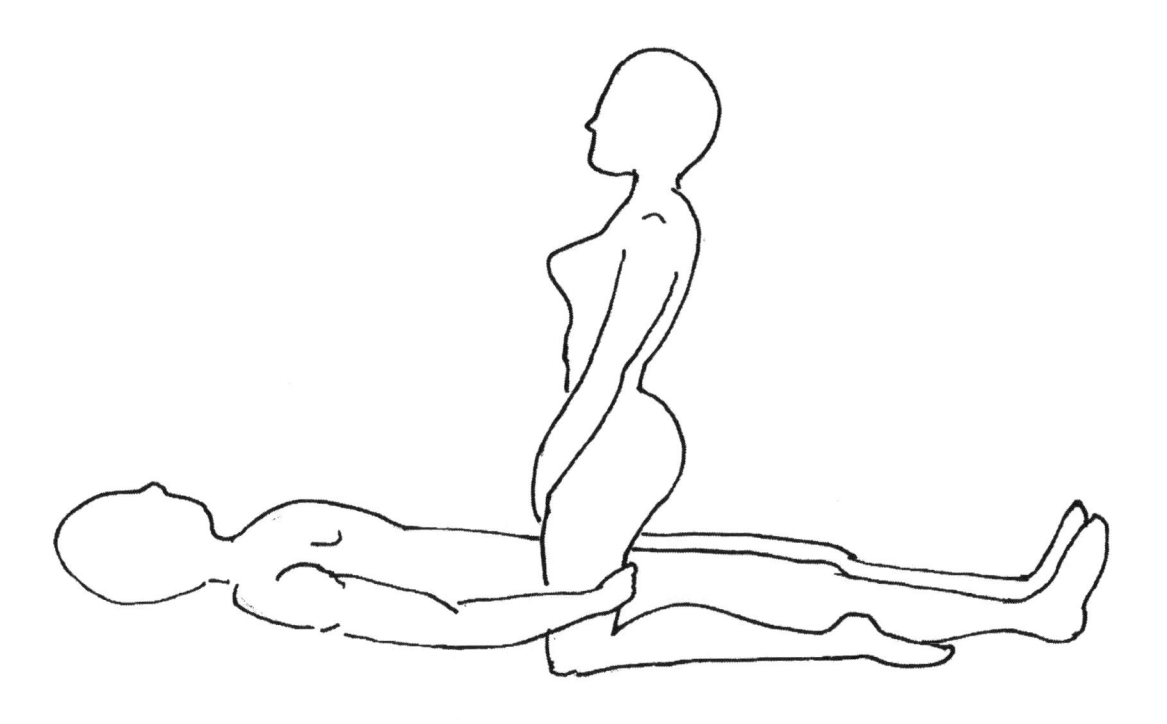

High and Low Blood Pressure in males.

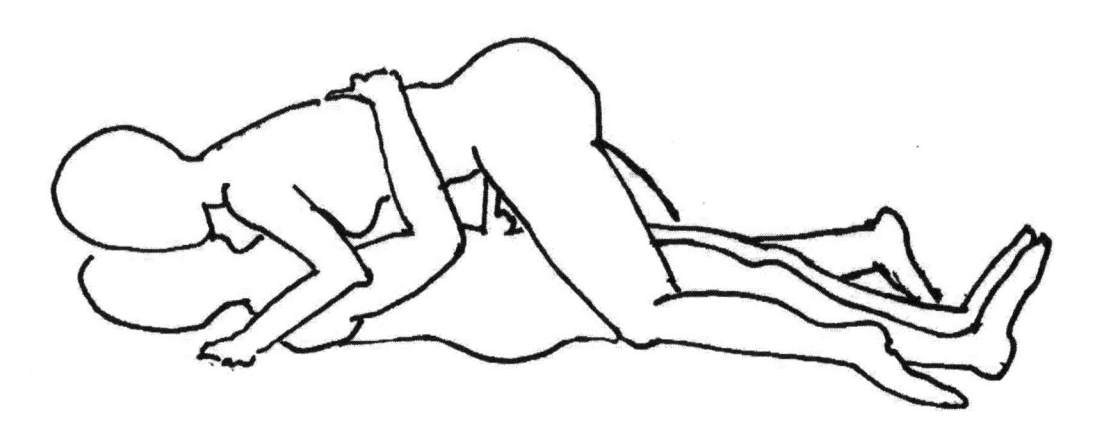

Decreased immunity, lymphatic problems

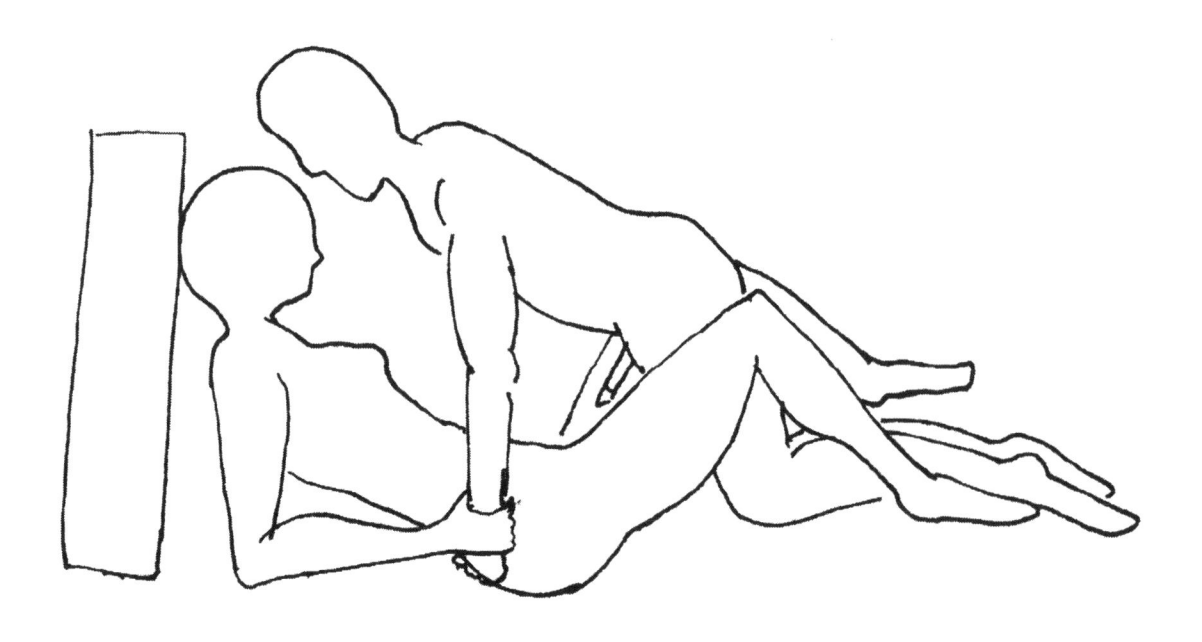

Internal organ problems, increased blood to female pelvic area

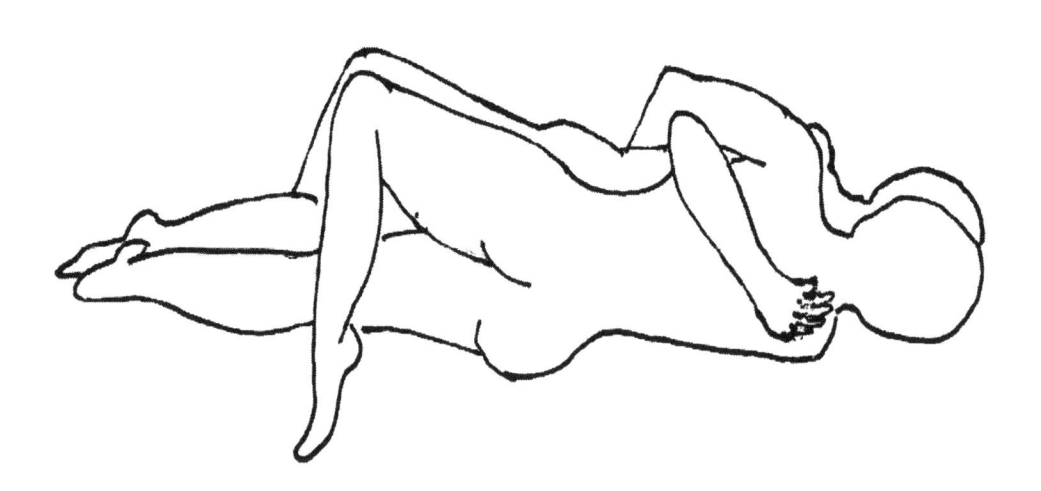

Stimulation and strengthening of the liver and kidney

274

High and Low blood pressure, various veins, hardening of arteries

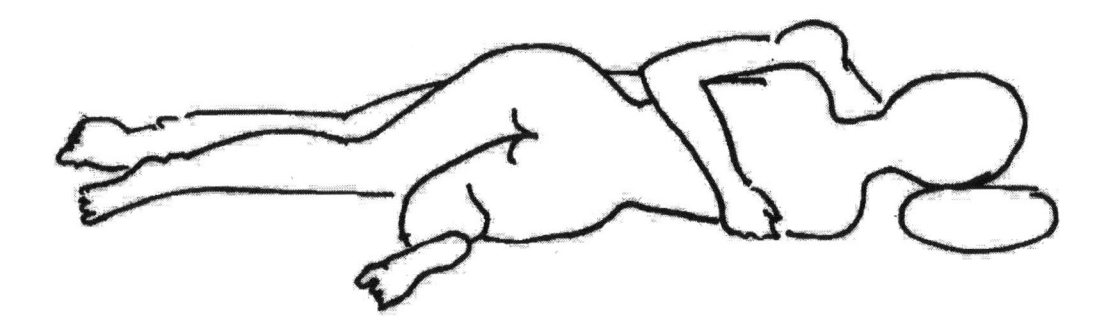

Bone deterioration, arthritis, bone marrow disease, broken bones, anemia, and leukemia

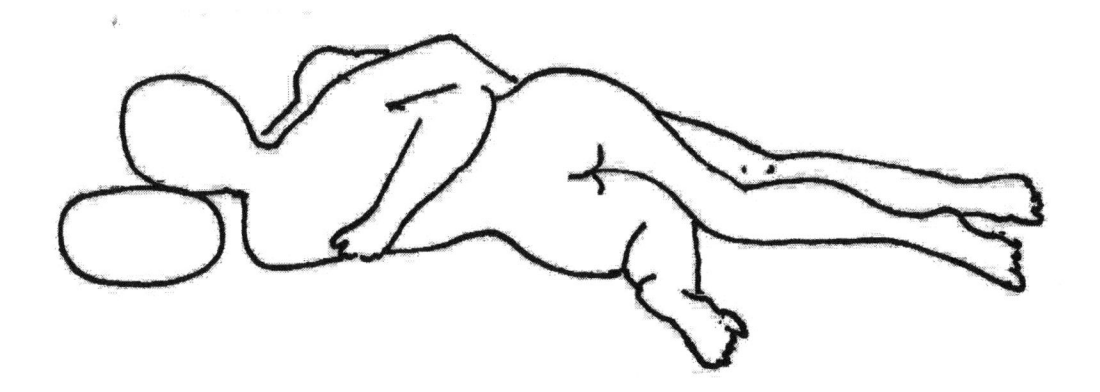

Stimulates wellness

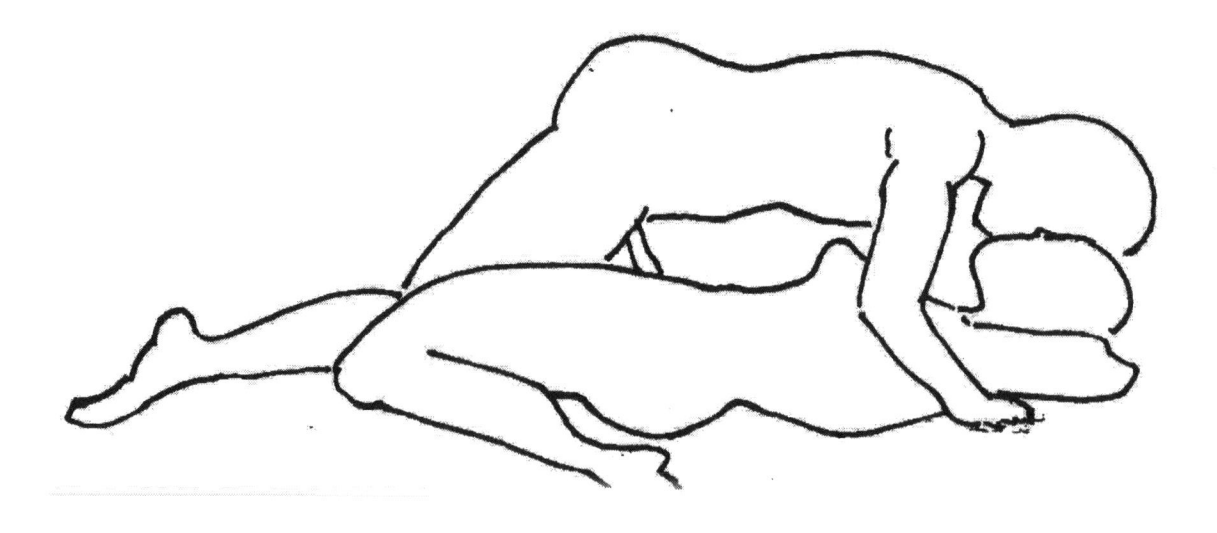

Digestive difficulties of stomach, liver, pancreas (diabetes) and spleen, Female organ problems

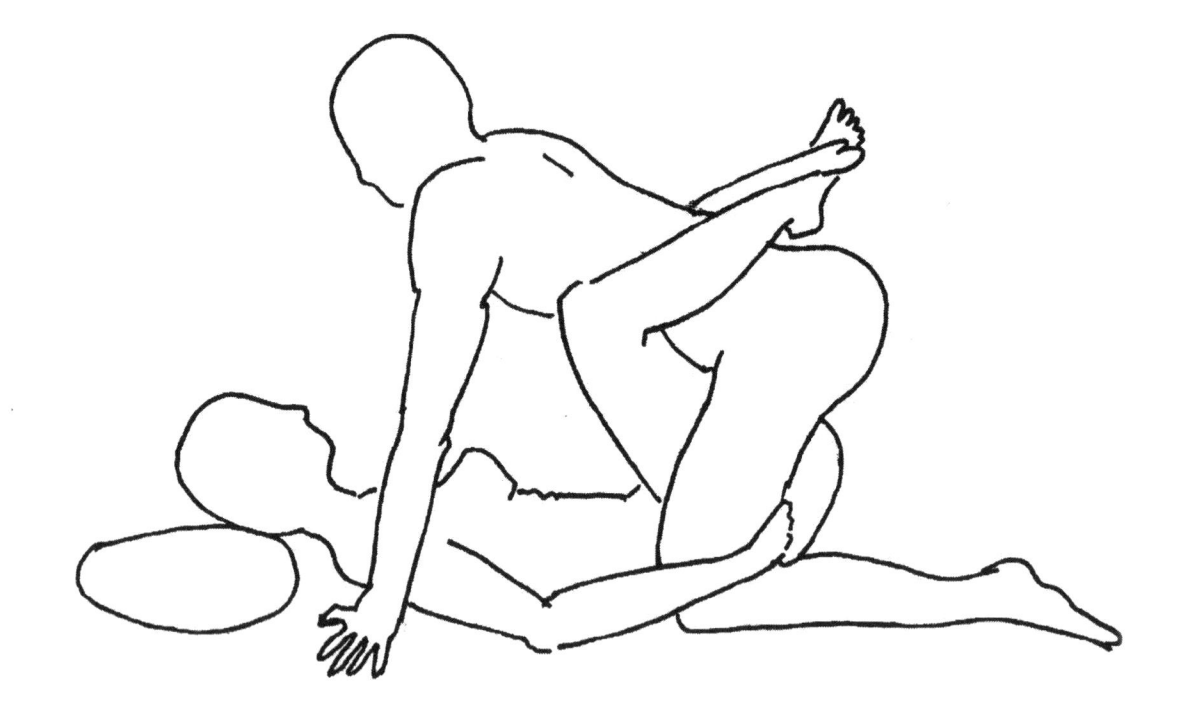

276

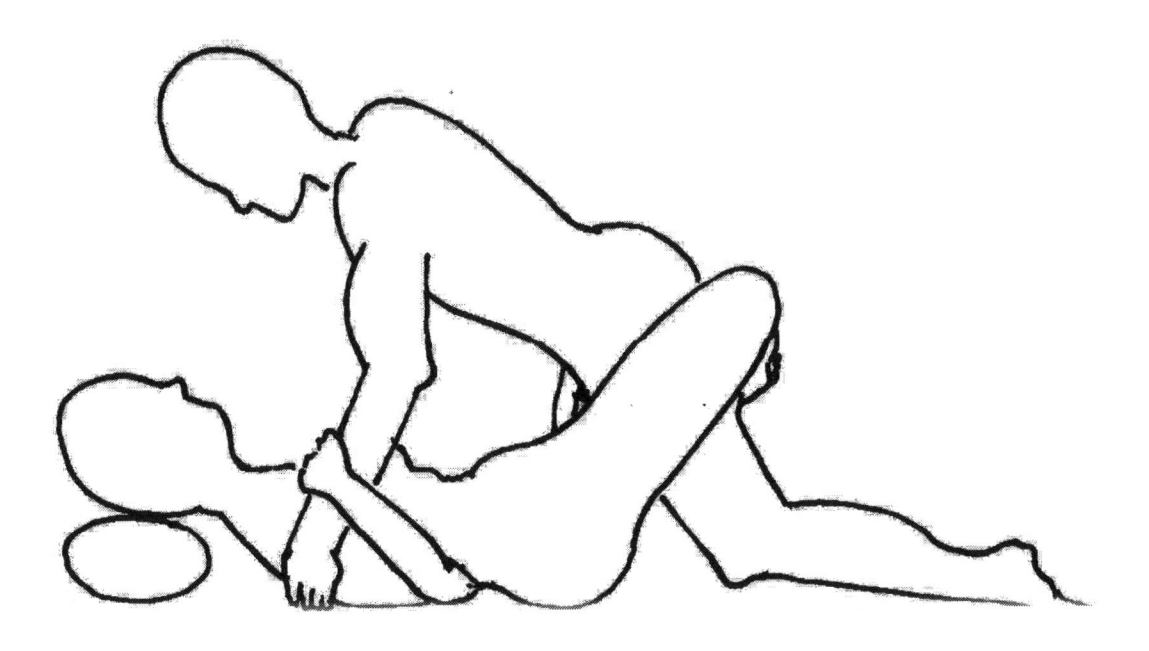

Hot Flashes, paining feet and knees, diabetes, liver problems

Nutritional Disorders Diagnosis

Body system or region	Sign or symptom	Indicates
General	- Weakness, fatigue - Weight loss	- Decreased calorie intake or increased calorie use - Anemia, electrolyte imbalance - Inadequate nutrient intake or absorption
Skin, Hair, Nails	- Dry, flaky skin - Thinning, dry hair - Rough scaly skin with bumps - Petechiae or ecchymoses - Sore that wont heal - Spoon-shaped, brittle, or ridged nails - Dry skin with poor turgor	- Vitamin A deficiency - Vitamin A, vitamin B-complex, or linoleic acid deficiency - Iron deficiency - Dehydration - Protein, vitamin C, or zinc deficiency - Vitamin C, or K deficiency - Protein deficiency
Eyes	- Night blindness; corneal swelling, softening, or dryness; Bitot's spots (gray triangular patches on the conjunctiva) - Red conjunctiva	- Vitamin A deficiency - Riboflavin
Throat, mouth	- Soft spongy, bleeding gums - Swollen neck (goiter) - Cracks at corner of mouth - Magenta tongue - Tongue reddish	- Riboflavin of niacin deficiency - Riboflavin deficiency - Vitamin B12 deficiency - Vitamin C deficiency - Iodine deficiency
Cardiovascular	- Edema - Tachycardia, hypotension	- Protein deficiency - Fluid volume deficit
Gastrointestinal	- Ascites	- Protein deficiency
Musculoskeletal	- Bone pain, bow leg - Muscle wasting	- Vitamin D or calcium deficiency or Boron - Protein, carbohydrate, and fat deficiency
Neurologic	- Mood swings - Altered mental status - Paresthesia	- Dehydration; thiamine, or vitamin B12 deficiency - Vitamin B12 pyridoxine, or thiamine deficiency

Body Posture Diagnosis

Posture Against Gravity

A person's body aligned correctly moves freely with gravity. There is no resistance to gravity. The correct alignment posture develops vitality into our bones tissues and muscles.

Posture Backward Bowing

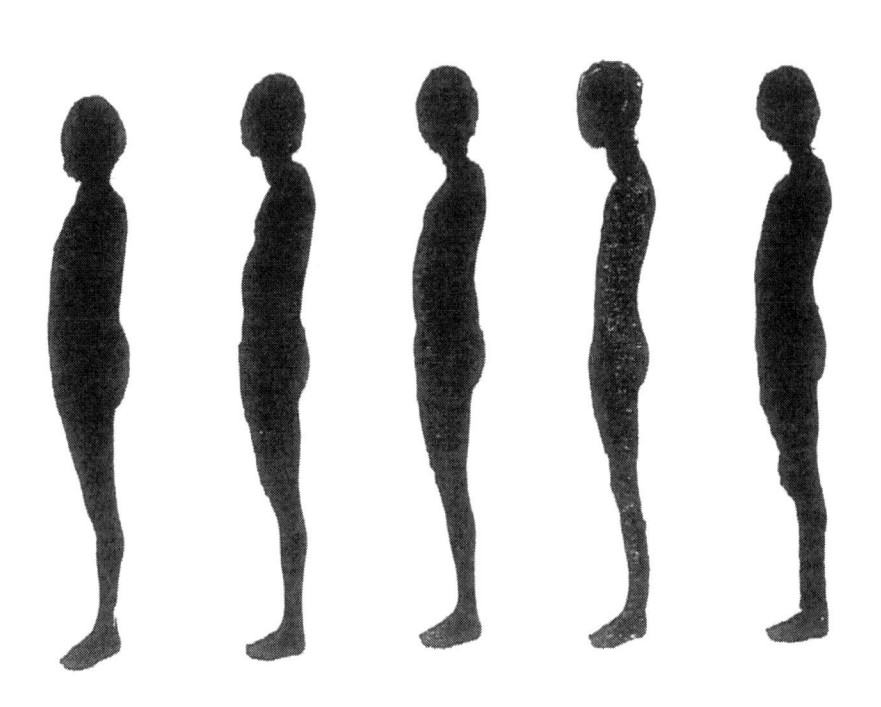

Each body indicates a different degree of backward bowing. All are shorter along the back than the front. With significant bowing, each will have attitudes of rigidity. They tend to be determined in their directions, with rigid ideas about right and wrong. They tend to push towards what they perceive that they want and guard their feelings by suppressing them.

Postural Alignment

The ideal axis for balance is that which aligns points at the top of the head, middle of the ear, middle of the shoulder, midpoint of the hip, center of the knee, and center of the ankle joints. This line should pass through the juncture of the lower backbones and the sacrum at the base of the spine. With these points aligned, each segment supports those above it. Considering that our muscles make up a large part of our total body weight, and consume a major portion of our energy, it is easy to see that their efficient functioning impacts alignment. When out of alignment extra amounts of energy are used to stand, move, and hold erect posture. When you are out of balance, movements tend to be weighted down by gravity. With balance, gravity is our helper and when out of balance you are working against gravity. Our nervous system is stressed when our muscles tend to be pushed down or weighted down. Many people who feel overburdened have bodies that are bent forward toward the ground. People that feel life is a struggle tend to have bodies that are bent backward, resisting and pushing against gravity.

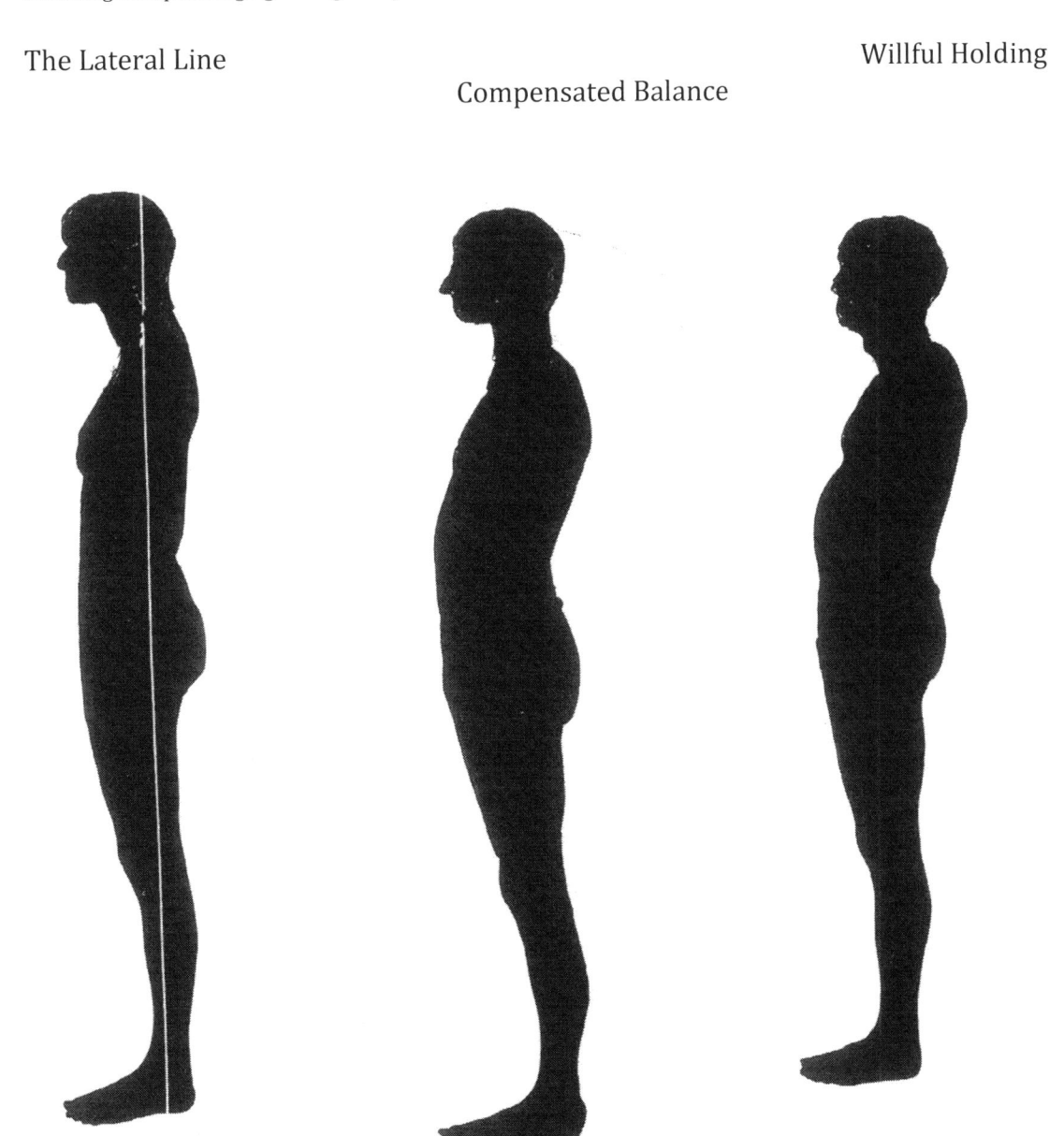

The Lateral LineWillful Holding

Compensated Balance

Posture Misalignment

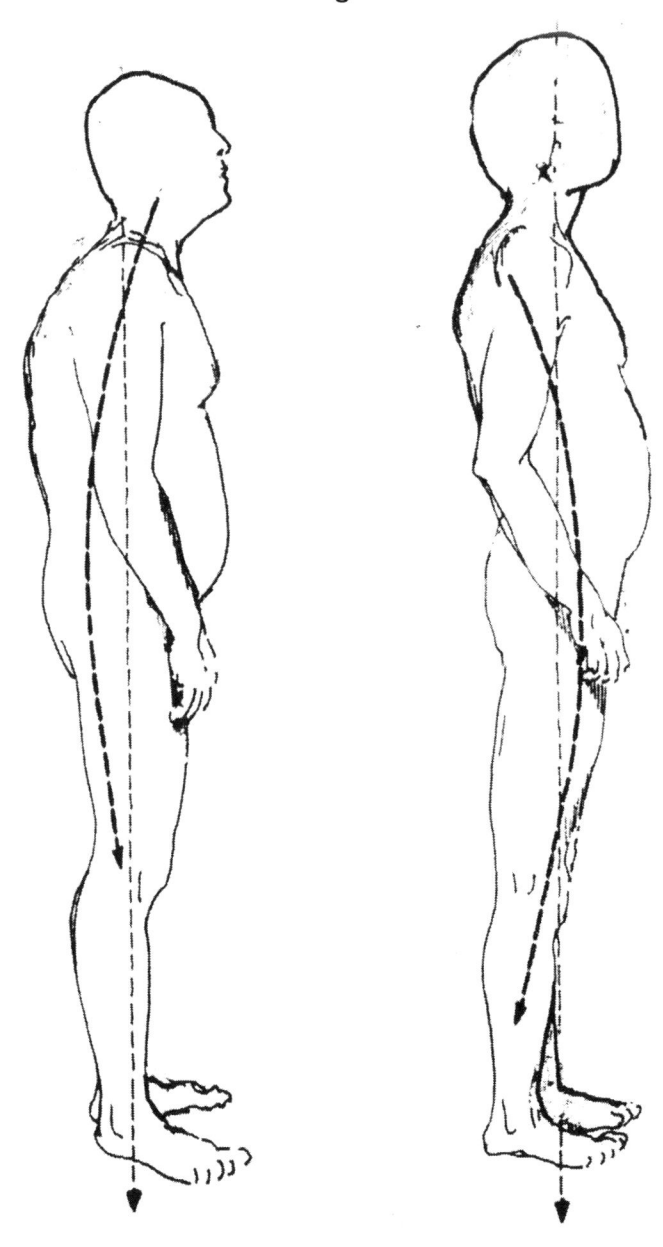

Posture Needy and Rigid Types

The bodily posture reveals the spiritual, mental, and emotional attitudes of a person. The posture and attitude may develop because of a negative dysfunctional experience or emotional trauma. There are basically two types of posture types.

The **Needy Types** tend to seek rewards and punishments from others (i.e. love, caring, attention). They seem to be asking the world to support them. The **Rigid Type** tends to contract their musculature personality in order to resist others from giving them rewards and punishments. They seem to be blocking emotional interpersonal interactions with a rigid wall of resistance.

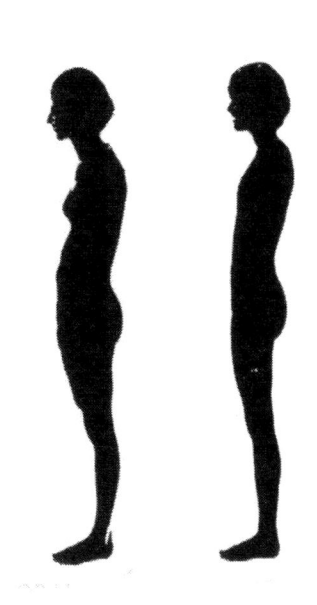

Female Pelvis

The pelvis is the cradle for the upper body. The pelvis should be able to move freely in all directions. While walking it should swing backward and forward. There is a normal swing of the pelvis in females. The female pelvis is wider than males. A pelvis that swings exaggeratedly from side to side (typical switching wiggle of females) is abnormal and was developed as a reaction to social sexual influences. The exaggerated side-to-side wiggle indicates over acidity and a pooling of emotional energy in one area, which blocks the flow of energy to all areas.

Positions of the Female Pelvis

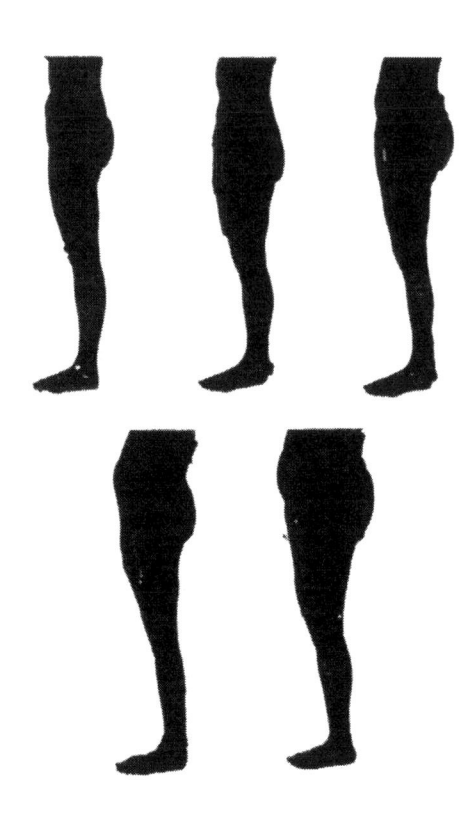

Locked Knees

Misaligned Angle of The Knee Joint forces weight off the anatomical center of gravity and puts stress on the body. Locked knees drain the body of energy.

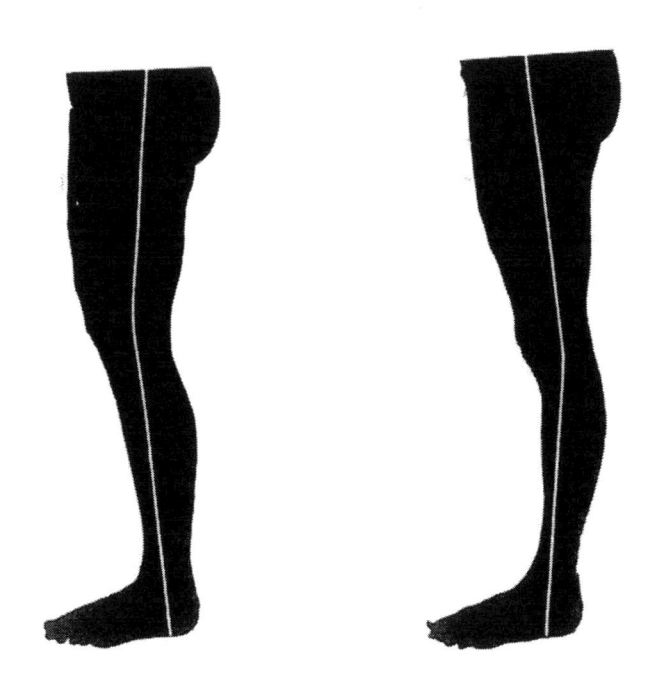

Locked knees can emotionally indicate:
- Allow you to stand your ground no matter what—" I won't be put down!"
- A defensive reaction to avoid being suppressed or subjugated—"I will stand up!" "I wont give in!"
- Maintaining a structure from collapsing and falling--"This is all I can do to hold myself up." "You should help me!"
- Keep a hold on reality—" I must hold myself together."

Sabotaging Self Posture (knees, legs and emotions)

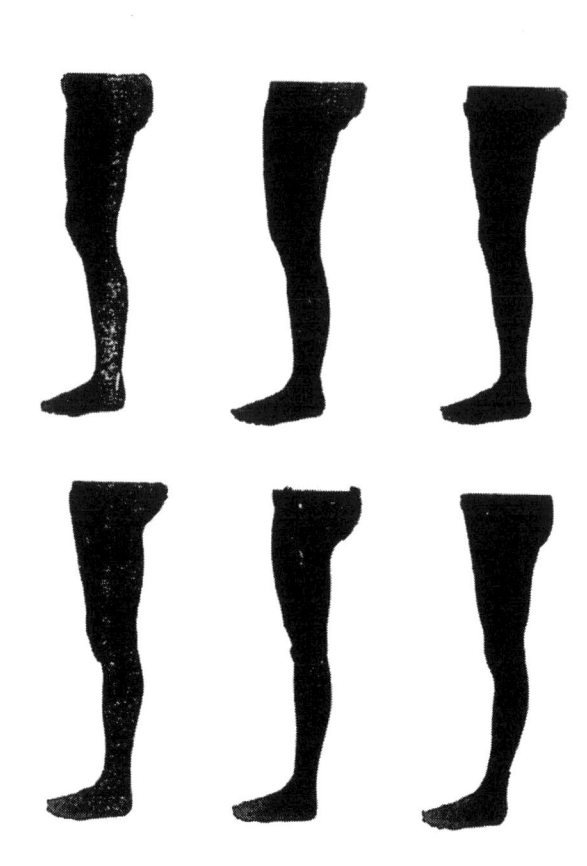

People emotionally sabotage themselves when they voluntarily hold onto a negative lifestyle and /or emotional position that will harm them. Sabotaging Self Posture mirrors their inner emotional contradiction. The body is bowed backward, feet are grasping the ground, and knees are locked. An emotional force is acting on the body and the person is fighting against the forces. This emotional influenced posture is a constant effort to stand on the ground or move forward.

The muscle energy in the legs is being tightly contained, and blood flow constricted. The blood flow between the ground and the body is blocked and limited. There is no flexibility in the ankle and knee joints. The lower extremity moves as a single rigid block. Below the locked knee there is muscle tension in the leg, and muscle rigidity in the feet. People with rigid legs can barely move their toes backward and forward. The muscle in the lower leg causes the movement of the toes to be stimulated.

Knees are associated with feelings of fear, humbleness, and begging.

Grounding

Our health is determined by how well we align ourselves to the ground. Correctly aligned posture, allows you to be fully in contact with the ground. Properly Aligned posture means you are "grounded," and stable in your contact with reality. Correct posture indicates that we accept "where we stand." Bad posture means we resist positive pressure to change and maintain a dysfunctional reality, lifestyle, love relationship despite recurring physical and emotional destructiveness. Misaligned individuals are rigid and in chronic emotional pain. Misaligned contact with the ground is misaligning contact with reality. This causes a fear of becoming aligned resulting in panic. They are functionally addicted and in desperation they choose to hold on to the bad posture. Physically misaligned people are bent, and overburdened. They have broad, rounded, hunched shoulders; head drooped onto their chest, stiff pelvis and thighs, knees rigidly locked, and legs and feet tightly contracted.

The tension and stiffness in the lower half of the body, (legs, and feet), indicates reduced emotional and physical sensitivity. Instead of relaxing and regaining proper alignment they further tighten their muscles and emotions. Emotionally, this is a real or imagined fear of being exploited or taken advantage of, or of losing status, and not performing well enough. A loss of self-esteem or status is a reason for Self-Sabotage. This causes the need to be emotionally and physically stiff, and medicate emotions with many gadgets (foods, games, gambling, sex, drugs, or many gadgets) in order to "Ground" yourself.

Displacement

Displaced weight and shapes are depicted in a progression from the person on your left, who has excessive weight in his top half, through the fourth figure, who has good balance between top and bottom, and to the last figure whose bottom half has excessive weight. In bodies with larger weight displacements, energy is blocked and not evenly flowing the entire length of the body. The main area of blockage is at the mid-back. The excessive weight parts have mineral and electrolyte congestion and a large amount of electromagnetic energy. This can be the result of dysfunctional diets, emotions, mentality and pituitary stress and embryonic impaired velocity of growth. Their body mirrors a congested uneven flow of emotions, moods and thoughts.

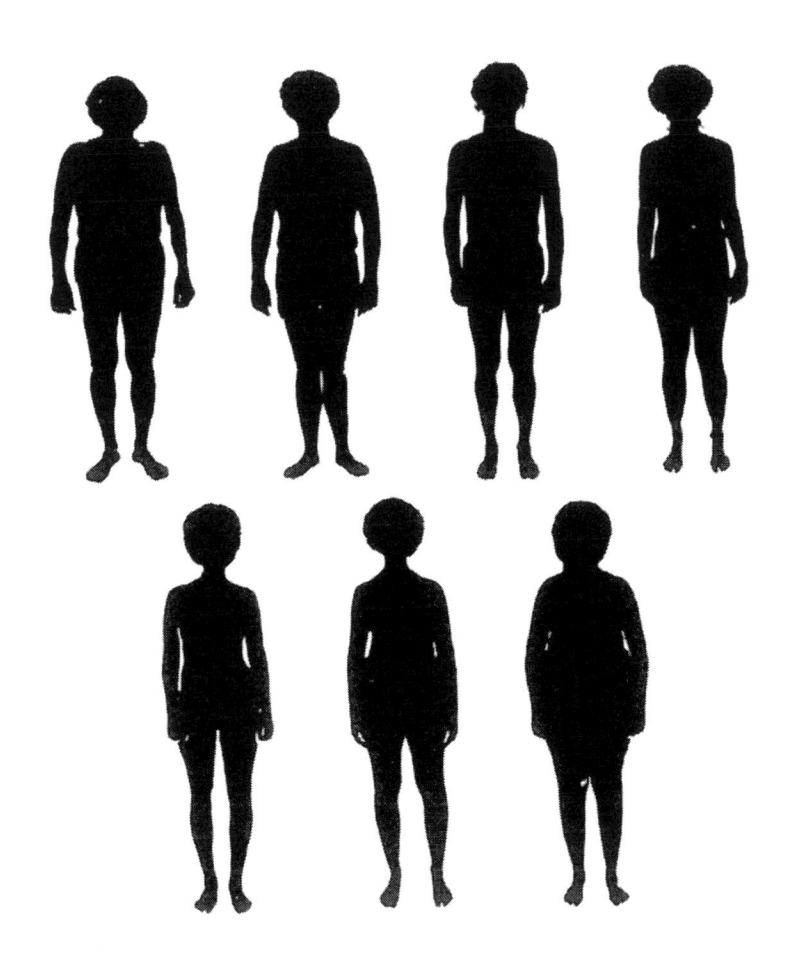

An Overburdened Individual

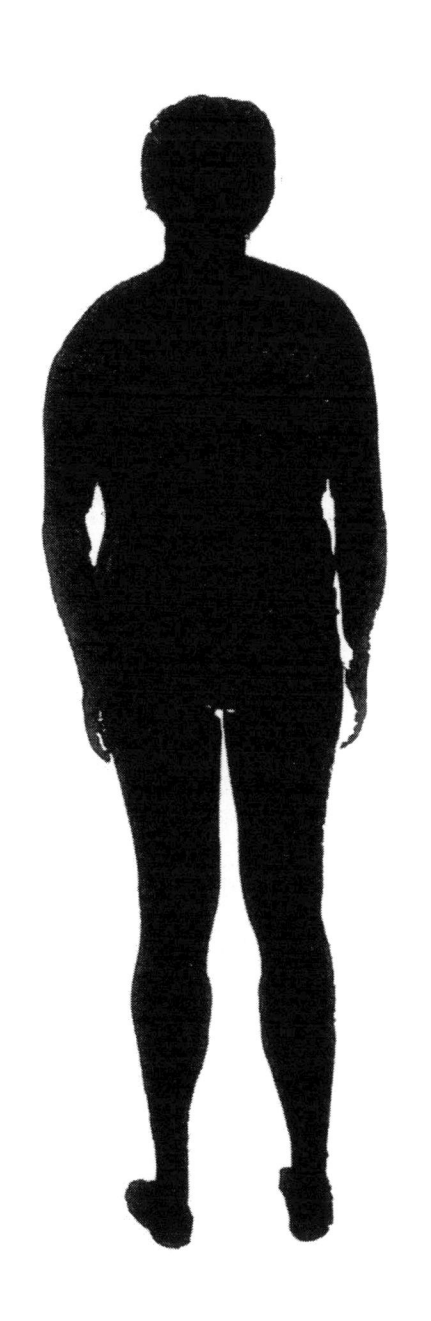

Pelvis Misalignment

The legs and pelvis join together and form particular shapes. The Arch shape indicates tension directed towards and into the perineum (center), which decreases blood flow to the genitals, buttocks, rectum, bladder, and anus. When the legs are close together or touching then tension is increased into and towards the organs in that are. This indicates that negative feelings, anger, rage, sex, self-esteem, and anxiety are related to this area. These postures can indicate dysfunctional emotions and feelings and problems with the organs in that area. In females the outer skin feels soft because of the natural layer of fat under their skin but there is tension deep within the muscles.

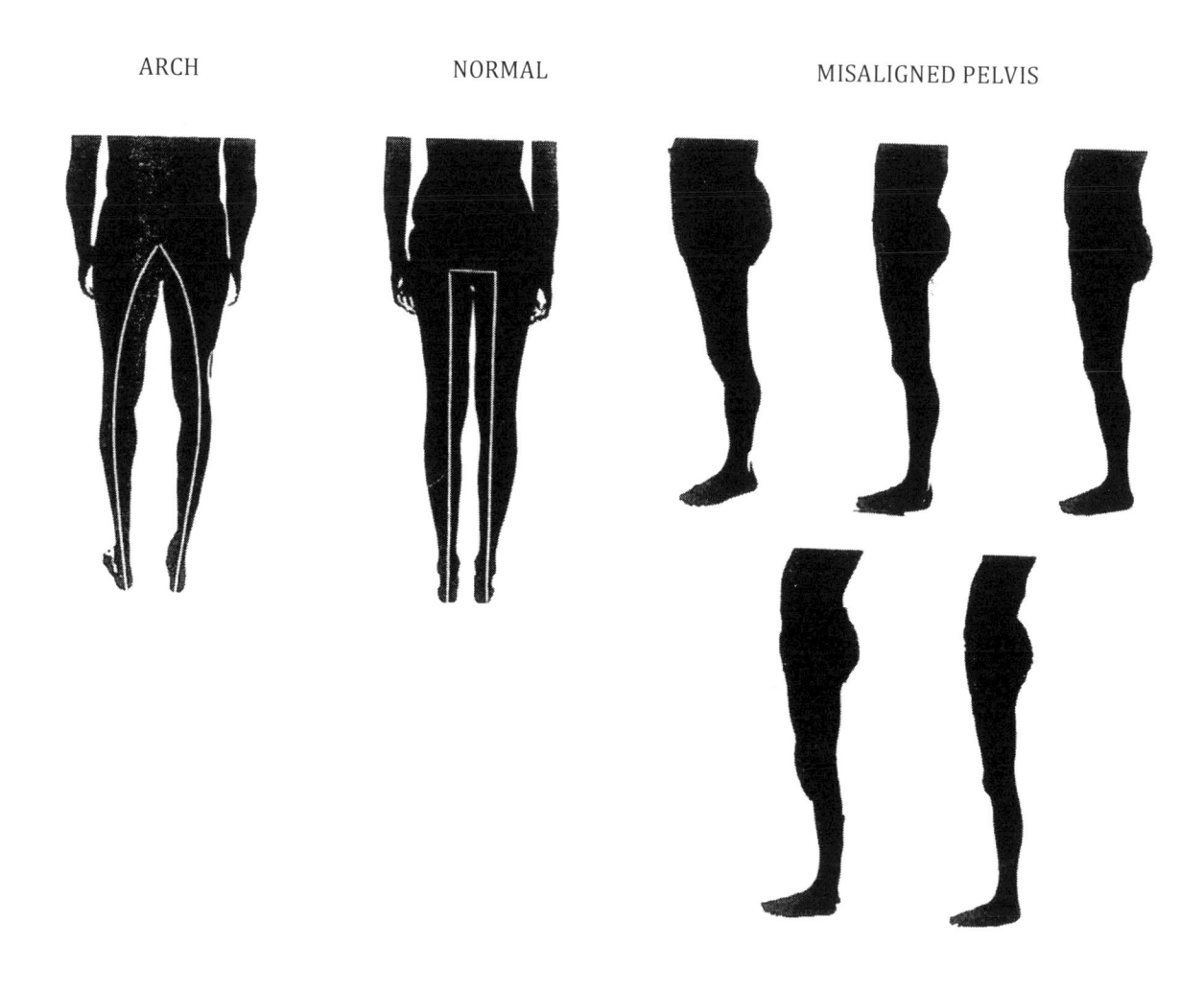

ARCH   NORMAL   MISALIGNED PELVIS

Normal Belly (abdominal)

In very young children it is natural to have belly posture. The normal belly bulges outward and expands with each breath. Adults tend to unconsciously assume the erroneous tucked in belly posture with the chest stuck out, belly drawn in tight and waist tight and small. This is against the flow of energy and does not allow the belly wall to relax outward and causes over and under inflation of the chest. It can cause the emotional expression to be limited and diffuses the natural emotional reaction to negative social conditions that warrant panic, anxiety, despair, hopelessness, and outrage.

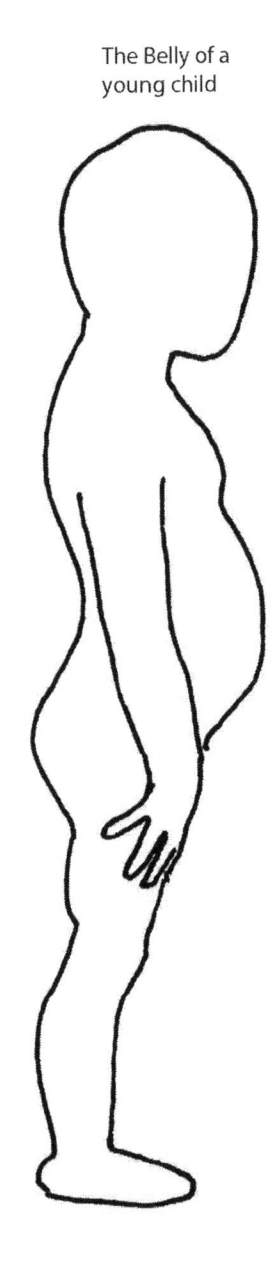

The Belly of a young child

Abnormal Belly (Abdominal)

The Belly of (Male)

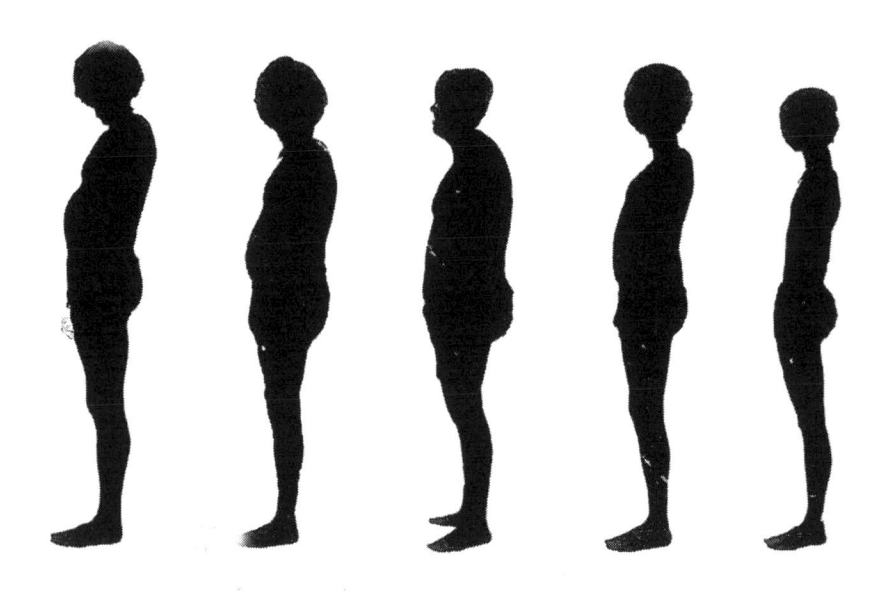

The Belly (Female)

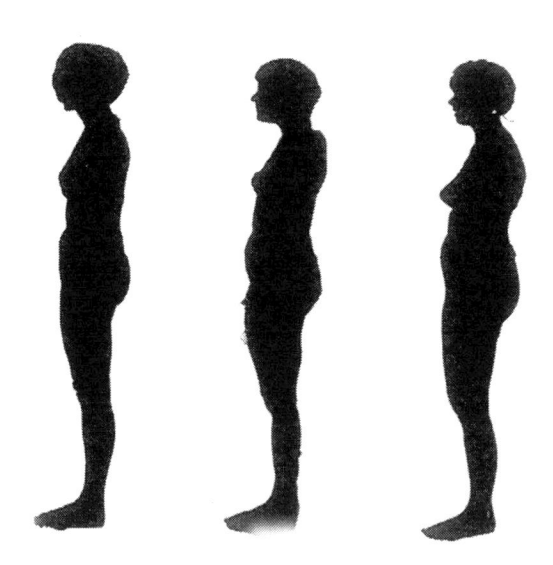

Neck in the hanged man posture indicating feelings that relationships, bills, children, your job/careers, economic status, disease, or society controls your life, It is also called the caught and hanged posture.

Left-Right Split Posture

The body's muscular structure should be equally developed on both sides of the body (symmetry). There is an unbalanced left – right split that indicates that the normal body symmetry is unequal. This is called asymmetric. The left side (your right) is larger, shoulder higher and left foot faces forward. The right side is smaller and the foot faces forward. The right side is smaller and the foot points outward. The energy does not flow evenly. The right muscles are strong and pull downward while the left muscle is too weak to counter balance by pulling downward. This unbalanced emotional person has a dysfunctional approach to themselves and mixed emotions to others. They resist and fear honest feelings and doubt they can overcome emotional crises.

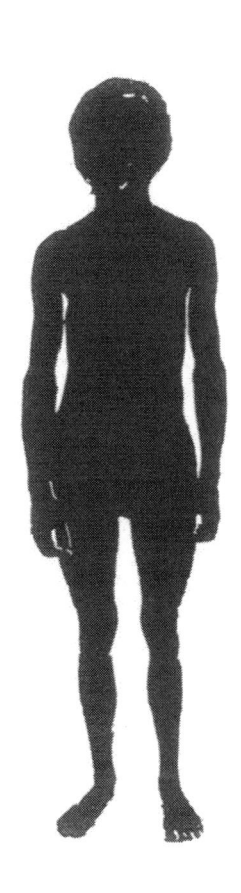

Head and Neck

The first silhouette (1) slightly forward tilted head of an emotional needy person, shoulder and body alignment. The second (2) silhouette has the head tilted back which puts the base of the skull close to the back. There is tension held in that area. The position indicates the holding back of true feelings. The tension radiates from the base of the skull over the top of the head to the face down to the jaw. This tension spreads to the eyes making them appear sharp with a hard stare. If the head is tilted to the left or right it indicates a one sided or indirect approach to life and themselves. The head tilted forward (3) it indicates that the person tends to be a thinker, aggressive, and may place their emotionally needy feelings in a secondary role.

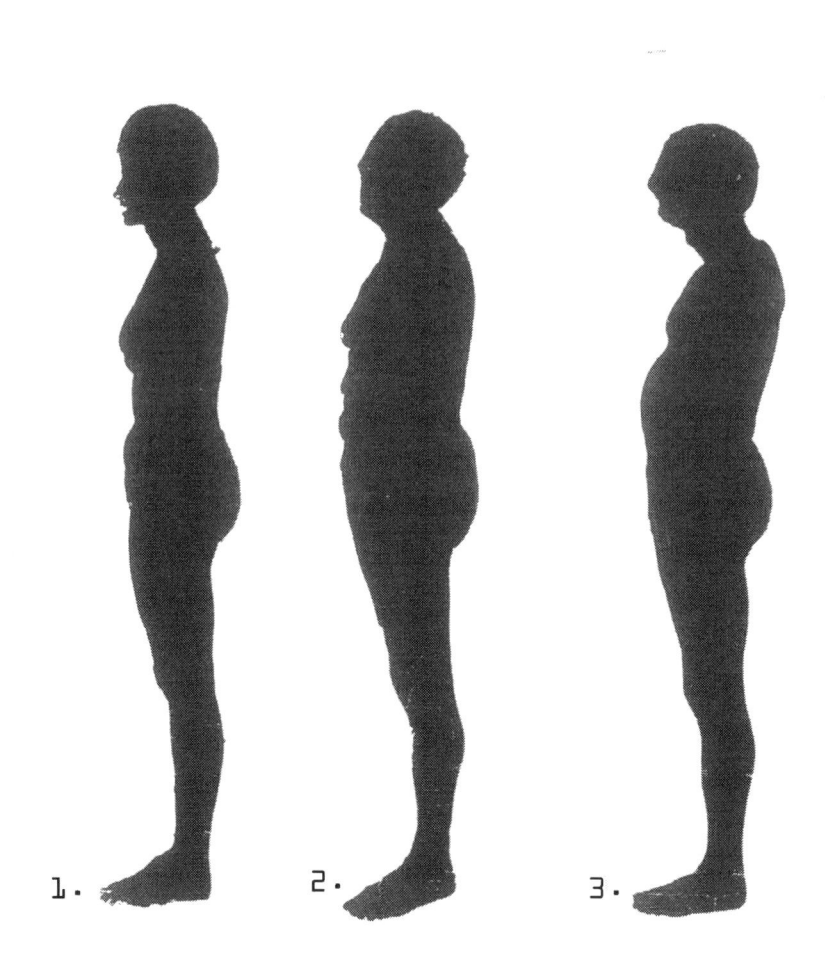

Pelvis Angle

The pelvis (1) is in proper alignment. The other pelvis (2) is retracted backward and there is displacement of the torso's weight. Displacement causes a loss of the correct self and holistic imbalances and they are emotionally untrue to themselves. A small pelvis is related to undeveloped feelings and holding back of emotions. In women a large or wide pelvis indicates a nurturing, loving and motherly attitude. A narrow pelvis in woman can indicate aggressive behavior and a need to be nurtured by others.

Being obese in the pelvis area indicates a passive and receptive personality masking a dominating type or a need to protect oneself with a wall of adipose (fat).

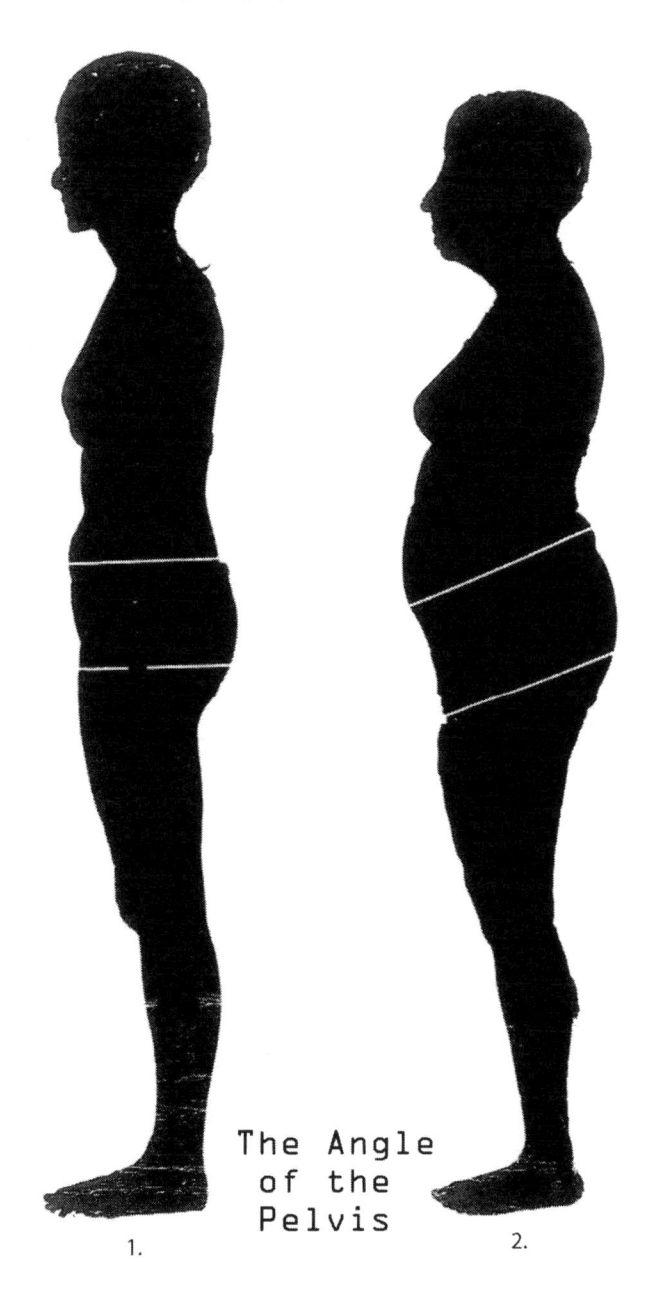

The Angle of the Pelvis

1.   2.

Burdened Posture

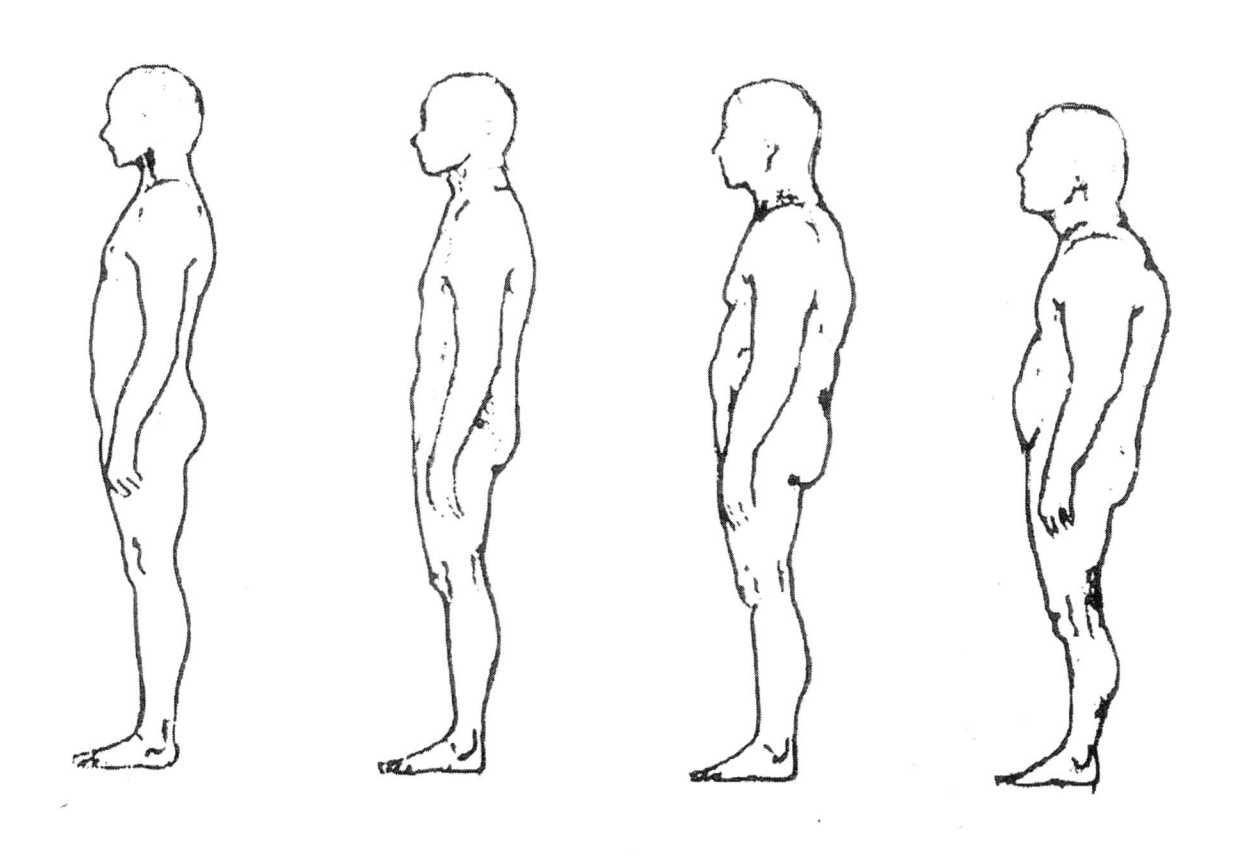

The Rigid Type

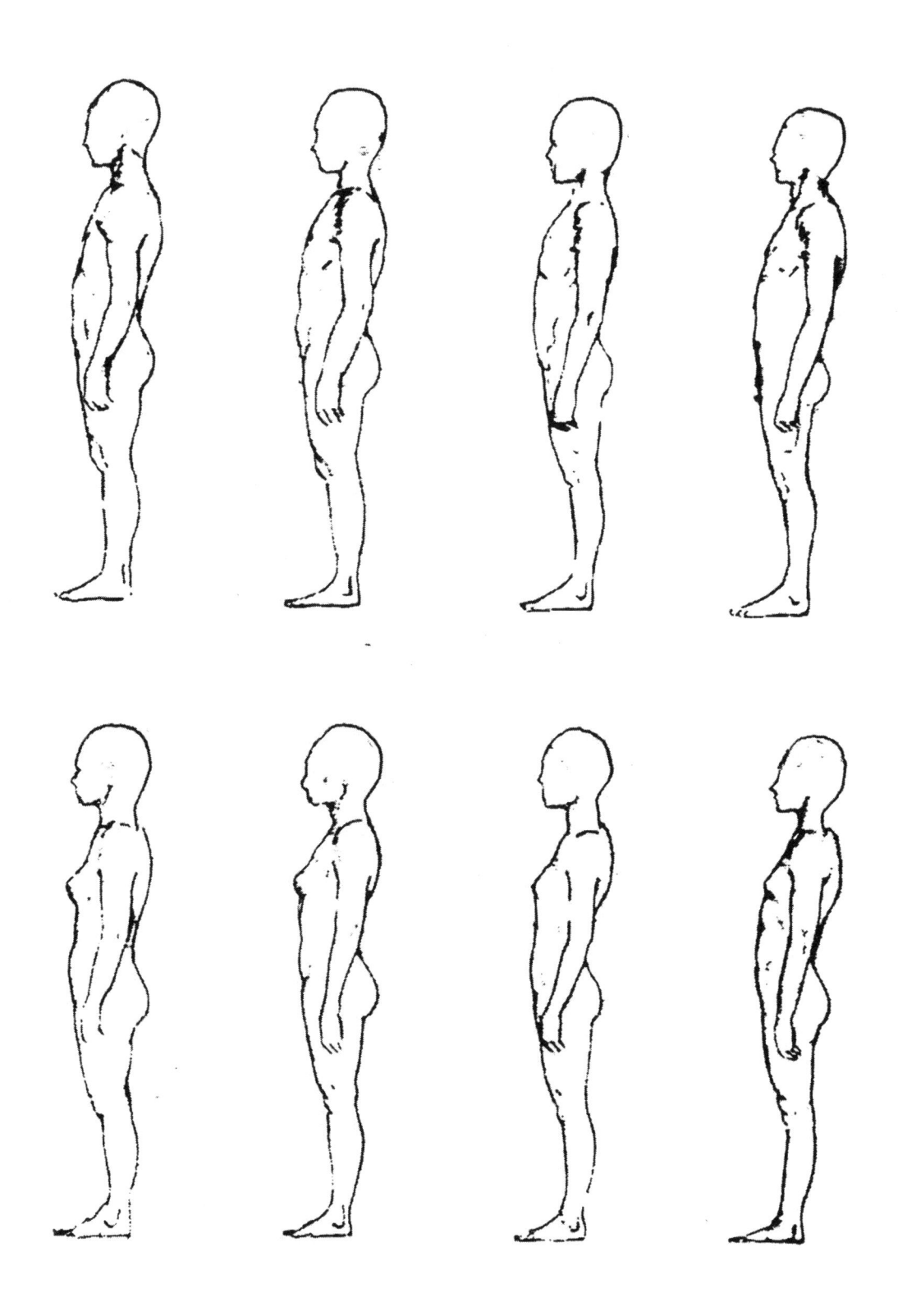

Posture Rules

- Women don't wear high heels which causes body posture to be misaligned
- Avoid exercise and activities, which arch or strain the low back (i.e. backward bends or forward bends to touch toes).
- When you cough or sneeze, round your back and bend your knees slightly.
- When making a bed, do so from a kneeling position.
- Avoid bending from the waist only; bend the knees and hips.
- Avoid lifting heavy objects higher than your waist.
- In mopping, vacuuming, raking, hoeing, etc. always work with the tool close to the body. Never use a "giant" step and a long reach in these activities.
- Sit down to dress: put on shoes and socks etc. Don't bend from the waist while trying to balance on one foot.
- Always turn and face the object you wish to lift.
- Avoid carrying unbalanced loads.
- Avoid sudden movements. Learn to move more deliberately.
- Change positions frequently.
- Hold heavy objects close to your body.
- Never carry or move anything, which you cannot handle with ease.

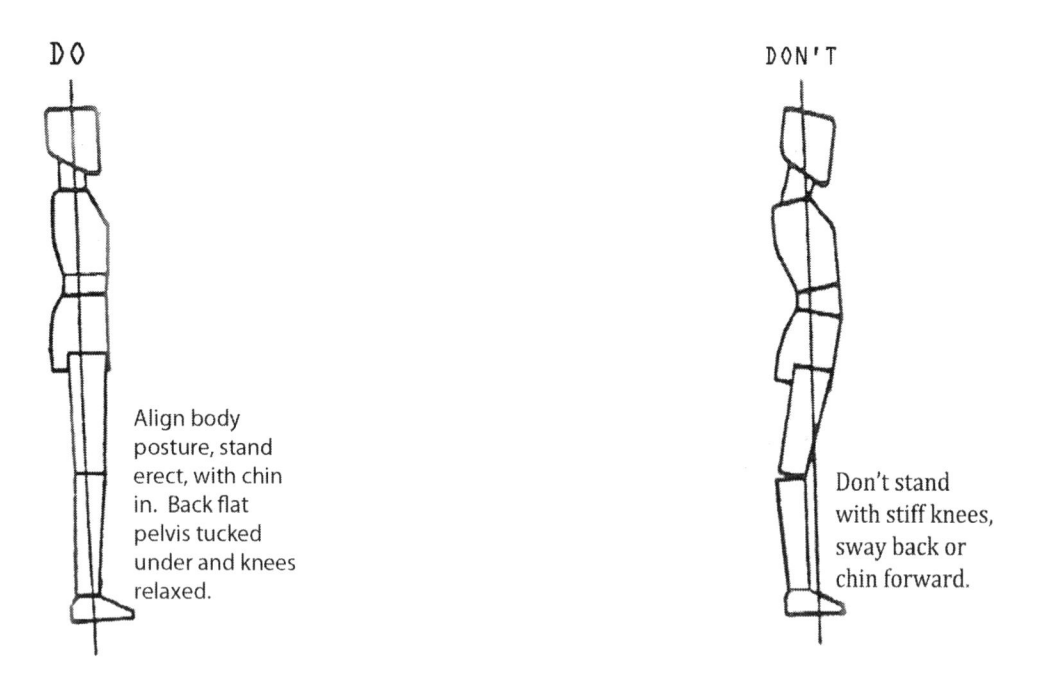

DO

Align body posture, stand erect, with chin in. Back flat pelvis tucked under and knees relaxed.

DON'T

Don't stand with stiff knees, sway back or chin forward.

Posture Do's and Don'ts

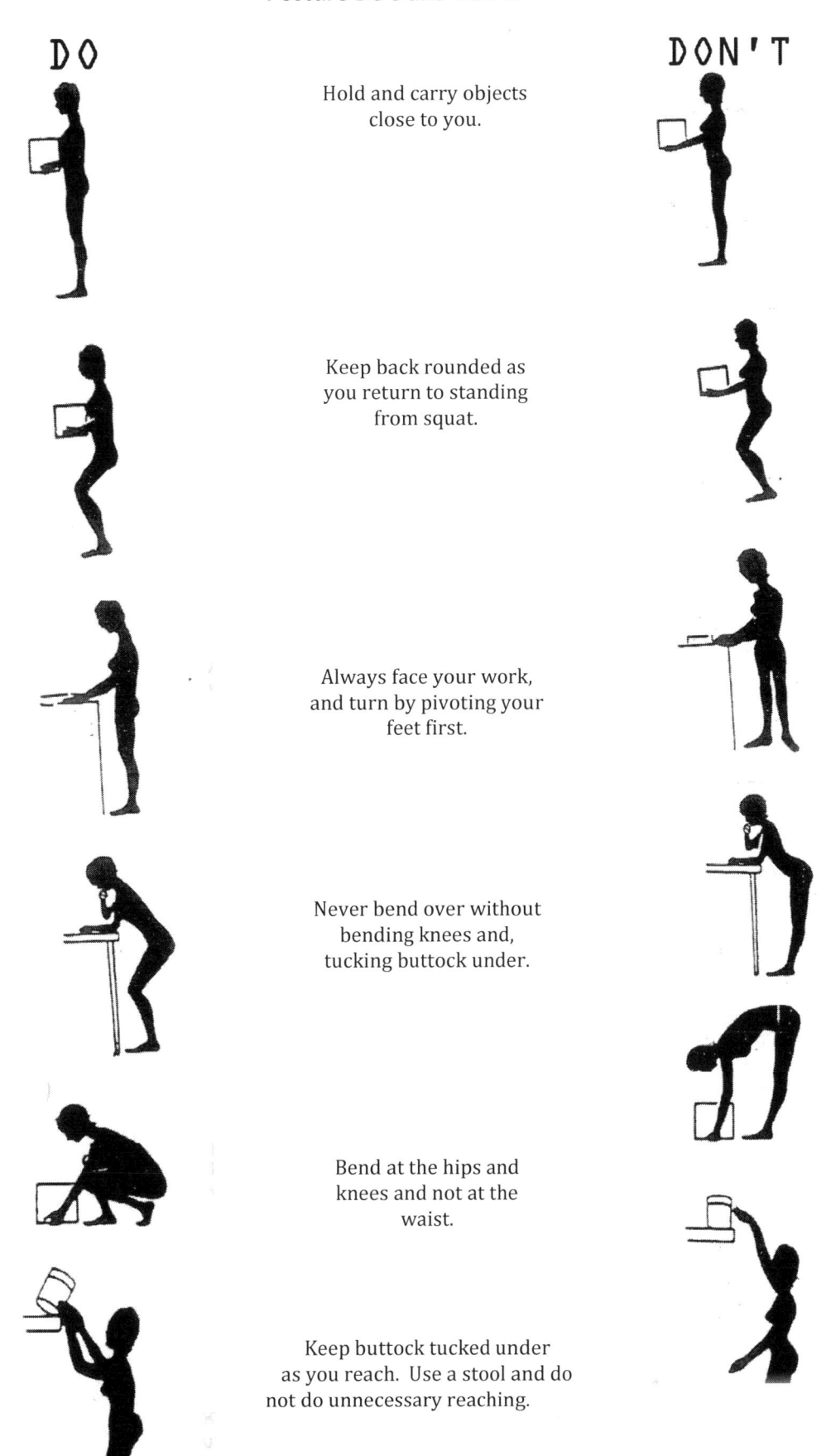

DO — DON'T

Hold and carry objects close to you.

Keep back rounded as you return to standing from squat.

Always face your work, and turn by pivoting your feet first.

Never bend over without bending knees and, tucking buttock under.

Bend at the hips and knees and not at the waist.

Keep buttock tucked under as you reach. Use a stool and do not do unnecessary reaching.

299

Shoulder Angles

Shoulders that are imbalanced (one side lower than other) indicate that the muscles on the side of the higher shoulder side are weaker than the muscles on the side of the lower shoulder. The organs on the lower shoulder side can be pushed too close together and violating cellular electronegativity.

The Female Principle is indicated by sloping shoulders. Square shoulders indicate the Male Principle. They are physical and social and intellectual. Shoulders with a round shape and balanced muscles, indicates a balanced between mental, emotional, and physical activities as well as esthetic and intellect.

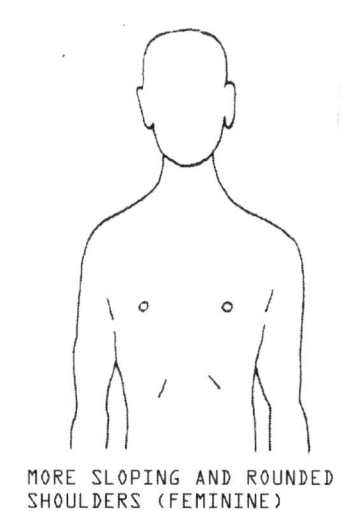

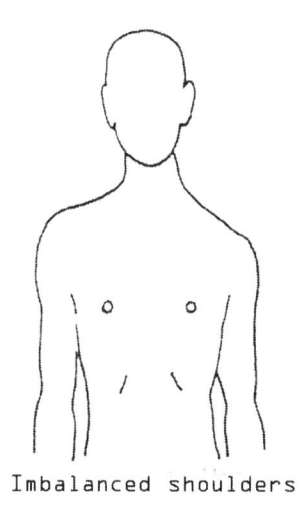

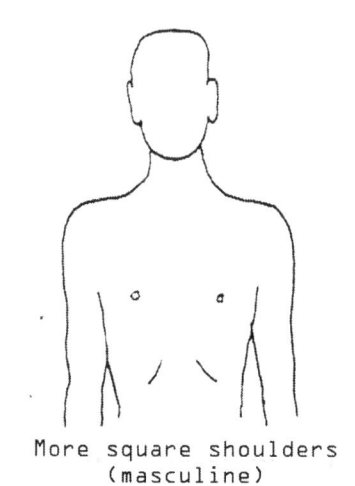

MORE SLOPING AND ROUNDED SHOULDERS (FEMININE)

Imbalanced shoulders

More square shoulders (masculine)

Anatomy And Body Types

Torn Ligaments Symptoms

Ligaments are stiff dense bands of fibrous tissue that attach one bone to another bone at the joint. Tendons attach muscles to bones. Inflexible malnourished weak overheated and/or over stretched ligaments will tare. Weak ligaments and /or damaged ligaments can cause bones to slide out of alignment. A torn ligament is painful. Tendons can be torn off the bone and immobilize a joint as well as cause pain.

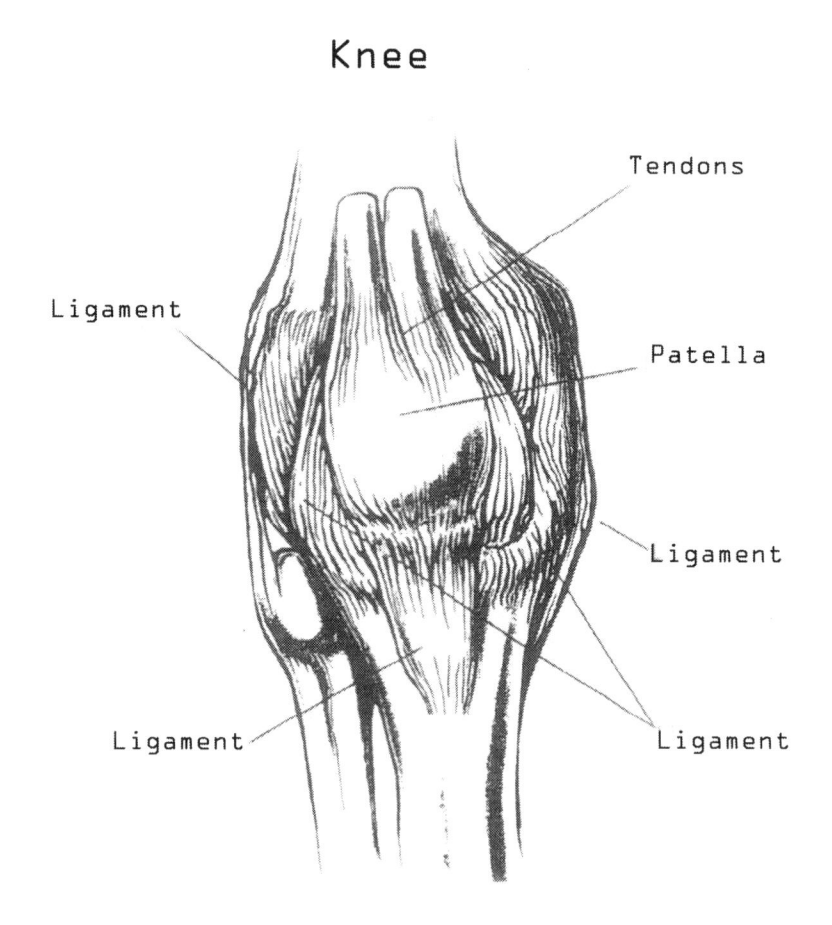

Knee

Muscles, Deep Layer, Front View

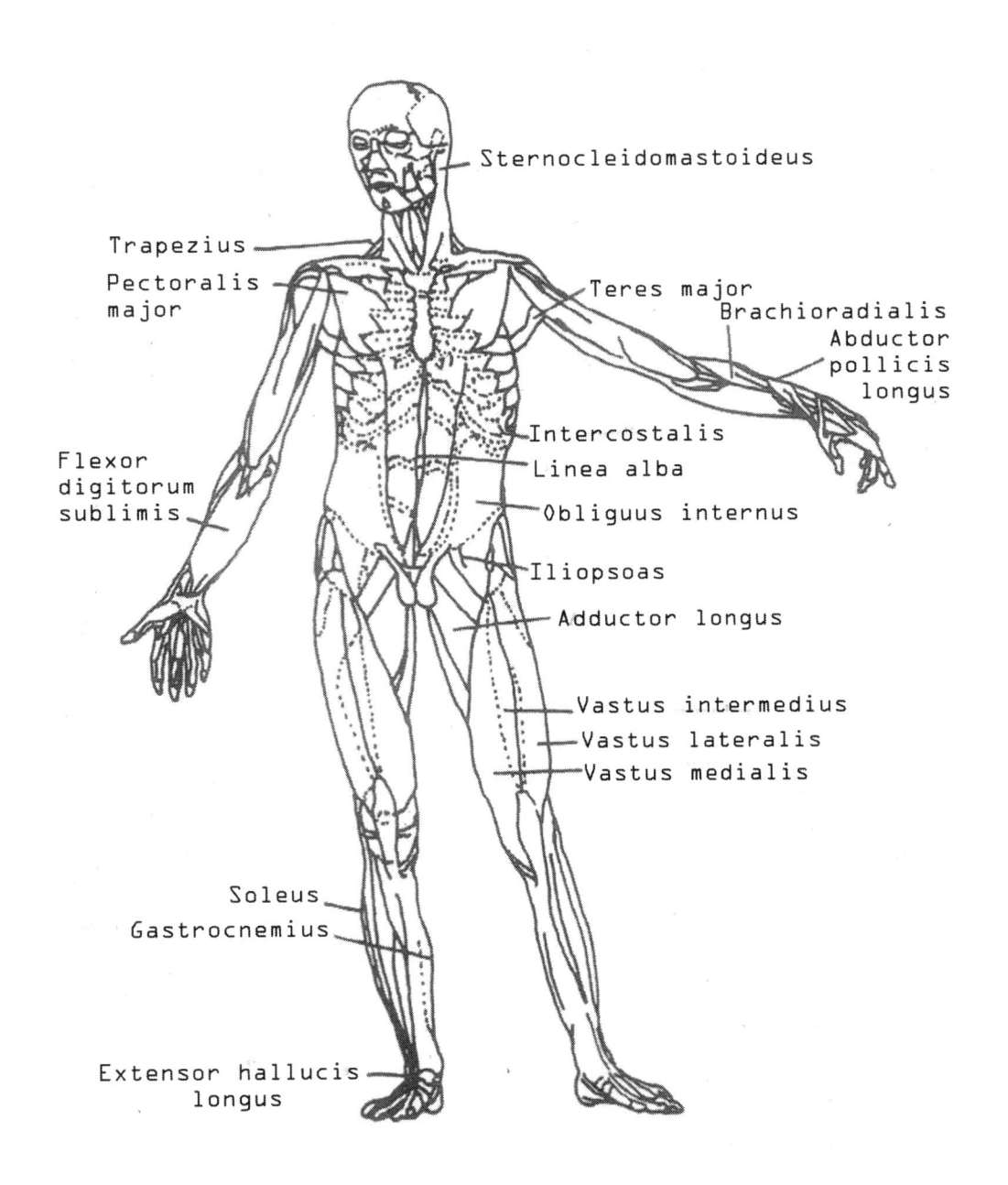

- Sternocleidomastoideus
- Trapezius
- Pectoralis major
- Teres major
- Brachioradialis
- Abductor pollicis longus
- Flexor digitorum sublimis
- Intercostalis
- Linea alba
- Obliquus internus
- Iliopsoas
- Adductor longus
- Vastus intermedius
- Vastus lateralis
- Vastus medialis
- Soleus
- Gastrocnemius
- Extensor hallucis longus

Muscles, Deep Layer, Back View

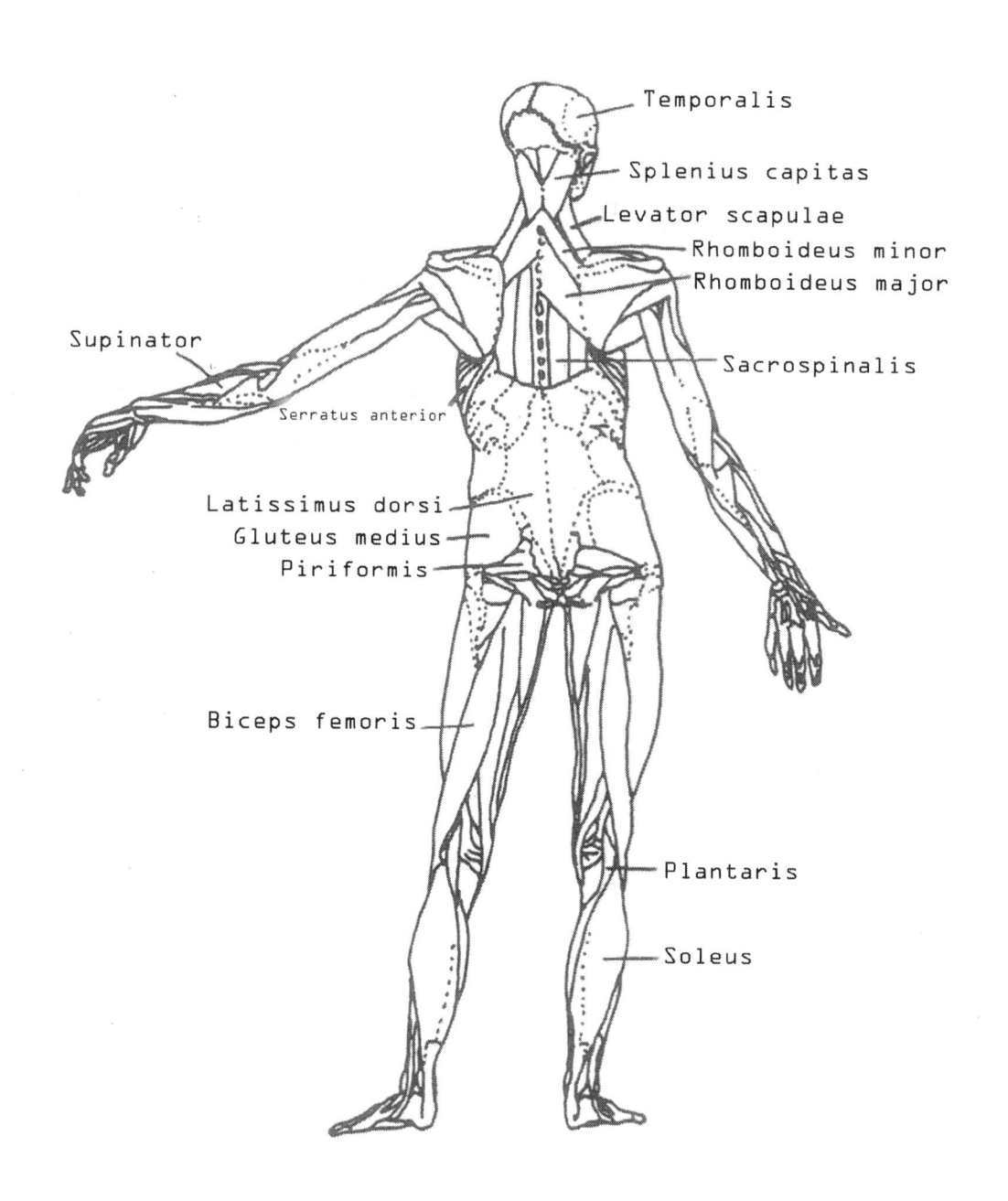

Muscles, Superficial Layer, Front View

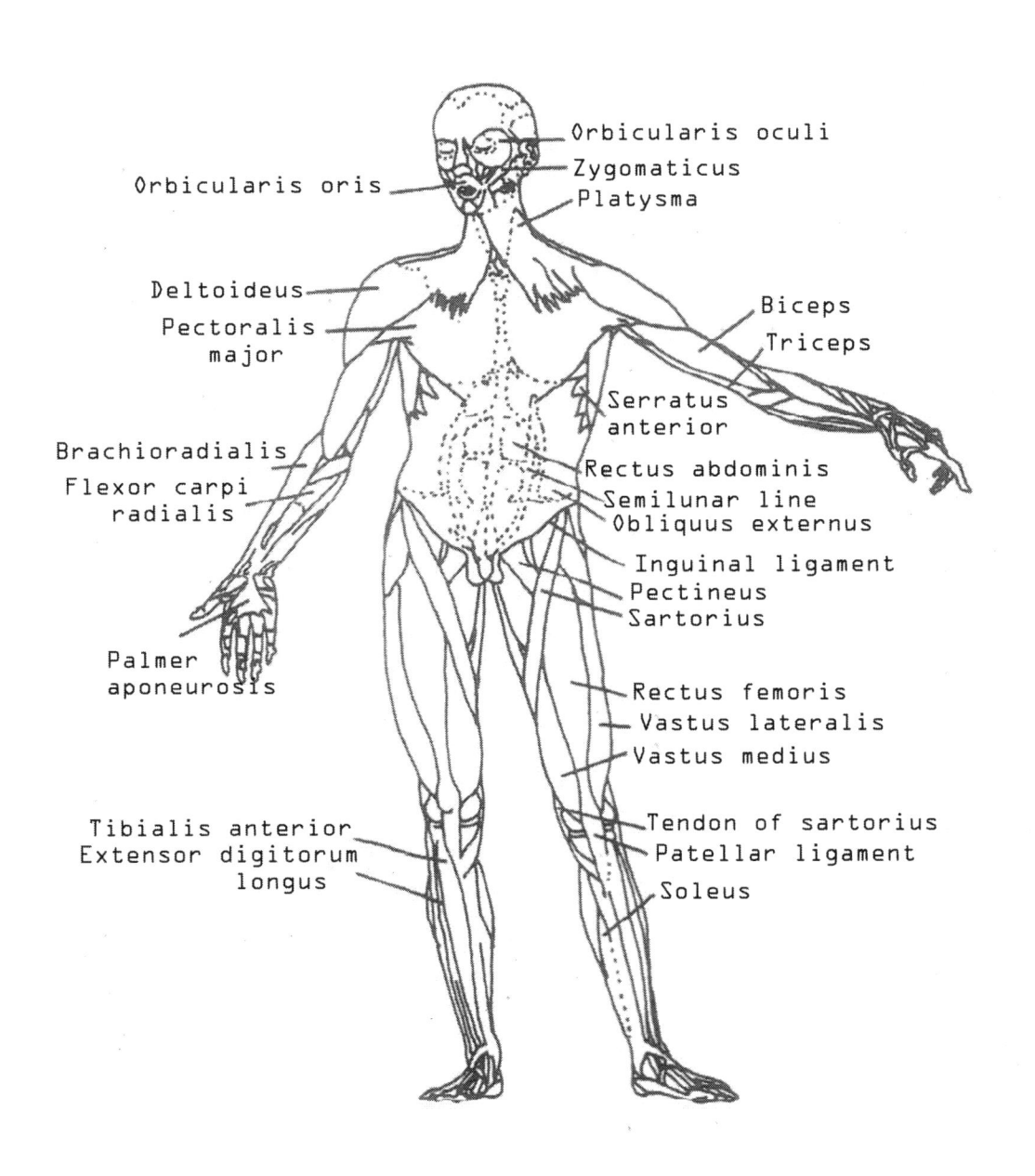

Muscles, Superficial Layer, Back View

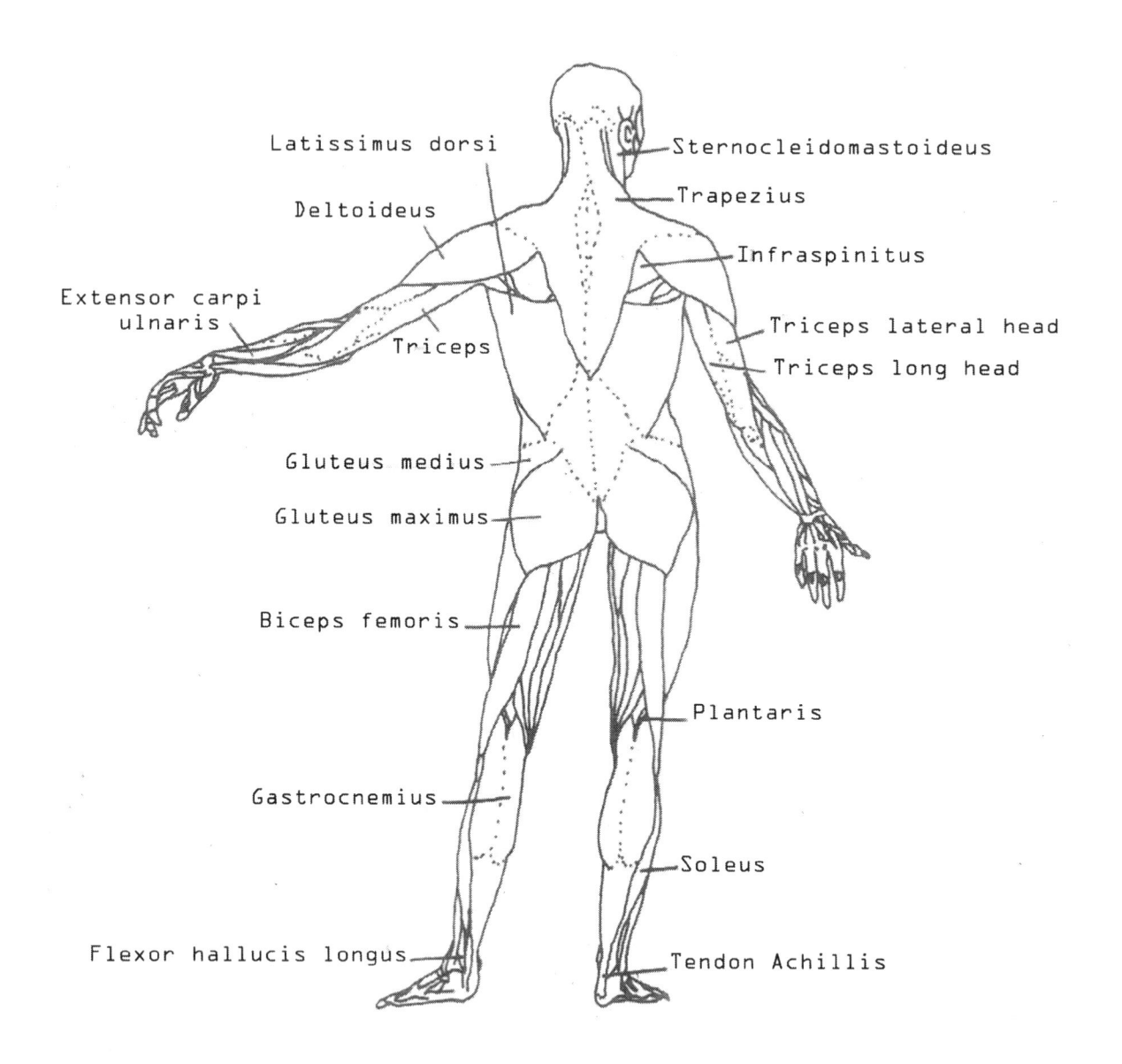

- Latissimus dorsi
- Deltoideus
- Extensor carpi ulnaris
- Triceps
- Sternocleidomastoideus
- Trapezius
- Infraspinitus
- Triceps lateral head
- Triceps long head
- Gluteus medius
- Gluteus maximus
- Biceps femoris
- Plantaris
- Gastrocnemius
- Soleus
- Flexor hallucis longus
- Tendon Achillis

Skeleton

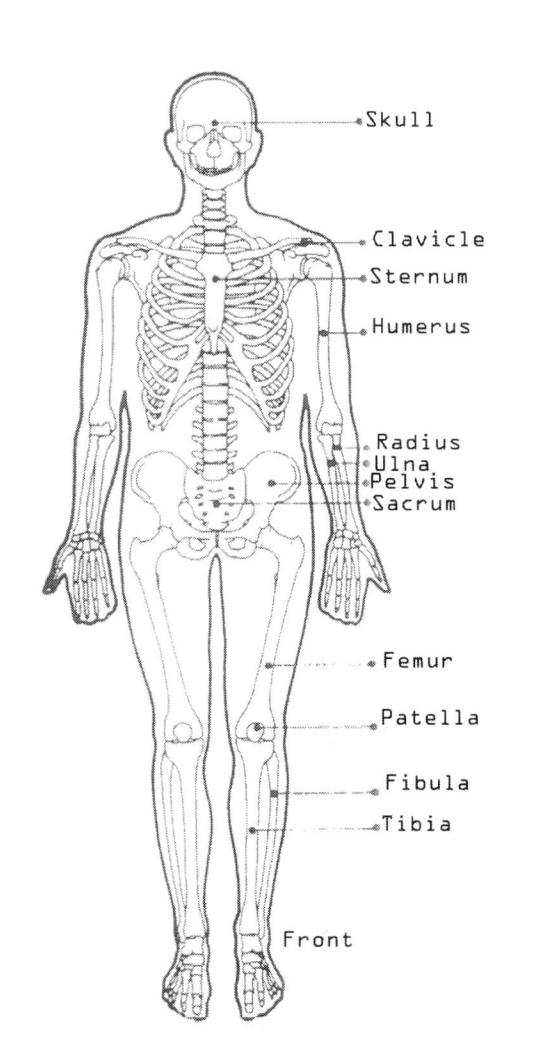

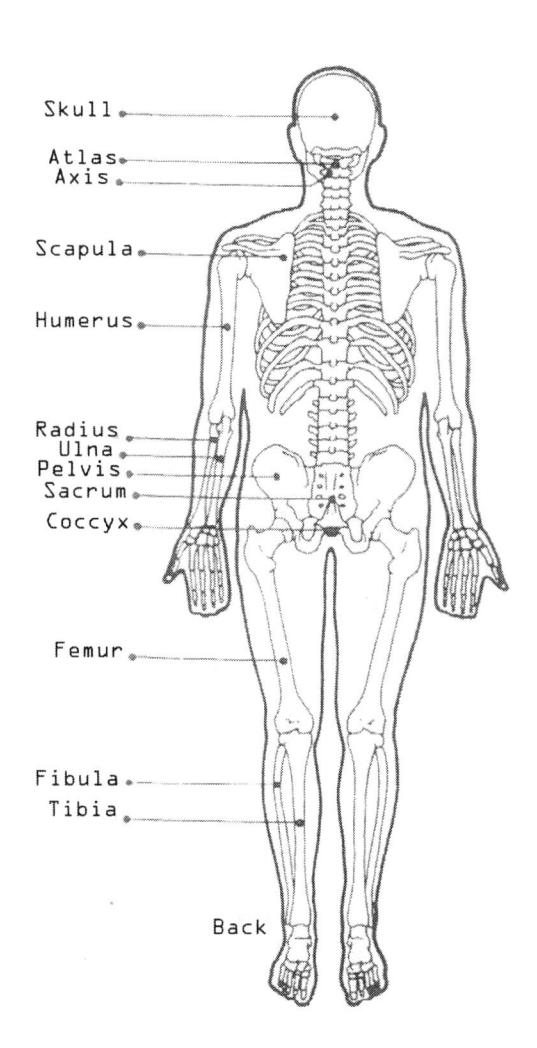

Front:
- Skull
- Clavicle
- Sternum
- Humerus
- Radius
- Ulna
- Pelvis
- Sacrum
- Femur
- Patella
- Fibula
- Tibia

Back:
- Skull
- Atlas
- Axis
- Scapula
- Humerus
- Radius
- Ulna
- Pelvis
- Sacrum
- Coccyx
- Femur
- Fibula
- Tibia

Bones Of The Foot, Right Inside View

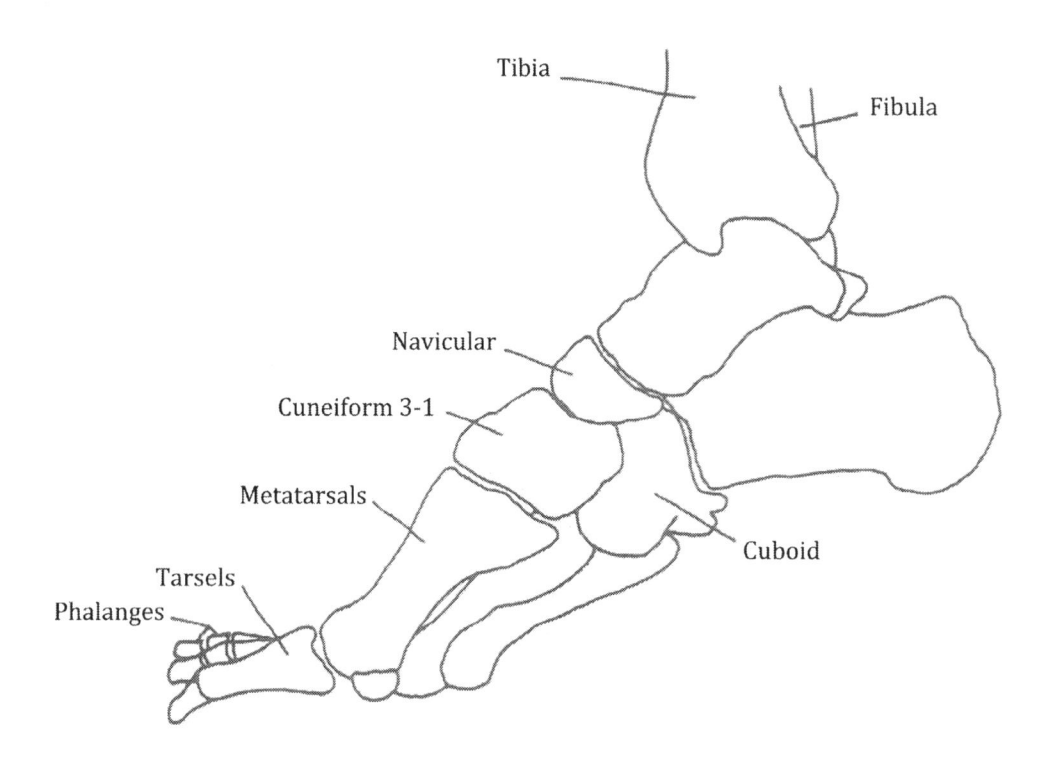

- Tibia
- Fibula
- Navicular
- Cuneiform 3-1
- Metatarsals
- Tarsels
- Phalanges
- Cuboid

Top View

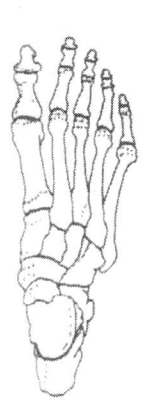

308

Bones of The Hand, Right Palm

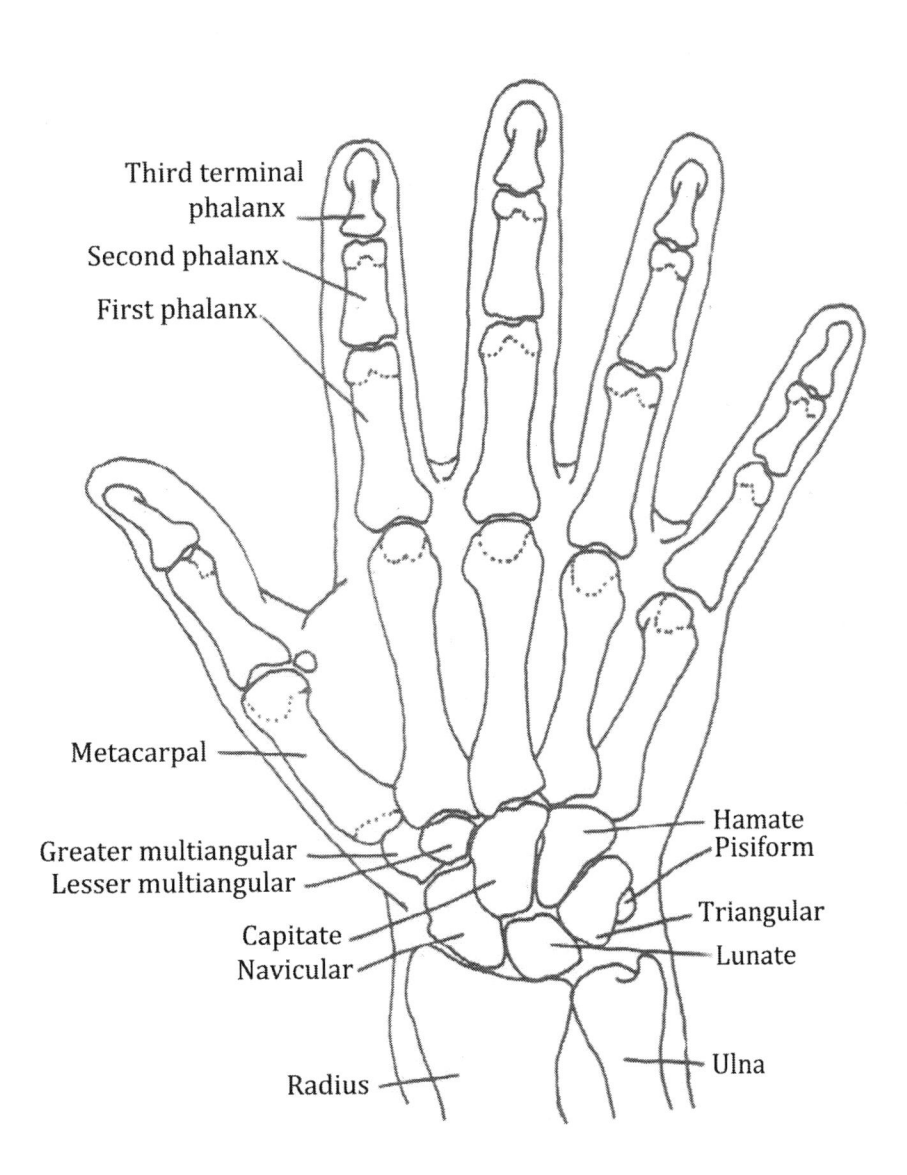

Skeleton, Front View

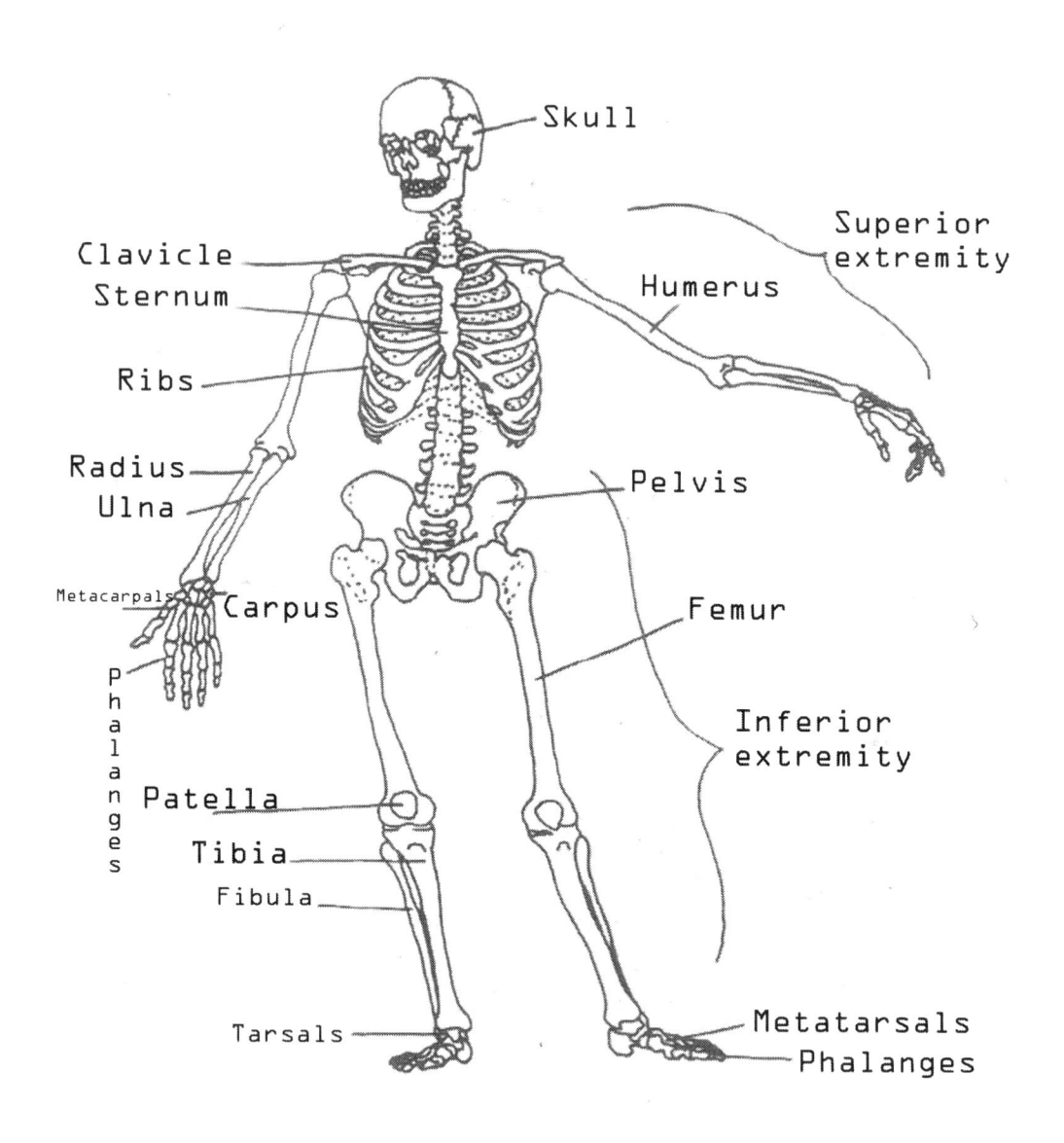

- Skull
- Clavicle
- Sternum
- Ribs
- Radius
- Ulna
- Metacarpals
- Carpus
- Phalanges
- Patella
- Tibia
- Fibula
- Tarsals
- Superior extremity
- Humerus
- Pelvis
- Femur
- Inferior extremity
- Metatarsals
- Phalanges

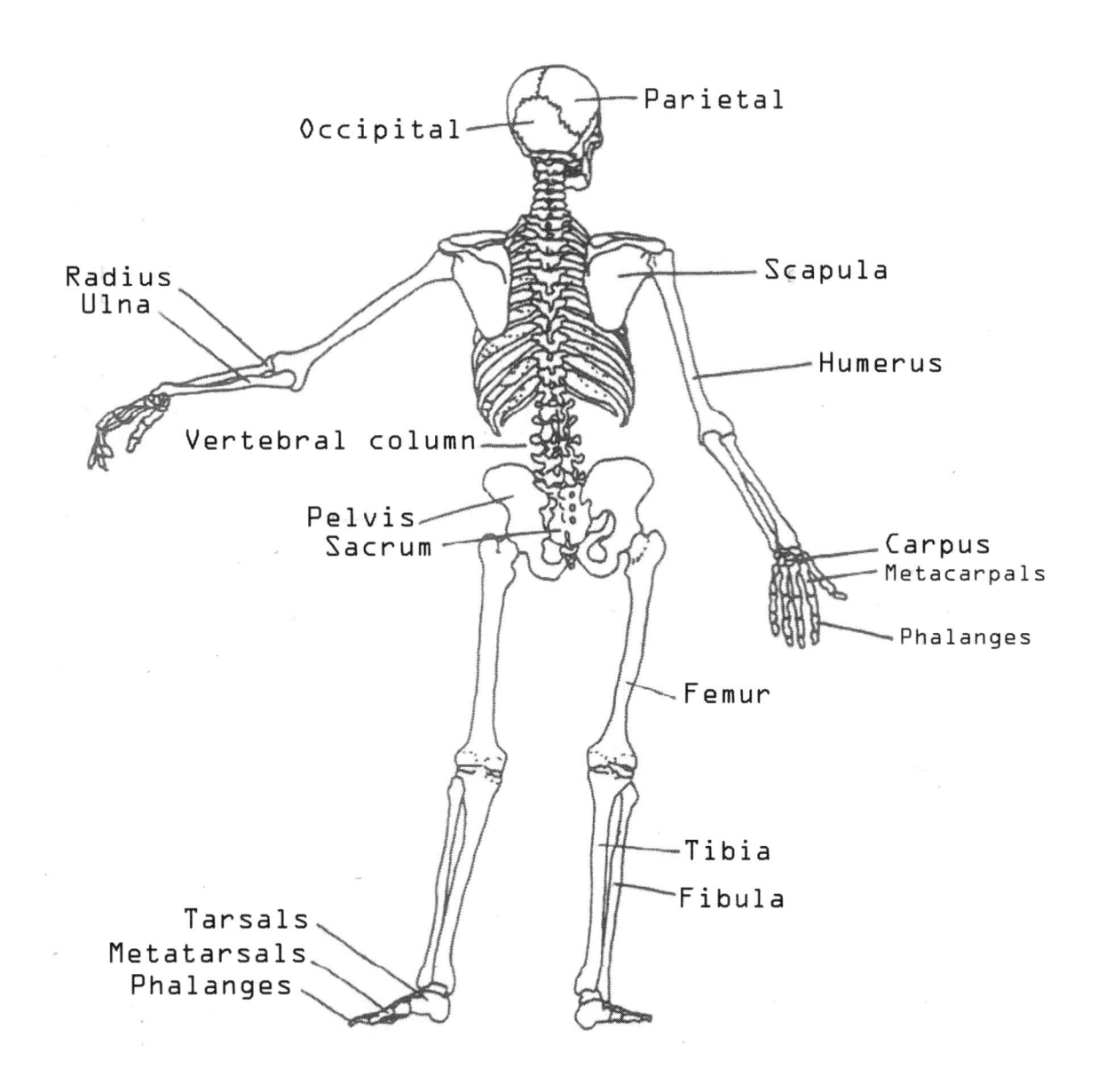

Skeleton, Back View

- Occipital
- Parietal
- Radius
- Ulna
- Scapula
- Humerus
- Vertebral column
- Pelvis
- Sacrum
- Carpus
- Metacarpals
- Phalanges
- Femur
- Tibia
- Fibula
- Tarsals
- Metatarsals
- Phalanges

Skeleton, Side View

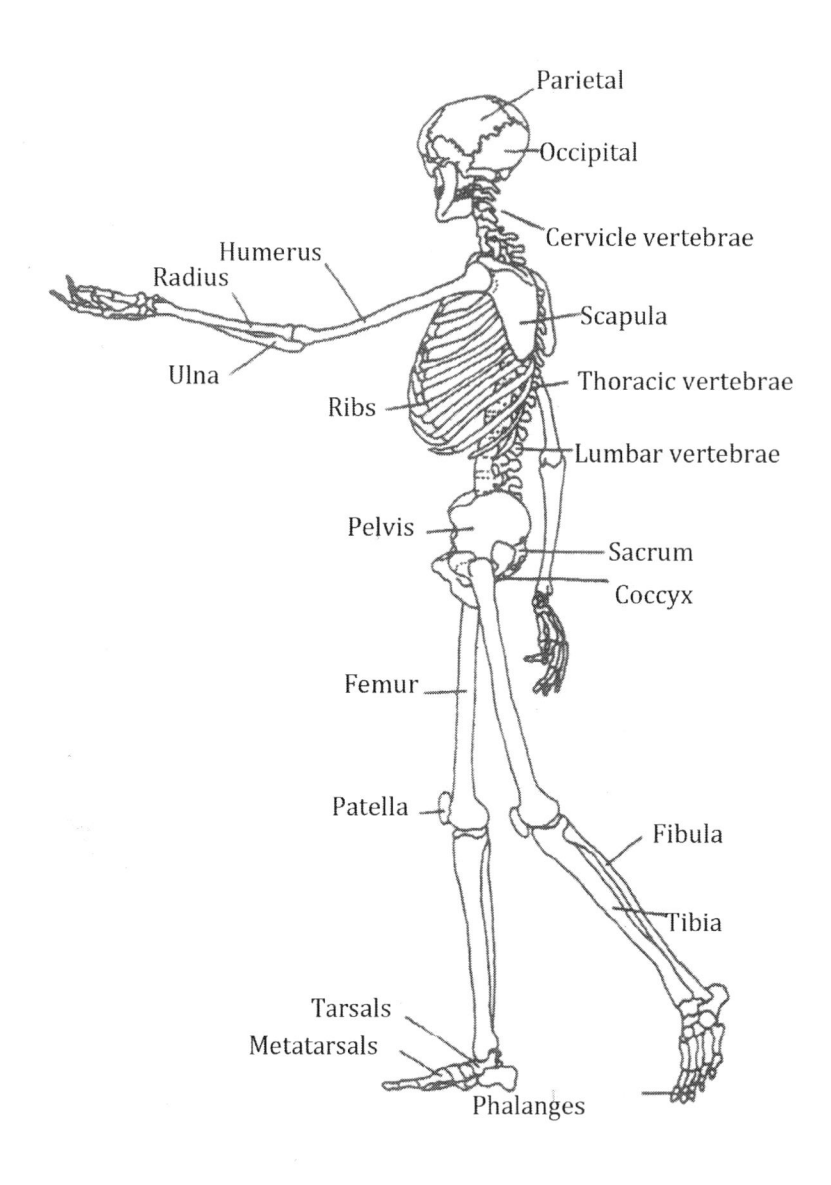

- Parietal
- Occipital
- Cervicle vertebrae
- Humerus
- Radius
- Scapula
- Ulna
- Thoracic vertebrae
- Ribs
- Lumbar vertebrae
- Pelvis
- Sacrum
- Coccyx
- Femur
- Patella
- Fibula
- Tibia
- Tarsals
- Metatarsals
- Phalanges

Muscle Exercise

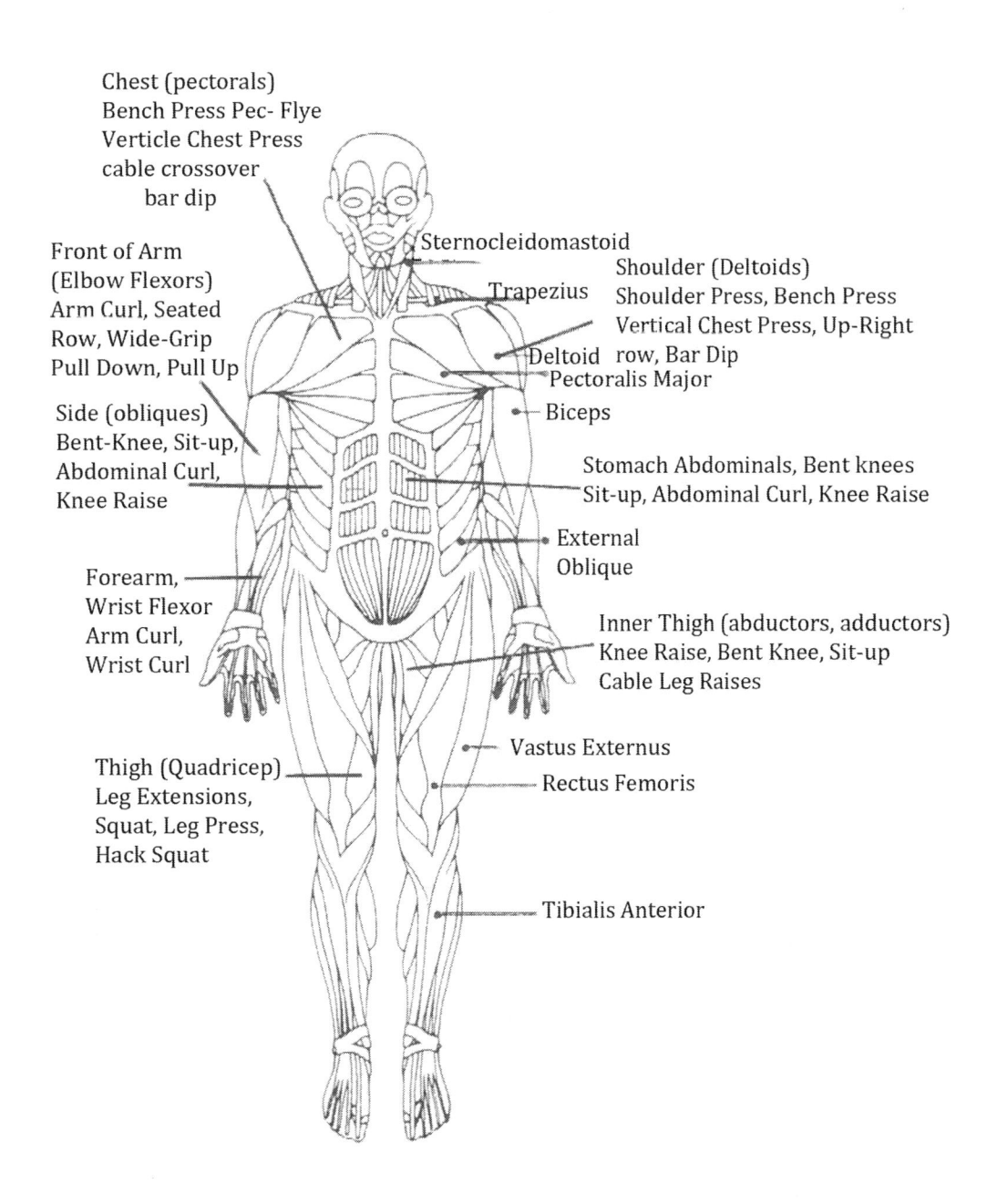

Chest (pectorals)
Bench Press Pec- Flye
Verticle Chest Press
cable crossover
bar dip

Front of Arm
(Elbow Flexors)
Arm Curl, Seated
Row, Wide-Grip
Pull Down, Pull Up

Side (obliques)
Bent-Knee, Sit-up,
Abdominal Curl,
Knee Raise

Forearm,
Wrist Flexor
Arm Curl,
Wrist Curl

Thigh (Quadricep)
Leg Extensions,
Squat, Leg Press,
Hack Squat

Sternocleidomastoid

Shoulder (Deltoids)
Trapezius   Shoulder Press, Bench Press
Vertical Chest Press, Up-Right
Deltoid row, Bar Dip
Pectoralis Major
Biceps

Stomach Abdominals, Bent knees
Sit-up, Abdominal Curl, Knee Raise

External
Oblique

Inner Thigh (abductors, adductors)
Knee Raise, Bent Knee, Sit-up
Cable Leg Raises

Vastus Externus
Rectus Femoris

Tibialis Anterior

Back Muscles and Exercise

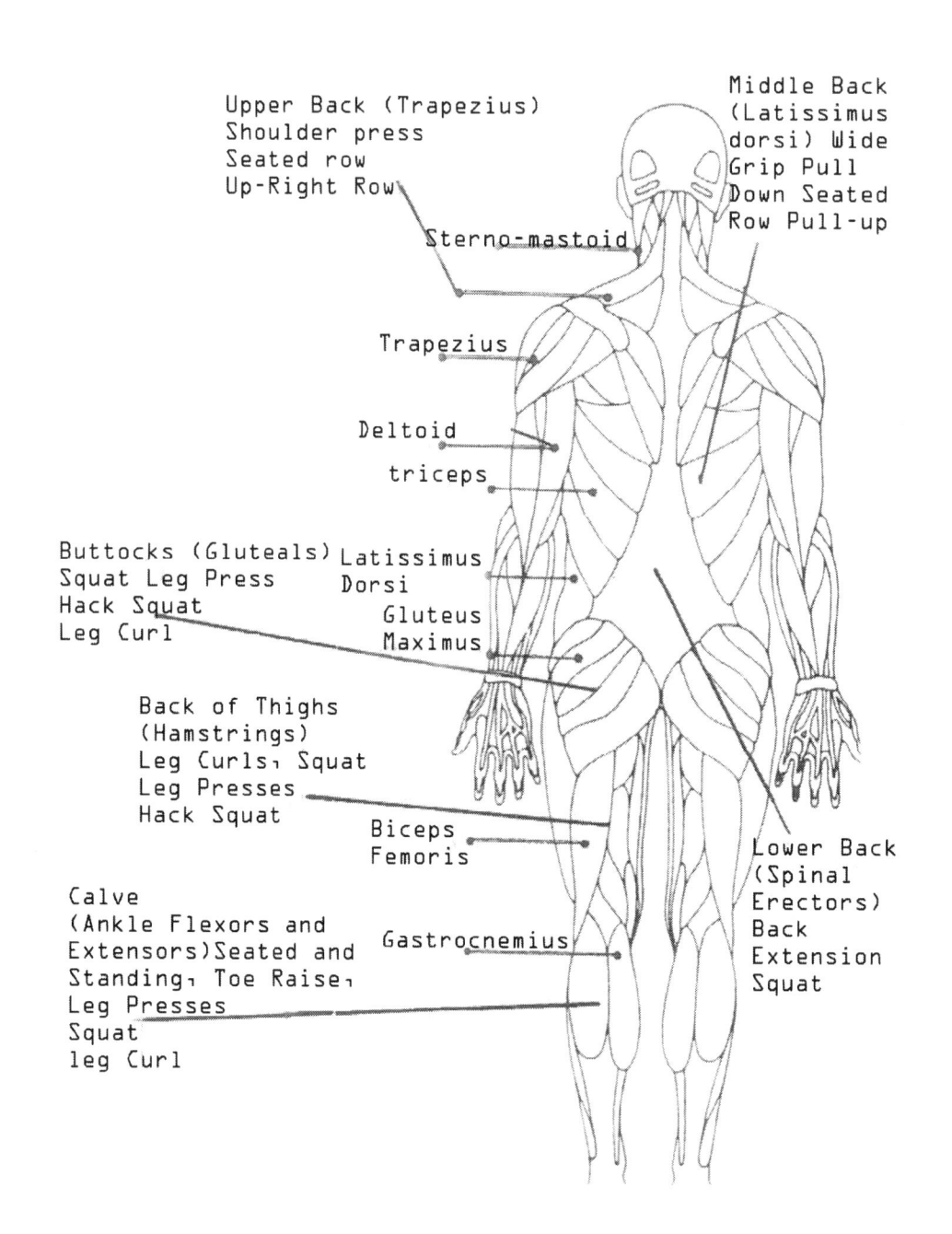

Upper Back (Trapezius)
Shoulder press
Seated row
Up-Right Row

Sterno-mastoid

Middle Back (Latissimus dorsi) Wide Grip Pull Down Seated Row Pull-up

Trapezius

Deltoid

triceps

Buttocks (Gluteals)
Squat Leg Press
Hack Squat
Leg Curl

Latissimus Dorsi

Gluteus Maximus

Back of Thighs (Hamstrings)
Leg Curls, Squat
Leg Presses
Hack Squat

Biceps Femoris

Lower Back (Spinal Erectors)
Back Extension
Squat

Calve (Ankle Flexors and Extensors) Seated and Standing, Toe Raise, Leg Presses
Squat
leg Curl

Gastrocnemius

Muscle of the Hand, Palm View

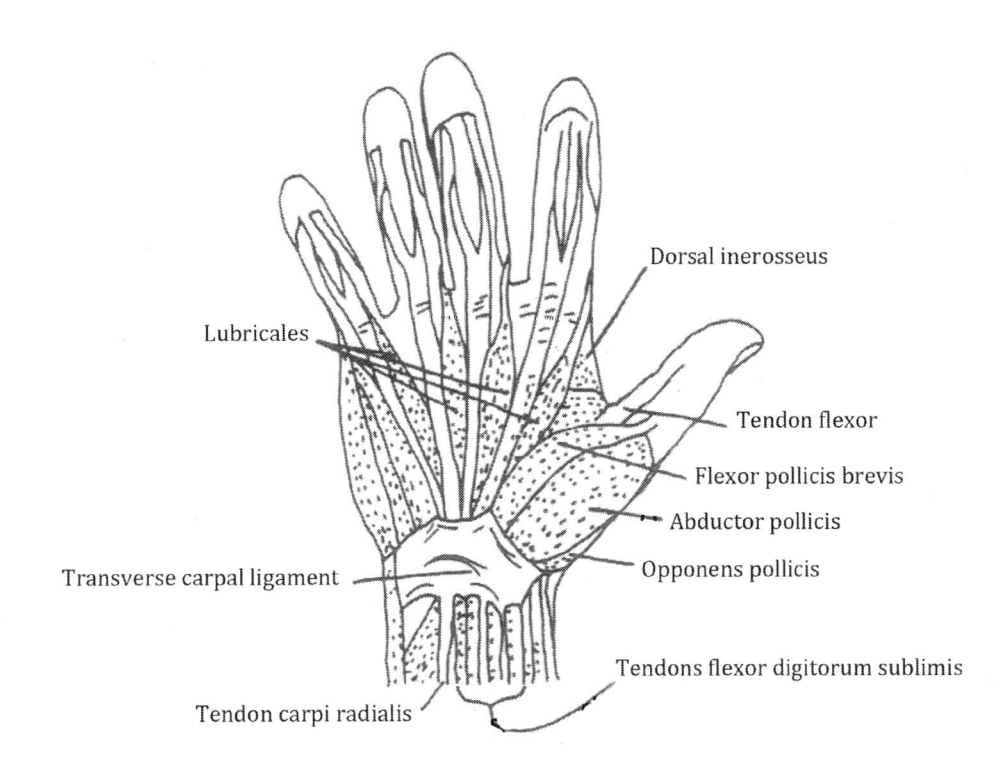

- Lubricales
- Dorsal inerosseus
- Tendon flexor
- Flexor pollicis brevis
- Abductor pollicis
- Transverse carpal ligament
- Opponens pollicis
- Tendons flexor digitorum sublimis
- Tendon carpi radialis

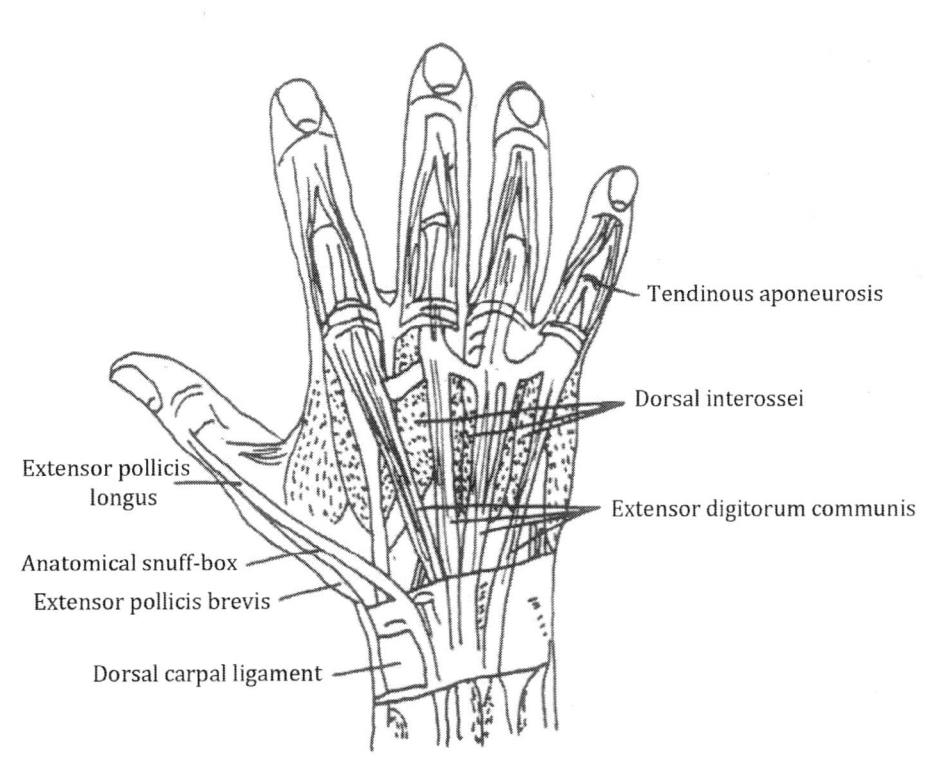

- Tendinous aponeurosis
- Dorsal interossei
- Extensor pollicis longus
- Extensor digitorum communis
- Anatomical snuff-box
- Extensor pollicis brevis
- Dorsal carpal ligament

Muscle of the Foot, Outer View

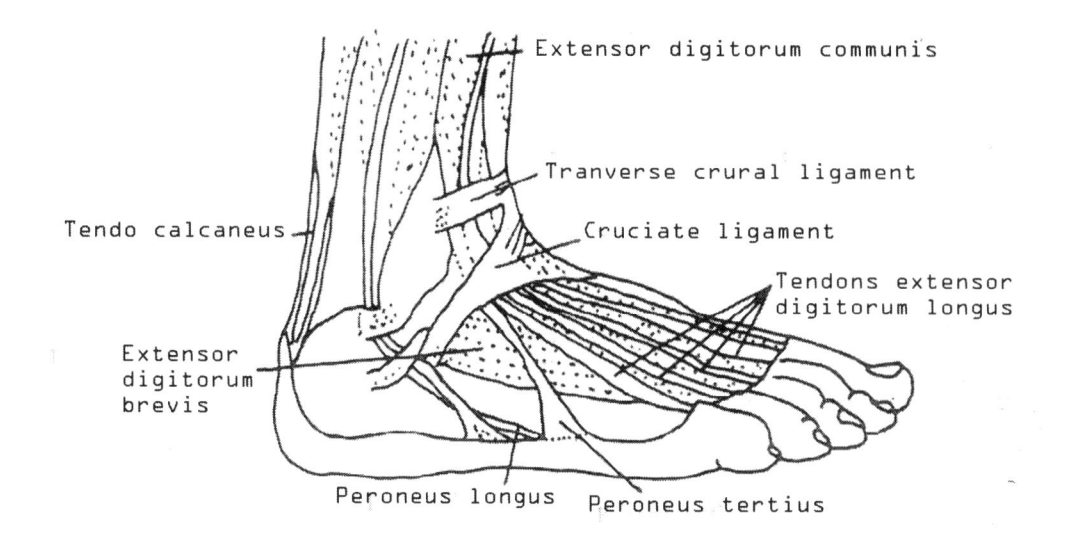

Muscles of the Foot, Inner View

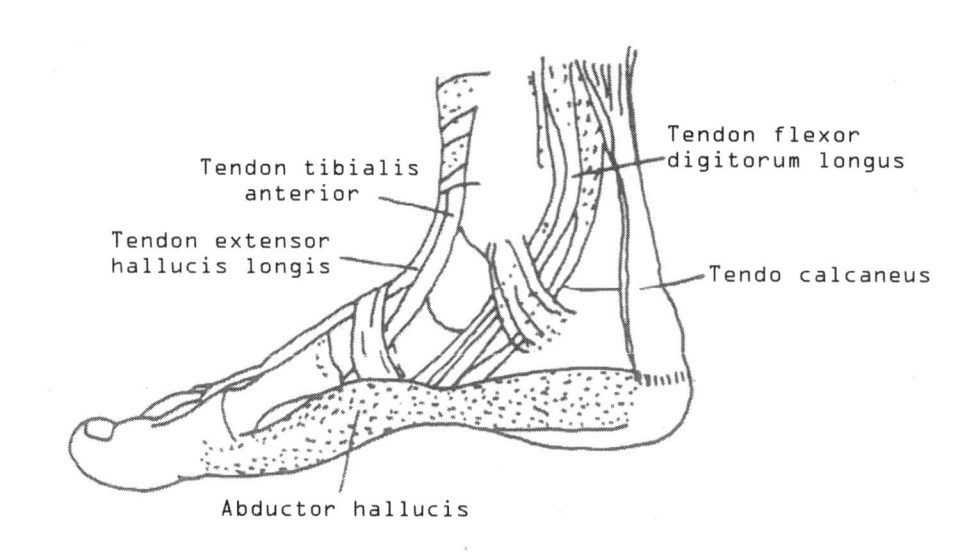

pH and the Body

SOFTEST, LOW DENSITY, SMALLEST, HIGHEST MICRONAGE, LOWEST CALCIUM

```
pH 8.0 Brain
        Lungs
            Testes – Ovaries – Placenta
            Stomach Lining – Uterus Lining
            Eyes
            Penis – Vagina – Breast
            Liver
                Fat
        Capillaries
            Muscles – Diaphragm – Skin – Spleen
pH 6.4 Transformer Glands
            Arteries – Veins – Intestinal Wall – Pancreas
            Thyroid – Esophagus
            Kidney – Heart
            Skin of Palms – Soles of Feet – Knee Caps
            Hair – Villi of Small Bowel – Mucosa of Colon
            Ligaments
            Cartilage
            Nails
            Teeth
pH 4.8 Bones
```

HARDEST, HIGH DENSITY, LARGEST, LOW MICRONAGE, HIGHEST CALCIUM

pH of Fluids and Tissues

FLUIDS	pH
Saliva	6.0 - 7.4
Food entering stomach	5.0 – 6.0
Stomach secretions	1.5 – 4.0
Digestive secretions from liver and liver bile	7.1 – 8.5
Bile from gallbladder	5.0 – 7.7
Pancreatic and biliary secretions into small intestine	7.5 – 8.3
Urine	4.5 – 8.0
Blood	7.35 – 7.45

- Most of the fluids in the body have a wide pH range. These fluids can shift their pH to maintain the alkalinity of the blood pH.
- The liver and pancreas have alkaline fluids for digestion of food and the stomach has acid fluids.
- The body is healthy when the pH of these tissues and fluids are within an optimal range.
- Diseases occur when the optimal acid – alkaline levels are not maintained.
- The average body has 1 gallon of blood and 1 teaspoon of unprocessed sugar. An additional teaspoon of sugar causes Hyperglycemia, which is the result of a high carbohydrate (starch) centered diet.

Fluids in the Body

The estimated amount of water in the human body, averaging 65percent, and varies considerably from person to person. A man may have 70 percent of his weight in water, while a woman because of her larger proportion of fatty tissues may be 52 percent water. The kidneys monitor the fluid content in the body. The lowering of the water content in the blood triggers the hypothalamus, the brains thirst center to demand the consumption of more fluids. What is commonly called blood and/or water in the body is a mixture or fats, proteins, amino acids, lymph fluid, white blood cells, red blood cells, plasma, albumin, platelets etc.

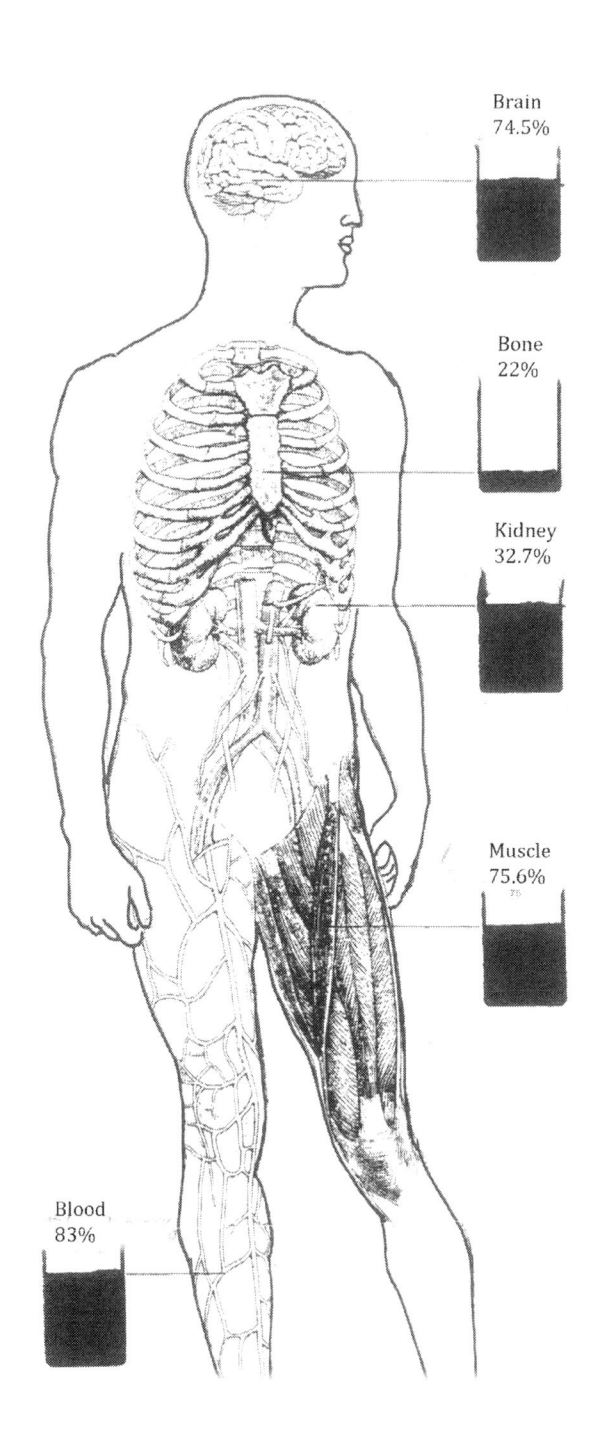

Brain 74.5%

Bone 22%

Kidney 32.7%

Muscle 75.6%

Blood 83%

Body Types

Amylase Deficient	Lipase Deficient
(Thyroid Problem)	(Gonadal Problem)
Craves: Carbohydrates, cakes, pasta, sweets, chocolate, coffee	**Craves**: Fats, creamy, rich tasting foods, oil droplets in smoke, oily Chinese and Mexican foods, chocolate, rich deserts

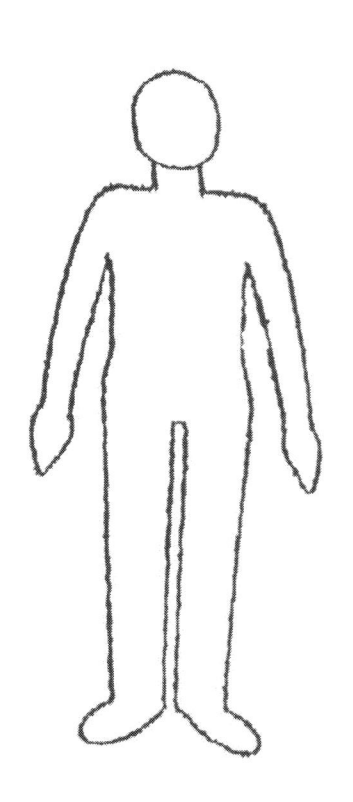

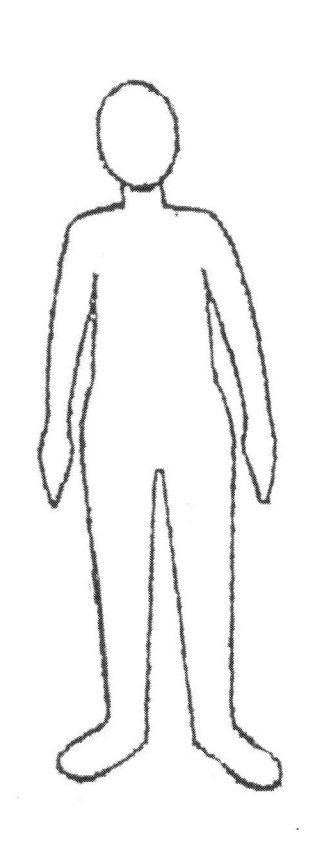

Underarms and hips are the Same width.	**Hips are wider than underarms.**
Weight is equally distributed.	Lower half of the body carries more weight
Disease Tendencies: Allergies, cold hands & feet, Depression, Fatigue, Headaches, Hemorrhoids, Low Blood Pressure, Neck & shoulder aches, PMS, Pancreatitis, Skin Eruption, Sprue (Wheat Intolerance), Upset Stomach, Ulcer	**Disease Tendencies:** Aching feet, arthritis, bladder, Breast Lumps, Breast Tumors, Bypass Surgery, Cataracts, Cirrhosis, Cystitis, Eczema, Gallbladder Problems, Gallstones, Hay Fever, Hepatitis, Hives, Urinary Problems

Protease Deficient	**Combination Deficient** (Amylase, Lipase, Protease)
(Adrenal Problems)	(Thyroid Problems)
Craves: Proteins, beef, bacon, and vegetable protein texturized meat substitute.	**Craves:** Dairy, sweets, and carbohydrates.

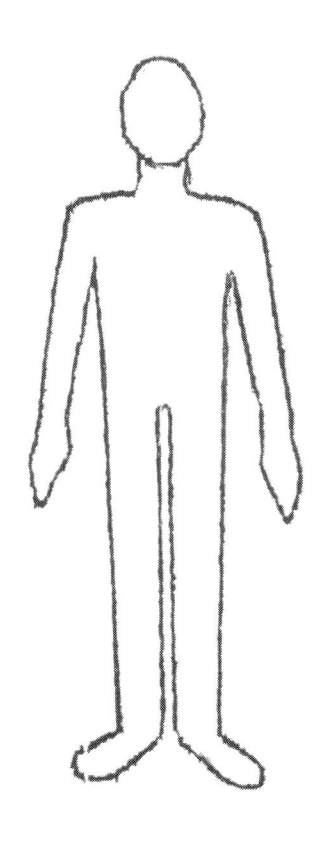

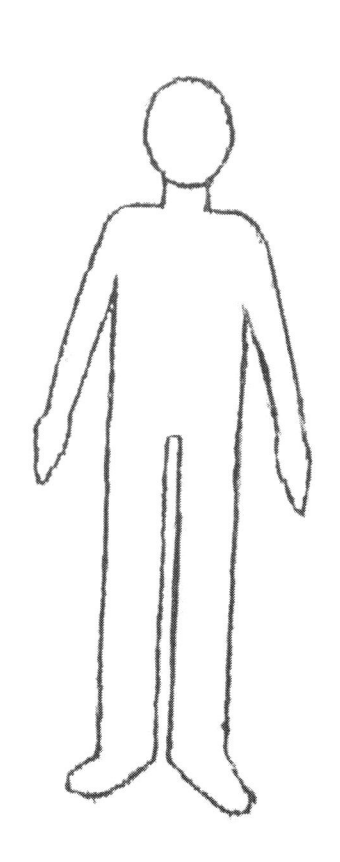

Underarms are wider than hips.	**This body type looks younger than**
Develops muscularly.	Shape is similar to teens.
Tends to carry weight above the waist.	Difficult to develop muscularly.
Disease Tendencies: Arteriosclerosis, Back Problems, Candidiasis, Constipation, Ear Infections, Heart Disease, Herniated Disc, High Blood Pressure, Insomnia, Kidney Disease, Lower Back Ache, Loss of Hearing, Osteoporosis, Sciatica	**Disease Tendencies:** Aching Knees, Chronic Allergies, Colds, Colitis, Chron's Disease, Diarrhea to Constipation, Irritable Bowel, Milk Intolerance, Frequent Colds

Lymphatic System, Blood System

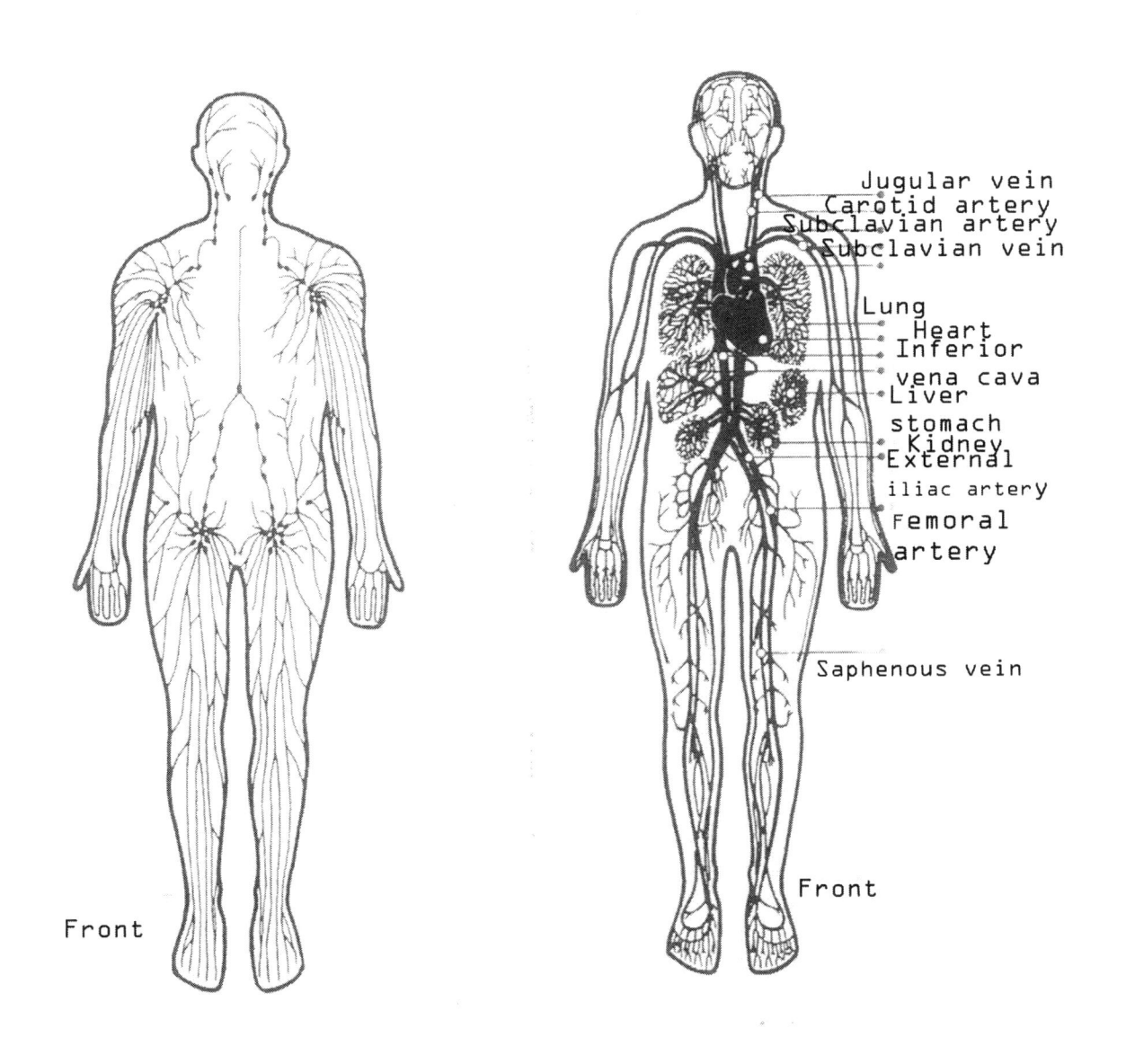

Front

Jugular vein
Carotid artery
Subclavian artery
Subclavian vein
Lung
Heart
Inferior
vena cava
Liver
stomach
Kidney
External
iliac artery
Femoral
artery

Saphenous vein

Front

Organs

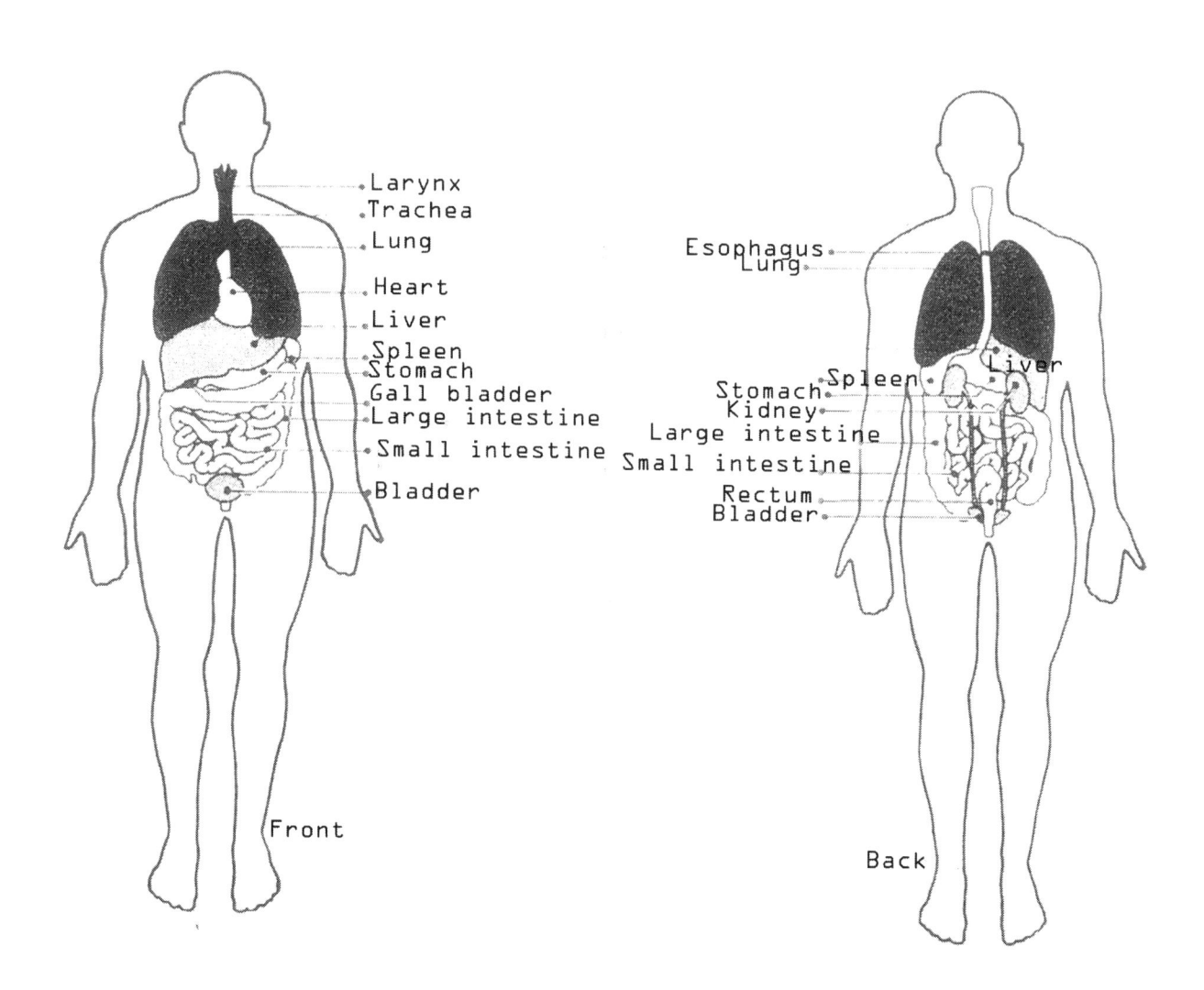

Front:
- Larynx
- Trachea
- Lung
- Heart
- Liver
- Spleen
- Stomach
- Gall bladder
- Large intestine
- Small intestine
- Bladder

Back:
- Esophagus
- Lung
- Spleen
- Liver
- Stomach
- Kidney
- Large intestine
- Small intestine
- Rectum
- Bladder

Nervous System, Endocrine Glands

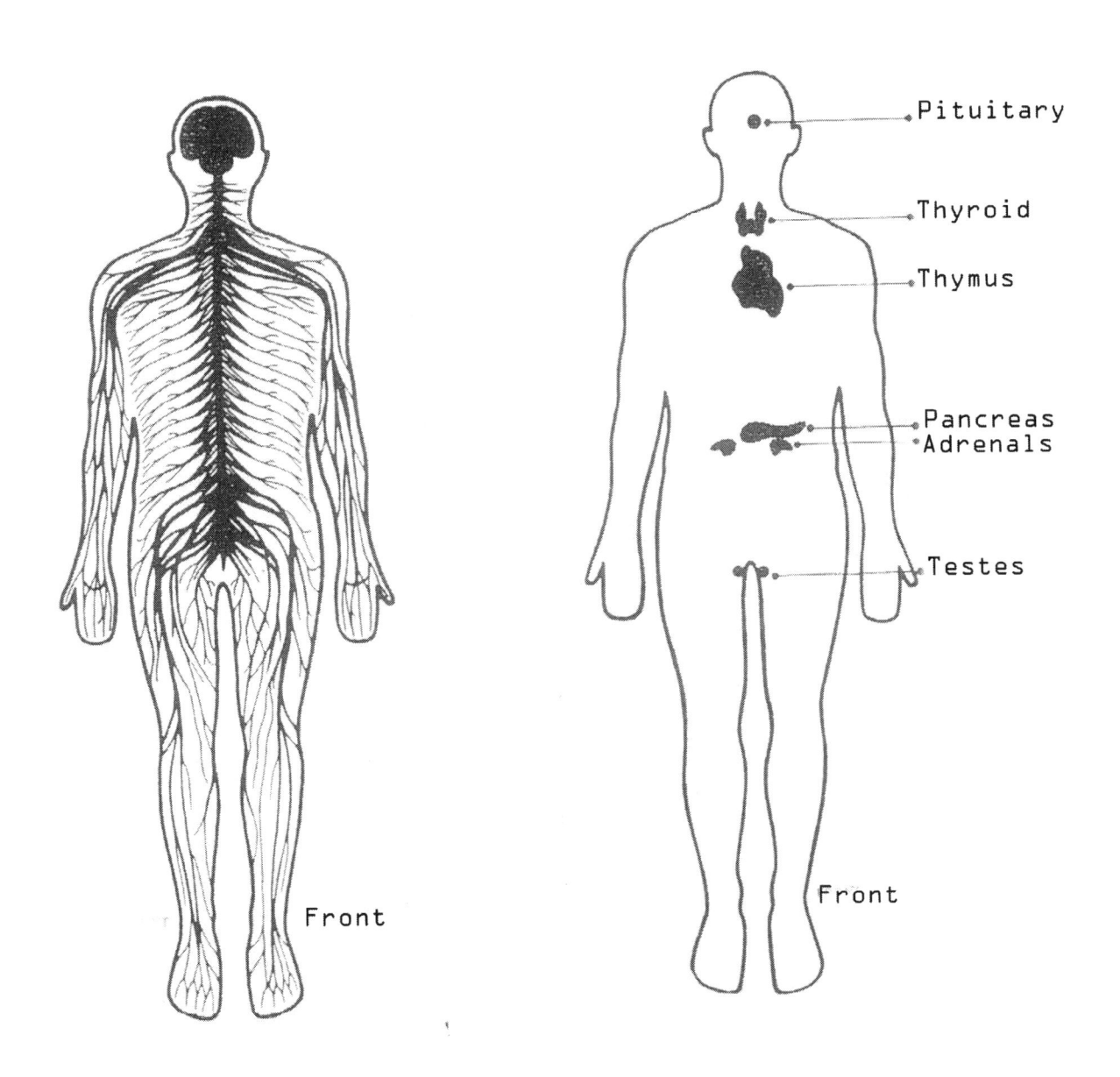

- Pituitary
- Thyroid
- Thymus
- Pancreas
- Adrenals
- Testes

Front

Front

Brain Centers

Brain Centers each part controls different functions.

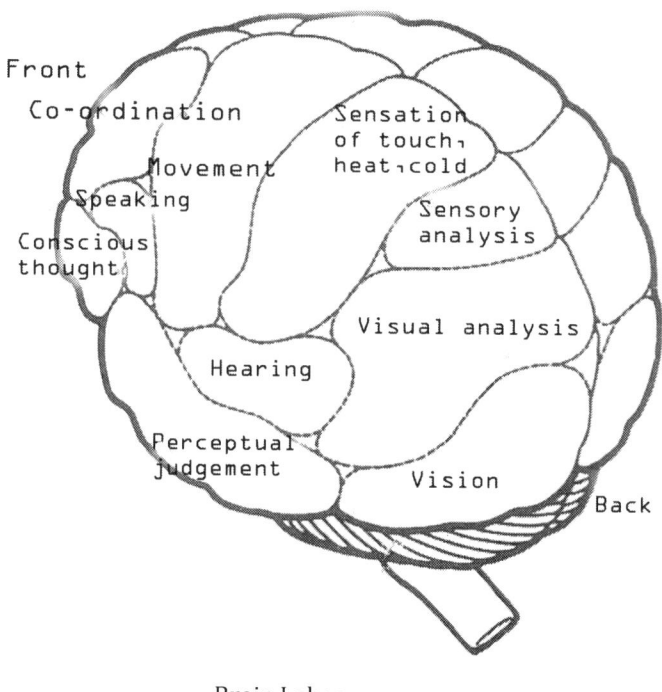

Brain diagram labels: Front, Co-ordination, Movement, Speaking, Conscious thought, Sensation of touch, heat, cold, Sensory analysis, Visual analysis, Hearing, Perceptual judgement, Vision, Back

Brain Lobes

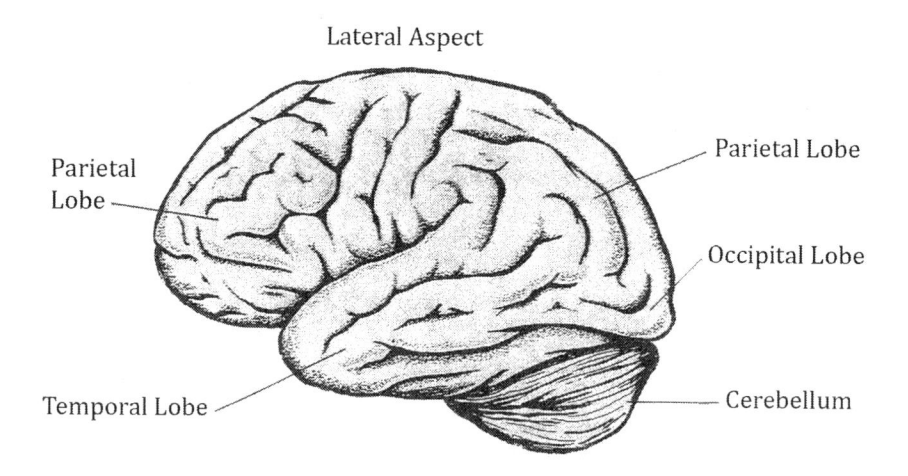

Lateral Aspect

Labels: Parietal Lobe, Parietal Lobe, Occipital Lobe, Temporal Lobe, Cerebellum

The brain is 15% neurons (transmit signals) and 85% glia cells, which nourish, repairs, store and communicate. Brain signals start in the brain stem and flow outward to the cortex. Intellectual and/or emotional overwork, drugs, and nutrient deprivation resulting in negative changes in moods and thoughts cause brain stress. Image machines (computers etc.) increase the interconnecting wiring size of the Audio/Visual centers and decrease the wiring of the Frontal Lobe (morals, Sensorship). The brain has a signal pathway. It starts with 1) Brain Stem (Pons) of the spinal cord (influences heart, breathing, digestion, etc.), 2)Limbic System (thirst, physical and emotional cycles, sex etc.) parts are; Amygdala (grades emotions, fear, joy etc.) Hippocampus (regulates emotions, long term memory etc.) Locus Cerulus (nucleus of Limbic-System) 3) Corpus Callosum (connects logic and emotions) 4) Para-Limbic Cortex (adds emotional value to signals) 5) Cerebral Cortex (so-called gray matter, morality, evaluates) parts are; Left Hemisphere (analytical, sequential emotions) Right Hemisphere (artistic, spiritual, emotions, random logic, and rationales). Females Language Center and Corpus Callosum are over 25% larger than males.

Brain Parts

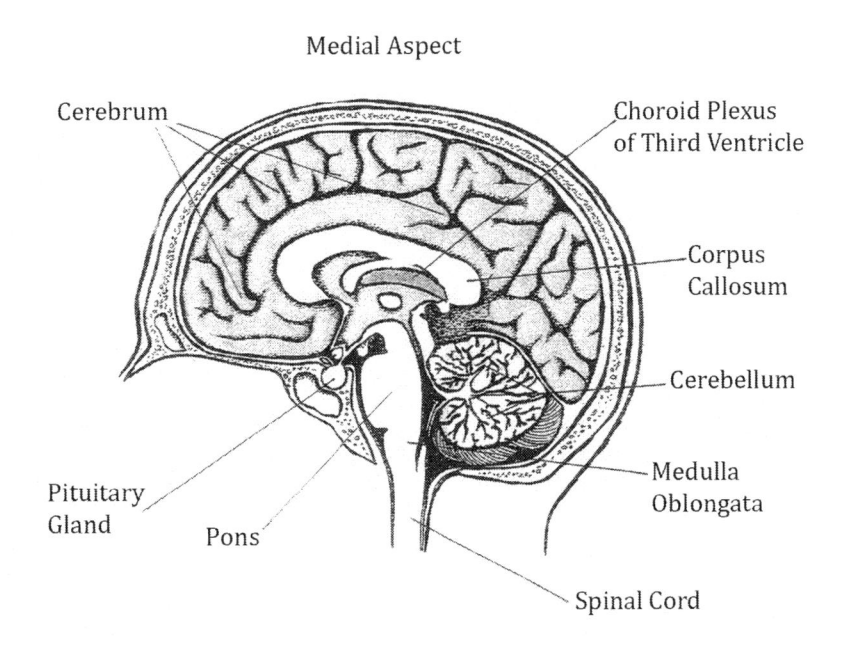

Medial Aspect

- Cerebrum
- Choroid Plexus of Third Ventricle
- Corpus Callosum
- Cerebellum
- Medulla Oblongata
- Pituitary Gland
- Pons
- Spinal Cord

The brain is stimulated by sex hormones progesterone, estrogen, and testosterone. When these hormones are altered it alters emotions and thoughts. The brain requires insulin and glucagon. Insulin helps the brain's neurons get glucose while glucagon helps convert fat into sugar from fat cells of the outer cell's skin. Impaired Glucose Tolerance/Insulin Resistance, Metabolic Syndrome (Syndrome X) are different names for the same disease which causes the brain to have Type 3 Diabetes (ADHD, Alzheimer's). The brain cells cannot get sugar and the brain cells die which is why Type 2 Diabetes causes a decrease in the brains size (volume of cells).

Gland and Organ Test

This evaluation determines which glands or organs are stressed, diseased or needs nutritional support. For each statement mark:
1) If mildly true.
2) If moderately true.
3) If totally true.
If a statement does not apply, leave it blank.
A score higher than 4 points can indicate a nutritional, hormonal, or malfunctioning problem.

Pituitary
___Pain in upper left neck or little finger
___Overweight from waist down
___Overweight from waist up
___Cold hands, feet/cold all over
___Headaches behind eyes or affecting one half of head
___Disease of bones, ligaments, or tendons
___Excessive urination
___Water swelling below eyes or in ankles, fingers, feet, etc.
___Difficult pregnancy or delivery
___Delivered with forceps
___History of head injury
___Infertility or impotency

Thyroid: Underactive
___Muscles stiff in morning, muscles become stiff after sitting for long duration
___Feel dizzy or nauseated in morning
___Motion sickness, dizzy when changing up and down positions
___Problems working under stress
___Emotionally unstable, cry easily
___Gain weight easily
___Difficulty concentrating, attention deficit
___Heart occasionally misses beats or unstable beats
___Coughing, hoarseness, or muscle cramps that get severe at night
___Sleeplessness, restlessness, forgetful, and memory problems
___Energy is low in the mornings, energy increases in afternoon

Thyroid: Overactive
___Energy goes up, then down
___Eats and cannot gain weight
___Thin skin and hair
___Rapid heartbeat when resting (more than 90 beats per min)
___Tongue shakes, hand shakes

Liver
___Skin oily on nose and forehead
___Digestion problems with fats or greasy foods, nausea, headaches
___Digestion problems and/or gas from sulpher in onions, cabbage, radishes, cucumbers
___Stool appears yellow, clay colored, and foul odor
___Bad breathe, bad taste in mouth
___History of constipation
___Feet and/or body odor

Adrenals: Underactive
___Salt cravings
___Excessive perspiration
___Eyes sensitive to bright lights
___Tightness or lump in throat
___Blood pressure fluctuates, has been too low on occasion
___Forms "gooseflesh" easily, cold sweats
___Voice rises to high pitch during stress
___Easily shaken up, startled, heart pounds hard from unexpected noise
___Extrovert tendency
___Allergies: skin rash, dermatitis, hay fever, sneezing attacks, or asthma
___Avoid and evades complaints, discomforts, and inconveniences

Adrenals: Overactive
___Persistent high blood pressure
___Female: Excessive hair on face, arms or legs/masculine aspects
___Males: Baldness, excess hair on arms or back,
___Extroverted
___Stronger than average physically
___Strong feelings, tends to be emotionally explosive

Pancreas
___Pain on inside of left shoulder blade or left side of abdomen
___White spots on fingernails
___Blurry vision in left eye
___High blood pressure
___Asthma
___Shingles on trunk of body
___Poor circulation, cold hands/ feet
___Arthritic pain, swelling, rheumatism
___Feel cold sweaty, shaky
___Psoriasis or acne

__Wounds heal slowly
__Lower bowel gas 2 hours after eating
__Blood clots rapidly, history of phlebitis or embolism

Kidney
__Swelling of hands and/or feet
__Burning sensation during urination
__High diastolic blood pressure
__Back near lower rib and/or leg pains
__Anemic
__Joint pain
__Urinary incontinence
__Prostate problems
__Urine has burning sensation

Heart
_Left shoulder pain that travels to the left arm
_Chest pain that radiates to shoulder and arm
_High Blood Pressure
_Unsteady heart beats
_Dizziness, nausea, unexplained headaches
_Rapid heart rate (above 90 bpm) or Slow heart rate (below 50 bpm)

__Chest pain radiating to left arm
__Heart beats not steady
__High blood pressure
__Rapid heart rate (above 90 bpm)
__Unexplained headaches, dizziness, nausea
__Slow heart rate (below 50 bpm)

Thymus
__Swollen glands in armpits and groin
__Easily susceptible to infections
__Soreness on both sides of neck and shoulder level
__Flu-like symptoms often occurs
__Unexplained sweating
__Feelings of puffiness in throat

Backbone (vertebrae) and Illness

Problems, discomfort, pain, and or illness affecting organs, glands, body parts or areas can indicate vertebrae misalignment or deterioration.

Parts of the body and areas	Vertebrae
Back of head	{1cervical}
Various areas of the head	{2cervical}
Side and front of the neck	{3cervical}
Upper back of neck	{4cervical}
Middle of neck and upper part of arms	{5cervical}
Lower part of neck, arms, and elbows	{6cervical}
Lower part of arms, shoulders	{7cervical}
Hands, wrists, fingers, thyroid	{1thoracic}
Heart, its valve and coronary arteries	{2 thoracic}
Lungs, bronchial tube, pleura, chest	{3 thoracic}
Gallbladder, common duct	{4 thoracic}
Liver, solar plexus	{5 thoracic}
Stomach, mid-back area	{6 thoracic}
Pancreas, duodenum	{7 thoracic}
Spleen, lower mid-back	{8 thoracic}
Adrenal glands	{9 thoracic}
Kidneys	{10 thoracic}
Ureters	{11 thoracic}
Small intestines, upper/lower back	{12 thoracic}
Illiocecal valve, large intestines	{1 lumber}
Appendix, abdomen, upper leg	{2 lumber}
Sex organs, uterus, bladder, knees	{3 lumber}
Prostate gland, lower back	{4 lumber}
Sciatic nerve, lower legs, ankles, feet	{5 lumber}
Hipbones, buttocks	
Rectum, anus	

Spinal Column

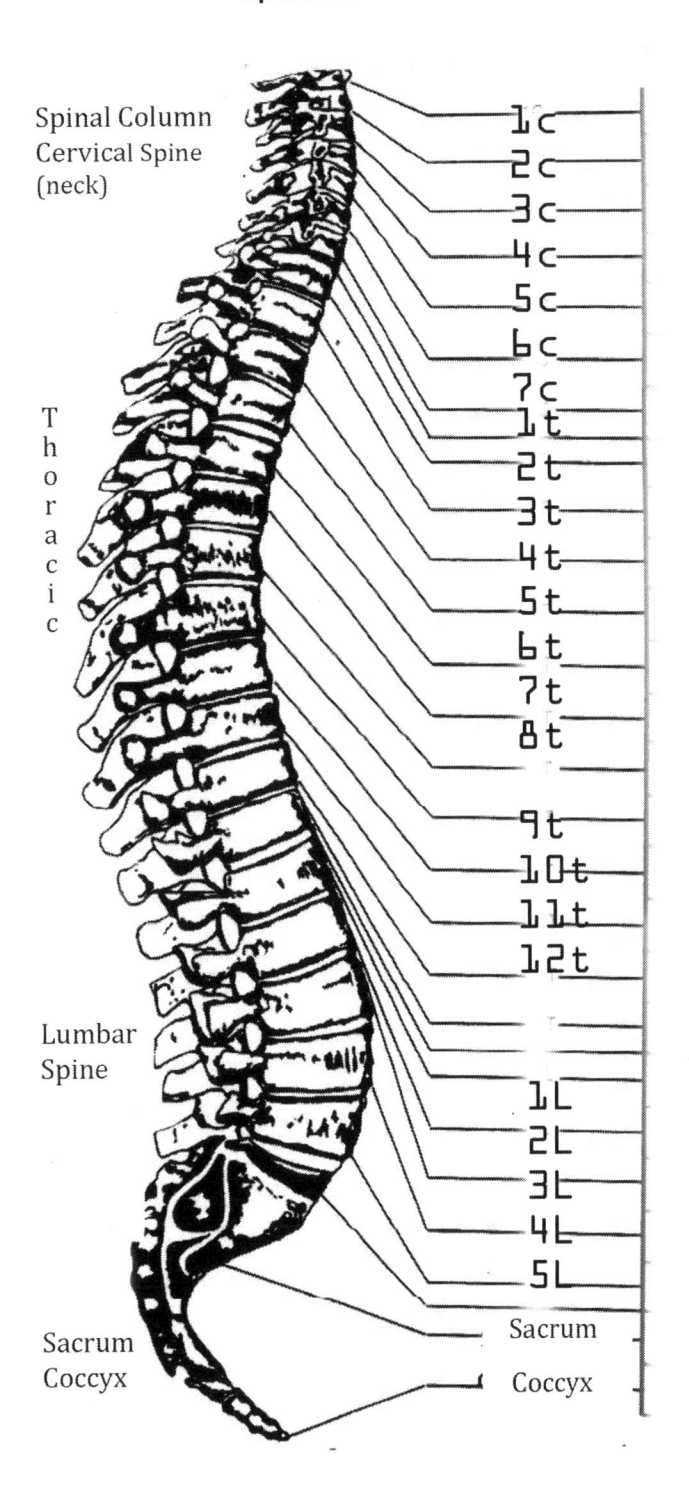

Spinal Column
Cervical Spine
(neck)

Thoracic

Lumbar Spine

Sacrum
Coccyx

- 1c
- 2c
- 3c
- 4c
- 5c
- 6c
- 7c
- 1t
- 2t
- 3t
- 4t
- 5t
- 6t
- 7t
- 8t
- 9t
- 10t
- 11t
- 12t
- 1L
- 2L
- 3L
- 4L
- 5L
- Sacrum
- Coccyx

Organs and Feelings

Organs that have inconsistencies in function tend to cause an emotional reaction.

Lungs
Sadness, denial, bonding difficulties, righteousness

Heart
Cruelty, impatient, mood swings, irregular beats, irregular lifestyle, thoughts, eating, and/or moods, honor, joy.

Kidney
Anguish, fear, unresolved, issues, gentleness.

Liver
Depression, unstable energy, kindness

The Elements, Organs, Senses, and Action

Parts of the body that have inconsistencies in function tend to have an effect on the senses.

ELEMENTS	SENSES	SENSE	ACTION	Parts of the body
Emotional, Spiritual	Hearing	Ear	Speech	Organs of Speech (tongue, vocal cords, mouth)
Air	Touch	Skin	Holdings	Hand
Fire	Seeing	Eyes	Walking	Feet
Water	Taste	Tongue	Procreation	Genitals
Earth	Smell	Nose	Excretion	Anus

Abdomen

Abdomen and Organs

Inconsistency of the abdomen's skin such as discoloration, textures, dryness, oiliness, bumps, rashes, blotches, sores, white or dark spots, excessive vertical and horizontal wrinkles, hair growth, tenderness, slight temperature variation, sensitivity to touch as well as weak muscle testing response can indicate that the organ related to the area has problems.

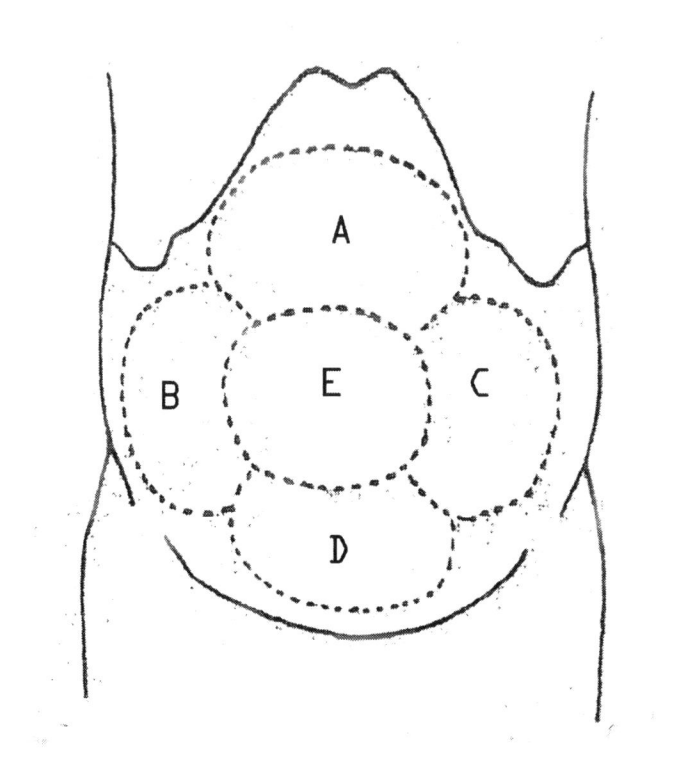

Area E: The central part of the abdominal region relates to the health of the spleen, pancreas, and stomach.
Area A: The upper abdominal region relates to the health conditions of the heart, and small intestines.
Area B: The right side of the abdominal region relates to the health of the lungs, and large intestines.
Area C: The left side of the abdominal region relates to the health of the liver, and the gallbladder.
Area D: The lower abdominal region relates to the health of the kidneys, and bladder.

Abdomen

Skin covers the abdomen. A slight outline of the substratum can be seen. The midline groove runs between the straight muscles down to the umbilicus; the lower border of the healthy small intestines convolution reaches only to linea interspinalis (imaginary connecting line of the ventral iliac spine = spina ilica ventralis). The slight bulging of the abdomen caused by the small intestine convolution is bounded below by a U-shaped depression: the U-valley. If these shapes are not visible, it can indicate damage to the digestive system, manure impaction and/ or fermenting gas.

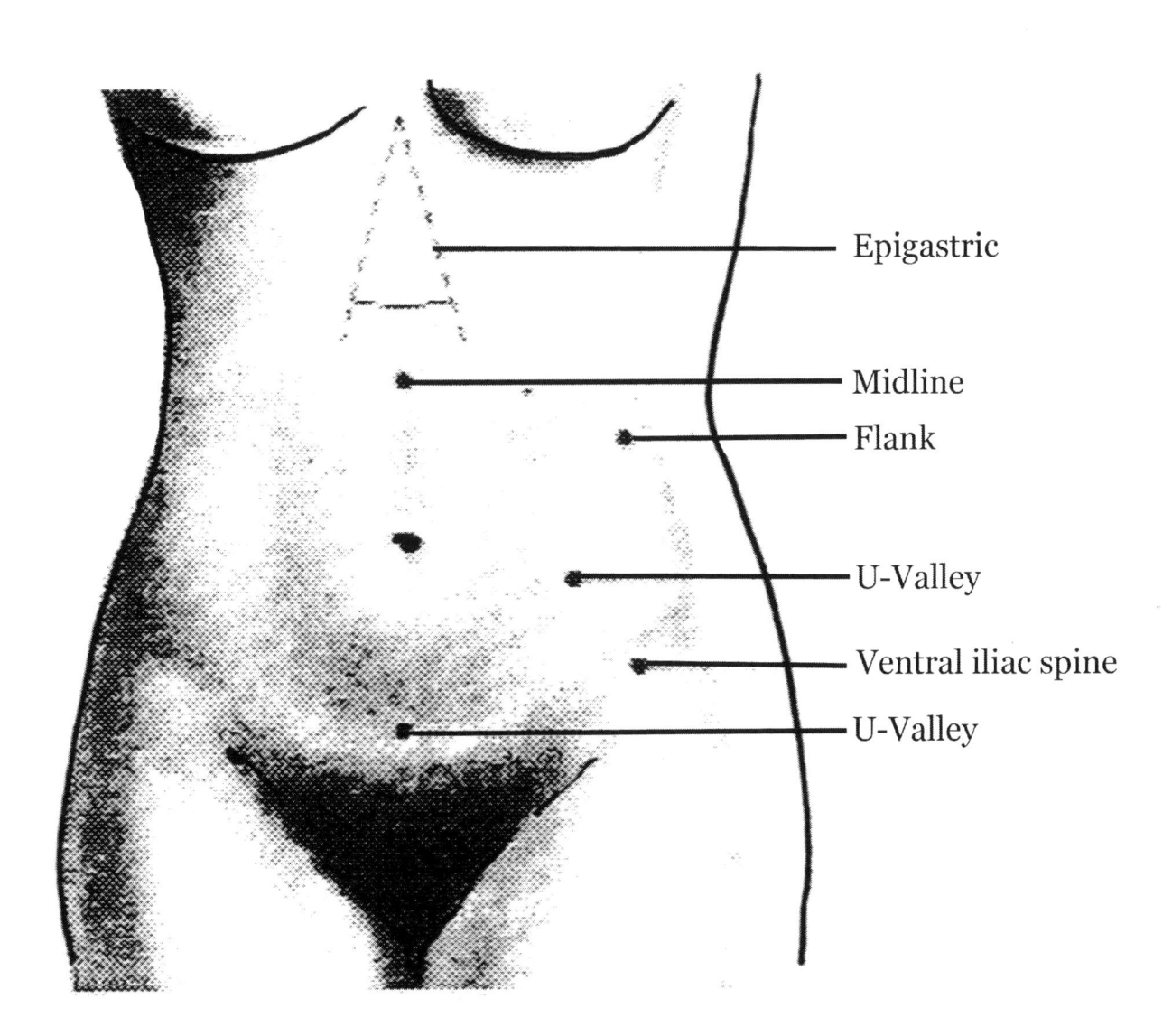

- Epigastric
- Midline
- Flank
- U-Valley
- Ventral iliac spine
- U-Valley

Abdomen Test

The purpose of the test is to locate areas, which are painful, tender and/or pulsate. An organ or organ system weakness, malfunction and/or disease can cause a pounding sensation/pulse. If there is a layer of fat or fatty tissue beneath the skin, then a deeper rub may be required in order to feel for sensation.

When testing yourself, put the palm of either hand on the abdomen. The abdomen or solar plexus area extends from the top of the hip bone to the area just beneath the sternum (breastbone) and includes the sides of the torso (area between lower ribs and sternum). With your fingers, feel the sides of the abdomen by rubbing up and then down. Feel for pulsation around the naval area. Areas of the skin are related to the internal organs and organ systems. Each area has acupuncture meridians that are specific to the organs.

A light pressure touch of the fingers that causes a sensation indicates parasympathetic stress and/or under-activity (hypoactive) of the function of organs or systems. If the light touch does not result in a sensation, then use a heavy pressure to touch. If this stronger pressure enables your fingers to locate tenderness, pain or pulsation then, it indicates disease. Heavy touch indicates sympathetic stress and the overworking (hyperactivity) of an organ and/or system. Hypo-activity or hyper-activity is stressors, which are usually caused by a malfunction or disease of an organ or system.

Small Intestine Measurement

Small Intestine

The measurer's right hand is placed, using no pressure, but only the hand's own weight, inside of the Spina, in the region of the U-valley; this is done on both sides. The finger widths, which can be laid between the spina ilica ventralis and the small intestine convolution are counted 4 finger widths on each side are normal; the smaller the U-valley, the smaller the intestine. This measurement shows the side and lower boundary of the small intestine to be determined. Hypertonus increases; hypotonus decreases this measurement, down to 0.

Abdominal Measurement

Normally it is possible to insert a finger width between the tips of the thumb or the index finger and the costal arch.

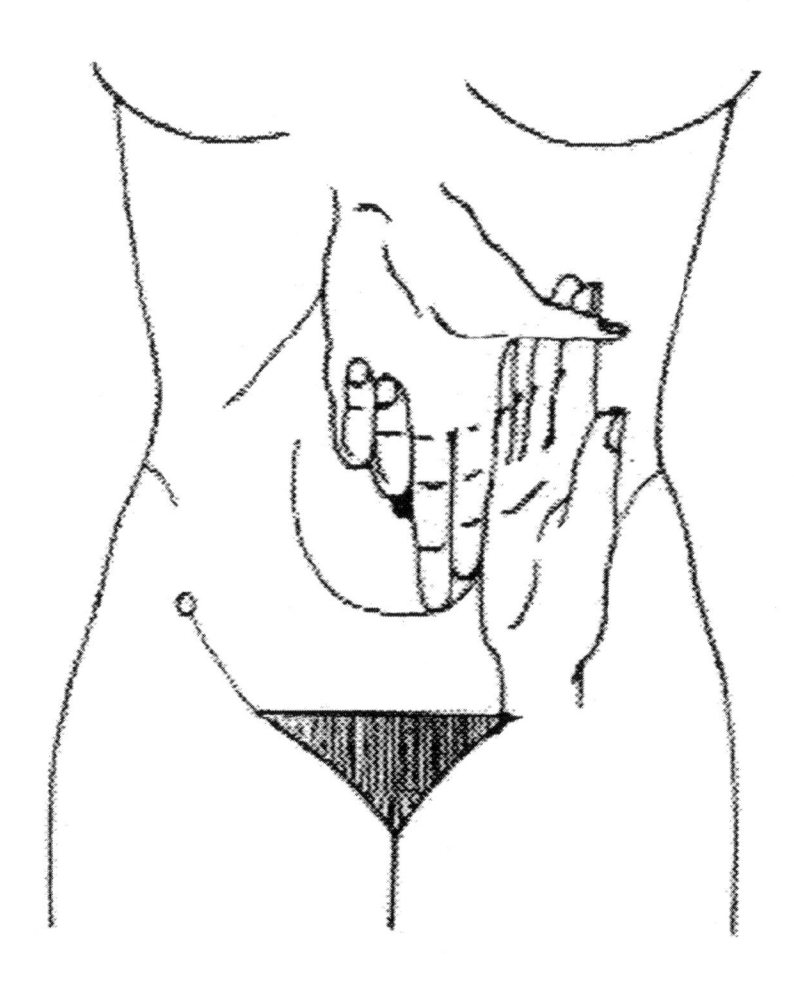

Umbilicus

This measures the lateral widths of the small intestine convolution on both sides. The left hand, should be gently placed vertically along the abdomen, touches and marks the right-hand boundary of the small intestine; then the number of finger widths, which can be inserted from that point to the umbilicus, is determined. The same measurement is performed on the left side. The normal measurement is 2 finger widths on either side. A large umbilicus area, indicates the weak muscles of the small intestine.

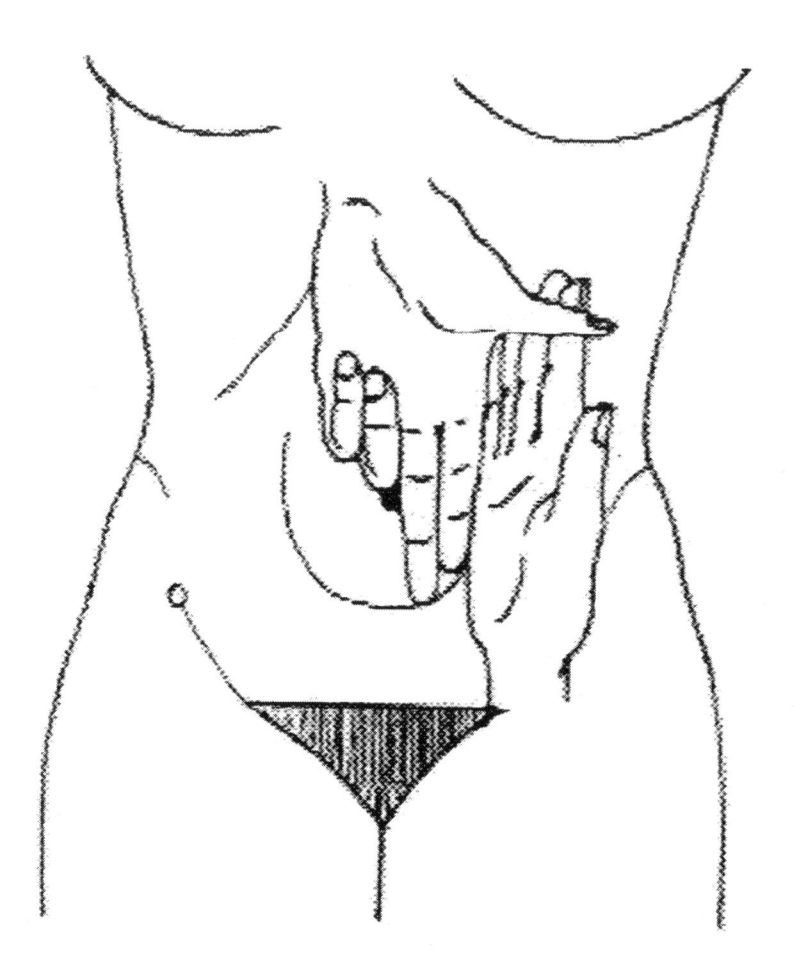

Measurement: Umbilicus Mesurement. Normal is 2 fingerwidths on each side.

Abdominal Measurement

The fingers of the right hand are spread as wide as possible and laced on the linea interspinalis, the distance from tip to the little finger to the left spina ilica ventralis should be equal that from the saddle joint of the thumb (metacarpo- carpal joint) to the right spinal ilica ventralis. Do not confuse the basal joint of the thumb (metacarpo-phalangeal joint) with the saddle joint! In a normal size abdomen, the tips of the thumb and index finger will touch the costal arch on the left and right: if they do not, the abdomen, and the abdominal cavity and its contents, are enlarged. This occurs when there is no "belly" (pronounced bulging). The abdomen can be symmetrically or asymmetrically enlarged. Right-side enlargement indicates the liver or right flexure of the colon, while left –side enlargement indicates the stomach, transverse colon or left colon flexure. The enlargement is measured by counting the finger widths, which can be inserted on each side between the costal arch and the thumb and the fingertips.

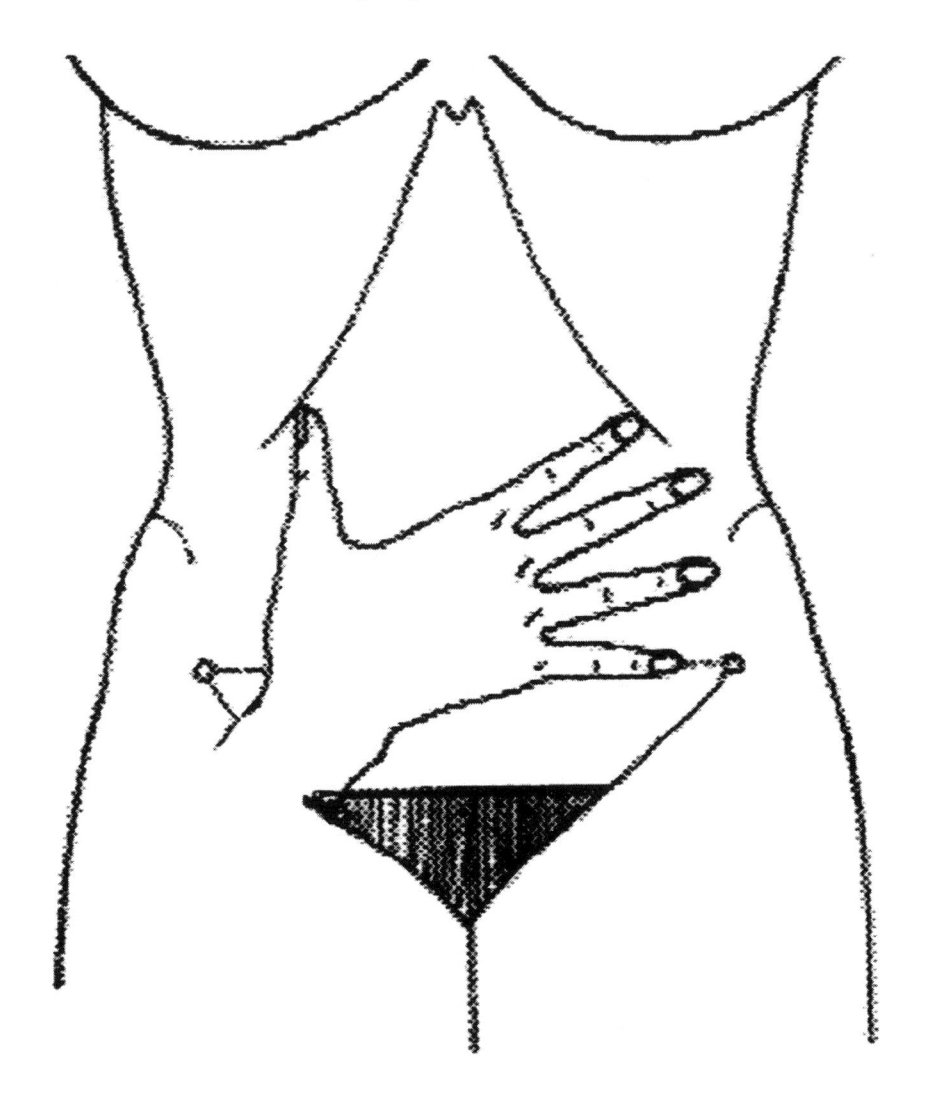

The measurement is the number of finger widths between the base of the outstretched hand and the right spina ilica ventralis.

Childhood and Adult Disease Symptoms and Signs

Childhood Disease Symptoms

Asthma
Spasm of the lungs (bronchial tubes) and/or swelling to lung tissue (mucous membrane). Usually, an over stimulated nervous system and an allergic reaction causes attacks.
Season: Varies
Most Susceptible: Children, young adults.
Symptoms:
1. Shortness of breath
2. Panting, Wheezing
3. Difficulty breathing – may hunch over to get air

Causes: Allergens such as dust, pollen, eggs, shellfish, chocolate, drugs, stress, fatigue and emotions.
Develops: Varies from a few moments to a few days.
Duration: Attacks vary.

Bronchiolitis
(Inflammation of the smaller branches of the bronchial tree leading to the lungs).
Season: For respiratory type winter and spring; for para influenza type, summer and fall.
Most Susceptible: Those under 2 years (especially under 6 months); those with an allergy.
Symptoms:
1. Cold symptoms
2. A few days later: Rapid, shallow breathing; wheezing on breathing out; 3 days with a low-grade fever.
3. Sometimes: Chest expansion, difficult on breathing, loss of appetite, dehydration, bluish fingertips and nails.

Causes: Mucous congestion, dairy, junk foods, cellular waste.
Transmission: Usually via respiratory secretions, person-to-person contact, or by contact with contaminated household objects.
Develops In: 2 to 8 days.
Duration: Acute phase may last only 3 days, cough from 1 to 3 weeks or more.

Bronchitis
(Inflammation of the bronchial tree and often the trachea, or windpipe).
Season: Varies.
Most Susceptible: Children under 4 years.
Symptoms:
1. Usually: Cold symptoms
2. Abrupt onset of: Fever, about 102°F (38.9°/c); harsh cough, worse at night, wheezing, bluish lips and fingernails, greenish or yellowish sputum, whistling on breathing out and periodic coughing episodes.

Cause: See Bronchiolitis
Duration: Fever lasts 2 or 3 days; cough 1 to 2 weeks or more.

Cat Scratch Disease
Season: More frequent in fall and winter.
Most Susceptible: Anyone, but 80% of cases occurs in those under 20.
Symptoms: Usually: Swollen lymph glands under arms or in the jaw or neck 1 to 4 weeks after contact. The glands may be tender, warm, red hard (sometimes) and can discharge pus.
Sometimes: Fever (100.4°F to 102.2°F, or 38°C to 39°C): also, malaise, and fatigue.
Occasionally: Loss of appetite, vomiting, and headache. Only indicates fever with no apparent cause and possibly abdominal pain. Also, visible rash and red pimple at site of scratches or bite, 1 to 2 weeks before other symptoms.
Transmission: Usually kitten scratch, bite or lick: sometimes, older cat or other animal; rarely no contact.
Develops in: 7 to 12 days from scratch to skin lesion (rash); then 5 to 50 days (a median of 12) to swollen glands.
Duration: Usually 2 to 4 months; fever about 2 weeks; gland tenderness, 4 to 6 weeks; swelling, several months can last a year.
Prevention: Keep away from cats, declawing the cat.

Chickenpox, (Varicella)
Season: Late winter and early spring in temperate zones.
Most susceptible: Anyone.
Symptoms: Slight fever, malaise and loss of appetite. Flat red spots turn into pimples, then blister, crust and scab and continue to develop for 3 or 4 days.
Itching is usually intense.
Transmission: Person-to person; and air droplets from respiratory secretions. Very contagious from 1 to 2 days before onset until sores get a scab (about 6 days).
Develops in: 11 to 20 days most often 14 to 16 days.
Duration: First vesicles crust I 6 to 8 hours, scab in 24 to 48 hours; scabs last 5 to 20 days.

Colds
(See Bronchiolitis)

Conjunctivitis
(Pinkeye)
Inflammation of the conjunctiva, the membrane lining the eyelids and the eyes.
Season: Not seasonal
Most Susceptible: Anyone
Symptoms: Can include: Bloodshot eyes; tearing; eye discharge (lids may be crusted after sleep), burning, itching; light sensitivity. Usually begins in one eye and can go to the other.
Cause: Many, include bacteria, chlamydia, parasites, fungi, allergens, irritants, chemicals.
Transmission: For infectious organisms, eye-hand-eye, towels, bed linens.
Develops: Quickly.
Duration: Varies with cause; viral, 2 days to 3 weeks (can become chronic); bacterial, about 2 weeks; others, until allergen or irritant is removed.

Croup
(See Bronchiolitis)

Encephalitis
(Inflammation of the brain)
Symptoms: Fever, drowsiness and headache.
Sometimes: Neurological impairment (confusion, moody, swimmy head, altered consciousness, muscle weakness), progression to coma at a late stage. In late stages, can cause a coma.
Cause: Bacteria usually a complication of another disease.
Transmission: Depends on cause.
Development: Depends on cause.
Duration: Varies.

Epiglottis
(Inflammation of the tongue – the upper part of the larynx, or voice box)
Season: Winter months in temperate climates.
Most Susceptible: children 2 to 4 years old.
Symptoms: Sudden onset of fever over 102°F or 38.9°C (lower 1 tots under 2); drooling, difficulty swallowing, hoarse cough (croupy in under 2's); noisy breathing (stridor) and sore throat.
Sometimes: Protruding tongue, retractions, bluish nails, and lips.
Symptoms: Worsen rapidly, child seems ill, restless, agitated, and irritable, and wants to sit upright, will lean forward with mouth open in order to get air. The tongue usually is extremely red and swollen.
Cause: Bacteria most often, hemophilia influenza; sometimes group A Streptococcus. See Bronchitis.
Transmission: Can be person-to-person, or the inhalation of respiratory droplets (remote possibility).
Duration: 4 to 7 days or longer.

Fifth Disease
(Erythema Infectiosum)
Season: Early spring
Most Susceptible: Children 2 to 12 years old.
Symptoms: Sometimes: Fever. Rarely: Joint Pain.
   1. Intense flush on face (slapped-cheek look).

2. Next day: Rash on inner surfaces, fingers, toes, trunk, and/or buttocks.
3. Rash may reappear on and off with exposure to heat (bath water, sun) for 2 to 3 weeks, even months.

Cause: Cellular waste, mucus congestion.
Transmission: Probably, respiratory secretions and blood; can be contagious before onset of illness.
Develops in about: 4 to 14 days but as long as 20 days.
Duration: Initial rash, several days to a week; rash can continue to recur for weeks to months.

German Measles
(Rubella)
Season: Late winter and early spring.
Most Susceptible: Any person
Symptoms: In 25% to 50% of cases – no symptoms
1. Sometimes: Slight fever and swollen glands.
2. Small (1/10inch) flat, reddish pink spots on face.
3. Rash spreads to body and sometimes, roof of mouth.

Cause: Cellular waste, mucus congestion.
Transmission: Can be contact or droplets from respiratory secretions. Usually contagious from a few days before 5 to 7 days after rash appears.
Develops in: 14 to 21 days, most often 16 to 18 days.
Duration: A few hours to 4 or 5 days.

Hand-Foot-Mouth Disease
(Vesicular stomatitis)
Season: Summer and fall in temperature climates.
Most Susceptible: Babies and young children.
Symptoms
1. Fever; loss of appetite. Difficulty swallowing, sore throat and mouth.
2. In 2 or 3 days: Sores in mouth (which can blister).
3. Then, sores on fingers: sometimes, buttocks, feet, legs, arms, less often on face.

Cause: Cellular waste, mucus congestion.
Transmission: Mouth-to-mouth, feces-to-hand-to-mouth.
Develops in: 3 to 6 days.
Duration: About 1 week.

Herpangia
(Mild herpes bumps)
Season: Mostly summer and fall in temperate climates: any time in tropical regions.
Most Susceptible: Babies and young children.
Symptoms:
1. Fever: 100°F, occasionally to 106°F; (7.8°C to 40°C or 41.1°C), sore throat. A seizure caused by a fever in the beginning.
2. Painful swallowing. Sometimes: Diarrhea, loss of appetite, lethargy, abdominal pain, and vomiting.
3. Distinct grayish white papules in back of mouth or throat (5 to 10 in number) that blister and ulcerate.

Cause: Cellular waste.
Transmission: Mouth-to-Mouth, feces-to-hand-mouth.
Develops in: 3 to 6 days.
Duration: 4 to 7 days but healing can take 2 to 3 weeks.

Hydrophobia
(Fear of water)

Impetigo
(Skin inflammation)
(See Encephalitis)

Influenza
(See Bronchitis)

341

Kawasaki Disease
(Mucocutaneous lymph node syndrome, MLNS- swollen glands)
Most Susceptible: Infants and children under 5; more boys than girls, more children of Asian (especially Japanese) than of other origin.
Symptoms:
1. Fever, usually last 7 days but can be between 5 to 39 days.
2. Within 3 days of onset of fever: Skin of nose, mouth and/or throat gets red, can have cracked lips, swollen neck gland, throat swollen, strawberry colored tongue, conjunctivitis in both eyes, with no discharge.
3. Flat red rash on body; redness and/or swelling or hardening of palms of hands and soles of feet.
4. Palms and soles may peel during second to third week.

Cause: Cellular waste, mucus congestion, junk food, dairy.
Duration: Without treatment, fever last about 12 days; appetite loss and irritability con last 2 to 3 weeks. Complications last longer.

Lyme Disease
(Borrelia burgdoferi)
Season: May 1 to November 30, with most cases in June and July.
Most Susceptible: Anyone
Symptoms:
1. Usually a bulls-eye-shaped red rash (erythema migrans) where tick bite occurred; it usually spreads in a few days and expands over days to weeks to form larger red rash.
2. Sometimes: Multiple rashes develop when it spreads. Pains, fatigue, aches, problems with nervous system involvement and headaches. If untreated: Chronic arthritis, central nervous system damage and painful knees, rarely heart damage.
3. Weeks to year are later, if untreated: Deformed joints. None of these symptoms alone, however, is diagnostic; see under Rash.

Treatment: See cat scratch disease.
Cause: A spirochete, borrelia burgdorferi
Transmission: Spread by the bite of a pinhead-size deer tick, and (carried by deer, mice, and other animals) can be caused by other ticks, and flying insects. It takes 24 to 48 hours for an attached tick to transmit Lyme disease.
Develops in: 3 to 32 days, typically 7 to 10 days.
Duration: Without treatment, possibly years.

Meningitis
(Inflammation of the membranes around the brain and/or the spinal cord)
Season: Varies.
Most Susceptible: Mostly infants and children under 3, usually city dwellers, African Americans, and children in day-care centers.
Symptoms: Fever, bulging soft spot on head (fontanel), high-pitched cry, vomiting, drowsiness, loss of appetite, and irritability. In older children: sensitivity to light blurred vision and neurological problems and/or stiff neck.
Cause: Bacteria, cellular waste.
Transmission: Can be person-to-person, possibility of direct contact through inhalation of droplets from respiratory secretions.
Develops in: Less than 10 days.
Duration: Varies.

Meningoencephalitis
(Combined meningitis and encephalitis) See Meningitis.

Mumps
Season: Late winter and spring.
Most Susceptible: Anyone.
Symptoms:
1. Sometimes: Vague pain, loss of appetite and fever.

2. Usually: Swelling of parotid (salivary) glands on one or both sides of jaw, below and in front of ear; pain on chewing; ear pain; swelling of the salivary glands. No symptoms in about 30% of cases.

Cause: Junk food.
Transmission: Can be direct contact with respiratory secretions from 1 or 2 (but as long as 7) days prior to onset until 9 days after.
Develops in: 16 to 18 days may be as few as 12 or as many as 25 days.
Duration: 5 to 7 days.

Nonspecific Viral (NSV) illnesses
Season: Mostly summer.
Most Susceptible: Young children.
Symptoms: Can vary and may include: loss of appetite, diarrhea and fever. Different type of rashes.
Skin Problems: See Cat Scratch Disease.
Cause: Cellular waste.
Transmission: Feces-to-hand-to-mouth, possibly mouth-to-mouth.
Develops in: 3 to 6 days.
Duration: Usually 6 weeks or longer

Pertussis
(Whooping Cough)
Season: Late winter, early spring.
Most Susceptible: Infants and young children.
Symptom:
1. Catarrhal stage: Cold symptoms with dry cough, irritability, and low-grade fever.
2. Paroxysmal stage 1 to 2 weeks later: Thick mucus, coughing in explosive bursts with no breaths between. Often: Vomiting, bulging eyes, protruding tongue, exhaustion, pale or reddened skin, sweating. Sometimes; Hernia, from coughing
3. Recovery stage; Whooping and vomiting stops, reduced coughing, less moodiness, and improved appetite.

Cause: Bacteria.
Transmission: Can be respiratory droplets, most communicable during catarrhal stage.
Develops in: 7 to 10 days, rarely more than 2 weeks.
Duration: Usually 6 weeks or longer.

Pharyngitis
(See sore throat)

Pinworm Infection
(Enterobiasis)
Season: Not seasonal
Most Susceptible: School age children and their mothers. Anyone that eats junk food, meat, processed sweeteners, cooked oils, uses wrong food combining, dairy, or suffers from constipation or gas.
Symptoms:
1. Pinworms enter and live in lower digestive tract; females lay eggs around anus and on buttocks. They can crawl out of the rectum at night or during the day to lay eggs. The eggs cannot hatch inside the body.
2. Itching begins around the anus. Children may cry at night; be irritable; restless and fatigued. Check for eggs with flashlight in the middle of night or before your child wakes up. You will see a little dark spot inside the egg. Anal area can be raw and red.
3. Occasionally, in girls, itching of the vulva. If worms enter the vagina, they can cause vaginitis and a slight vaginal discharge.

Cause: A tiny (¼ to ½) grayish, thread-like parasitic worm, Enterobius vermicularis.
Transmission: Letting animals lick you in the face, walking bare foot in dirt where dogs or cats had bowel movements, hand-to-mouth, thumb sucking after scratching or wiping or using an unclean toilet seat. If swallowed, eggs hatch and worms move down to rectum. You can have worms and give them to others as long as the females are laying eggs; eggs remain ineffective for 2 or 3 weeks.
Duration: If you do not treat it, you can keep worms forever.

Pneumonia
(Inflammation of the lungs)
Season: Varies.
Most Susceptible: Anyone.
Symptoms: A child with a cold or other illness that seems to suddenly get worse. There can be increased fever; pain; heavy mucus; unproductive cough; shortness of breath; wheezy, raspy and/or difficult breathing; chest reaction, abdominal bloating and rapid breathing.
Cause: Protozoa, fungus, mycoplasmas, allergens, inhalation of a chemical.
Transmission: Varies.
Development: Varies.
Duration: Varies.

Respiratory
Synctial Virus

(RSV) Illness
(Includes pneumonia; bronchiolitis and the common cold).
Season: Winter and early spring in temperate climates; rainy season in the tropics.
Most Susceptible: Anyone, most cases occur before age 3.
Symptoms: Can be like a mild cold, pneumonia or bronchiolitis. There can be a cough; sore throat; painful breathing; inflammation of the nose and throat, malaise, and wheezing. Sometimes: A long pause between breathes (apnea), mostly in premature infants.
Cause: Cellular waste.
Transmission: Direct or close contact with respiratory secretions (fluids of others) or contaminated articles, it takes from 3 days to 4 weeks for it to begin.
Duration: Varies.

Reye Syndrome
Season: Not seasonal.
Most Susceptible: Children who are given aspirin during illness.
Symptoms:
  1. 1 to 7 days following an upper respiratory infection: Persistent sporadic vomiting every hour or two, all day; lethargy; irritability, rapid heartbeat, confusion, and delirium.
  2. Can have seizures if untreated.
Cause: Unknown, can be related to a reaction to aspirin.
Transmission: Unknown.
Develops in: Unknown, it seems to develop within 6 days or onset of viral infection.
Duration: Varies.

Rocky Mountain Spotted Fever
(RMSF)
Season: Spring and summer.
Most Susceptible: Adults and children under 15 years old.
Symptoms:
  1. Fever; nausea, vomiting, muscle pain and weakness; headache. Sometimes; abdominal pain, cough.
  2. Usually before the sixth day: Flat red spots or splotches appear on the soles of the feet and palms, spreads to wrist, arms, legs, ankles and then trunk.
  3. Later bumps can develop. Occasionally: No rash or late-developing rash.
Transmission: The bite of a tick.
Develops in: 1 to 14 days, usually 1 week.
Duration: Up to 3 weeks.

Sore Throat
(See Bronchiolitis)

Tetanus
(Lockjaw)
Season: More frequent in warmer climates and months.

Symptoms: Localized: Spasm and increased muscle tone near the entry wound. Generalized: Uncontrollable muscle contractions, which can arch the back, twist the neck and lock the jaw; convulsions; children have difficulty sucking the breast and the nipple on the bottle; profuse sweating; low-grade fever; rapid heartbeat.
Cause: Cellular waste toxins, junk food, dairy.
Transmission: Infection or contamination of a cut, scrape, puncture, burn, open skin, or wound.
Develops in: 3 days to 3 weeks but an average of 8 days.
Duration: Several weeks.

Tonsillitis
(See Bronchiolitis)

Upper Respiratory Infection (URI)
(See Bronchiolitis)

Whooping Cough
(See Bronchiolitis)

Delivery of Baby Affects Emotions

Babies delivered by hospital births suffer from emotional injuries and scars, which become part of their adult life and is permanently imprinted on their Limbic (Emotional) System. In hospitals the medical model treats birth as well as menopause as an illness. In medical facilities during birth the lights are bright, noise level is high, umbilical cord is cut before it stops pulsating, rooms too cold, technology and drugs alter the natural process, the baby is not immediately placed on mother's breast, baby is separated from mother and the baby is surrounded by strangers (hospital personnel) and isolated.

Type of Delivery	Emotions and Behavior	Symptom
Analgesic, Anesthesia	Feeling of confusion, and helplessness, difficulty bonding to task and/or relationship, sense of emptiness, unable to focus, feelings of loneliness, self destructive emotions violence insensitivity, dull mind, stress prone, easily irritated and/or bored, needs high level of simulation, Learning and behavioral problems, emotionally paralyzed when stressed.	Psychosomatic illness, lacks consistency with healing, easily stressed.
Forceps	Inability to receive nurturing, does not like to be touched.	Prone to headaches, sees wellness as a difficulty. Under stress neck and/or shoulder pain.
C-Section	Desires to nurture others, Excessive desires to be touch, problems with success, hypersensitive cuddle hunger, wants to be rescued from their life, fears abandonment, feels helpless, feels things are blocking them, gets into conflicts and difficulties.	Problems completing task, skin problems, weak digestion.
Breech	Feels they are doing something wrong, stubborn, determine, wants things their way, and obsesses with control, difficulty accomplishing goals and/or solution.	Needs positive re-enforcement during healing easily gets confused about disease and healing.
Episiotomy	Feeling of guilt, problems getting into and out of situation.	Delayed response to healing, slowly reacts to wellness.
Premature/ Short Labor	Lacks emotional maturity, emotional weakness, and High Corticotrophin Releasing Hormone (CRH) indicator of premature birth.	Problems absorbing nutrient weak immunity, hyperactivity stress, anemic tendency, respiratory problems.
Late Delivery/Long Labor	Procrastinator, tendency to lag behind, tires easily.	Lack of energy, hypoactive problems changing behavior
Umbilical Cord around Neck	Hesitant, to participate fear of suffocation, does not like face covered, fear of injury, does not like interruptions, Vocal problems	Respiratory problems, Cold/Flu tendency.
Induced Labor	Resentful of authority and/or control, rebellious without reason, difficulty-controlling emotions.	Disease linger, immune stress.

Not Breastfeed after Delivery	Defensiveness rationalized as common sense, revenge rationalized as justice, lack heart to heart stimulation, moral and ethical problems, lack visual brain awareness, lack phoneme synchronicity, confused with separating emotional and intellectual differences (Negative Cerebrum Limbic Loop)	Digestive problems, relationship to health
Mother did not nurture after birth	Over reacts to perceived unfairness, feelings they can not get ahead, feels social relationship holds them back, over reacts to rejection.	Depression tendency, obsessive behavior

Baby's Emotion in Hospital

Baby's Reaction	Tendency (from Childhood to Adulthood)
Intense fear, anxiety emptiness	Hyperactivity, Depression, Needs over Stimulation Tends to be in a hurry to get well. Can develop negative attitude towards wellness.
Isolation, abandonment, un-nurtured stress	Obsessive Compulsive Problems When following healing protocol, can take excessive amounts. Will sometimes have problems discontinuing bad habits.
Emotional and/or physical traumatized	Post Traumatic Stress Problems Nerve damage, can have fragile feelings about wellness, and past efforts to be well.
Disappointing loss, sadness, unfulfilled	Depression Doubts ability to be well. Can have negative feelings about health.

Diaper Rashes

Type	Signs and Symptoms	Cause
Atopic Dermatitis	Itching with redness	Allergy or sensitivity
Candidal (fungal) Dermatitis	Bright red, tender rash increases between abdomen and thighs, bumps spreading uncomfortable	Candida albicans (a fungus); Candida often infects a skin rash usually last 3 days or longer
Chafing Dermatitis	Redness where there is the most friction, no discomfort	Moisture rubbing
Impetigo		Bacteria
Intertrigo	Poorly defined reddened areas where skin rubs together, can ooze white to yellowish pus, can burn when in contact with urine	Rubbing of skin on skin
Seborrheic Dermatitis	Deep red rash, can have yellow scales; may start on or spread to scalp; no discomfort.	Cellular waste, mucus waste, dairy, junk food

Fevers in Children and Adults

Common Causes of Fever & Sore Throat		Rare Causes of Fever	
Smallpox	Typhoid fever	Brucellosis (Bang's disease)	
Syphilis	Herpes simplex	Bubonic plague	
Chickenpox	Herpangina	Hemolytic-uremic syndrome	
Coxsackie virus	Infectious mononucleosis	Kawasaki disease	
Enterovirus	Influenza	Malaria	
Gingivostomatitis	Scarlet fever	Mycotic infection	
Toxoplasmosis	Tonsillitis	Tuberculosis Typhoid Fever	
Rare Causes of Fever & Sore Throat		**Rare Causes of Fever & Rash**	
Diphtheria	Peritonsillar abscess	Erythema nodusum	Polyartesitis nodosis
Hand, foot & mouth disease	Retropharyngeal abscess	Leptospirosis	Rat-bite fever Rickettsial disease
Infectious lymphocytosis		Listeria monocytogenes	Septicemia
		Lupus erythematosus	
Common Cause of Fever & Rash		**Causes of Fever & Severe Headache**	
Chickenpox	Measles	Cavernous sinus thrombosis	Mononucleosis
Enterovirus	Roseola		Ethmoiditis
Erythema infectiosum	Rubella	Encephalitis	Meningitis
Exanthems chart	Rubeola	Viral	Poliomyelitis
Infectious mononucleosis	Scarlet fever	Herpes	Reye's disease
		Mumps	
Fever & Skin Sores		**Fever & Joint Pain**	
Cat-scratch disease	Polyarteritis nodosa	Arthritis	
Mycotic infection	Rat-bite fever		

Skin Eruptions in Children and Adults
(Bump, Rashes)

Disease	Symptoms	Skin Characteristics	Duration
Entererovira Exanthemas	Temperature of 101°F to 103°F, pharyngitis, gastrointestinal symptoms.	Rash starts with the fever or after fever drops; non-itchy bumps on the chest and face, and can be on the palms and soles.	5 days or less
Erythema Infectiosum	Low-grade fever, pharyngitis, headache.	Flushed cheeks; reticulated erythema on extremities (often itch) exacerbated by sunlight, pressure, and heat.	2 to 5 weeks
Infectious Mononucleosis	Temperature to 101°F, malaise, sore throat, enlarged lymph nodes, enlarged spleen, upper pharyngitis	Rash occurs in less than 15% of the cases. Small dark red bumps, or papules on trunk and arms. Tonsillitis, enlarge spleen.	1 to 2 days
Roseola	High fever for three to four days resolving by crisis, convulsions can be caused by fever.	When fever drops, dark reddish bumps appear on trunk spread to neck and behind ears and may not appear on face or extremities. Swollen lymph nodes at the back of neck. (95% in children under 3 years)	3 days or less
Rubeola (Measles)	Temperature of 103° to 104°F, inflammation, conjunctivitis, cough small red spots with bluish center on the mouth.	Temperature is usually highest on the fourth day. Bumps develop on forehead and neck; spread to face and trunk, and by the third day it appears on the feet. Rash becomes brownish, and patchy.	5 days or more
Rubella	Low-grade fever, eye and throat inflammation, lymph nodes behind ears are sensitive.	Pink-red macules around mouth, spreading to trunk.	Less than 5 days
Scarlet Fever	Temperature of 101° to 103°F, for 3 to 4 days, headaches, tonsillitis, vomiting, and sore throat.	Rash develops one to two days after the fever begins. Starts on neck, underarms, and chest: rapidly spreads. Skin on hands and feet peel.	5 to 7 days
Warts	Raised, Indented lesions and bumps.	Common warts: Brownish, rough, raised lesions, often including genitals (common warts are not sexually transmitted). Flat warts: Multiple small, slightly raised lesions, flesh-colored to tan, on face, neck, arms, legs. Plantar Warts: Speckled raised, or indented sores, often painful. Genital Warts: Soft, flesh-colored bumps on genitalia.	Without treatment, warts resolve in 6 months to 3 years

Sleeping Disorders of Children
(Wakeful at night, problems falling asleep)
Possible Causes

Age	Won't go to Sleep	Awakening after going to sleep
Birth to 6 months	Colic, Over-stimulated, hunger	Colic, hunger, sickness, lost pacifier, bed too small, urinary infection, cutting teeth, earache, urine contacting open sores
6 months to 15 months	Fear of separation. Used to staying up late. Naps too long. Low calcium over stimulated.	Croup, ear infection, pinworms, fever, diaper rash, gas, low calcium, allergic to blanket, pillow, or toy
15 months to 3 years	Playing a "game". Fear of separation. Naps too long. Anxiety.	Sickness, pinworms, teething, refused to have a bowel movement during day, relaxes and has it at night, bed too small, diaper rash
3 to 5 years	Naps too long. Fears ghosts in room. Family arguments or sex in next room. Over stimulated	Pinworms, sickness, fell out of bed
5 years and older	House too noisy. Doesn't need much sleep. Parents fighting. Use to staying up late.	Pinworms, seizure, sickness, full bladder

Test for Disease, Examinations, and Symptoms

Abdomen Palpation Exam

Palpate (feel) the abdomen. Locate the organs on the right and left side. If you are examining someone else keep in mind where their left is your right and their right is you left. Imagine a cross on your abdomen, the center of the two imaginary lines are on your navel (one vertically and one horizontally). This divides the abdomen into four quadrants. For the examination lay on your back this will relax the abdomen area. Put the flat parts of the fingers of your left hand on your abdomen. Use your right hand to press down on top of your left fingers. Your right hand should be used to apply pressure while your left fingers do the feeling.

Aneurysms in Blood Vessels Test

Arteries have thicker and muscular walls and more pressure inside them than veins. Arteries may develop atherosclerosis (hardening of the arteries) and/or aneurysms and blockages. Aneurysms are ball-like swellings that develop in weak walls of an artery. Any artery can develop an aneurysm. However they usually occur in the brain and in the aorta (big artery that runs through the chest and abdomen down the legs). A weak spot in the wall of an artery can swell and the swelling causes the vessel wall to become weaker. Eventually the swelling will break open (aneurysm), leaking blood into surrounding tissues. In both the brain and the aorta, the leaking blood can cause death. Aneurysms of the brain are usually detected with Magnetic Resonance Imagining (MRI). An aneurysm in the aorta can be detected with a chest x-ray. An aneurysm farther down the aorta, in the abdomen, can be detected in an x-ray, or it can be felt by palpating the abdomen (pressing firmly into the abdomen and feeling with the fingers).

Aortic Aneurysm in the Abdomen

In order to feel for an aneurysm the person should be flat on their back and have a relaxed abdomen. If there is excessive abdominal fat to feel through the detection may be difficult. Palpate (feel) in the centerline of the abdomen down from just below the breastbone to the pelvic area. You should palpate by using the flats of the fingers of your left hand on your abdomen. Press down with your right hand on the fingers of the left hand. The right hand applies the pressure while the fingers of your left hand do the feeling. An aneurysm feels like a round mass, and can be as large as the size of a golf ball. It pulsates regularly with the heartbeats. A normal aorta may feel like a pulsating tube-like pipe structure.

Appendicitis Symptoms

Lower right side of the abdomen can have tenderness when touched (palpated), no tenderness on left side.
- Pain begins near the naval and travels to the right lower quadrant of the abdomen.
- Low fevers -100 degrees Fahrenheit to 101 degrees Fahrenheit or a little higher.
- Slight muscle spasm on the right side, which can be felt with no pain the left side. If the pain is severe and constant it can indicate diverticular disease (pouches forming on the descending colon).

Astigmatism Test

Astigmatism is a faulty curvature of the cornea lens or shape of the eyeball. It causes visual images to be blurred and distorted. It causes tension and headaches because the eyes try to cope with focusing different images in different planes.

- Place the chart in good light about twenty feet away from you. If you can't see the lines on the chart at twenty feet, move closer until you can see the lines. Cover one eye and see if any sets of lines look darker, sharper, or clearer, than the set of lines at right angles to it. Next cover the other eye. If there tends to be a difference in the darkness and clarity of one set of lines at right angles to it, then there is a degree of astigmatism. Most astigmatism can be corrected with eye exercises and exercise pinhole eyeglasses.

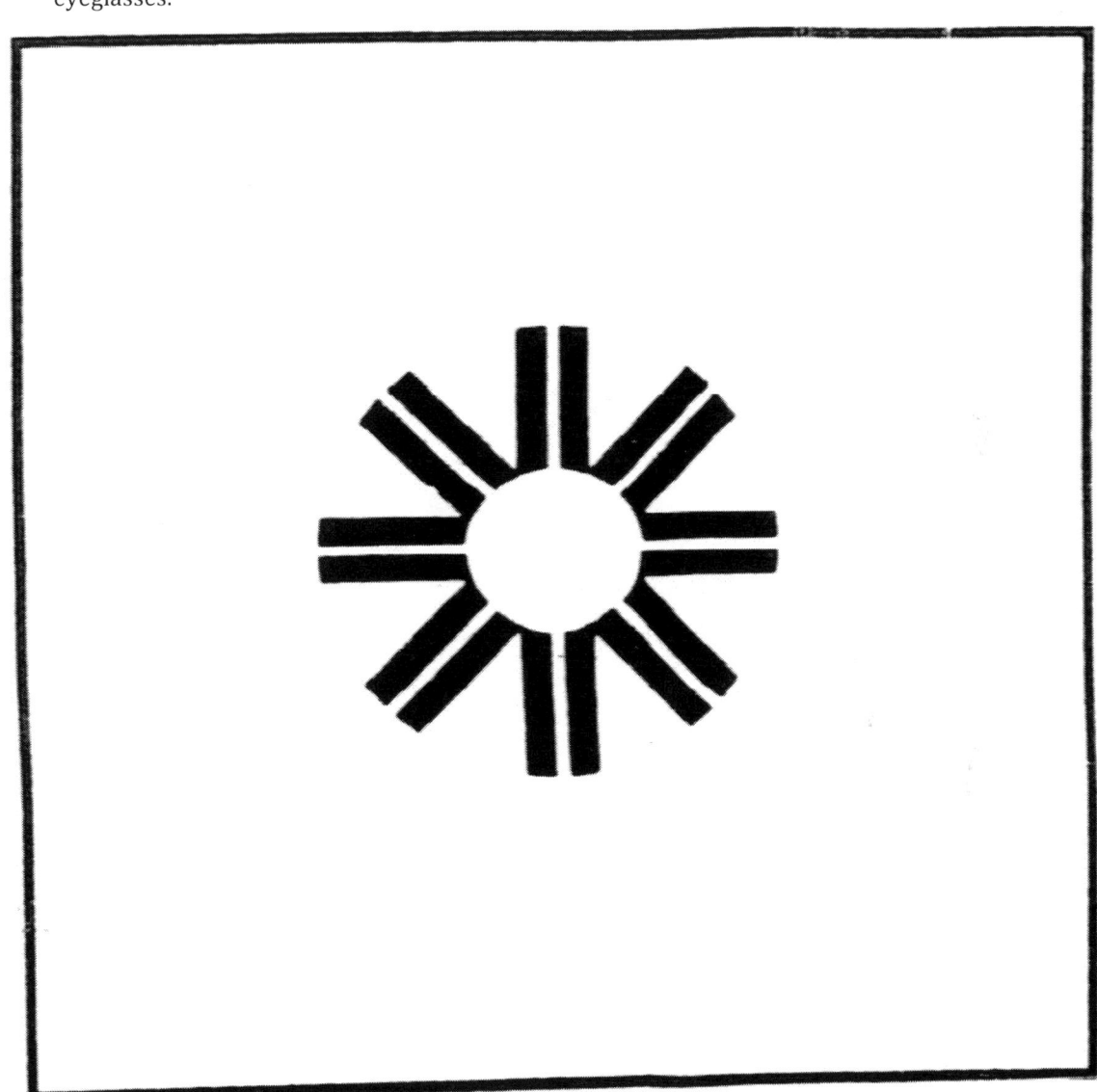

Auditory Nerve Test

The auditory nerve has two functions, which are 1) hearing and 2) the balance and position sense. Balance and position sense require feedback from the muscle system. The following simple test will help assess the auditory nerve.

- Stand with your feet together and your arms down at your side and eyes closed. The person testing you should give you a sudden push backward, forward, or to one side. The push should not knock you over.
- If you have normal balance mechanism, you will immediately regain balance from the unexpected shove. Symptoms of disorders of this function of the auditory nerve can be slight hearing loss and feelings of dizziness.

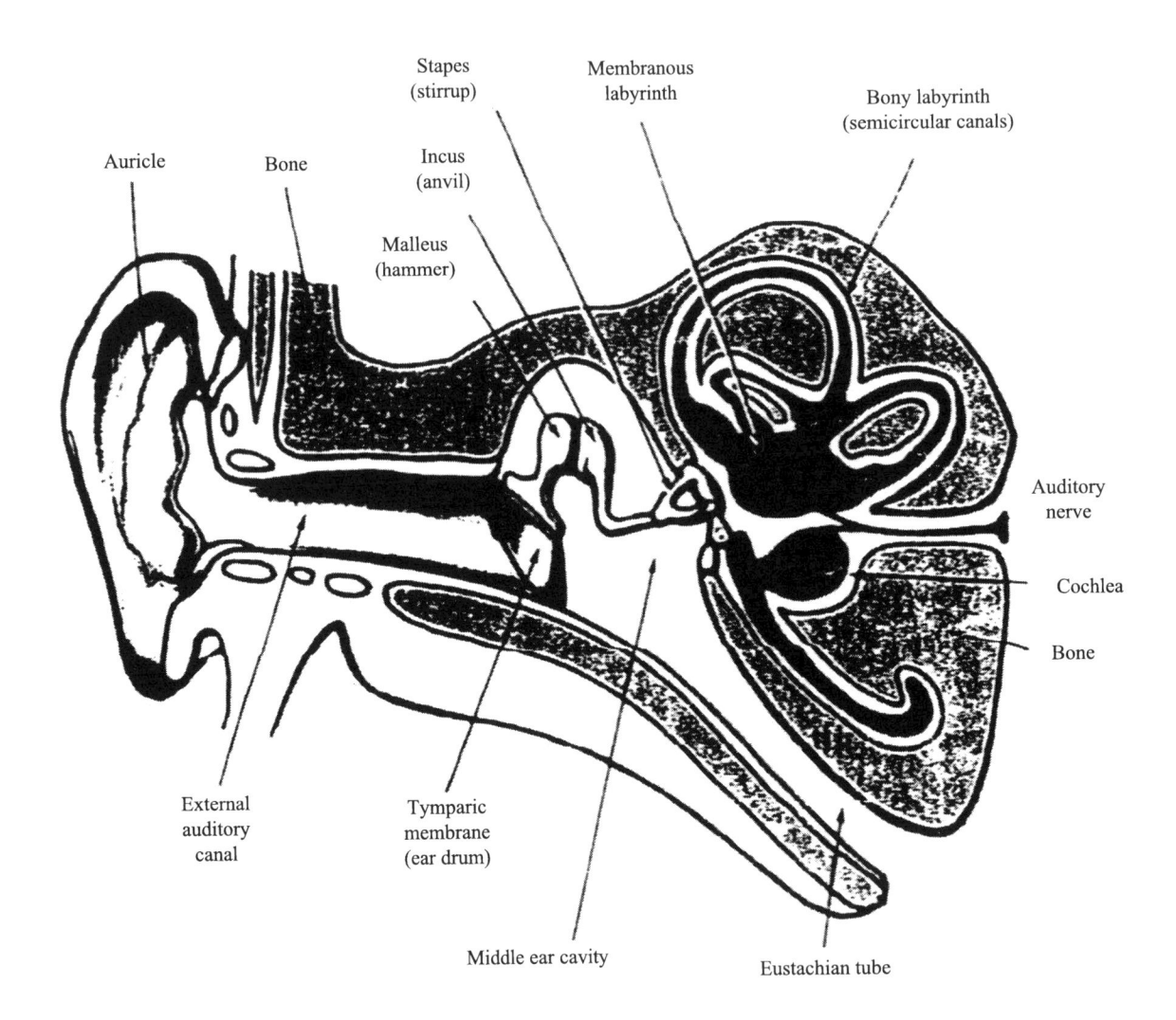

Dominant Eye Examination

Usually the right eye is dominant. Right-handed people usually have right eye dominance while left-handed people have left eye dominance. One eye fixes (dominates) itself on an image then the other eye turns to fix on the same object. The first eye to fix on an image is the dominant eye. The eyes work in a sequence to see a single image. If this doesn't happen it could result in double vision.

- Cut a one-inch circle in the center of a piece of paper or in an index card. It doesn't have to be perfectly round.
- Hold the circle about a foot away from your eyes, and with both eyes open, look through the circle at some distant object.
- Hold your index finger so that it lines up with the center of the hole and on any object you choose to look at. Hold your finger like sighting a rifle at a target.
- Close your left eye. Look at the circle, your finger, and the object. If they are lined up, your are fixing with your right eye because you are right eye dominant. If the opposite is true everything is lined up while looking with your left eye and the right eye is shut, you are left eye dominant.

Make a half-inch diameter black spot on a piece of stiff paper. A 3 by 5 index card works fine. About three inches to the left of the spot make a pyramid or a star.

Blind Spot Test

Images and light impulses travel from the retina of the eye to the brain by the optic nerve. Where the optic nerve inters the eyeball is called the optic disc. The disc has nerves that travel from it to points on the retina where they make contact with the photoreceptor cells (rods and cones). The optic disc itself contains no rods or cones and is, therefore, a blind spot. Each eye has a blind spot.

Test Procedure

- Close your right eye and hold the paper at arm's length with the pyramid in front of your left eye. Look at the pyramid and bring the paper slowly toward your face. At some point the black round spot will disappear. The black round spot disappears because the image of the spot has fallen on the blind spot of your left eye.
- Move the paper a little more closely and the spot reappears. To find the blind spot of your right eye, look at the spot with the left eye closed and make the pyramid disappear in the same way.

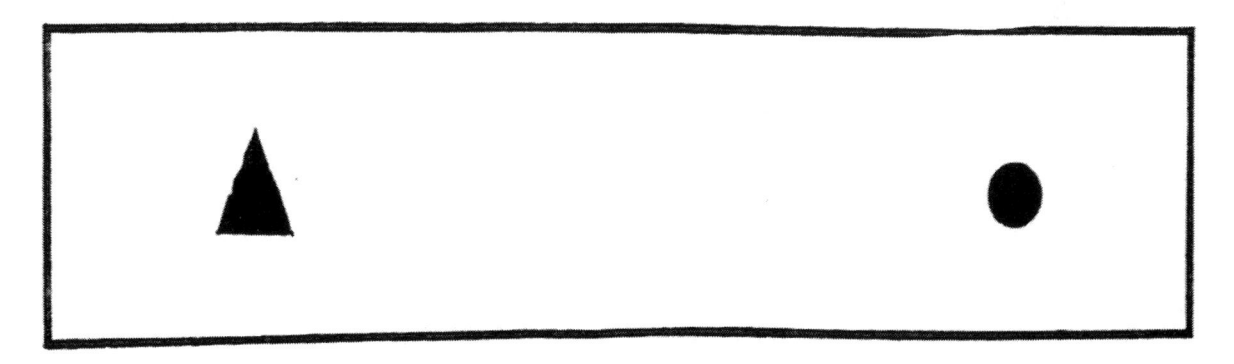

Facial Nerve and Taste Sensation Test

The facial nerve controls the taste sensation in the front two-thirds of the tongue. There are seven tastes that each taste bud is capable of sensing, salt, sour, sweet, bitter, pungent savory (pleasant) and a taste sensation for protein called Glutamate. Check the taste aspect of the nerve function by identifying the primary tastes of sweet, sour, bitter, and salty.

- Prepare separate solutions of each of the four primary taste sensations in cups: a strong solution of honey in water, a strong solution of ordinary sea salt in water, use extracts or make a tea of a quassia, or wormwood, calamus, angelica, cubeb, hops horehound or snakeroot herb for a bitter taste (1 tablespoon to a cup), Kombu mushroom form Glutamate and either lemon juice or lime for sour. It is best to rinse your mouth with water before beginning the test and after each of the four primary tastes. The taste sensation/ taste buds are located under the tongue, roof of mouth, cheeks, throat and in the lungs.

- Take a cotton-tipped swab; dip it in one of the solution and touch far forward but not at the tip. When doing this test, it is necessary to put the solution-dipped swab on one side of the midline of the tongue. If a small amount of fluid seeps across to the other side, then you can taste the solution with the other side of your tongue.

- Test each of the primary-taste (sweet, bitter, salty, sour) and glutamate sensation on one side of the tongue, and then repeat and test on the other side. Each solution should be tasted correctly and separately on each side of your tongue. Failure to distinguish between any two of them can indicate a problem with the facial nerve.

Facial Nerve and Blinking

The trifacial (trigeminal) nerve is the sensory nerve of the face and head. The following is a way to test it.
- The person to be tested must close their eyes.
- Use a soft piece of cotton. Touch the face with cotton (purchase from pharmacy cotton balls) at different points, ask the person to tell you if they felt the touch of the cotton
- If the person is unable to sense two or more touches it is considered abnormal.

The trigeminal helps to control the feeling of sensation over the white part of the eye, which makes you, blink when the eyeball is touched.
- Twist the piece of cotton to a point.
- The person being tested must look straight ahead a object.
- Bring the pointed cotton in toward the eye from the very outer edge. Make sure the person is looking straight ahead so as not to see the cotton coming.
- If the eye blinks when the cotton touches the white of the eye, trigeminal nerve is normal.

When the trigeminal has impairment, the person will not feel the cotton against the eye that is touched and the blink response will not occur in the eye. If the eyelid of the opposite eye closes when one eye is touched; there is a possible lesion or impairment of a facial nerve.

Phlebitis Symptoms

- Unexplained pain in one leg, usually in the calf.
- A heavy feeling with the leg. The leg feeling sensitive to the touch.
- Squeeze the affected calf gently with both hands. Then squeeze the unaffected calf. The calf with the phlebitis is usually very sensitive and tender.
- Measure the widest part of both calves with a tape measure. Move the tape measure up and down a bit to make sure you are measuring the fattest part of the calf. When the affected calf is a quarter inch or more larger than the unaffected side.
- There is swelling, with heaviness in the leg and sensitive to touch.

Phlebitis Test

Phlebitis usually occurs in the legs.
- Gently squeeze the painful or sensitive calf with both hands, and then gently squeeze the non-painful calf. Phlebitis usually occurs in the legs. It usually starts after a long period of sitting or rest or inactivity.

Venous blood flow in the legs depends upon muscle contraction of the leg muscles around the veins. When the muscles contract they put pumping pressure on the veins and cause the blood to flow. Slow or loss of movement of the muscles causes the blood flow to be slow and sluggish and a clot can form. Clogged veins inflamed, harden or deteriorated veins or rough spots caused by minor damage can cause the blood to move slow and clot.

Blockages in Vein

Veins have thin walls and less pressure inside them than arteries. Veins can develop thrombophlebitis, or phlebitis, and varicose veins. (Thrombos is a clot; "phleps" means blood vessel; and the suffix "itis" means inflammation).

Plaque Test

Plaque is sticky film that consists of bacteria, saliva, and food debris that sticks to the tooth's surfaces. It will cause tooth decay and gum disease. You can check your teeth for plaque by using "Disclosing Tablets". These tablets contain dye that will turn plaque bright red. The red stain will disappear within a few hours. Drugstores have the tablets.

- Brush and/or floss your teeth then chew a disclosing tablet, let it dissolve in your saliva, and swish it around in your mouth; then spit it out.
- Look at your teeth using a penlight and dental mirror or while looking in a mirror. Look at the tooth's inner and outer surface. The red stain appears on deposits of plaques, which can be removed with thorough brushing and flossing.

Position Sense Test

Position sense is the ability to know where various parts of your body are without looking. Nerve impulses from sensory cells send signals to the central nervous system that let you know you have raised your arm or moved your leg.

Position Arm Test

With your eyes closed, touch the tip of your nose with you index finger, first with one hand and then with the other. Extend your arm straight out and bring your arm slowly in so that the index finger can touch the nose. Coming near to touching the nose indicates that you have position sense.

Position Leg Test

Sit in a chair with your eyes closed, touch the heel of one foot to the shin of the opposite leg and move the heel up and down a little. Position sense is normal accurately with each foot.

Pupillary Eye Reflex Test

1. Look into a mirror. Use a penlight to shine light diagonally into the eye from the outside corner. Do not shine the light directly into your eye. A quick flash of light is all that is needed.
2. When the light strikes your eye the iris instantly contract which makes the pupil smaller. When you take the light away, the pupil becomes larger. The pupillary reflex should be fast.

Disease and injuries can affect the functioning of the irises. This causes response to light to change or be altered. The pupils may appear to be unequal in size due to illness, or injury, nerve damage or an un-noticed Stroke.

Rheumatoid Arthritis Symptoms

Rheumatoid Arthritis (RA) is a systemic (bodily) disease, which can cause a slight fever, joint and muscle pain, general fatigue, weakness, confinement in bed and loss of appetite. It is a crippling disease that affects children and adults.

Symptoms:
- Morning stiffness of long duration and/or stiffness from sitting.
- Swollen, inflamed joints in the hands, wrist, elbows, knees, ankles, or feet
- Muscle weakness and deterioration of muscle.
- Bilateral involvement – same joint affected on both sides of the body
- Inflamed or reddish skin over the affected joints.

Rib Fracture Test

Symptoms:
- A rib fracture can alter and interfere with breathing. A person with a fractured rib tends to "splint" the injured side of the chest so that when they breathe in, the injured side of the chest will rise less than uninjured side.
- To test for a rib fracture put one hand on the injured person's backbone and the other hand on the breastbone (sternum). Then press your hands together gently, as if attempting to press the

breastbone toward the backbone. If there is no fracture there will be little discomfort. If the rib is fractured pressing will cause a sharp pain at the fracture site.

Scoliosis Test

Scoliosis is an abnormal side-to-side curvature of the spine.
Have the person being examined to stand up straight with their back bared to the waist. The spinous process or knobby protrusions of the backbone running down the center of the back should line up in a straight vertical column that does not curve from side to side. Look at the vertebral column for signs of lateral curvature. If you can not see the spinous process, then have the person to bend forward slightly from the waist; this will make the boney knobs of the spinous process visible. Use a Black felt-tip pen to make a dot on the skin directly over each of the twenty-four spinous process. After you have made the dots have the person stand straight. The dots should form a straight line up the back. Curving dots is scoliosis. **Dropped shoulder** is another indication of scoliosis. Have the person stand up with their back to you, bared to below the waist. Look to see if one shoulder drops lower than the other. They should be equal. A dropped shoulder indicates scoliosis. Have the person being tested stand with their feet slightly apart and then bend forward slowly at the waist while letting the arms hang down in front and keeping the knees straight. Looking from behind the person watch as the upper body drops downward. Look to see if one side of the torso is higher than the other at any time. Both sides should remain equal. If they are not, it is scoliosis.

Slipped Disc Test

Slipped discs usually is in the area of the lower five lumbar vertebrae which support most of the body's weight. A slipped lumbar disc irritates the sciatic nerve. The sciatic nerve goes down the back of the legs. The sciatic is the largest nerve in the body. The following tests can indicate either directly or indirectly sciatic nerve problems.
- Lie down on your back, keeping your legs straight, raise first one leg then the other up as high as possible. Normally, the leg can be raised about 90 degrees, so that the bottom of your foot is facing the ceiling. If there is a slipped disc, you will be unable to raise one leg more than 45 degrees from the floor without pain. If pain is experienced, do not try to force the leg higher because this will irritate the inflamed sciatic nerve.
- Stand with your legs straight, then bend down to touch your toes with your fingertips. Usually a person can get within a few inches of their toes or at least to their knees. A person with a slipped disc probably will not reach the knees because of a painful pulling in the back of one leg. If a person with a slipped disc were to try to touch their toes one leg at a time, they would probably do better on one side than the other.

An untreated slipped disc can cause deterioration of the nerves resulting in a tingling, weakness, numbness, and/or decreased reflexes in the affected leg. Test such as "Tactile Sensation Test", "Superficial-Pain Sensation Test", "The Knee Jerk Reflex Test", and "Ankle –Jerk Reflex Test", can indicate disc problems.

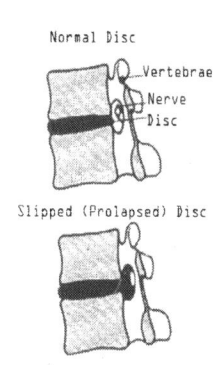

Back Problems

The possibility of having back problems is increased if you have some of the following behaviors or symptoms.
- Are your stomach muscles weak or flabby?
- If you feel pain when stand with your heels and shoulders against a wall, and slip your clenched fist between the wall and the small of your back is just above the buttocks.
- Do you exercise less than three times a week?
- Do you regularly sleep on you stomach or spend long periods of time lying on your stomach?
- Do you pick up items from the floor without bending your knees?
- Do you participate in sports activities that require quick, severe or sudden twisting of the back?
- Are you overweight or obese?
- Do you constantly lift items from a shelf or platform that is above your head?
- Do you stand or sit for long hours without back support?
- Do you bend forward from the waist with your knees stiff when you lift items?
- Do you spend long hours in a chair where you upper legs slant downward from your hips to your knees?
- Do you have to lift heavy objects and twist your body to place the object somewhere?

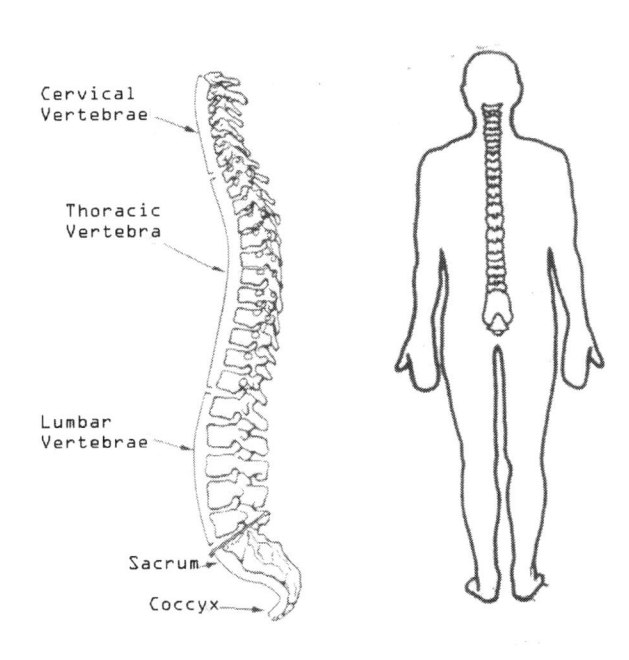

Bilateral Muscle Strength Test

Muscles disease affects muscle strength. The muscle or the nerves that serve a weaker or inadequately functioning muscle can lose muscle tone and then muscle strength and this affects bilateral muscle movement. It can be caused by muscle disease nerves attached to the area whether nutritional, emotional reactions to problems real or imagine, injury, diseases etc.

The following can help detect the problem.
- In order to detect muscle weakness in one leg, lie on your stomach with your knees bent and your legs forming a 90-degree angle.
- The person testing the muscle should grasp one ankle with both hands and use as much strength as possible to bring the leg down to the floor while you use your strength to resist.
- Do this with both legs. The tester should find it equally difficult (or easy) to bring either leg down to the floor. The resistance in both legs should be equal.

Breast Exam

The breast contains fat that give them their shape and ligament structures that stop them from sagging. The milk glands are deep in the fat structure. They cannot be felt on the surface of the breast tissue. The breast glands can be tender to the touch and their size remains the same from month to month. Most breast tumors grow either in the milk glands or in the milk ducts. Men get breast cancer and diseases. All men and women should examine their breast on a regular monthly basis. Women should examine the breast about once a week after the end of the menstrual period. After the cycle, the breasts are neither tender nor swollen. The swelling and tenderness of the breast can be caused by cyclic hormonal changes. After menopause or hysterectomy the exam should be done on a regular calendar basis, such as on the first of each month. If the hysterectomy did not include the removal of both ovaries, the breasts should not be examined during the swollen, tender period.

Fractured (Broken) Collarbone Test

Collarbone fracture is common. The two collarbones (clavicles) are located just above the first rib, at the base of the neck, one on each side. The test for a fractured collarbone is a follows:
- The two slender collarbones extend from the sternum (breast bone) in the center of the chest outward to each shoulder. When it is injured a fracture of this long bone is indicated by immediate pain in the shoulder. The pain increases with movements of the upper arm.
- Hold the upper arm on the injured side tightly against the chest and support it upward a little. If this position relieves the pain and discomfort there is probably a fractured collarbone.

Fractured Limb Signs and Symptoms

A fractured limb causes pain and stops you from using the injured part. Immediately after a fracture there can be numbness, which will gradually disappear and leaving intense pain. If the fractured limb is moved the pain will increase. Pain generally increases until a cast or splint has immobilized a fracture.

The following are indications of a fracture:
- An unnatural angle or deformity of a bone
- Tenderness at the fracture site
- The sound of grinding when moving a limb
- Discoloration caused by bleeding into the tissue
- A tense and hard muscle spasm
- False motion or motion not at a joint
- Swelling, inflammation and/or redness at fractured bone

A fracture is simply a break in the bone. This break can be a hairline, double, fracture, an open fracture that a bone protrudes through the skin or segmented.

Gallbladder Symptoms

Gallbladder problems are indicated by severe knife-like pain in the upper right quadrant of the abdomen. The pain usually starts when a greasy, oily, fried food, or fatty meal has been eaten. The pain can last several hours and then gradually decrease and stop and then occur when another fatty meal is eaten. The pain can travel up into the chest and is usually felt in the area of the right shoulder blade. The pains of both gallbladder inflammation and a Heart Attack can occur in the shoulder. This causes a Liver Attack (gallbladder) to be confused with a Heart Attack.

Glossopharyngeal Nerve Test

The ninth cranial (glossopharyngeal) nerve regulates two functions, which are taste on the back of the tongue, and the sensation in the back of the throat. Use the taste buds on the front part of the tongue.

- Use the five solutions used for the test on the front two-thirds of the tongue- solutions of honey, sea salt, quassia, kombu (glutamate test), and lemon or lime.
- Using a cotton- tipped swab, to put drops of solution on the rear third of the tongue. Test both sides of the tongue avoid being test too close to the midline. Each solution should be tested separately and correctly on each side of the rear third of your tongue. If you fail to distinguish between any two of them, then there can be a problem with the ninth cranial nerve.

Gum Disease Signs

Healthy gums have basics characteristics:

- Gum tissue forms a "v" between the teeth.
- Gum should be firm and fit snugly around the tooth
- The gum tissue forms a collar around the base of the tooth
- Gums are pink to dark pink or purple or whitish pink or a mixture of colors
- Gums have stippling (dot like indentations) usually in the areas closest to the teeth

To identify gum stippling and collars you will need to blot dry with a sterile gauze a section of gum tissue and look at the gums with a penlight.

The following are signs of gum disease:

- Inflamed Gums are red and swollen and puffy. Look at the base around each tooth for this abnormal reddening.
- Bleeding Gums that bleed during brushing or while eating are not normal. To check for bleeding gums floss between two tenth and against the area you are checking. If this causes the gum to bleed it indicates some degree of gum disease. Healthy gums do not bleed.
- Painful Gums have a burning sensation tender to touch and have stinging, are usually diseased.
- Receding Gums- Gums should be attached to the enamel (white part) of the tooth. If the gum seems to be moving away from the tooth and exposing the bottom of the tooth and/or the root it is receding gums. If the tip of the gum between the teeth looks white and pus-filled, put your finger on the gum and press inward and upward to squeeze pus or blood out of the gum. Pus coming out the tip of the gums in not normal.

Gum disease can caused bad breathe and a slight fever.

Hearing and Loss Test

Hearing is measured by pitch. Pitch is low and high tones. Pitch measurement uses cycles per second. Normal conversation registers about 1,000 cycles; a 6,000- cycle sound is a very high squeak. Average hearing ranges from a low of 20 to a high of 20,000 cycles per second. Poor health can cause a decrease in hearing at age 50, hearing can be reduced to 8000 cycles per second and at 60 years 6500, 70 year 5,000 cycle etc.

Indication of Hearing Loss

- Difficulty hearing on the telephone
- Seeming inattention when someone speaks
- Talking louder than necessary
- Continually saying, "What?" or "Huh?" "What you say?"
- Difficulty in learning to speak

Hearing loss Test

A ticking watch or clock and tape measure is needed for this test. Test someone who has good hearing by seeing how far away from a ticking clock the ticking can be heard by the person known to have good hearing. Start at a distance that the watch is too far away to be heard and gradually bring it closer to the person being tested.

Hypoglossal *(Tongue) Nerve Test*

The test for the hypoglossal (from hypo= under and glossa =tongue) called the twelfth cranial nerve. Stick your tongue out and look into a mirror. The tongue usually can have a very slight deviation to one side. A tongue that protrudes crookedly to one side of the mouth indicates lesions of one side of the twelfth cranial nerve or a stroke. When it is difficult to stick the tongue out both sides of the nerve is affected. Clumsiness when using the tongue can affect speech, this indicates twelfth cranial nerve problems.

Nose Examine

Examine the inside of the nose with either a penlight or a nasal speculum. Otoscopes have a nasal speculum (largest of the little funnels).

- Press the tip of the nose inward to widen the openings and look upward into the nasal cavity. If you are using a nasal speculum, never insert the instrument up the nostril without looking to see whether there are foreign objects that could be pushed farther into the nasal cavity by your speculum.
- Look at the skin (mucous membrane) that is inside of the nose. It is normally pinkish in color and is covered with a number of fine hairs. If you have a cold this skin becomes inflamed, swollen and reddened. The mucous membrane becomes swollen due to allergic reactions such as hay fever. The swollen membrane tends to be pale in color and the discharge is profuse and watery.
- Look at the central nasal septum (wall between the two nostrils). The septum should be straight and smooth and the skin pinkish.
- Locate the three small, shellfish protrusions (turbinates) high up in the nasal cavity. The nasal turbinates are on either side of the septum and are covered with mucous membrane tissue. You may not be able to see the turbinates without a nasal speculum.
- Look for swollen, mushroom saclike masses (polyps) that can block air passages and sinus channels. They resemble little mushrooms and can be small or as large as a grape. Polyps are often found in cases of allergies

Kidney Pain and Kidney Stones Test

You can find where your kidneys are by feeling for the edge of the lowest rib on your back. The kidneys are on both sides of the spinal column. This point is known as the costophrenic angle. The prefix "costo" refers to the diaphragm. The costophrenic angle is the corner formed by ribs and the diaphragm. Kidney disease can cause pain in this costophrenic angle area.

Test procedure

- Make a fist and reach back and lightly hit yourself a few times behind the right and left kidney in the costrophrenic angle. A sharp light blow will do. Do not hurt yourself.
- If thee blow causes pain, it can indicate kidney disease. There may be pain on one side as only one kidney is involved, and only that one hurts. In the past, you may have experience kidney pain while running, riding a train that bounced, an airplane hitting an air pocket or landing, or a car riding over a pot hole or railroad track or while exercising.

Kidney disorders are painless. Therefore the absence of costophernic- angle pain does not mean that there is no kidney disease. But if you do have pain in the costrophrenic- angle this suggests a kidney disorder. The muscles of the back can be painful or ache in the kidney area. Don't confuse a muscle ache with the sharper pain originating in the kidneys. Kidney pain can be caused by kidney infections and kidney stones. Kidney pain can occur when the kidney stone passes down the ureter (tube that goes from the kidney to the bladder). Stones can cause intense and agonizing pain. Passing a stone or stones may feel like a severe cramp that starts in the side or back and moves toward the genital region and inner thigh. The pain may last for several minutes or hours. Once the kidney stone gets out of the ureter and into the bladder, the pain usually stops quite suddenly. The stone, however, may remain in the bladder anywhere from a few minutes to a few days. When kidney stones are in the bladder, there is the constant urge to urinate and there are frequent attempts to urinate but only very small amounts of urine pass out. Also kidney infections can cause the urge to urinate. However if the urge to urinate occurs after severe pain in the back, it is probably a kidney stone. Kidney stones can scrape and cut the kidney's ureters and/or bladder resulting in blood in the urine. The amount of blood in the urine is very small and not enough to make the urine look red or even pink.

Large Intestine Examine

The large intestine (colon) is the last part of the digestive tract. Undigested food residue accumulates in the colon. In the colon water nutrients are taken out the food residue leaving waste, then the waste is moved into the rectum.

- Put your finger on the vertical midline of the abdomen about halfway between the navel and the top of urinary bladder (is about 4 finger widths below the navel). Move your fingers to the right until they touch the pelvis (hip bone). The large intestine begins in this location. It lies in the inside hollow of the right pelvic bone.
- Under the edge of pelvic bone, the small intestine connects to the large intestine (colon) ascends (goes up) to the bottom of the liver. Therefore this section of the colon is called the ascending colon. There is a small section of colon called the Cecum. The Appendix can be from two to six inches long. It extends inward and slightly to the left from the Cecum (your right side of the lower abdomen).
- Upward from where the liver was felt is the ascending colon. It makes a right –angle turn in this location and goes across (tranverse) the abdomen to the same site under the left rib cage. This section is the Transverse Colon.
- The descending colon makes a right angle turn down the center of the left pelvis where it turns and moves inward. This section is called the Sigmoid Colon. It travels a short way to the rectum.

Liver and Gallbladder Exam

- Feel the bottom tip of you breastbone (sternum), it feels like a little lump just before you get into the soft fleshy part of the abdomen. This is the Xiphoid (zy'-foidz) Process of the sternum. The Xiphoid is on the vertical midline that extends straight up through the naval. The diaphragm is just above this point at the upper limit of the abdomen. Part of the liver is underneath.
- From the Xiphoid Process, move your fingers down diagonally to the right along the bottom of the right of your rib cage. At the bottom of your rib cage, where the last rib turns towards the back, are the lower right limits of your liver. It is the largest in your body and generates the most heat. The remainder of the liber is up under the right rib cage and the top of liver lies against the diaghram.
- At the bottom of the rib cage down from your right nipple is the gallbladder. It cannot be felt unless there is a problem with it.
- With the flat part of your left hand on your abdomen with the index finger just rubbing against the rib cage. Apply pressure with your right hand on top of the left fingers.
- Exhale the air out of your lungs, press down with your hand, and then take a deep breath. While you breathe in, you can feel the edge of your liver pass under the fingers of your left hand either right under the rib cage or two to three finger widths below it. Feeling your liver depends on your built and the sensitivity of your hands.

Lumber Lordosis Test

Lordosis is excessive lumbar curve that is called swayback. This can also be caused by weak muscle groups that support the back or a genetic (structural) defect. It can cause backaches and disc problems. The following are ways to detect it:

- Use a full-length mirror or have someone look at your posture from one side. Excessive lumbar Lordosis can be seen.
- The lumbar curve, as explained previously. Is the inward curve of the spine in the small of the back just above the buttocks? Look to see that the abdomen extends forward excessively in front, or the pelvis protrudes out in the back.
- If you or the person being tested stands with their back against a wall, you should barely be able to slip your hand into the space between your lower back and the wall. In Lordosis the space between the lower back and wall is large or has a wide distance between the lumbar curve and the wall. Strengthening the muscles of the buttocks, abdomen and back will reduce Lordosis.

Spine Exam

The spinal column of an adult should be vertical, with a slight "S" shaped curve when viewed from the side. The "S" shaped curve is the four (4) natural curves in the back:

1. The cervical backward curve of the neck curves in at the neck to the shoulders;
2. The thoracic forward curve reverses the cervical curve, curving outward
to just under the shoulders;

3. Then the lumbar backward curve is an inward curve at the small of the back slightly above the buttocks;
4. The sacral curve is an outward curve at the buttocks.

Lung Vital Capacity and Peak Air Flow Test

When you inhale and exhale you never completely fill the lungs with all the air or completely empty your lungs of air. The vital capacity is the maximum amount of air that you can take into your lungs (inhale) and then expel completely (exhale). You can check your peak airflow with the match test.

Match Test

- Light an ordinary match and hold it arms length of the person being tested
- You or the person being tested should take a deep breath and try to blow the match; failure to blow out the match indicates respiratory problems.

Lymph System Test

Lymph fluid is plasma like and drains from body tissue in a system of vessels called lymph vessels, or lymphatics. The lymph fluid enters into the bloodstream through a large vein in the neck. Lymph nodes are round beanlike structures that are clustered along the lymph vessels. The nodes absorb infecting organism, cellular waste, toxins or foreign particles. The nodes fluid neutralize toxins, and attacks harmful substances. The body has many lymph nodes in the neck, groin, and hollow of the collarbones, behind and above the elbows and behind the ears. When the lymph nodes enlarge it indicates an infections. Nodes in the neck and jaw areas usually swell as a reaction to a toothache, respiratory infection and sores in the mouth. Swollen nodes behind the ears can indicate skin disease (German Measles), an ear infection or sore on the scalp. While enlarged nodes in front of the ears indicate toxins in the area of the face and eyes. Swollen armpit nodes usually indicate infections or an injury to the legs or feet. If all the lymph nodes in the body are swollen it can indicate a generalized infection (.i.e. mononucleosis) or systemic diseases.

Neck Lymph Nodes Exam

Feeling for swollen lymph nodes in the neck, armpits and groin follows the same procedure.
- Hold the fingers together, use the fleshy pads of the fingers and feel for the lymph nodes along the neck and the back of the neck, up under the chin, and at the angle of the jaw. Relax the neck muscles during the exam.
- A swollen lymph node can feel soft or hard and usually feels painful when you press it. The lymph node absorbs toxins and enlarges during an infection.

Malocclusion (improper bite) Test

An improper bite (malocclusion) is one in which the teeth do not come together uniformly and evenly. A common form is jaw-to-jaw mismatch in which either the upper or the lower jaw protrudes. Malocclusion can be caused by crooked teeth and high fillings. A high filling is slightly higher than the teeth on either side. Therefore when you bite, the teeth will be hitting first on this high spot. The constant impacting on the high spot when chewing can damage a tooth. A high spot can be detected by closing the teeth gently, then rub the teeth together from side to side. If there is a high spot it will be felt.

Minimum Strength and Flexibility Test

The musculoskeletal system should be strong enough to cope with the normal routines of daily living. The musculoskeletal system test is as follows:
- Lie down on your back with your hands on the floor, palms up, next to your neck. Keep your legs straight, and raise the legs approximately ten inches off the floor and hold them there for ten seconds.
- Lie down on your back with your knees bent and your feet secured.
- Lie down on your stomach with a pillow placed under your hips and the tester should hold down your feet. Put your hands behind your neck and raise your head and chest off the floor. In this position you should be able to keep your legs straight and raise your legs off the floor, and hold them in the raise position for ten seconds
- Keep your legs straight and feet together, bend from the waist and touch the floor with your fingertips.

If you fail to do any of these test, then you need to exercise.

Motor Functioning

The nervous system controls motor functioning (body movements) by signaling muscles to relax or contract. The nerves send impulses from the brain or spinal cord to the muscles through motor cells. The fibers of each motor cell branch off at their endpoints and touch strands of muscle. The impulses sent through these motor fibers stimulate the release of neurotransmitters (messenger chemicals) that start the muscle contracting. When the impulses stop stimulating the muscles they will relax. Motor function is controlled by motor nerves that direct muscle action. An abnormality of the motor system can cause a problem with the muscles. The neurological tests, called the knee-jerk reflex, test the nerves of the knee, or patella (knee cap) tendon. The knee-jerk reaction is called a Simple Reflex Arc because the nerves that received the tap from the handle end of a screwdriver send the afferent signal to the spinal cord; the signal is processed in the spine and the efferent nerve message directing the muscles to jerk is sent right back. A person that does not have the kneejerk reflex usually has nerve damage.

Movement Sense Test

- The tester should passively (gently) move one of your fingers or toes while you have your eyes closed. The tester must not touch one of the adjacent digits (fingers) during the examination.
- Each time a movement is made, you should respond and tell the direction of the movement. You should be able to distinguish a movement of less than a quarter of an inch in any direction.

Muscle Spasm Symptoms

Leg cramps, a "pinch" in the side, swimmer's cramp, a stiff neck, or the pain that can "lock" your back as you bend over to tie your shoe lace are all examples of a muscle spasm. A muscle spasm is a severe contraction of a muscle which indicates that a muscle of the nerves serving it are irritated: The muscle can be full of waste and/or lactic acid, fatigued from overuse; have insufficient oxygen and can not support the muscle's activity. The muscle can have an injury to the tendon. A muscle spasm in a thigh or somewhere in the back can be caused by a vertebrae disc problem. A shin splint is a spasm of the front lower leg. Runners and joggers get shin splits. Cramps in the calves of the legs or in the stomach, are muscle spasm caused by muscle fatigue, decreased blood circulation, varicose veins and/or clogged arteries that disrupts metabolism in the muscle cells.

Myasthenia Gravis Test

Myasthenia Gravis is a disorder of nerve and muscle function that usually begins by affecting the muscles of the eyes, tongue and the swallowing muscles. Myasthenia Gravis in its early stages causes a drooping of one or both eyelids muscles.

- Sit in a chair with your head held in its normal position, facing straight ahead.
- Without tilting your head move your eyes upward to look at the ceiling. Look for about two to three minutes.
- If you have Myasthenia Gravis, you will not be able to keep the eyelids open. Your eyelids will slowly droop until they cover most of the eye. Stop and rest the eyes for five to ten minutes. The eyelids strength will return. When the test is repeated the person being tested will have eyelids that droop because they are unable to keep the eyelid up and stare at the ceiling for a sustained period of time.

Tooth Nerve Damage

Stains on the teeth can be of various colors (orange, red, green, brown, and even yellow). Usually stains can be removed with cleaning. Dark stains in a tooth that was white and healthy looking can indicate damage to the nerve root. Discoloration in a tooth or in two adjacent teeth that were recently white and healthy looking should be investigated especially if there has been a blow to the mouth. A well-placed blow to the mouth does not have to be hard to kill the nerve in the tooth. A child can forget that they got hit in the mouth while playing. Therefore, their teeth have to be checked periodically. If the nerve root is damaged, the tooth will die. A dying tooth changes color from gray to yellow to brown or black.

Oculomotor (Eye) Nerve Test

The oculomotor nerve controls the opening and closing of the eye's pupil.

- Shine a flashlight into one eye and then the other of the person to be tested. Shine the light from the side; do not shine the light directly into the eye. Shine the light from the side for one side for one or two seconds.
- The pupils of both eyes will get smaller (constrict) in response to light shined into either eye.

- If the pupil remains wide open (dilated) and unresponsive to light, the oculomotor nerve can have a problem.
-

Olfactory (Smell) Nerve Test

- The olfactory nerve controls the sense of smell. Use a variety of small bottles of flavor extracts, the kind you find in the spice section of the supermarket. (cherry, vanilla, almond, peppermint etc.)
- Cover the bottles so that only the mouth of the jar is exposed.
- Smell each of them. If all four scents can be identified correctly, the olfactory nerve is intact and functioning.

Optic Nerve and Eye Movement Test

Check the nerve that controls eye movement by doing the following:
- The person being tested should look at a small object (tip of a pencil).
- Ask the person being tested to follow the object, (pencil) with their eyes while keeping the head still. Move the object (pencil) from side to side and up and down and observe how the eyes move to follow it.
- The eyes should fully move and be in coordination with each other.

If double vision should occur during this test, it indicates that some degree of malfunction of one of the muscle that moves the eyes. It is difficult to determine whether one or more nerves are malfunctioning or if it is a muscle weakness.

Osteoarthritis Symptoms

Arthritis is the inflammation of the joint. The suffix "itis" means inflamed and "arthr" means joints. If there is stiff joints in the morning and/or after sitting for a long period.
- Aching pain in a weight-bearing joint (knee or hip).
- If the fingers are affected they can develop deformities characterized by a knobby, twisted appearance. Knobs (Herbden's nodes) can be at the base of the finger joints.
- Joints that swell (i.e. knee).

Overactive Thyroid Test

An overactive thyroid is called hyperthyroidism and is characterize by nervousness, moist skin, "pop eyes" (exothaphthalmia), constant weight loss, increased food intake; excessive sweating, and a rapid heartbeat.
Testing Procedure:
- The person being tested should hold one hand out in front of them with the backside up with all the fingers stretched out as far as they will go.
- Next lay an 8 ½ by 11-inch sheet of paper on the back of the outstretched hand. Watch the edges of this paper; there can be a slight wiggle of the edges. If the thyroid is overactive, the edges of the paper will vibrate quite violently.
- There can be other factors that can cause the paper edges to wiggle.

Sensation in the Throat (Vagus Nerve) Test

Stroking the back of the throat causes gagging. The Gag Reflex indicates that the tenth cranial nerve (vagus) is functioning. Parts of the vagus nerve extend down to the stomach and are involved in the secretions of the stomach acid. The vagus nerve has branches that control some of the muscles in the palate that help form normal speech sounds. If during a period of weeks or months, the speech uncontrollably develops a slightly nasal quality, this can be an indication of a problem with the vagus nerve. If this occurs, the uvula will deviate to one side and if there is a nasal quality to the speech it indicates a vagus nerve disorder. This test is of the many vagus nerve functions. A thin straw with a bit of cotton attached to one end is needed to test for sensation of the throat and back wall of the pharynx.
- The person being tested should open their mouth wide while the tester gently rubs the piece of cotton attached to the straw against the back of your throat.
- The person being tested should say "aah" in order to get the tongue out of their way. A light touch is needed to determine if there is sensation in this area.
- In some people the Gag Reflex is very sensitive and they will react to the lightest touch. Others can tolerate more stroking. A failure to respond can indicate vagus-nerve malfunction.

Scrotum, Testicles, and Inguinal Exam

Feel the scrotum to see that both testicles have descended into the scrotal sac. If there is only one testicle it is called an undescended testicle. Compare the plum size to the testicles- they should be approximately equal. The left testicles hang slightly lower than the right. Gently palpate both testicles and the entire scrotum for lumps or extreme sensitivity. Any lump or mass within the scrotum is abnormal. Hard small lumps that suddenly appear within the scrotum can be a malignant tumor. Small lumps that appear in the inguinal area (crease where the legs join the body) are probably swollen lymph nodes. Lymph nodes can swell due to an infection in a leg or foot. If lumps persist there can be a problem. However, the swelling of lymph nodes usually has nothing to do with the sex organs.

Small Intestine Exam

The abdomen cavity is filled with twenty to thirty feet of tubing called the small intestine. It starts at the bottom right end of the stomach and winds around until it connects to the large intestine on the lower right side of the abdomen (above the hip bone). The area across the bottom edges of the rib cage, down to the pelvis on each side, across to the top of the urinary bladder is filled with the convoluted folded small intestine. When pressing into this area it should feel soft with no hard spots or any discomfort.

Spinal Accessory Nerve Test

The spinal accessory (eleventh cranial) nerve, controls certain muscles in the shoulders. The test of this nerve function is as follows:
- The person being tested raises both of their shoulders as if shrugging them and holds them elevated.
- The tester simultaneously pushes down hard on both shoulders with an equal amount of force on both sides.
- If one shoulder can be pushed down with relative ease while the other cannot, there can be impairment of the eleventh cranial nerve.

Sport Injuries

Sports injuries to joints, ligaments, tendons and muscles are caused by prolonged, repetitive over exercise activities that the body was not built to constantly perform. The same type injuries can occur from chopping wood, scrubbing floors, and using computer keypads etc. The symptoms for these injuries are pain, stiffness, inflammation, and some degree of incapacitation of the affected joint. Sports-related injuries are tendinitis, bursitis, torn ligaments, arthritis, strains, over exertion or some combination of these.

Stereognostic (Decoding) Sense Test

The stereognostic sense is the ability to "decode" sensory information. Stereognostic sense identifies an object by touch only. Using an assortment of small objects such as a key, coin, marble, ring, a staple, penny and/or a safety pin can test this sense.
- The tester places these objects in the person hand one at a time.
- The person being tested must close their eyes and be able to identify the object put in their hands. If they can do this, they have normal stereognostic sense. The two-point discrimination sense is the awareness of being touched at two nearby places at the same time. You should be able to tell the difference between being touched by one finger or two.

Stomach Exam

- Place your fingers on the xiphoid process. This is the site where the esophagus (a tube) enters the stomach.
- Imagine a slight downward line from the xiphoid process to a point on your left rib, which is about two inches below your left nipple. This is usually the location of the limit of your stomach. Part of the stomach, and liver are located under the dome-shaped diaphragm and they are partially protected by the rib cage.
- Move your fingers down and circle to the right across abdomen to the location on your right rib cage where you felt your liver. This is usually the right lower limit of the stomach. This is where the stomach connects with the small intestine. The stomach and small intestine can be under the bottom edge of the liver at this location.
- After a meal push in with your fingers and you will feel fullness and discomfort in the same area more than pushing in to the abdomen lower down, around the navel or below. There are normal stomachs that descend as low as the naval or further. The spleen is located behind the left rib cage under the

left nipple area between the stomach and the left side of the rib cage. The spleen is not part of the digestive tract. It is a filter and storage center for blood cells. Blood diseases or infections can cause the spleen to become enlarge, in which case the tip of it can be felt around the left rib cage.

Stroke Symptoms

- A change in mental ability; loss of ability to concentrate.
- Loss of vision, double vision, or dimness, particularly in one eye.
- Weakness, numbness, or paralysis of arms, legs, or face often on just one side.
- Sudden severe headache that is different from other headaches normally experienced.
- Unexplained dizziness, unsteadiness, or confusion.
- Problems speaking or loss of the ability to speak.
- Decreases consciousness.
- Tongue favoring on side of the mouth.

Strabismus Eyes

When both eyes do not turn and work together, the condition is known as strabismus. When one eye has much better visual acuity than the other it can cause the brain to suppress vision in one of the eyes. The brain avoids the disparate and confusing images and uses vision in one eye; When the brain constantly suppresses the vision in one eye during normal seeing, the suppressed eye eventually will lose its ability to see. This occurs with young children. Infants eyes tend to dissociate, or do not work together until they are about six months. After six months, the eyes should be developed to work together. Vision in a suppressed eye can be rapidly lost so the sooner it is treated the better.

- Eyes that do not work together (children over 6 months).
- Divergence or crossing of eyes.

Superficial (Slight) Pain Sensation Test

Superficial-pain sensation is a distinct sensory input to the nervous system. Superficial (slight) pain is a brief reaction to slight irritation of the surface of the skin. Superficial pain is not a throbbing or deep pain similar to that of a cut or a minor burn. A light pinprick is used to check superficial-pain sensation. A large hatpin with a little knob at one end is used for this test. The person being tested must close their eyes.

- The tester uses the pin knob and pointed pin end to lightly touch various places on the legs and arms.
- The person being tested must report each time they feel a sharp or dull touch.
- The tester should retest any areas where an incorrect response was given. Areas where there was inconsistent or incorrect response or failure to distinguish a sharp pin from a pin knob should be noted.

Tactile (Touch) Sensation Test

Superficial (light) touch is very different from the firm touch.

- Use a piece of a cotton ball. The tester should lightly touch one side on the person being tested arms and legs, then test the other side.
- The person being tested must close their eyes and say when a light-touch sensation is felt. The tester should rate the responses and compare the degree of sensitivity on each side of the arm or leg. Not being able to detect light touches on one side of the body is more significant than random misses on both sides.

Throat and Tonsils Exam

Examining the throat and tonsils requires using a penlight and the handle of a spoon or a wooden tongue depressor. The person you are examining should open their mouth wide and relax the tongue. Usually the throat can be seen clearly without the aid of a tongue depressor. However, if their is difficulty seeing past the tongue, place the spoon handle (or tongue depressor) on the surface of the tongue about two-thirds of the way back and gently yet firmly press down the tongue. If the spoon handle is too far forward, you will not be able to press down enough of the tongue to clearly see the throat. Shine your flashlight into the mouth. With the tongue pressed down, you should be able to see the throat clearly. The wall at the very rear of the mouth is part of a tube called the pharynx. It connects to the stomach. You will see the uvula, which is tongue tissue that hangs down from the roof of the mouth to the center of the throat. It is a flap that closes off the passage to the nasal cavity and allows the food you have swallowed to go down the pharynx instead of up into your nose. Your tonsils are located on both sides of the uvula behind little curtains of tissue (tonsillar pillars). The

tonsillar pillers are on each side of the rear wall of the mouth. The tonsils slightly protrude out from behind the tonsillar pillars one on each side.
- The skin (membranes) inside the mouth and nose, the tonsillar pillars and the tonsils are pinkish in color. The tonsils are normally about the size of a cherry and the tonsils are covered with a series of irregular, barely visible grooves. Healthy tonsils are usually behind the tonsillar pillars.
- The tonsils get enlarges when the throat becomes infected and inflamed especially in children.

Infected tonsils can have white patches of material in the normal cracks and grooves of the surface. White patches on the tonsils indicate strep throat (streptococcal infections). If there is a fever, a sore throat, enlarged tonsils with white patches, swollen lymph nodes at the angle of the jaw and along the front of the neck, then treatment is needed immediately. A streptococcal infection, which spreads throughout the whole body (scarlet fever) as well as valvular heart disease, usually follows a strep throat. Untreated valvular heart disease can cause extensive damage that may require open-heart surgery. The kidneys can be affected by untreated strep throat.

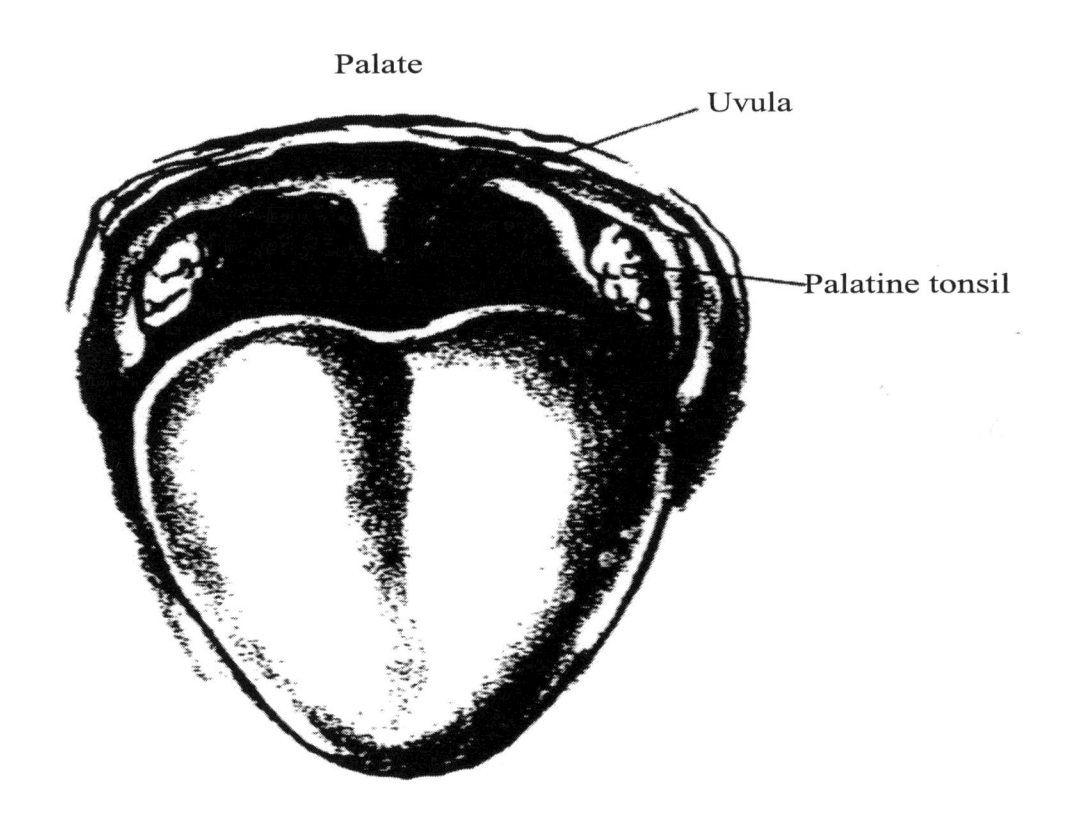

Temperature Sensation Test
Temperature sensation can be tested using two small glass bottles or a drinking glass.
- Fill one bottle (or glass) with cold water and the other with hot water.
- The tester should lightly touch each of the bottles to various parts of the body alternating between the hot and cold.
- The person being tested must close their eyes and distinguish between the hot and the cold bottle. A person with a neurological disorder can lose the sensation of cold but still be able to sense warmth. In this type of disorder ice cubes placed on the skin will feel warm.

Tendinitis Symptoms
Tendons are the tough fibrous cords that attach muscle to bone. When a muscle group is stressed by constantly over exercising, using a hammer, hitting a tennis ball, soccer or baseball, or walking on concrete the shock to the muscle stops abruptly in the tendon. Too many constant shocks irritate the tendon and the bone where the tendon is attached. This causes a inflammation and irritation at the site of attachment deterioration, in the tendon or the muscle tissue and other types of tissue damage. The tendon can tear away completely pulling with it a portion of the bone or joint covering to which it is attached.

Tooth Sensitivity Test
- Healthy teeth should not be sensitive to pressure, heat, or cold. If a particular tooth is unsound, gently tap its upper surface with a spoon handle. If the tap causes moderate sensitive or hurts there can be something wrong with the tooth. Normally a tooth does not hurt when you tap it with a spoon handle. If you are uncertain concerning the response of a tooth, tap the same tooth on the other side of the jaw for comparison.
- Swish some hot water and then cold water around in your mouth. Neither the hot or cold water should cause undue discomfort. Constant temperature sensitivity in one or more teeth is not normal.

The mouth, ears, and nose are related. Therefore pain in one area can travel to another nearby area. Tooth pain can be felt in the ear, or a sinus problem can travel to the upper teeth.

Underactive Thyroid Test
The thyroid is a butterfly shaped gland with one "wing" on each side of the windpipe (trachea). It moves when you swallow. Press your fingers lightly but firmly below your Adam's apple and swallow, or drink water, you will feel the thyroid move. An enlarged gland is called a goiter. A goiter can feel hard or soft, smooth or lumpy, and vary in size from slightly visible to distended. The thyroids hormones for metabolism may become either underactive or overactive in production. A thyroid hormone deficiency (hypothyroidism) is indicated by depression, increased in the amount of sleep-required daily, dry skin, chronic fatigue, a moderate weight gain with no increased food intake, brittle and coarse hair, and a tired sluggish feeling. The following test can identify a thyroid hormone deficiency. The person being tested should have their legs relaxed. Tap each knee with the handle of a screwdriver or a rubber flex hammer at the point marked "x". The tap should not be a blow.

Testing Procedure
This test involves the knee-jerk reflex.
- The person being tested must have bare knees and sit on a table so that their legs swing freely from the knee joint.
- Locate the kneecap with your fingers. This is the rounded bone that sits right over the knee.
- Then locate a bony protrusion about an inch below the kneecap. This is the top end of the large bone (tibia) in the lower leg. In the very front part of the leg you will feel a stiff cord in a short space between the bottom of the kneecap and the top of the leg bone. You should be able to put your thumb and index finger on each side of this cord. This is then tendon to test. Mark this point with an "x" using a felt tip pen.
- The person being tested should have their legs relaxed. Tap each knee with the handle of a screwdriver or a rubber flex hammer at the point marked with an "x". The tap should not be a blow.
- After the point marked "x" is tapped the lower leg will immediately give a little jerk. Then the lower leg will quickly relax. Observe closely the relaxation stage of the reflex, which occurs when the lower leg returns to its normal position. A sluggish relaxation phase of the deep-tendon reflex indicates an underactive thyroid.

Visible Field Test

Light impulses are transmitted to the black and white sensitive rods and the color sensitive cone cells are located on the retina at the back of the eye. The retina is about the size of a postage stamp, and as thin as onionskins, and has rods and cones, (150 million or more). The Fovea is the most sensitive point on the retina and is a small spot located near the center. It is almost one-fiftieth of an inch in diameter and has many cones. Fovea is where the sharpest vision and most color vision occur. In the center of the fovea is a deposit of very small yellow fat. This fat requires the hormone insulin to absorb light messages. Vision can be altered by blood sugar levels, and diabetes. The eyes stay in constant motion in order to keep the image you are looking at focused on the Fovea. Diseases can reduce the visual field.

Test Procedure

- Stand approximately an arm's length away from a wall with the right shoulder pointing toward the edge of a window or picture frame or an object on the wall.
- Choose an object in front of you that is a distance away, and look at it. Cover your left eye with your left hand.
- Next, hold your right hand out from your right side at eye level and point at the edge or object on the wall.
- Move you arm slightly back from the mark and loosely point your fingers forward. Wiggle your fingers and slowly move your arm forward. Constantly continue to look at the object in front of you. Do not look forward.
- After you have moved your arm slightly forward, your wiggling fingers will come into view while you are staring straight to the front. It will not be a clear image of your fingers, but the motion will be perceived. This is your right eye's edge of the visual field on your right side.
- Stop as soon as you see your fingers and look to see where your arm is. It should be about 85° (degrees) to 90° from a line straight in front of you. Touch the wall. You will be less than six inches from your marker. This means you can perceive objects almost in back of you.
- Do the same test with your wiggling fingers from several angles (from the nose side above your head, from below and diagonally). You will have to change hands when doing the test from the nasal side. The visual field from above will be about 50° and slightly more from the bottom. This is because the eyebrows and cheekbones obstruct your vision. Test both eyes in the same manner. If your visual field is getting smaller it indicates trouble. Test your visual field at least once a year.

Blood Pressure Interpretation

Blood Pressure and Pulse Table

SYSTOLIC PRESSURE			
92 - 110	112 - 140	140 - 190	192 - 280

PULSE

		50-70(2)(3)(6) 72-86(3) 88-120(1)(17)	50-70(2)(3)(6) 72-86(30 88-120(1)(17)	170-110	
	72-86(1)(3) 88-120(1)(11)	50-70(2)(3) 72-86(3) 88-120(1)(17)	50-70(2)(3)(6) 72-86(10)(13) 88-120(1)(17)	110-90	DIASTOLIC PRESSURE
50-70(7) 72-86(6) 88-120(4)(15)	60-85 NORMAL	50-70(6)(13) 72-86(10)13 88-120(10)	50-70(13) 72-86(10)(13) 88-120(10)	90-74	
50-70(2)(7) 72-86(4)(5)(14) 88-120(4)(5)14)	50-70(8)	72-86(9)		74-50	
50-70(2)(12) 90-120(14)				50-10	

1. Alkaline imbalance.
2. Acid imbalance
3. Electrolytes, cellular debris, unbounded elements and mineral precipitating and congesting heart and vascular, kidney weakness.
4. Nerve deterioration, problems metabolizing starches, blood sugar problems.
5. Overworked heart; hypertrophy, heart muscle degeneration.
6. Heart failure tendency.
7. Sympathetic stress, decrease circulation to skin and sex organs, hypertension, rheumatism, weak immunity, weak digestion.
8. Problems absorbing minerals, difficulty with hormones, enzymes.
9. Heart failure tendency.
10. Parasympathetic stress, respiratory, circulation, alkaline problems, inadequately building and growing tissue, arthritis problems, hypertension, rheumatism, weak immunity, weak digestion.
11. Heart staying in acid phase too long with a decrease in alkaline phase, heart muscle weakness, problems dilating, problems with valves.
12. Blood congested with waste causing flow to decrease, sluggish blood; precedes cardiac failure, cellular toxic waste fight or flight reaction can result in shock.
13. Neuritis, menopause, mental overwork, worry anxiety, real or imagine emotion stress, hormones altered.
14. Anemia, cardiac weakness, under nutrition, digestion decreased.
15. Infections, waste, toxicity, heart inadequately functioning.
16. Biochemical reaction to waste accumulating faster than it can be disposed, physical and emotional stress, neurosis, nerve stress, and/or pain.
17. Nervous system impaired and becoming weak, heart failing, minerals clogging bones, nerves and tissues.

How to use the Blood Pressure and Pulse Table

A battery operated Blood Pressure Monitor (that also reads pulse rate) should be used. With the results use this table. The Systolic Pressure numbers (i.e. 92-110) are located in the horizontal box at the top of the table. The Diastolic numbers (i.e. 10-50) are located in the vertical box located on the side of the table. The pulse rate numbers (i.e. 50-70) are located in square boxes labeled Pulse and are below the Systolic Pressure numbers are located horizontally. Next to the Pulse rate numbers are the numbers in parenthesis [i.e. (2)(3)(6)]. The numbers in parenthesis are found under Interpretations. Locate the Systolic Pressure numbers and select the range (i.e.92-110), which your systolic number coincides.

1. Locate the Diastolic Pressure numbers (i.e.10-50) and select the range, which your number coincides.
2. Draw a vertical line down from the Systolic box and then draw a horizontal line form the Diastolic box until it connects to the vertical line of the Systolic. Where the lines meet is in a Pulse box.
3. In the pulse box the range of numbers (i.e.50-70 etc.) that correlates with your pulse number is selected. Next to the Pulse number are numbers in parenthesis. The numbers in parenthesis are found below the table under Interpretation. These numbers explain the causes of your blood pressure numbers.

Blood Pressure Chart

The Blood Pressure Chart is used when the pulse rate is unknown. You must determine whether the systolic or diastolic numbers is the furthest out of normal range. It can be above normal (High) or below (Low). For Example;
Normal Blood Pressure is 120/80. You have a blood pressure of 160/90. Subtract systolic 120 (normal) -160 (your number)=40, then subtract diastolic 80 normal – 90 (your number)= 10
The systolic is the furthest from normal; it is a High Systolic read interpretation for High Systolic. Another Example normal 120/80, your Blood Pressure is 100/50. Subtract 120– 100= 10, then subtract diastolic 80 – 50= 30 the diastolic is the furthest out of range. It is a Low Diastolic

Systolic BP High	Diastolic BP High
• Minerals congesting tissue and bones • Electrolyte stress • Alkaline imbalance • Sympathetic stress • Heart and veins weakening due to waste • Kidney not diluting minerals fluids • Testosterone low level • Fertility and growth (posterior pituitary) problems	• Electrolyte stress • Minerals congesting tissue and bones • Alkaline imbalance • Heart, Kidney, arteries weakening due to waste • Kidneys not diluting minerals and fluids properly • Testosterone stress
Systolic BP Low	**Diastolic BP Low**
• Not able to absorb minerals • Acid imbalance • Poor heart muscle functions • Glandular and Kidney problems • Progesterone level low • Testosterone level low	• Not able to absorb minerals • Acid imbalance • Poor heart muscle functions • Kidneys inadequate • Testosterone level low • Problems with estrogen level • Kidney's glandular function poor

Normal (average)
120 Systolic,/ Male Principle,/ Active, Mental, / Conscious, / Willing Spirit, /Carbohydrates, /Acid
80 Diastolic, / Female Principle, / Rest, / Emotional, / Subconscious, / Forming Spirit, / Fats, / Alkaline
A Systolic or Diastolic number the farthest out of normal range indicates a type of holistic stressor

pH Test Procedure

pH means Potential of Hydrogen to be acid or alkaline. It is an electrical measure of the speed (acid), slowness (alkaline) and magnetism of a liquid. This test normal number is 6.4.

- Do not eat or drink water or any liquids for at least 1 hour before the test (pH and multistix).
- Put urine and/or saliva in appropriate glass or plastic container (i.e. bottle, cup etc.).

pH Test

- Dip one pH test paper or strip into the urine sample.
- Shake off excess fluid and immediately read results.
- The pH paper should change color.
- Look at the color of your test paper with the color on the pH color chart.
- Record the results.
- Follow the above procedure for the saliva test.

How to Read Symptoms

The further the number of the pH test results are above or below the normal number of 6.4 the more the symptoms associated with the result. For example 6.6 (alkaline tendency) and 6.2 (acid) is associated with two symptoms, while 5.0 is associated with three or more and 4.0 with all of the symptoms.

Urine pH
(Liver function, left lung, left side of body)

Alkaline 6.4-8.5
Liver stress   Menstruation
Weak enzymes   Energy loss
Gas, indigestion   Toxicity
Gallbladder stress   Hemorrhoids
Diarrhea (8.0) Poor oxygen assimilation

Acid 6.4- 4.0
Uterus/prostrate weak
Arthritis tendency
Arteriosclerosis tendency
Liver and colon toxic
Muscle weakness
Inadequate calcium and vitamin C use
Loss of energy, Rheumatism
Food moving too fast
Energy loss as heat

Saliva pH
(Liver biles, right lung, right side of body)

Alkaline 6.4-8.5
Weak hydrochloric acid
 Degenerative arthritic changes
Gallstones and/or heavy metal poisoning
Calcium deposits
Kidney Stress
Slow digestion
Emphysema

Acid 6.4-4.0
Liver Stress
 Cellular waste
Gas
Inadequate Vitamin C
Parasites
Constipation
Poor digestion, Energy loss

pH Disease Progression
The two pH numbers indicate the severity of the disease

Normal Number	Mild	Acute	Chronic	Degenerative
6.4 Urine	Alkaline (above 6.4)	Acid (below 6.4)	Alkaline	Acid
6.4 Saliva	Alkaline	Alkaline	Acid	Acid

$$\frac{2 \text{ (saliva pH)} + \text{urine pH}}{3} = \text{AVERAGE pH}$$

Multistix 10SG Test Procedure

- Do not eat or drink water or any liquids for at least 1 hour before test (pH and multistix).
- Put urine in appropriate glass or plastic container (i.e. bottle, cup, etc.).
  - Do not touch the test paper attached to the plastic multistix.
  - Hold the end of the plastic stick that does not have attached test paper of various colors.
  - Look at the urine's color and clarity/ transparency (free of particles) and observe the odor. Record your results.

- Dip the Multistix in the urine (lightly blot excess urine off the Multistix with unscented white tissue, white paper napkin, or white paper towel).
- The individual test paper squares attached are chemically treated to react to substances, which can change color.
- Wait approximate indicated specified time for each paper square to change color.
- Record normal (negative) and abnormal (positive) Findings.
- There are various degrees of abnormal findings, note which color on the Multistix matches the abnormal findings. After the stipulated time, match the color. Do not go back and read it again. It is too late.

Multistix Urinalysis 10SG (SG=Specific Gravity)
(Urine Reagent Strip Urinalysis)

Test	Normal	Abnormal Findings
Color	Straw to amber	colorless milky red yellow blue green orange brown black
Clarity	Clear	low turbidity high turbidity mucous
Odor	Odorless	sweet ammonia offensive medicinal
Glucose	Negative	100 250 500 1000 2000 mg/dl
Bilirubin	Negative	small (=1) moderate (+2) high (+3)
Ketones	Negative	trace (5) small (15) moderate (40) high (80) very high (160)
Sp. Gravity	1.015	1.005 1.010 Low | High 1.020 1.030
Blood	Negative	hemolyzed: trace moderate high non-hemolyzed: trace moderate high
pH	6.0	5.0 6.5 7.0 8.0 8.5
Protein	Negative	trace 30(+1) 100(=2) 300 (=3) over 2000(=4) mg/dl
Urobilinogen	0.2 1mg/dL	2 4 8mg/dl
Nitrate	Negative	positive
Leukocytes	Negative	positive

Interpretations

Color (Straw to amber)	Normal
Colorless	Large volume of water consumed. Consider diabetes, chronic kidney inflammation. Severe iron deficiency, alcohol ingestion.
Blue	Food dyes/ certain medications. Pseudomonas infection.
Orange	Concentrated urine from dehydration, fever, heatstroke, laxative, bile, drugs, carrots, carotene, riboflavin, food dyes.
Milky	Can indicate bacterial infection. UTI, vaginitis. Some food. RBC's.
Green	Food dyes/ certain medications. Pseudomonas infection.
Brown	Consider acute hepatitis or cirrohosis. Blood, bilirubin, urobilinogen, melanoma. Addison's disease, sulfonamides.
Yellow	High concentration of supplements. Dehydration.
Red	Beets/ berries. Consider blood from infection or menses, or lesion. Porphyria (port wine). Cascara, senna, aniline dyes.
Black	Possible liver/ kidney disease. Having problems breaking down amino acid (tyrosine), which builds muscle (protein). Kidney problems due to infection.
Transparency (clear)	Normal
Low turbidity (smoky, opaque, unclear)	Low infection or poor diet.
High turbidity	Stronger infection, vaginitis, UTI, Chylomicrons.
Mucous	Discharge due to infection of UTI or vaginal tracts.
Odor Very low odor	Normal
Sweet	Can indicate diabetes or liver blockage or obstruction. Sugars in urine.
Ammonia	Loss of alkaline buffers or bacterial growth.
Offensive	Toxicity, possible inflammatory response.
Medicinal	Medications altering the urine chemistry.
Glucose (sugar)	(75-125mg/dl) Indicates glucose spill in urine. Check for diabetic tendencies or kidney disease.
Bilirubin (reddish, yellow color of digestive liver fluid).	(0.4-0.8mg/dl) Red blood cells weak due to poor nutritional absorption. Possible liver inflammation, liber malfunction or blockage, cirrhosis, liver cancer. Look for jaundice. Congestive Heart Failure.
Ketone (fats turn to sugar)	Body unable to use carbohydrates, switches to using fats as energy. Possible diabetic acidosis. Kidney disease and kidney failure. Can be unable to use carbohydrates properly, high protein diet, or fasting. Can indicate below normal water consumption or dehydration. Kidneys can't eliminate ketones efficiently. >HGH,> cortisol,> glucagon. They mediate release of fatty acids.
SPECIFIC GRAVITY (weight of urine caused by minerals in it) Above 1.015	Healthy specific gravity <Minerals or extremely high intake of water or < kidney stress.
Below 1.015 Above 1.015	Dehydration or possibly too much salt. Diabetes, over active adrenal glands (i.e. stress)
Very below= Kidney damage	

Blood Hemolyzed (split red blood cells)	Allergies
Non-Hemolyed (unsplit red blood cells)	Can indicate kidney infection or inflammation. Possible urinary tract infection. Can indicate stress/ hypertension. If female patient, can be having a menstrual cycle do not test.
pH (Speed of digestion) 6.0 to 6.8 Normal	Normal urine pH.
Alkaline 7.0 to 8.0	Infection from urea- splitting microbes: proteus. Pseudomonas, slow digestion
Acid 5.0 to 6.0	Digestive & absorption problems, Consider stress/ hypertension, kidney problems, undigested food.
Protein	Can indicate kidney damage or inflammation. Possible allergies to food. Look for edema. Consider stress / hypertension.
Urobilinogen 0.2 – 1.0 mg/dl (Intestinal bacteria acting on bile from the liver)	Possibility of the liver losing ability to make digestive enzymes. Consider blockage in liver. Possible inflammation of liver (Hepatitis). Can indicate spleen dysfunction. Consider > red blood cells dying due to toxicity or infection. Check for all conditions that affect blood break- down.
Nitrates (Regulates blood pressure, dilates veins and arteries, help muscle spasms)	Indicates gram- negative bacterial growth proliferation in urinary tract. (E Coli, Enterobacteria, Pseudomonas).
Leukocytes (White blood cells are used for infections)	Possible infection. Possible signs that white blood cells are put together poorly because of inadequate diet. Can indicate infection of urinary tract. In female, may be contaminated by the skin or mucus from vaginal contact.

Pulse Pressure

Pulse Pressure is the difference between systolic and diastolic. The normal pulse difference range is 31-35.
P/R Quotient 4 and higher indicates sympathetic stress with similar symptoms as a high systolic.
P/R Quotient 3 and less indicates parasympathetic stress with similar symptoms as low diastolic.

Low Pulse	Disease State	High Pulse
27 - 30	= Acute =	46 - 50
24 - 26	= Chronic =	51 -54
23 or under	= Degenerative =	55 -57
	Failing Health =	58 or above

Pulse Pressure Low

Parasympathetic stress

Poor heart muscle function

Glandular and/ or kidney problems

Progesterone level low

Testosterone level low

Pulse pressure High

Sympathetic stress

Pineal insufficiency

Pulse/ Respiratory Quotient
Count the number of times the pulse beats per minute and count the number of breaths taken per minute.

P (pulse)   P = 80   80 divided by 20 = 4
RR (Respiratory Rate)   RR=20

Blood Test Interpretation

Glucose

This test is a measure of the metabolization (breakdown) of carbohydrates (i.e. vegetables, starches). Glucose is stored (storage form is glycogen) in the liver and other tissue. The sugar cell – Glycohemoglobin HBG A1C can indicate glucose metabolic problems. It can be used to predict diabetes up to a year of its onset.

Glucose is the primary source of energy. A level above 105 in someone who has fasted for 12 hours indicates a diabetic tendency. If the level is elevated in non- fasting setting, there is a risk for developing diabetes. This test can predict diabetes ten years or more before on develops strict definition of diabetes which is levels greater than 120.

Primary Causes of Increase: Diabetes, poor carbohydrate utilization, Syndrome X, Thiamine deficiency can cause an increase in glucose levels.

Secondary Causes of Increase: Cerebral lesions, uremia, pregnancy, intracranial pressure, Cushing's Disease, hyperthyroidism, chronic nephritis, infections, first 24 hours after a severe burn, pancreatitis, early hyperpituitarism.

Primary Causes of Decrease: Fasting Hypoglycemia, fasting can cause a low normal decrease, reactive hypoglycemia will cause a LDH decrease.

Secondary Causes of Decrease: Liver damage, pancreatic adenoma, Addison's Disease (adrenal insufficiency), starvation, late hypopituitarism, Carcinoma of islet tissue.

Clinical Adult Range	70 -115 mg/dL
Optimal Range	85 – 100mg /dL
Disease Range	<50 or >250 mg/L

Sodium

This element maintains water balance in your body. Sodium is in fluids of the body; lymph serum and lowest concentrations are in tissues. It helps maintain balance between calcium and potassium, which regulates normal heart action and the equilibrium of the body, regulates osmotic pressure in the cells and fluids, act as an ion balancer in tissue, helps buffer blood and combats excessive loss of water from the tissues. Do not confuse Sodium (salt) with table salt or sea salt because they are Sodium Chloride= salt and bleach combine. Bleach is a poison- do not eat it.

Clinical Adult Range	135 – 145
Optimal Adult Range	140 – 144
Disease Range	<125or >mmol/L

Primary Causes of Increase: Nephritis (kidney problems), eating salt, dehydration, hypercorticoadreanalism (increased adrenal function), water softeners, and inadequate water drinking,

Primary Causes of Decrease: Reduced kidney filtration, diarrhea, heart problems, Addison's disease, adrenal hypo-function, too much water intake, kidney failure, vomiting, weakness, loss of weight, disturbed digestion, and nerve damage

Potassium

This element is found primarily inside the cells of the body. It helps the regulation of osmotic pressure and acid alkaline balance, helps conduction of nerve signals, and muscle activity.

Clinical Range	3.5 – 5.0
Optimal Range	4.0 – 4.6
Disease Range	<3.0 or 6.0 mmol/L

Magnesium

An element found in soft tissue, arteries, nerve, teeth, heart and body fluids. It activates enzymes that help the reaction between phosphate ions and Adenosine Triphosphate (ATP energy). Helps synthesis of protein, neuromuscular contractions.

Clinical Adult Range	1.7 – 2.4
Optimal Adult Range	2.2 – 2.6
Disease Range	<1.2 mg/dl, <2.0 mg/dl (erythrocyte magnesium test or magnesium loading test is needed)

Primary Causes of Increase: Kidney problems, heart disease, and constant use of antacids.

Primary Causes of Deficiency: Anxiety, aching muscles, disorientation, low body temperature, easily angered, hyperactivity, insomnia, muscle tremors, nervousness, rapid pulse, sensitivity to noise and loud sounds, epilepsy, chronic diarrhea, disease related to absorption, and fibromyalgia (usually low CO2)

Chloride

This is a compound of chlorine (bleach). It is a salt of hydrochloric acid used in digestion. It is needed for the production of hydrochloric acid of the skin and stomach.
This electrolyte is controlled by the kidneys and can be affected by diet. It is involved in maintaining acid – base balance and helps regulate blood volume and artery pressure.

Clinical Adult Range	96 – 110mmol/L
Optimal Adult Range	100 – 106mmol/L
Disease Range	<90 or >115mmol/L Hypochondria (with <2.4 total globulin an<3.0serumphosphorus)

Primary Causes of Increase: Renal (kidney) problems, metabolic acidosis, excess water-crossing cell membrane.

Secondary Causes of Increase: Hyperventilation, anemia, prostate problems, salicylate poisoning, excess intake of salt(sodium chloride), dehydration.

Primary Causes of Decrease: Kidney problems, metabolic alkalosis, hypochondria (too little acid in stomach).

Secondary Causes of Decrease: Diabetes, pneumonia, intestinal obstruction, pyloric spasm, Adrenal hypo-function.

Blood Urea Nitrogen (BUN)

A waste product made from the breakdown of protein in the liver. When kidney function is impaired by disease, the excretion of urea can be decreased and BUN increased.

Clinical Adult Range	10 – 26mg/dL

Optimal Adult Range	13 – 18mg/dL
Disease Range	<5 or>mg/dl <mg/dL with low specific gravity can indicate posterior pituitary function dysfunction. >25mg/dL kidney disease if creatine is 1.1 or below can indicate dehydration, hypochlorhydria, pituitary problems

Primary Causes of Increase: Renal disease, gout, Boron Deficiency, synthetic diuretics, excessive protein intake, drugs, exercise, weak pancreas digestive enzymes, kidney disease, low fluid intake, heart disease, fever.

Secondary Causes of Increase: Metallic poisoning, pneumonia, ulcers, Addison's Disease, increased protein catabolism, dysbiosis, congestive heart failure, intestinal bleeding.

Primary Causes of Decrease: Pregnancy, liver damage, malabsorption, inadequate protein intake.

Secondary Causes of Increase: Acute liver destruction, dysbiosis, celiac sprue.

Creatinine

Creatinine is a by-product of protein breakdown. Its level is a reflection of the body's muscle mass. It is formed from creatine and provides energy for muscles. It is the by-product of muscle metabolism (not made from muscle). It is a non-protein part of blood and is an alkaline constituent.

Clinical Adult Range	0.7 – 1.5mg/dL
Optimal Adult Range	0.7 – 1.0mg/dL
Disease Range	>1.6mg/dL 2- 4mg/dL kidney disease nephritis 4 – 35mg/dL severe nephritis >1.2mg/dL in males over 40 years old, rule out hypertrophy

Primary Causes of Increase: Kidney problems, gout, and kidney damage.

Secondary Causes of Increase: Renal Hypertension, dehydration, uncontrolled diabetes, congestive heart failure, urinary tract infection.

Primary Causes of Decrease: Amyotonia congenital, inadequate protein intake, kidney damage, pregnancy, liver disease.

BUN/Creatinine Ratio

BUN/Creatinine Ratio: The BUN, urea in blood provides an estimate of kidney function, when compared (ratio) to Creatinine it reflects overall kidney health.

Clinical Adult Range	6 -10
Optimal Adult Range	10 -16
Disease Range	<5 or >30

Primary Causes of Increase: Kidney problems, poor circulation, congestive heart problems, urinary tract obstruction, and mild to severe kidney failure.

Secondary Causes of Ratio Increase: Catabolic states, prostatic hypertrophy, high protein diet, dehydration and shock.

Primary Causes of Decrease: Low protein/ high carbohydrate diet, pregnancy and over hydration.

Uric Acid

Uric acid is the end product of purine metabolism. It is formed from purine bases derived from nucleoproteins. It is a constituent of urinary and kidney stones

Clinical Female Range	2.4 – 6.0mg/dL
Clinical Male Range	3.4 – 7.0mg/dL
Optimal Female Range	3.0 – 5.5mg/dL
Optimal Male Range	3.5 – 5.9mg/dL
Disease Range	<2mg/dL or >9.0mg/dL

Primary Causes of Increase: Gout, infection, arteriosclerosis, kidney problems, exercise, arthritis, heart disease, pneumonia, glycogen storage disease, acute articular rheumatism.

Secondary Causes of Increase: Intestinal obstruction, malignant tumors, metallic poisoning (mercury, lead), polycythemia, diuretic drugs, Lesch-Nyhan (mental retardation), aspirin, theophylline.

Primary Causes of Decrease: Chronic B12 or folate anemia, high protein diet, pregnancy, piperazine (worm medicine), anticoagulant drugs (i.e. coumarin), high amounts of ascorbic acid, nephritis, chlorosis, lead poisoning, liver damage, protein, molybdenum deficiency (If the uric acid is low with normal MCV and MCH), overly acid kidney.

Phosphorus

Phosphorus is closely associated with calcium in bone development. Most of the phosphate is found in the bones. Phosphorus levels in the blood are important for muscle and nerve function. However, the blood must be drawn carefully as improper handling may falsely increase the reading.

Clinical Adult Range	2.5 – 4.5
Optimal Adult Range	3.2 – 3.9
Disease Range	<2.0mgldL or >5.0mg/dL <3.0mg/dL and >3.0mg/dL or <2.4mg/dL total serum globulin consider hypochlorhydria

Primary Causes of Increase: Parathyroid dysfunction, kidney dysfunction, excessive phosphoric acid in soft drinks, broken bones (fractures) can cause an increase, normal bone growth in children can increase phosphorus.

Secondary Causes of Increase: Bone tumors, edema, ovarian hyper-function, diabetes, and excess intake of vitamin D.

Primary Causes of Decrease: Parathyroid Hyper-function, osteomalacia, rickets, malnutrition, muscle weakness, vitamin D deficiency.

Secondary Causes of Increase: Diabetes, liver dysfunction, protein malnutrition, neurofibromatosis, myxedema, starvation, a diet high in concentrated sweeteners (sugars).

Calcium

Calcium is the most abundant mineral in the body. It is involved in acid-alkaline balance, permeability of membranes, in activating enzymes, bone metabolism, protein absorption, fat transfer, muscular contraction, lactation, transmission of nerve impulses, blood clotting, and heart function. It's used in hormonal activity,

Vitamin D levels, CO2 levels and many drugs. The hormone from four tiny glands (parathyroid) within the thyroid (but distinctly different from the thyroid) controls the body's calcium with calcitonin hormone. Circadian cycle abnormality can cause calcium levels to be either above or below normal.

Clinical Adult Range	8.5 – 10.8
Optimal Adult Range	9.7 – 10.1
Disease Range	<7.0mg/dL or >12.0mg/dL

Primary Causes of Increase: Hyperparathyroidism, excess protein causes increase, while decrease protein decreases calcium.

Secondary Causes of Increase: Tumor of the thyroid, antacids, hypervitaminosis (excess Vitamin D), multiple myeloma, neurofibromatosis, osteoporosis, ovarian hypo- function, adrenal hypo-function.

Primary Causes of Decrease: Hypoparathyroidism, pregnancy, hypochlorhydria, kidney dysfunction, weak bones.

Secondary Causes of Decrease: Vitamin D deficiency, diarrhea, celiac disease, protein malnutrition, chemical/heavy metal toxicity, HPA – axis dysfunction, heart problems, hyperirritability, dental caries, decreased albumin will give decreased calcium, poor fat intestinal absorption, and pancreatic enzyme deficiency may be suspected with low levels of calcium, triglycerides, increased levels of LDH.

Albumin

It is made in the liver and is the most abundant plasma in the blood, an antioxidant, protects tissues from free radicals, binds waste products, toxins and dangerous drugs that can damage the body, a major buffer in the body, regulates the content of water tissues, helps transport vitamins, minerals and hormones.

Clinical Adult Range	3.0 – 5.5
Optimal Adult Range	4.0 – 4.4
Disease Range	<4.0g/dL

Primary Causes of Increase: Dehydration, high albumin ratio with high calcium indicates visceral protein loss or malnutrition.

Secondary Causes of Increase: Thyroid and adrenal hypo function.

Primary Causes of Decrease: Liver decreases, decreased albumin with decreases serum phosphorus indicate an inflamed digestive system.

Secondary Causes of Decrease: Acute nephritis, malnutrition, acute cholecystitis (gall bladder), multiple sclerosis, vitamin B-12 or folic acid, anemia, albumin 3.5 or below with 1500 or less lymphocyte count indicates disease.

Globulin

Globulin is the main plasma protein in blood. Provides nutrition for tissues. There are four different globulins; the largest in number are the gamma globulins, which carry the immune cells that fight disease. Globulins have many diverse functions such as, the carrier of some hormones, lipids, metals, and antibodies. Albumin and globulins maintain osmotic pressure of the blood that keeps a balance between the percentage of chemicals and plasma.

Clinical Adult Range	2.0 – 4.0

Optimal Range	2.8 – 3.5
Disease Range	<2.0g/dL or > 3.5g/100ml

Albumins and Globulin Ratio

They are an important indicator of disease states. Usually there is almost twice as much albumin as there are globulins and when the amount is divided by the amount of globulins, the normal A/G ratio is two to one (2:1).

Clinical Adult Range	1.1 – 2.5
Optimal Adult Range	1.2 – 1.5
Disease Range	<1.0

Primary Causes of Increase: Elevated A/G ratio, elevated protein and cholesterol may indicate too high protein consumption.

Primary Causes of Decrease: Kidney disease, liver disease, cirrhosis, burns, multiple myeloma, ulcerative colitis.

Alkaline Phosphatase

Alkaline phosphatase is an enzyme that is found in all body tissue. The most important sites are bone, liver, bile ducts and the intestines. Different forms of this enzyme are produced in the liver, bone cells, and intestines. It is usually high in children under 18 years old and high with bone fractures.

Clinical Adult Range	30 – 115
Optimal Adult Range	60 – 80
Disease Range	<30U/L or > Laboratory Range

Primary Causes of Increase: Primary bone lesion, invasive liver lesion, biliary (liver) duct obstruction, osteomalacia, Paget's Disease, rheumatoid arthritis, cancerous and noncancerous bone disease, drugs, birth control pills/patches, antiarthritics, tranquilizers, gallbladder problems, male hormonal drugs.

Secondary Causes of Increase: Excess consumption of Vitamin D, Rickets, Cirrhosis of liver, adrenal hyper-function, shingles, thyroid problems, Hodgkin's Disease, osteogenic sarcoma, alcoholism, multiple mycelia, jaundice, cholesterol drugs.

Primary Causes of Decrease: Anemia, too little Vitamin C, hypothyroidism, celiac disease, poor nutrition.

Secondary Causes of Decrease: Adrenal hypo-function, Vitamin C deficiency, progesterone deficiency, malnutrition, Zinc deficiency.

SGPT/ALT & SGOT/AST

(Serum Glutamic Pyruvic Transaminase SGPT, Alanine Amino Transferase ALT and Serum Glutamic Oxalacetic Transaminase SGOT, Aspartate Amino Transferase AST)

Transaminases (SGTP/ALT)&(SGOT/AST) are enzymes that are primarily found in the liver. SGPT values are higher than SGOT in hepatitis and liver obstruction. Hepatitis can raise these levels. SGOT values are higher then SGPT in jaundice, cirrhosis and liver cancer. Low levels of SGPT and SGOT can indicate deficient of Vitamin B6. These enzymes are released into the blood when there is heart muscle damage. They are extra large in size bacteria (Rickettsial) infection, liver cell destruction or hepatitis. There are very small amounts of these enzymes in the brain, kidney, lungs, and other body tissues.

Clinical Adult Range	0 – 41
Optimal Adult Range	18 – 26
Disease Range	>100 U/L

SGOST/AST: Problems with heart, skeletal muscles, brain, liver, kidneys.

Primary Causes of SGOT/ASTL Increase: Myocardial infarction, pulmonary embolism, congestive heart failure, myocarditis, hepatitis, liver cirrhosis, liver disease, pancreatitis.

Secondary Causes of SGOT/AST: Liver neoplasm
Nutritional Note: Low levels of SGOT/ AST and SGPT/ALT can indicate a Vitamin B-6 deficiency.
SGPT/ALT: Indicates problems with the liver, kidneys, heart, skeletal muscles.

Primary Causes of SGPT/ALT Increase: Acute hepatitis, cirrhosis of liver, mononucleosis, heart problems.

Secondary common Causes of SGPT/ALT Increase: Pancreatitis, biliary dysfunction, diabetes.

GGT (Gamma-Glutamyl Transerase)

GGT: An enzyme that is associated with glutathione, metabolism and helping the amino acids get into cells. When GGT values are five times greater than clinical range suspect pancreatitis. If GGT is higher than 150 u/L with serum bilirubin over 2.8mg/dL suspect blocked liver biliary with biliary dysfunction suspect food allergy/sensitivity.

Clinical Adult Range	0 - 55U/L
Optimal Adult Range	10 – 30U/L
Disease Range	>90U/L

Primary Causes of Increase: Biliary obstruction, alcoholism, liver disease, cholangitis/cholecystitis (bile duct and gall bladder inflammation), excess magnesium.
Clinical Note: If GGT is greater than 15 U/L with serum bilirubin of over 2.8 mg/dL, strongly suspect biliary obstruction. Seek immediate medical attention.

Secondary common Causes of Increase: Brucellosis, hepatitis, mononucleosis, bacterial and viral infection, malignancy, congestive heart failure biliary.
Primary Causes of Decrease: Vitamin B-6 deficiency.

LDH (Lactate Dehydroenase)

LDH is an enzyme found in the blood, organs and all tissues. When tissue and cells are diseased or damaged, the enzyme is released into the blood serum. LDH helps in carbohydrate metabolism LDH helps carbohydrates metabolism. There are five forms (isoenzymes) in varying amounts in muscle, organs, the heart and liver. A high level in the blood can result from a number of different diseases such as hepatitis, anemia etc. Slightly elevated LDH levels in the blood are common and usually do not indicate disease. The most common sources of LDH are the heart, liver, muscles, and red blood cells.

Clinical Adult Range	60 -225 U/L
Optimal Adult Range	140 – 220 U/L
Disease Range	>250U/L

Primary Causes of Increase: Liver/biliary dysfunction, pulmonary embolism, myocardial infarction, tissue inflammation, tissue destruction, hepatitis, malignancy anywhere in the body, several types of anemia's (folic acid, Vitamin B12 etc.), infectious mononucleosis, heart disease, low thyroid function, birth control drugs.

Primary Causes of Decrease: After x-ray, reactive hypoglycemia (Check glucose).

Total Protein

Total Protein is a measurement of the total amount of protein in your blood. Total protein is the combination of albumin and total globulin. A low or high total protein does not indicate a specific disease. It indicates that additional tests may be required to determine if there is a problem. When protein and calcium are found to be on the low part of the optimal range suspect poor protein absorption.

Clinical Adult Range	6.0 – 8.5 5g/dL
Optimal Adult Range	7.1 – 7.6g/dL
Disease Range	<5.9g/dL or >8.5g/dL

Primary Causes of Increase: Dehydration, "early" carcinoma, multiple myeloma (should be correlated with serum protein electrophoresis).

Secondary Causes of Increase: Malignancy, diabetes, rheumatoid arthritis.

Primary Causes of Decrease: Protein malnutrition, digestive inflammation (colitis, gastritis), decrease protein, cholesterol and SGPT can indicate fatty liver congestion.

Secondary Causes of Decrease: Hypothyroidism, leukemia, adrenal hyper-function, congestive heart failure.

Iron

Iron is used to make hemoglobin and to transfer oxygen to the muscle. The test is a measure of the total iron-binding capacity. It reflects the iron's availability to pick up oxygen from the lungs and deliver it to the tissue. Iron has a particular effect on adults and brain cells in children. Females that have menstrual cycles should consider a Ferritin test if Iron is low.

Clinical Adult Range	40 – 150ug/ml
Optimal Adult Range	50 -100ug/ml
Disease Range	<25ug/ml or >200ug/ml

Primary Causes of Increase: Hemochromomatosis, liver dysfunction, iron therapy, pernicious and hemolytic anemia, after surgery, intrinsic factor deficiency when hemocrit (HCT) decrease and iron increase.
Secondary Causes of Increase: Cooking with iron utensils.

Primary Causes of Decrease: Pruritis(itching skin) pathologic bleeding (especially in geriatric population) iron deficiency anemia, infections, steroid, birth control drugs, inherited intestinal iron absorption disease.

Secondary Causes of Decrease: Chronic infection, kidney and liver problems, cancer.

Ferritin

Ferritin is a measurement of the blood and body iron, the serum iron-binding capacity (Transferrin) is the specific amount of iron that can be carried in plasma; and the ferritin level or the amount of iron stored in the body. It is stored primarily in the bone marrow. This test is considered the main test for documenting iron deficiency anemia. Arteriosclerosis has been associated with high iron levels. Iron overload has has been associated with dementia, stroke, diabetes, infections and cirrhosis.

Clinical Male Adult Range	33 – 23ng/mL
Clinical Female Adult Range	(before menopause) 11 122ng/mL
Clinical Female Adult Range	(after menopause) 12 – 263ng/mL

Optimal Male Adult Range	20 – 200ng/mL
Optimal Female Adult Range	(before menopause) 10 –110ng/mL
Optimal Female Adult Range	(after menopause) 20 – 200ng/mL
Disease Range	<8ng/mL or >500ng/mL

Primary Causes of Increase: Iron overload, hemochromatosis, infections, chronic kidney disease.

Secondary Causes of Increase: Inflammation, liver disease, rheumatoid arthritis.

Primary Causes of Decrease: Iron deficiency anemia. Levels below 25ng/mL indicate a need for iron supplement.

Secondary Causes of Decrease: Free radical pathology.

Triglycerides

Triglycerides are fats used for metabolism, energy, and fuel by the body. The test measures primarily three major lipids (fats) in the blood serum, phospholipids, triglycerides and cholesterol (not a true fat). Triglycerides have the highest amount by weight of all fats. It is in foods and made by the liver.

Clinical Adult Range	50 – 150mg/dL
Optimal Adult Range	70 – 110mg/dL
Disease Range	<35mg/dL or >350mg/dL

Primary Causes of Increase: Hyperlipidism, diabetes, alcoholism, alcohol and carbohydrates more than fatty foods cause high levels of triglycerides.
Secondary Causes of Increase: Hypothyroidism, early stages of fatty liver, malnutrition, malabsorption.

Primary Causes of Decrease: Synthetic Chemicals/Heavy metal overload, liver dysfunction, hyper thyroid function

Cholesterol

Cholesterol is a group of fats vital to cell membranes, nerve fiber, bile salts, and a necessary precursor for the sex hormones. Cholesterol is an alcohol and not a true fat but still is medically categorized as a fat. The liver makes about 80% of the cholesterol that the body needs.

Clinical Adult Range	120 – 200 mg/dL
Optimal Adult Range	150 – 180mg/dL
Disease Range	<50mg/dL or >400mg/dL

Primary Causes of Increase: Early stages of diabetes, fatty liver, arteriosclerosis, hypothyroidism, a diet high in cooked fats/ oils ,carbohydrates, concentrated sweeteners and processed sugars.

Secondary Causes of Increase: Biliary obstruction, multiple sclerosis, pregnancy.

Primary Causes of Decrease: Liver dysfunction, Synthetic Chemicals, Heavy metal overload, hyperthyroidism, viral hepatitis, free radical pathology, low raw fat diet, malabsorption, anemia, carbohydrate sensitivity.

LDL Cholesterol (Low Density Lipoproteins)

LDL Cholesterol is Lipoproteins, which are substances that transport cholesterol in the blood. LDL transport cholesterol from the liver to the cells that need it. LDL is the cholesterol rich remnants of the lipid transport vehicle VLDL (very low density lipoproteins). If LDL becomes oxidized (rust, oxygen combines with a substances and is a harmful free radical) and attaches to artery walls this will lead to inflammation of arteries, resulting in hardening of the arteries and decreases blood flow.

Clinical Adult Range	<130mg/dL
Optimal Adult Range	<120ng/dL
Disease Range	>180mg/dL

Primary Causes of Increase: Arteriosclerosis, diabetes, Syndrome X.

HDL (High Density Lipoprotein)

HDL transports excess cholesterol from the cells and takes it back to the liver, where it is broken down and reprocessed or excreted from the body. HDL is the cholesterol carried by the alpha lipoproteins. A high level of HDL is an indication of a healthy metabolic system if there is no sign of liver disease or intoxication. HDL offers protection against chronic heart disease because HDL inhibits cellular uptake of LDL.

Clinical Adult Males Range	>50mg/dL
Clinical Adult Female Range	>55mg/dL
Optimal Adult Male Range	>55mg/dL
Optimal Adult Female Range	>60mg/dL
Disease Range	<35mg/dL

Primary Causes of Decrease: Arteriosclerosis, diabetes, Syndrome X, processed saturated fats, animal products, refined carbohydrates.

Secondary Causes of Decrease: Cigarette smoking, steroids, beta-blockers.

Cholesterol/ HDL Ratio

Cholesterol/HDL Ratio affects how cholesterol is transported into the arteries and tissues. A high ratio puts you at risk of dying from a heart attack. The ratio indicates cardiovascular health. A ratio <4.0 is considered adequate. A ratio <3.1 is ideal.

CO2 (Carbon Dioxide)

The CO2 level is related to the exchange of carbon dioxide for oxygen in the lungs. It is part of the body's buffering system. Carbon dioxide levels indicate pH or acid/alkaline balance. Carbon dioxide and water are the result of oxygen metabolic processes. CO2 is eliminated through the lungs. A small amount of CO2 is changed into bicarbonates (buffer, reduces acidity) and is excreted in the urine. Respiratory problems, acidosis, alkalosis and metabolic disorders change CO2 levels in the tissues.

Clinical Adult Range	24 -32 mmol/ L
Optimal Adult Range	26 – 30mmol/ L
Disease Range	<18mmol/L or >38mmol/L

Primary Causes of Increase: Alkalosis, hypochlorhydria, diuretic drugs, steroid hormones, antacids.

Secondary Causes of Increase: Acute vomiting, fever, adrenal hyper function, emphysema (respiratory distress), asthma, intestinal obstruction, hyperactivity, starvation.

Primary Causes of Decrease: Acidosis, aspirin, liver disease, kidney problems.

Secondary Causes of Decrease: Diabetes, sleep apnea, severe diarrhea, hyperventilation, thiamine deficiency.

White Blood Cell (WBC)

The WBC's kill bacteria. An increase indicates infection. WBC's are round with edges occasionally broken, nucleated, granular, and grayish in color and sometimes clumped. WBC's act as scavengers to fight infection. They constantly change shape (pseudopodia), which allows them to move and penetrate tissue, and then return to the blood stream. There are two types: granulocytes (grains in cells) and agranulocytes (does not have grains). When destroyed by bacteria, the dead leukocytes form pus. The relative increase or decrease of a WBC is indicated by adding the suffix "philia" for increase or the suffix "penia" for decrease (ex. neutrophilia, neutropenia). An increase in the total WBC with a lymphocyte count below 20 and serum albumin below 4.0 is associated with the development of neoplasm tumors. The WBC count measures the total number of white blood cells in a given volume of blood and the percentage of each type (differential count).

Clinical Adult Range	24 – 32mmol/l
Optimal Adult Range	26 – 30mmol/L
Disease Range	<18mmol/L or >38mmol/L

Primary Causes of Increase: Active infections, leukemia, childhood diseases (measles, mumps, chickenpox, rubella, etc.)

Secondary Causes of Increase: Asthma, emphysema, adrenal dysfunction, intestinal parasites, severe emotional stress.

Primary Causes of Decrease: Chronic viral or bacterial infectious, lupus (SLE), Vitamin B12, B6 and folic acid deficiencies.

Secondary Causes of Decrease: Hepatitis, immune dysfunction, synthetic chemical/heavy metal toxicity.

Neutrophils

Neutrophils are type of WBC that is granulated and a phagocyte (eats bacteria). It indicates an acute infection. They tend to increase with chronic bacterial infection and decrease with chronic viral infection.

Clinical Adult Range	35 – 65 percent of total WBC
Optimal Adult Range	40 – 60 percent of total WBC
Disease Range	<30 percent of total WBC or >80 percent of total WBC

Primary Causes of Increase: See WBC
Primary Causes of Decrease: See WBC

Monocytes

Monocytes are a type of WBC that does not have grains in the cell (agranulocyte). It is a lymphocyte. They are formed from cells lining the capillaries in various organs and probably in the spleen and bone marrow. They are elevated in bacterial infections, protozoal infections.

Clinical Adult Range	0- 10 percent of total WBC
Optimal Adult Range	<7 percent of total WBC
Disease Range	>15 percent of total WBC

Primary Causes of Increase: Bacterial infections, parasitic infections, prostate disease, female reproduction diseases increase basophils (>1.0) and increase eosinophils (>3.0), indicate intestinal parasites.

Primary Causes of Decrease: High doses of corticosteroids will depress monocytes.

Lymphocytes

Lymphocytes are a type of leukocyte (WBC) that attacks bacteria and foreign particles. It is not a phagocyte. B-lymphocytes produce antibodies and T-lymphocytes produce antigens, which gives cellular immunity. It is elevated in acute and chronic infections. Decreased in viral infection and immune deficiency.

Clinical Adult Range	20 – 40 percent of total WBC
Optimal Adult Range	2 – 40 percent of total WBC
Disease Range	<20 percent of total WBC or >55 percent of total WBC

Primary Causes of Increase: Chronic viral or bacterial infection, childhood diseases (measles, mumps, chicken-pox, rubella, etc.), HIV, hepatitis, when increased to a point that equals or exceeds the neutrophil level, it can indicate viral infection.

Secondary Causes of Increase: Synthetic Chemical/ heavy metal toxicity.
Primary Causes of Decrease: Active infections.

Eosinophils

Eosinophils are a type of leukocyte (WBC), which is a corpuscle. It has grains (granules) in the cell (granulocytes). It eats small particles and bacteria (phagocyte). It is formed in the bone marrow. It is elevated in allergic conditions, skin diseases, parasitic diseases, respiratory problems, etc.

Clinical Adult Range	0 – 2 percent of total WBC
Optimal Adult Range	0 – 1 percent of total WBC
Disease Range	<5 percent of total WBC

Primary Causes of Increase: Inflammation, childhood diseases (measles, mumps, chicken-pox, rubella, etc.) acute trauma and parasites.
Secondary Causes of Increase: Chemical/heavy metal toxicity

Red Blood Cells (RBC)

RBC's transport oxygen, nutrients, and waste products such as carbon dioxide. RBC's regulate the acid-alkaline balance of the blood. When RBC's are broken down and disintegrated (decomposed) the hemoglobin (made of iron and protein) is removed from the blood (by the liver, spleen etc.). The globin (protein) is broken down into amino acids and reused, iron (hematin) is removed and stored in the liver and spleen and the other pigments are changed into bilirubin. RBC's are also made in the spleen. RBC's reveal the oxygen carrying ability of the blood. The iron carries oxygen from the lungs to the tissues.

Clinical Adult Male Range	4.60 – 6.0 million cu/mm
Clinical Adult Female Range	3.90 – 5.50 million cu/mm
Optimal Adult Male Range	4.20 – 4.90 million cu/mm
Optimal Adult Range	3.90 – 4.50 million cu/mm
Disease Range for Men	<3.90 or >6.00 million cu/mm
Disease Range for Women	<3.50 or >5.00 million cu/mm

Primary Causes of Increase: Polycythemia, dehydration, respiratory distress (asthma, emphysema).
Secondary Causes of Increase: Acute poisoning, cystic fibrosis, adrenal hyper function.
Primary Causes of Decrease: Iron deficiency anemia, internal bleeding, Vitamin B12, Vitamin B6 and/or folic acid deficiency.

Secondary Causes of Decrease: Excessive exercise, salicylate toxicity, lead poisoning.

Hemoglobin

Hemoglobin is a conjugated protein made of iron (hematin) and a simple protein (globin). It combines with oxygen and forms a loose unstable compound called oxyhemoglobin. Hemoglobin transports oxygen into the blood and carbon dioxide out of the blood. It is composed of "globin", a group of amino acids that form a protein and "heme", which contains iron. It is an important determinant of anemia (decreased hemoglobin) or poor diet/nutrition or malabsorption. In the tissue, oxygen is low and carbon dioxide is high, the hemoglobin gets rid of its oxygen in exchange for carbon dioxide.

Clinical Adult Male Range	13.5 – 18.0g/dL
Clinical Adult Female Range	12.5 – 16.0g /dL
Optimal Adult Male Range	14.0 – 15.0g/dL
Optimal Adult Female Range	13.5 – 14.5g/dL
Disease Range	<10.0 or >17g/dL

PRIMARY CAUSE OF INCREASE: Polycythemia, dehydration, emphysema, asthma, B12, thiamine and/or folic acid deficiency.
SECONDARY CAUSE OF INCREASE: Anemia, internal bleeding, digestive inflammation, overhydration.

Hematocrit

Hematocrit is the measurement of the percentage of red blood cells in the total volume. The test measures the viscosity (thinness and thickness) of the blood as well as the amount of fluid in the blood.

Clinical Adult Male Range	40.0 – 52.0 percent
Clinical Adult Female Range	36.0 – 47.0 percent
Optimal Adult Male Range	40.0 – 48.0 percent
Optimal Adult Female Range	37.0 – 44.0 percent
Disease Range	<32.0 or >55 percent

Primary Causes of Increase: Same as hemoglobin.
Primary Causes of Decrease: Same as hemoglobin; indicate iron anemia if serum iron hemoglobin and hematocrit are low; Vitamin B12 and folic acid anemia. It there is low hematocrit with high MCH, MCV, and iron; Vitamin B6 anemia if MCT, hematocrit, and iron are low, look for low SGOT.

Reticulocyte Count

Reticulocytes are immature red blood cells. The reticulocyte count is a measurement of the productions of erythrocytes (RBC). The count increases when bone marrow is stimulated. Bodily processes (kidney disease, infection) can limit red blood cell production and limit reticulocyte numbers. This test can confirm chronic microscopic bleeding.

Clinical Adult Range	0.5 – 1.5 percent
Optimal Adult Range	Same as clinical range
Disease Range	>2.0 percent

Primary Causes of Increase: Internal Bleeding.

Primary Causes of Decrease: Vitamin B12, B-6 and folic acid anemia.

Platelets (Thrombocytes)

Platelets are essential for the clotting of the blood. They are made in the marrow.

Clinical Adult Range	150,000 – 450,000cu.mm
Optimal Adult Range	200,000 – 300,000cu.mm
Disease Range	<50,000 or >600,000cu.mm

Primary Causes of Increase: Polycythemia, inflammatory arthritis, several types of anemia, arteriosclerosis, acute blood loss.
Primary Causes of Decrease: Leukemia, liver dysfunction, selenium, B12, Iron and/or folic acid deficiency.

Secondary Causes of Decrease: Synthetic chemical/Heavy metal toxicity

MCV (Mean Corpuscular Volume)

MCV is a ratio of the hematocrit to the red blood cell count. The MCV indicates the volume occupied by the average red blood cell.

Clinical Adult Range	81.0 – 99.0cu.microns
Optimal Adult Range	82.0 - 89.9cu.microns
Disease Range	<78.0 or >95.0cu.microns

Primary Causes of Increase: Vitamin B12/folic acid anemia.
Primary Causes of Decrease: Iron anemia, internal bleeding.

MCH (Mean Corpuscular Hemoglobin)

MCH is a ratio of the hemoglobin to the red blood cell count. The MCV indicates the volume occupied by the average red blood cell.

Clinical Adult Range	26.0 – 33.0 micro-micro grams
Optimal Adult Range	27.0 – 31.9 micro-micro grams
Disease Range	<24.0 or >34.0 micro-micro grams

Primary Causes of Increase: Vitamin B12/folic acid anemia.
Primary Causes of Decrease: Iron anemia, Internal bleeding.

Thyroid Function

The thyroid gland function tests are the measurement of the amounts of Triiodiothyronine (T3) and Thyroxin (T4), which make the thyroid hormone. The hormones are made by the thyroid gland from the amino acid tyrosine and the element iodine. T3 is four times stronger than T4. If T3 is believed to be a "true" thyroid hormone and T4 is believe to be a precursor of T3.

Thyroid hormones are necessary for the making of other hormones (i.e. insulin, glucagon, sex hormones), growth and development, and control of oxygen metabolism and the speed of Food metabolism and use of energy. The thyroid gland is located in the base of the neck on both sides of the lower part of the larynx and upper part of the trachea. The axillary (underarm) temperature is usually lower than 97.8F in hypothyroidism. Axillary temperature can be low with adrenal stress, protein malnutrition, thiamine deficiency and diets low in unprocessed fatty acids. Thyroid problems can be indicated with headaches that start in the morning and lessen during the day, difficulty losing weight, dry or scaly skin, lack of motivation, impaired hearing, low blood pressure, ringing in the ears, constipation, difficulty working under stress, fatigue and sensitivity to cold.

T3 (Tri-Iodthyronine)

T3 is a thyroid hormone. The Majority of it is made from the peripheral conversion of thyroxin (t4).

| Clinical Adult Range | 22 – 33 percent |
| Optimal Adult Range | 26 -30 percent |

Primary Causes of T3 Increase: Hyperthyroidism
Primary Causes of T3 Decrease: Hypothyroidism
T4 is the major hormone secreted by the thyroid gland.

| Clinical Adult Range | 4.0 -12.mcg/dL |
| Optimal Adult Range | 7.0 – 8.5mcg/dL |

Primary Causes of T4 Increase: Hyperthyroidism
Primary Causes of T4 Decrease: Hypothyroidism, anterior pituitary hypofunction.

T7 (FTI-Free Thyroxine Index)

T7 is an estimate, calculated from T4 and T3 uptake.

| Clinical Adult Range | 4.0 – 12.0mcg/dL |
| Optimal Adult Range | 7.0 – 8.5mcg/dL |

Primary Causes of T7 Increase: See T3 uptake.

Primary Causes of T3 Decrease: See T3 uptake.

T3 Uptake

T3 uptake measures the unsaturated binding sites on the thyroid binding proteins.

Clinical Adult Range	22 – 36 percent
Optimal Adult Range	27 – 37 percent
Disease Range	<20 percent of uptake or > 39 percent of uptake

Primary Causes of T3 UPTAKE Increase: Thyroid hyperfunction.
Secondary Causes of T3 UPTALE Increase: Kidney dysfunction, salicylates toxicity and protein malnutrition.
Primary Causes of Decrease: Thyroid hypo-function.

TSH (Thyroid Stimulating Hormone)

TSH is used to validate or dismiss suspected hypothyroidism when T3, T4, T7 are in a normal range and clinical signs suggest hypothyroidism.

Clinical Adult Range	0.4 – 4mlU/L
Optimal Adult Range	2.0 – 4.0mlU/L
Red Flag Range	<0.3mlU/L or >10.0mlU/L

Primary Causes of TSH Increase: Thyroid hypofunction.

Secondary Causes of TSH **Increase**: Liver dysfunction.

Primary Causes of TSH **Decrease**: Thyroid hyper-function, anterior hypo-function.

ESR (Erythrocyte Sedimentation Rate)

ESR (Erythrocyte Sedimentation Rate) is a measure of how red blood cells cling together, fall and settle. The cells group together and then form sediment. It can document organic disease with vague symptoms.

Clinical Adult Male <50Range	0 – 15mm/hour
Clinical Adult Male <40 Range	0 – 20mm/hour
Clinical Adult Male <50 Range	0 – 25mm/hour
Clinical Adult Female >50Range	0 – 30mm/hour
Clinical Adult Male Range	<5mm/hour
Optimal Adult Female Range	<10mm/hour
Disease Range	>45mm/hour

Test (Nutrients, Biochemical Actions)

Breathe – Hold Test

This test indicates acid/alkaline imbalances. It should not be taken if there are cardiovascular, pulmonary, or respiratory tract infections. In an <u>acid</u> condition oxygen has a decreased uptake and transport, which causes a decreased breath holding time. In an <u>alkaline</u> condition oxygen has an increased uptake and transport and a compensatory suppression of the respiratory center, which results in an increased ability to hold the breath.

Directions
This test measures the length of time breath is held after a deep breath. It is best to have a family member or friend do the timing. The person must be seated and should take a deep breathe and hold it as long as possible. A watch that can indicate seconds must be used to time the breath holding. When a person finishes taking in a deep breath and holds their breath as long as they can and then exhale, the seconds the breath was held should be recorded.

Results
Normal: 40 – 65 seconds

Increased Breath-Hold Time

Clinical Implications	Causes
Metabolic Alkalosis Respiratory Alkalosis	Alkalosis causes an increased oxygen uptake and transport. Resulting in an increased ability to hold ones breath.

Decreased Breath-Hold Time

Clinical Implications	Causes
Metabolic Acidosis Respiratory Acidosis	In Acidosis a decreased transport and uptake of oxygen by the body causes a decreased breath holding time.
Anemia	Decreased oxygen-carrying capacity of red blood cells caused by anemia results in decreased breath hold time.
Other Causes include:	Antioxidant deficiency, emotional stress, anxiety.

Pulse Challenge Food Sensitivity Testing

The taste buds, (papillae), on the tongue sense the organic and non-organic chemicals in foods and transmits sensory information to the digestive system, central nervous system and brain. It is best to test organic non-GNO foods. People assume that they are allergic to a particular food because the food allergy list was created using commercial synthetic chemicalized non-organic foods. Therefore, the allergy test should be done with organic non-GMO foods and then on the chemicalized food. If the organic food is intolerant or the synthetic chemical in and on the non-organic food is intolerant, then the sympathetic nervous system reacts by increasing blood flow (increase pulse and heart beat) to fight the intolerant substance. Acute Phase Response is stimulated making the person feel sick and sending white blood cells to fight the intolerant substance. The pulse increases when foods are consumed that cannot be tolerated or increases sensitivity or have an allergic response. A sympathetic (Fight/Flight) stress reaction to foods causes the pulse to increase and heart to beat faster. The pulse test can help eliminate symptoms and conditions by identifying and eliminating food from the diet, which are intolerant. The advantage of the pulse test is that you can do the evaluation of intolerant foods at home. As health recovery proceeds, some foods to which you are sensitive to can be reintroduced in moderation using the pulse to monitor their acceptability.

- ❖ This test helps you find out the foods you are intolerant to.
- ❖ This test helps you find environment toxins you are sensitive to.

Directions
Pulse Challenge Food Sensitivity Testing has two methods of assessing food sensitivities.
1. The initial pulse testing procedure identifies food combinations that may or may not include foods that can cause an allergic, intolerant or sensitive reaction. This technique can be used with gluten, diary and or GMO foods.
2. The second pulse testing procedures identifies individual organic or non-organic foods that cause sensitive reaction. You can perform a simple 2-minute self-test to determine if a particular food causes a stressful reaction. You can either choose your own foods to test, or specific suspected foods could be tested. The Pulse testing method can be used to determine whether or not a particular supplement is causing stress to the system.

Diet /Pulse Record

1. Ideally you should take your pulse 14 times across three days (assuming you eat 3 meals).
   a. Once before getting out of bed.
   b. Before each meal.
   c. After each meal, and finally
   d. Before bed.
2. You should record what foods were in the meals and bodily reactions, feelings, activities, and cravings across the day.
3. Avoid snacks between meals. If a snack is eaten, the type of snack must be noted.
4. For accuracy a full one-minute pulse should be taken.
5. You should avoid alcohol, artificial sweeteners and smoking for the three-day test. They can make the test invalid.
6. By the end of the three days there will be adequate data to begin the using pulse testing to find individual foods.

Pulse Testing Individual Foods

1. You should be relaxed, sit down and take a deep breath.
2. A baseline pulse should be established by counting the pulse.
3. You should then place a sample of food in your mouth or on the tongue. You will need to taste it for approximately one-half minute without swallowing.
4. It is important to test only one food or ingredient in a food at one time. Testing individual ingredients will yield specific information, compares with testing foods containing multiple ingredients.
5. You should retake your pulse while the food remains in the mouth and record the "after" pulse on the pulse test record form.
6. You must discard the tested ingredient, do not swallow it.
7. If a reaction occurs, you must rinse your mouth out with some distilled water and spit the water.
8. Wait two minutes, and then you should retest the pulse to see if it has returned to its baseline. If it hasn't, then wait a few minutes more and retest.
9. You should continue to retest until the pulse has returned to normal.
10. Once the pulse has returned to its normal rate test the next food.
11. The procedure can be repeated as frequently as necessary, as long as you let your pulse return to its baseline before testing the next food.

Diet /Pulse (3-day test record)

Result	Interpretation
Pulse greater standing than sitting	Food or environmental sensitivities.
Daily maximal pulse rate varies more than two beats (i.e. Monday 72, Tuesday 78, Wednesday 76).	Signs of sensitivities.
Minimum pulse-rate that does not regularly occur "before rising" but at some other time of day.	Sensitivity to dust, dust mites or chemical substance in the sleeping environment.
6 – 8 point or more increase after a meal.	Sensitivity to a chemical substance during that meal.
6 – 8 point or more increase 30 minutes after a meal	Sensitivity to a chemical or substance that is quickly absorbed (i.e. refined carbohydrates).
6 – 8 point or more increase 60 minutes after a meal	Sensitivity to proteins in that meal.
6 – 8 point or more increase 90 minutes after a meal	Sensitivity to proteins in that meal.
Pulse rate is constant for three days in a row	"Foods sensitivities" have been avoided on those days.
Ingestion of a frequently eaten food causes no acceleration of the pulse	Decreased allergic reaction or sensitivity to any food in that meal.

Acid-Alkaline Imbalance Interpretation

Pattern	Metabolic Acidosis	Metabolic Alkalosis
Systemic	Build-up of H+cellular fluids causes systemic acidosis	⇑ Excretion of H+ or retention of HCO_3 → systemic alkalosis
Respiration Rate	**Increased** The respiratory system compensates by the ↑ rate and depth of respiration to blow off CO_2 and ↓ Carbonic acid levels	**Decreased** Suppression of respiratory centers causes ↓ rate and depth of respiration to retain CO_2 and ↑ carbonic levels
Breath Hold Time	**Decreased** Acidosis causes a ↓ O_2 transport and uptake increases breath hold	**Increased** Alkalosis causes an ↑↑O_2 transport and uptake leading to a ↑ breath hold
Urine pH	**Decreased** Acidic urine-kidneys compensate by excreting H+ in urine and retaining bicarbonate	**Increased** Acidic urine-kidneys compensate by retaining H+ in urine and excreting bicarbonate
Saliva pH	**Increased** Alkaline saliva- ↑ respiratory rate lowers the dissolved carbonic acid levels resulting in alkaline saliva	**Decreased** Alkaline saliva- ↓ respiratory rate increases the dissolved carbonic acid levels resulting in acidic saliva

Pattern	Respiratory Acidosis	Respiratory Alkalosis
Systemic	Retention of H+ due to excretion of CO_2	Loss of H+ due to ↑ excretion CO_2 from lungs-hyperventilation
Respiration Rate	**Decreased as a 1° cause** ↓ Respiration rate (hypoventilation) causes acidosis in respiratory acidosis. Increased in compensation for metabolic acidosis. Rate and depth of respiration to blow off CO_2 and ↓ carbonic acid levels.	**Increases as a 1° cause** ↑Respiration rate (hyperventilation) is the cause alkalosis in respiratory alkalosis. Decreased in compensation The respiration rate is ↓ in respiratory compensation for metabolic acidosis. Rate and depth of respiration is ↓ to retain more CO_2 and ↑ carbonic acid levels.
Breath hold time	**Decreased** Acidosis causes an ↓ O2 transport and uptake leading to an ability to hold one's breath.	**Increased** Alkalosis causes an ↑ O_2 transport and uptake leading to an ↑ ability to holds ones breath.
Urine pH	**Decreased** Acidic urine- kidneys compensate by excreting H+ in urine and retaining bicarbonate.	**Increased** Alkaline urine- kidneys compensate by retaining H+ in urine and excreting bicarbonate in urine.
Saliva pH	**Increased** Alkaline saliva-↑ levels of CO_2 & carbonic acid due to hyperventilation	**Decreased** Alkaline saliva- ↓ levels of CO_2 & carbonic acid due to hyperventilation

Respiratory Rate

Respiratory rate can indicate acid/alkaline imbalances. The respiratory rate is determined by the brains respiratory centers. They measure the amount of oxygen in the blood that flows through the aortic and carotid arteries.

Directions

This test is a measurement of respiratory rate. The number of times you breath for one minute should be counted with a watch that has a second hand or digital clock. Do not count your breathing rate yourself, have someone else count for you, in a self test people tend to alter their breathing rate and invalidate the results. The person timing your respiratory rate can either watch the rise and fall of the chest, or place a hand on the abdomen and count the number of breaths in a full minute. Count one full cycle of inhalation and exhalation as one breath.

Results

Normal: 14-18 respiratory cycles/minutes

Increased Respiratory Rate

Implication	Interpretation
Metabolic acidosis	Metabolic acidosis causes an increase of the respiratory rate as a means of exhaling CO2, which lowers carbonic acid levels to decrease the acidosis.
Respiratory acidosis (compensation)	Increased respiratory rate indicates compensation by the body to overcome respiratory acidosis, which can be caused by hypoventilation. CO2 levels increase because the body increased respiration rate. This is the body's method of compensating. The breathing is rapid and often shallow.
Respiratory alkalosis (Primary cause/acute)	Respiratory alkalosis is caused by hypoventilation or and increased respiratory rate. In the acute or primary phase there is hyperventilation. This compensatory action helps the respiration rate decreases.
Sympathetic stress	Increased sympathetic output can cause hyperventilation.

Decreased Respiratory Rate

Implication	Interpretation
Metabolic alkalosis	Slowing of the respiration rate is caused by the suppression of the respiratory centers. This lessens the amount of CO_2 blown off to increase carbonic acid levels.
Respiratory alkalosis (chronic or compensation/ recovery stage)	Respiratory alkalosis is caused by hyperventilation. The reduced respiratory rate is to counter the alkalosis by slowing the breath, which increase the levels of CO_2 and carbonic acid.
Respiratory acidosis primary cause (usually accompanied by high blood pressure)	Blood pressure increases the aorta and carotid arteries ability to carry more oxygenated blood past the chemoreceptors, they lower the respiratory rate by changing the rate and depth of breathing. This results in respiratory acidosis.

Urine Vitamin C Test

Vitamin C increases the health of glands, teeth, organs, is an antibiotic, is needed to maintain healthy connective tissue, adrenal glands, red blood cells and capillary walls, and protects you from diseases, stomach disorders, and toxins. It is not excreted until the Vitamin C optimum level in the blood is too high above a certain value related to the degree of tissue saturated when Vitamin C is stored in tissues of the body, such as the kidneys, adrenals and lungs. If Vitamin C intake is too high the intestines do not absorb it. It is eliminated in the feces. If Vitamin C reserves in the body are low, then little will be excreted in the urine. It takes more drops of urine to decolonize the reagent indicating less Vitamin C in each drop of urine. The test measures a fragment of Vitamin C called ascorbic acid, which is the antioxidant fragment of the Vitamin C complex.

People taking the ascorbate form of Vitamin C may appear deficient in this test. Ascorbic acid is not Vitamin C; it is a fragment of it.

Normal Values: 1-5 drops of urine will decolorize the reagent

HIGH (>5 drops of urine to decolorize reagent)

Implication	Information
Dietary insufficiency or deficiency of vitamin C	Consumption of refined (junk) foods, immune suppressive drugs, people with two or more diseases, pregnant and breastfeeding women, children smoking, drinking alcohol

Low vitamin C is associated with the following
- Adrenal insufficiency, fatigue, exhaustion
- ↑ Capillary permeability: bruising, bleeding gums, gum disorders
- Joint pain, loss of bone mass, stiffness, aching joints
- Lowered resistance to infections, sore throat, laryngitis, and tonsillitis
- Slow healing of wounds and fractures
- Digestion problems
- Shortness of breath
- Scurvy
- Tissue and collagen disorders

Lingual Ascorbic Acid Test (Lingual-C)

This indicates the tissue levels of ascorbic acid in the body. The test uses an oxidation-reduction reaction between the ascorbic acid present in the lingual tissues and 2,6 dichlorphenol-indophenol, a dye that becomes colorless when reduced by ascorbic acid. Ascorbic acid converts into Hydro-L-Ascorbic Acid when it comes into contact with the lingual tissue and the dye. This test indicates for tissue levels of Vitamin C, antioxidants and plasma levels. Ascorbic acid is an antioxidant and high levels indicate antioxidant reserve in the tissue. The Vitamin C complex includes co- factors, such as bioflavonoids, chelated ascorbate minerals and copper, which help with its absorption and utilization in the body. Supplements that include isolated and/or synthetic ascorbic acid can cause long-term Vitamin C deficiency. Vitamin C supplementation should include co-factors, bioflavonoid, rutin, etc.
- This test is to assess tissue ascorbic acid levels and antioxidant reserves.
- This test is performed if there are symptoms of Vitamin C deficiency or are at a higher risk of developing Vitamin C tissue deficiency: pregnancy lactation, smoking, on prolonged antibiotic or cortisone therapy, on pain killers, alcoholism, deficient diets and under stress.
- The test is performed if you suspect high oxidative stress

Directions:
1. You should rinse their mouth thoroughly and the protruded tongue is grasped and held with a gauze pad.
2. With your mouth wide open, the anterior and middle third of the dorsum of the tongue can be observed.
3. Dry this area with a gauze pad stroking the taste buds (papillae) so that they stand erect.
4. Select and area with a papillae standing erect on the left or right of the midline of the tongue.
5. Drop 1 drop of the dye and begin timing immediately after the drop touches the tissue. Use a watch with a second hand or a digital clock with a second hand.
6. Continue timing until all the color has completely disappeared or 60 seconds has elapsed, and record the results in seconds.
7. After the test you must rinse their mouth vigorously with water.

Results:

1-10 seconds	Excellent tissue ascorbic acid status
11-20	Satisfactory tissue ascorbic acid status
>20 seconds	Indicates inadequate tissue ascorbic acid status and low antioxidant reserve

Implications
- A reading of 10-20 indicates satisfactory tissue ascorbic acid levels. Consider supplementing with antioxidants.
- >20 seconds indicates poor tissue ascorbic acid level and a low antioxidant reserve.
- Reasons for failing the test include:
    - High free radical load
    - Poor antioxidant status
    - Poor diet and deficiency in vitamin C
    - Mega dosing the wrong kind of vitamin C
    - Not taking co-factors especially bioflavonoid with ascorbic acid
- Supplement with a broad-spectrum antioxidant with bioflavonoid should be implemented and monitored with further tests.
- Check for oxidative stress in people with poor tissue ascorbic acid levels, use Oxidata test.

Interfering Factors:

False Positive and Negative Results
• Plaque coating on the tongue can prevent a proper interpretation • Wet tongue • Pooling of dye in midline of tongue or in small cracks and crevices • Lipstick on tongue • Medications • Mouthwashes • The eating of foods immediately prior to testing

Iodine Patch Test

Iodine is a nutrient that can be deficient. It indicates deterioration of the thyroid, or an enlargement of the thyroid (Goiter). Iodine is essential for thyroid function; begin an integral part of thyroxine (T4) and Triiodithyronine (T3) molecules. Iodine deficiency can cause an increase in the number and size of the epithelial cells resulting in an enlarged thyroid gland called a "goiter". Iodine is a structural substance for the thyroid. The majority of the body's iodine (20 to 30 mg in the average adult body) is stored in the thyroid in the form of thyroid hormone. Less than 1 mg is in the blood, and trace amounts are in the tissue. Iodine is a black, non –metallic element and a salt formerly a Halogen. It combines with hydrogen to form acids and with metal to form salts. The iodine patch test is a functional assessment for iodine status in the body. By painting the skin with a 2% solution of iodine indicates how quick the body absorbs available iodine. If there is a deficiency or a need for iodine then the iodine stain will fade in less than 24 hours. This indicates that there is not enough iodine to normalize thyroid secretions. The quicker the iodine fades, the greater the deficiency.

Symptoms of iodine deficiency
1. Lowered vitality
2. Inability to think clearly
3. Low resistance to infection
4. Teeth defects and deformities
5. Obesity
6. Cretinism
7. Circulatory disorders
8. Abnormal breast tissue growth

Functions of Iodine
1. Iodine helps to manufacture thyroid hormone
2. Estrogen can indicate the development of breast cancer (dysplasia) in women who are iodine deficient. Iodine helps regulate estrogen's effect on breast tissue.
3. Iodine aids the conversion of a group of hormones called estrogen (estrone, estradiol, and estroil)

This test is used when iodine deficiency is suspected, and when there are signs of hypothyroidism or low basal body temperatures.

Directions
1. You should paint your skin with a 2-inch square patch of 2% iodine solution.
2. You must avoid soaking in hot tubs or baths for 24 hours, as the chlorine or bromine in the water will cause the iodine patch to come off.
3. You must write down how soon after application the iodine patch has disappeared.

Results:
Color lasts for >24 hours   Sufficient iodine
Color fades in <24 hours   Deficient iodine

Implications
The quicker the iodine fades, the greater the deficiency can be assumed to be. The following protocol should be implemented until sufficiency is obtained i.e the strain remains for a minimum of 24 hours:
- 20-30 drops of liquid iodine (as potassium iodide) per day

Interfering factors:
You can have a reaction to the topical application of iodine or they can have symptoms of iodism (too much iodine) during iodine supplementation, such as tachycardia, skin irritation, thinning of secretions (water eyes, nose, saliva), nervousness and headache.

Related Test:
Use the following tests to further assess low thyroid function
1. Check for tenderness in the Chapman reflex for the thyroid located in the right second intercostal space near the sternum.
2. Check for a delayed Achilles return reflex, which is a strong sign of a hypo-functioning thyroid.
3. Check for general costochondral tenderness and pre-tibial edema, a sign of a hypo-functioning thyroid.
4. The person's blood chemistry test may have changes TSH, T4, T3, FTI, and T3- Uptake.

Iodine Patch Test Form
Iodine deficiency has increased because of the increased amount of synthetic chemicals such as chlorine, bromine and fluoride in our foods, environment and water supply. These chemicals can deplete iodine from the body and interfere with Iodine usage causing problems such as hypothyroidism, lowered vitality, cognitive dysfunction, lowered immunity and obesity. The iodine patch test is an easy method of assessing you iodine levels.

Instructions:
1. Use the topical iodine solution, which is used topically and not orally.
2. Paint the skin of the inside of the forearm or abdomen with a 2-inch square patch of 2% iodine solution. The solution can stain your clothes. Note the time you put the iodine onto the skin on the form below.
3. Air-dry the patch before putting clothes on.
4. Monitor and indicate how quickly the patch fades.
5. Avoid soaking in hot tubs or baths for 24 hours, as the chlorine or bromine in the water will cause the iodine patch to come off.
6. Note on the form below how soon after application the iodine patch has disappeared.

Time Iodine Put On Skin	Time Color Disappears	Number of Hours it Took to Completely Disappear

Zinc Taste Test

Background

Zinc is a trace mineral. It is used in the enzyme systems. A decrease causes a loss of appetite while liquid zinc can restore the appetite. Zinc is part of over 70 metalloenzyme complexes that catalyze biochemical reactions in the body. Zinc is part of carbonic anhydrase. It is an enzyme that stimulates the carbonic acid-bicarbonate buffering system. Zinc helps in the maintenance of the Basal Metabolic Rate. Zinc deficiency has been associated with a decreased Basal Metabolic Rate (BMR).

The major portion of the body's zinc is binded in bone and protein, which is one of the reasons that zinc deficiency is very common. Zinc deficiency is caused by impaired absorption, due to hypochlorhydria, inhibition by certain nutrients (iron), and drugs (birth control pills and steroids), and deficient zinc in the soil. Zinc deficiency decreases bodily and cellular function and metabolism. Zinc deficiency can cause a loss of taste and smell, reduced immunity, failure for a baby to live (thrive), slow healing, reproductive difficulties (especially in men), various skin disorders including seborrhea, scaling or flaking skin, and acne, and loss of appetite and gustatory sensitivity.

The test is a non-invasive, and helps determine the physiological zinc status. The test is a functional assessment instead of measuring the quantity zinc, such as serum or plasma zinc studies.

The test indicates the "functional" availability of zinc. Functional zinc can indicate deficiency in Vitamin B6 and magnesium, synergistic nutrients with zinc. If the zinc test is failed and there is no response to zinc therapy, an evaluation of B6 and magnesium status can indicate the cause of the problem.

Liquid zinc therapy is clinically more useful than tableted zinc, because hydrochloric acid production is zinc dependent and zinc tablets may not be absorbed due to hypochlorhydria. If there is a deficiency then this test can determine how deficient they are. 1 bottle of aqueous zinc (zinc sulphate) can be used to perform a full zinc challenge test.

Directions:

This test is done in two parts. The first part determines whether there is deficiency. The second part is a zinc challenge, which uses the same test to determine the level of zinc deficiency.

Test Instructions:
1. Your mouth should be free of any strong tastes
2. You then hold and swishes ¼ ounce of aqueous zinc in their mouth
3. Start timing and you should indicate when they first taste the solution
4. Have them swallow after 15 seconds
5. You should describe the strength to taste or presence of an after taste
6. Record strength of taste and seconds it took them to taste the solution

Ranges:

Level	Interpretation	Description
1	Optimal Zinc Zone	An immediate, unpleasant and adverse taste in a few seconds
2	Mild Zinc Deficiency	A definite but not strong unpleasant taste is noted in 4-6 seconds and tends to intensify with time (delayed metallic)
3	Moderate Zinc Deficiency	No taste noted initially, but develops in 7-13 seconds. May be described as sweet or bitter
4	Very Zinc Deficiency	Tasteless or "tastes like water"

Implications:
Levels 3 or 4 represent a zinc deficiency and should be treated by fallowing the following zinc challenge protocol.

Zinc Challenge

The zinc challenge evaluates the level of zinc deficiency you have and how much zinc therapy is needed. The zinc challenge uses repeated challenges with the aqueous zinc to determine the amount of aqueous zinc that is needed to begin supplementation.

Aqueous zinc can be used therapeutically in the initial stages of zinc supplementation. It is a low dose, and liquid is the optimal form to help zinc absorption. It is less dependent on optimal hydrochloric acid levels than other forms of zinc.

This test requires 1 bottle of aqueous zinc, which is used to perform a full zinc challenge test.

Zinc Challenge Directions
1. Begin with standard Zinc Taste Test as previously described.
2. Repeat the process successively, resting 30 seconds between tests, and noting changes in strength of taste.
3. Indicate how many taste test used for the person to reach a strong metallic taste indicating zinc saturation.

The number of taste test can equal the number of bottles of aqueous zinc that the person needs to begin a zinc maintenance program. Dosage for aqueous zinc supplementation is 1ounce 2x/day with meals. After the course of aqueos zinc begin supplementation with 45 mg of zinc 2 times a day for 60 days. At this time redo the ZTT.

If you are not able to achieve a metallic taste then:
1. Assume that zinc deficiency signs are present.
2. Screen with white blood cell zinc and magnesium levels (synergistic nutrients with zinc).
3. Rule out vitamin B6 deficiency with serum homocysteine.
4. If there is a vitamin B6 deficiency, then treat it.
5. There can be damage olfactory center, which comprise the ability to taste and smell (trauma, smoking).

Zinc is best taken with meals to prevent nausea. This behavior is seen in people who are both zinc deficient and hypochlorhydric. Vitamin B6 or magnesium deficiency can cause a false positive results.

Related Tests:
The following can be used if there are other mineral deficiencies:
1. Assess for mineral deficiency using the Tissue Mineral Assessment Test. Place a standard blood pressure cuff around the largest portion of calf muscle (sitting). Be mindful of when you feel the onset of cramping pain and gradually inflate the cuff. Stop and deflate immediately when threshold has been reach. Less than 200 mmHg is considered deficient in minerals. Use the neurolingual testing to challenge the body with several different types of minerals and other co-factors to see which combination of minerals and other co-factors to see which combination of minerals and co-factors increases the threshold above 200mmHg.
2. Assess for mineral insufficiency by using Dr. Kane's mineral assessment test.
3. Assess the impact of mineral deficiencies on the body's acid buffering capacities by using Dr. Bieler's salivary pH acid challenge.

HCl (Hydrochloric Acid) Challenge Test

The HCL challenge test can evaluate the stomach's ability to secrete adequate stomach acid. Stomach acid is secreted when the skin of the stomach is stimulated, such as thinking about food, chewing and the presence of certain foods (healthy or not) in the stomach e.g. proteins, milk, calcium salts, coffee, etc. Due to this stimuli gastrin, a hormone secreted by gastrin cells, is released in pyloric glands located in the antrum of the stomach. Gastrin stimulates the parietal glands to produce and secrete acid into the stomach. The histamine hormone stimulates acid production. Its effect is potentiated by the presence of gastrin. A deficiency of HCL is caused by hypochlorohydria or in more severe cases achlorhydria.

Functions of stomach acid include:
1. Sterilization of food we eat.
2. Killing ingested parasites, bacteria, etc.
3. Allowing for optimal absorption of B12.
4. Initiating the metabolic process for the food (chime) to be alkaline in the intestines.
5. Stimulating duodenal Cholecystokinin and secretin, which stimulates pancreatic secretions to be released.
6. Essential for optimum absorption of minerals.

Hypochlorhydria (low hydrochloric acid)

Can be caused by:
1. Excessive caffeine, sugar, refined foods, alcohol, chronic overeating, drugs, emotional stress, sympathetic dominant lifestyle, and inadequate sleep.
2. Antacid drugs e.g. Tagamet, Pepcid AC, Prilosec, Nexium, etc.
3. History of sodas, energy drinks, flavor water, or coffee drinking.
4. Abrupt diet changes: meat to vegetarian, or vegetarian to mean. Veganism
5. Autoimmune disease (antipariteal cell antibody)

Symptoms of Hypochlorhydria
1. Gas, bloating, eructation.
2. Food sits and doesn't digest, slow emptying time with heavy, long lasting, full feeling in stomach.
3. Trouble digesting proteins, may have food sensitivities to proteins.
4. Diarrhea /constipation
5. Bloating, gas, heaviness, fullness, worse after eating,
6. Heartburn and indigestion (may use OTC antacids) usually worse when food is in the stomach.
7. Easy satiety, functional dyspepsia: can indicate constipation, diarrhea or normal stools.
8. Symptoms worse ½ - 1 hour after meals from eating protein: there is inadequate acid to balance the alkali in the duodenum so there's reflux of alkali through the pyloric valve and alkali burns esophageal tissue (not unlike GERDs)

Hypochlorhdria is Indicated By
1. Joint aches and muscle weakness caused by protein improperly digested.
2. Chronic anemia: pallor, bruising, and fatigue.
3. Nervousness, insomnia.
4. Soft, brittle or peeling nails
5. Hair loss in women
6. Telangiectasia of the maxillary area/facial skin eruptions, acne

Gastric Reflux and Hyper-secretion of Stomach Acid
Weak or "excess" stomach acid causes Gastric Reflux. Hyper-secretion of stomach acid is not common, and can an irritated or inflamed digestive tract.
- The reflux of stomach content in the esophagus is associated with inadequate secretions of the stomach causing putrification of food and symptoms of gas, bloating, reflux and belching.
- Antacid therapy may provide temporary relief and decreases the digestion of food, and is suppressive in the long term.
- Treatments of this condition is to perform a stomach challenge by taking a small amount of supplemental hydrochloric acid during the middle of a large complex meal.
- If the dosage does not cause stomach pain, aggravation or burning, queasiness, abdominal or lower chest discomfort, then slowly increase the dosage over the course of the next few days.
- It is important to proceed as long as the acid supplement is well tolerated.

This test is used to:
1. Determine whether the person has sufficient HCL for digestion.
2. Determine the appropriate dose of supplemental stomach acid to use.
3. Assess for gastric inflammation by challenging the mucosal lining of the stomach.

Supplies you will need to give patient
10 HCl capsules or tablets, which are enough to challenge 4 meals

Directions
- The meals to challenge are high in protein and have combinations of foods.

- Do not challenge small meals or meals that consist of only fruit, or bowl of cereal or salads.
- Meals without protein can result in stomach irritation when challenged with supplemental HCl.

Meal 1: Take 1 capsule of HCl at the beginning of the meal, after the first few bites of a substantial complex meal (contains protein). Record if there is an experience of any mild burning or irritation. Stop the challenge and record the symptoms after 1 capsule. If no burning is experienced, then continue.

Meal 2: Take 2 capsules at the beginning of the next complex meal and record any mild burning or irritation. If burning reaction stop the challenge meal and record that 2 capsules produced symptoms. If no symptoms, move on to challenge meal number 3.

Meal 3: Take 3 capsules at the beginning of the next complex meal and record any mild burning or irritation. If no symptoms, proceed onto the last challenge.

Meal 4: This is the last meal to challenge. Take the remaining 4 capsules with a complex meal, recording any mild burning or irritation. If no symptoms, write no symptoms after 4 capsules of the form.

Stop taking the supplemental HCl if any of the following reactions occur;
1. Feeling of warmth or pressure in the stomach.
2. Irritation such as heartburn, stomach ache is experienced. If the above reaction drink a glass of water to relieve the symptoms. Take an antacid, or baking soda and water -½ tsp. per cup to neutralize the acidity.

Implications

Implications	Information
Burning with 1 capsule	Burning sensation with one capsule of HCL can indicate the following: 1. Gastric irritation or inflammation that needs to be treated before beginning needed HCl supplementation. 2. Adequate HCl secretions
Burning with 2 – 4capsules	Mild to moderate hypochlorhydria is likely. May have mild gastric inflammation. Bothe would indicate a need for HCl supplementation. Start at a dose below the amount that caused burning
No burning, even with 4 capsules	A need for aggressive HCl supplementation

The following can indicate digestive dysfunction with hydrochloric acid:
1. Check the stomach acid reflex point for tenderness. This is located 1 inch below the xyphoid and over to the left edge of the rib cage.
2. Check for tenderness in the stomach and upper digestion reflex located in the 6th intercostal space on the left.

HCl Challenge Test

This test indicates the integrity of the skin of the stomach and the amount of supplemental HCl (stomach acid) that is sufficient for good health. There relationship between a good test and a strong digestive function (i.e. acid and enzyme production).

Meal 1: Take 2 capsules at the beginning of the next complex meal.

Meal 2: Take 3 capsules at the beginning of the next complex meal and continue successive meals until you reach 4 capsules.

Stop taking the supplemental HCl if there is adverse reaction or the following symptoms:
1. Feeling of warmth or pressure in the stomach.

2. Irritation i.e. heartburn, stomachache.

If there is the above reaction, drink a tall glass of water to relieve the symptoms. Calcium carbonate (Tums), or baking soda and water-½ tsp. per cup, can be taken if necessary to neutralize the acidity.

If there is a current or past history of ulcers, or you are currently taking antacids or acid blocking medications. DO NOT TAKE THIS TEST.

Basal Body Temperature Test

The thyroid hormones, Thyroxine (T4) and Triiodothyronine (T3) help to maintain the metabolic rate. T3 stimulates and increase activity of the mitochondria. T3 and the catecholamine hormones from the adrenal glands stimulate the use of oxygen and increases energy use, resulting in increased heat production. A low body temperature is a symptom of the thyroid hormone and hypothyroidism.
The basal body temperature test measures the core body temperature over time. It assesses both axillary and oral temperature during the day which indicates the factors that contribute to basal metabolism.
A low armpit (axillary) temperature before getting out of bed in the morning can indicate hypothyroidism. The axillary temperature correlates with thyroid function.
Oral temperatures taken during the day can indicate the adrenal glands influence to basal metabolism and blood sugar swings, especially of the before and after lunch temperature are significantly different.
Axillary and oral temperature should be taken for two days and compared to verify the absence of oral lesions that can cause an elevated oral temperature unrelated to basal metabolic status.
A lowered basal body temperature can indicate low levels of essential trace minerals (zinc, copper, and selenium) rather than a deficiency of thyroid hormone. Trace minerals are essential for the peripheral conversion T4 into T3.

This test is used:
1. To assess the hormonal influences on metabolism
2. To identify sub-clinical hypothyroidism
3. To indicate adrenal and blood sugar influences on basal metabolism

Pre-menopausal women should start taking their temperature the second day of menstruation. A temperature rise occurs around the time of ovulation, which can lead to incorrect interpretation of the test.

A day can be missed, but they should be sure to finish the testing before ovulation.

Menopausal or post-menopausal women and men should not be concerned with the time of day temperatures are taken. However, they should not do the test if there is an infection or any other condition that would raise their temperature.
A basal body thermometer is needed for this test or a computerized Ovuscope device.

Directions:
1. A digital thermometer should be used. If a mercury thermometer is used the mercury has to be shaken down in the thermometer to 96 degrees or less the night before and put it by the bedside.
2. In the morning before they get out of bed, they must put the thermometer deep in their armpit for ten minutes and record the temperature 1 tenth of a degree. They should not have anything to eat or drink, or do any activity until they take their temperature. The lowest temperature of the day is in the morning, which correlates with thyroid gland function.
3. All of the temperature readings are recorded on the Basal Body Temperature Form.
4. They should record their axillary temperature for 2 days and then average it out.
5. Next, shake the thermometer down and immediately take an oral temperature for 3 minutes. Record this temperature as "a.m. by mouth" for 7 days. You can use an Ovuscope computer device.
6. Repeat the oral temperature at three-hour intervals for seven days.
7. Record the time when meals are eaten. The person should record foods eaten on back of the form. This can indicate foods that can be causing blood sugar swings.
8. Indicate change of activity (i.e. I went to the gym, riding a bike).
9. They bring the form filled out and the averages are figured.

<u>Optimal Results</u>

The normal axillary temperature should ideally be 97.8°-98.2°F
The normal oral temperature should ideally be 98.6°F
Axillary and oral temperatures should be within 1°F of each other

<u>Interpretation</u>

Low average auxiliary temperature

Results	Interpretation
If the average first morning axillary temperature is below 97.6°	Suspect hypothyroidism and low basal metabolism. Evaluate this with the other findings for hypothyroidism

Low average oral temperature

Results	Interpretation
If the average oral temperature is below 98.4°	Suspect hypothyroidism and low basal metabolic activity. Evaluate this with the other findings for hypothyroidism.

Oral temperature fluctuations during the day

Results	Interpretation
Oral temperature fluctuate across the day°	When activity levels are constant, variations of oral temperatures during the day can indicate blood sugar swings, particularly if the before and after temperatures are significantly different (i.e. low prior to lunch and higher after lunch}, often ½ to 1½ degree variation

Factors that can interfere with Results
1. Menstruation
2. Excess movement before taking the axillary temperature
3. Use of an electric blanket, hot water bottles
4. Fever
5. Some type of infections, inflammation: earache, toothache, oral lesions etc....
6. Medications: birth control pills, cortisone, prednisone, DHEA, progesterone, estrogen

The following test can indicate low thyroid function:
1. Check for tenderness in the Chapman reflex for the thyroid located in the right second intercostal space near the sternum.
2. Check for a delayed Achilles return reflex, which is a strong sign of a hypo-functional thyroid.
3. Check for general costochondral tenderness, a thyroid indicator.
4. Check for pre-tibial edema, a sign of a hypo-function thyroid.
5. Iodine patch test: Use a tincture of 2% iodine solution, and paint a 3 by 3 square on the person's abdomen. The person is to leave the patch unwashed until it disappears. The square should still be there in 24 hours. If it has disappeared, there is and indication of iodine need.

Basal Body Temperature Test
The body temperature indicates the metabolism, hormones secreted by the thyroid and to a lesser degree and the adrenal glands that control metabolism. There is evidence that the current tests for the diagnosis of hypothyroidism (low thyroid function) are not adequate and can lack in accuracy. The thyroid gland can be observed by measuring the body temperature. A thermometer is required.

INSTRUCTIONS:

1. Use a digital device or Ovuscope device or a glass mercury-filled thermometer that has been shaken down below 96.0°F the night before and put beside the bed or a good-quality digital thermometer. Ear and tape thermometers are inconsistent and do not give very accurate temperature measurements, but if necessary they can be used. A basal body thermometer is best.
2. Upon awakening, place the bulb part of the thermometer into the deepest part of your armpit (for 10 minutes) and record a temperature each morning for two days. Do this before you have gotten out of bed, had any physical activity, or had anything to eat or drink. Record this temperature to 1/10 of a degree in the chart below.
3. Next, shake the thermometer down and immediately take an oral temperature for 3 minutes. Record this temperature as "a.m. by mouth" for 7 days.
4. Repeat the oral temperature at three-hour intervals for 7 days.
5. Record the time when meals are consumed. Record the types of foods eaten on the back of this page.
6. Record when activity has changed (i.e. I went for a walk).

Note for women: **avoid recording temperature for 3 days prior to menstruation**

Date	Arising Underarm	Arising by Mouth	Meal Yes or No	At 3 hours by Mouth	Meal Yes or No	At 6 hours by mouth	Meal Yes or No	At 9 hours by mouth
Averages								

Bowel Transit Time

Elimination of waste involves the transient time of food digested. The Bowel Transit Time is a test to measure how long it takes for food to move from your mouth to the anus for elimination. It should take 18 to 24 hours for food to move through the digestive tract. A shorter time is associated with diarrhea, bowel irritation, bowel toxicity, malabsorption and increased peristalsis. A longer transit time can indicate low fiber and/or water in the diet and other digestive problems.

Enzymes in the small intestine do not digest the dietary fiber of food. Food is digested in the duodenum and absorbed in the small intestine. Dietary fiber is divided into insoluble and soluble fiber. Insoluble fiber speeds the movement of food through the digestive tract. This absorbs water and increases fecal bulk and helps maintain regularity. Insoluble fiber can prevent or decrease digestive disorders (colon cancer, irritable bowel syndrome, Chrohn's disease, ulcerative colitis). A high fiber diet usually has a transit time of 20 hours and a fecal weight of 500 grams. Poor food combining and a junk food diet low in fiber and has transit time of more than 48 hours and a fecal weight of only 100 grams. There is a correlation between transit time and stool weight and size. A larger, bulkier stool passes through the colon easily and requires less pressure and straining during defecation. A high fiber diet can increase lactobacillus bacteria (good ones) while inhibiting endotoxin-producing bacteria (bad ones) in the colon. The proper micro flora in the intestines aids elimination and protects against disease causing bacteria.

This test uses charcoal (an inert substance) to measure the transit time. Charcoal will strain the stool black or gray, and provides a visible, medium for measuring the transit time.

The test indicates changes in the stool. The presence of blood, mucous, or undigested food particles can indicate problems in the digestive system.

This test is used:
1. To assess the eliminative capacity.
2. To indicate constipation or diarrhea.
3. To indicate changes in stools. This test indicates gastrointestinal health.

8 charcoal capsules or tablets, which are enough for 2 tests is used.

Directions:
1. Swallow 4 charcoal capsules at the evening meal.
2. Record the date and time that they swallowed the capsules.
3. After every bowel movement, observe the stool under bright light.
4. When a black or charcoal grey stool is first seen it must be recorded the date and time under " The Color First Appears on the form".
5. Calculate the number of hours between the time recorded under "Time in" and the time recorded under "time Color First Appears" and write this time (in hours) in the form. This is the time it took for the charcoal to pass through the digestive tract.
6. Examine every stool and record the time and date when the color has completely disappeared.
7. Repeat the test by waiting five (5) days to allow the marker to clear fully from the intestines and then repeat the process again, following the same instructions.

Results:
Optimal Bowel Transit Time: 10-24 hours. The Bowel Movement (manure) should smell like the food eaten.

Implications	Information
Normal Transit Time with Residual color on next stool	This indicates an optimal transit time but can be lacking in fiber or water as the charcoal should be expelled in one bowel movement.
Fast Transit Time	A fast transit time can be associated with diarrhea, which can be acute or chronic. A fast transit time indicates a gastrointestinal infection from the following: Parasites (Giardia lamlia, Entamoeba histolytica, Cryptosporidium, Isospora), Viral infection (Enterovirus, rotavirus), Bacterial infection (Campylobacter jejuni, Shigella, Salmonella, Yersinia enterocolitica), Intestinal toxins (Clostridiun, E Coli, staphylococcus) A fast transit time can indicate the use of laxatives or other medications that cause an increased peristalsis within the gastrointestinal tract. The main concerns with chronic fast bowel transit time is malabsorption of nutrients, both fat and water soluble, and dehydration. The digested food matter must spend enough time in the small intestine for optimal absorption of nutrients. A rapid transit time does not allow for proper absorption. Consider conditions such as inflammatory bowel disease, irritable bowel, malabsorption, leaky gut syndrome, emotional stress, food allergies, carbohydrate sweeteners (maltitiol, sorbital etc.), ascorbic acid intake, insufficient bile output indicates gallbladder insufficiency causing fat malabsorption and steatorrhea, and laxative abuse.
Fast Transit Time with Residual color on the next stool	The implications for a fast transit time apply to this type. The person has a small stool volume causing residual color on the next stool.

Slow Transit Time	There are organic and functional reasons why a person has a slow bowel transit time: **Organic causes** include diverticulitis, fissures, weakness in the rectum or sigmoid colon (often caused by laxative abuse) impaction of fecal material in the bowel, a mass of some kind obstructing the bowel (tumor or pregnancy), inflammation or spasm from pain in the rectum or anal canal. **Functional causes** include a diet that is irritating to the colon, lack of bulk to the stool (fiber absorbs water making the stool soft and allows for enough bulk for the muscles of the large intestine to move the stool through the colon), lack of fluids, insufficient digestion (hypochlorhydria and/or pancreatic insufficiency), stress, hypothyroidism, infection, or even adrenal dysfunction. A slow bowel transit time can have a mental/emotional causes. It can be neurogenic constipation caused by a repeated voluntary resistance of the urge to have a bowel movement. This can increase under increased stress that increase sympathetic outflow, which causes the blood vessels of the colon to constrict.
Slow Transit time with residual color in the next stool	The implications for a slow transit time apply to this type. This person can have a delayed transit time and a diminished stool volume.

Change in Stool	Implications
Blood on Stool	This is abnormal. Blood streaked on the outer surface usually indicates hemmorrhoids or anal abnormalities: blood present in stool from higher in colon; if transit time is rapid, can be from stomach or duodenum as bright or dark red.
Undigested food	May be indicated insufficient HCL and/or pepsin production. An insufficiently acid bolus of chewed food moving into the intestines may not stimulate sufficient pancreatic enzymes causing pancreatic insufficiency. Inadequate chewing of food may also be indicated.
Mucus on the stool	Mucus on the stool is usually due to gastrointestinal irritation (colitis, food sensitivity, pancreatitis). A translucent gelatinous mucus clinging to the surface of formed stool occurs in: spastic constipation, mucous colitis: emotional problems; excessive straining at stool.
Loose stool	Loose but not watery can indicate mild intestinal irritation and malabsorption.
Hard stool	Can indicate increased absorption of fluid as a result of prolonged contact of luminal contents with the mucosa of the colon because of delayed transit time (lack of fiber, dehydration, hypochlorohydria).
Floating stool	Consider malabsorption (esp. fats), reduced transient time due to anxiety or irritation, and a high fiber diet. The stool can be described as slippery or greasy looking.
Ribbon-like stool	A ribbon like stool suggests possibility of spastic bowel, rectal narrowing or stricture (pencil shaped), decreased elasticity, or partial obstruction (uterus malposition, prostitis, polyp, tumor).
Larger caliber stool	Possibility of a high fiber diet or dilation of the viscus of the colon.
Small, round and hard	This is called scybala which is found with habitual or morderate constipation. Severe fecal retention can produce a large amount of impacted masses in the colon with a small, round and hard stool as an overflow.
Brown	A brown colored stool can be caused by Sterobulin (urobilin), a bile pigment derivative resulting from the action of reducing bacteria in bilirubin. It is a normal finding.
Dark brown	Consistently dark brown stools indicate an excessively alkaline colon that may indicate dysbiosis. A dark brown stool can be a normal finding indicating good bile flow and elimination of fat-soluble toxins.

Yellow	Can be seen with severe diarrhea, can be caused by intestinal flora and can occur from antibiotic use. Indicates excessive bile secretions caused by over stimulation or irritation to the small intestine.
Black	Can be the result of bleeding into upper GI tract (ulcer, Chron's, Colitis, cancer); can be caused by iron, bismuth, charcoal or heavy meat diet.
Tan or clay colored	Can indicate a blockage of the common bile duct (lack of bile pigments) as well as pancreatic insufficiency, which can produce a pale, greasy alcohol stool. Consider gall bladder insufficiency or hepatobiliary obstruction.
Offensive odor	Indole and Skatole, intestinal toxins formed from intestinal putrification and fermentation by bacteria, are primarily responsible for odor. **Usually offensive odor** can indicate malabsorption, food decay, dysbiosis. **Occasionally offensive**- consider intermittent malabsorption with food decay and dysbiosis.

Test indicate gastrointestinal dysfunction:

1. Check the stomach acid reflex point for tenderness. This is located 1 inch below xyphoid and over to the left edge of the rib cage.
2. Check for tenderness in the stomach and upper digestion reflex located in 6th intercostal space on the left,
3. Assess the pH of the stomach's gastric acid assessment using the Gastro test.
4. Check for tenderness in the Chapman reflex for the colon located bilaterally along the iliotibial band on the thighs. Palpate the colon for tenderness and tension.

Bile Transit Time Instruction for Self-Testing

Instructions:
1. Swallow 4 charcoal capsules at the evening meal. Record the date and time you swallowed the capsule under "Time In" on the form below.
2. After every bowel movement, observe the stool under "The Color First Appears" on the form below.
3. Calculate the number of hours between the time record under "Time In" and the time record under "Time Color First Appears" and write this time (in hours) in the form below. This is the time took for the charcoal to pass through the digestive tract.
4. Continue to examine every stool and record the time and date when the color has completely disappeared.
5. Wait five (5) days to allow the marker to clear fully from the intestines and then repeat this process again, following the same instructions.
6.

	Time and Date in	Time Color first appears	Transit time (hours)	Time completely cleared
1				
2				

Indicate on the form below if any of the following are noticed in your stool:

o	Blood on the stool	o	Undigested food in stool	o	Mucus on stool
o	Stool is loose	o	Stool is hard	o	Stool is floating
o	Ribbon like stool	o	Large caliber stool	o	Small, round and hard
o	Brown colored	o	Dark brown colored	o	Yellow
o	Black	o	Tan or clay colored	o	Offensive odor

Respiratory Rate

Respiratory rate can determine acid or alkaline imbalances. The respiratory rate is set from the respiratory centers in the brain and responds to oxygen levels of blood that flows through the aortic and carotid arteries.

This is used to indicate:
This test is a measurement of respiratory rate. It is not a self-test. It is for another person to time the respiratory rate because you may get self-conscious and alter your breathing rate and skew the results. The best method of taking another person's respiratory rate is to tell the person that you are going to take a pulse for one minute and count the pulse for the first 30 seconds and the respiratory rate for the latter. Use a digital clock or a watch with a second-hand, hold the person's wrist and gently place your hand on the upper abdomen and count the pulse and the number of respiratory cycles in 30 seconds. Multiply by two and record the number on the results form.

Results
Normal: 14-18 respiratory cycles/minute

Increased Respiratory Rate (hyperventilation)

Implication	Information
Metabolic acidosis	In metabolic acidosis the body increases respiratory rate as a means of blowing off CO_2 which lowers carbonic acid levels and relieve the acidosis.
Respiratory acidosis (compensation)	The increased respiratory rate is compensated by the body in dealing with respiratory acidosis, which has an etiology in hypoventilation i.e. CO_2 levels increase because the body is unable to blow it off (e.g. in asthma and emphysema). The increased respiration rate is the body's way if compensating. The breathing is rapid and often shallow.
Respiratory alkalosis (primary cause/acute)	Respiratory alkalosis is caused by hyperventilation or an increased respiratory rate. In the acute or primary phase there is hyperventilation, as the body begins to compensate. The breathing is rapid and often shallow.
Sympathetic stress	Increased sympathetic output can cause hyperventilation.

Decrease Respiratory Rate

Implication	Information
Metabolic alkalosis	A slowing of the reparation rate caused by the suppression of the respiratory centers (the body is attempting to lessen the amount of CO_2 blown off to increase carbonic acid levels)
Respiratory alkalosis (chronic or compensation/recovery stage)	Respiratory alkalosis is caused by hyperventilation. The reduced respiratory rate is the body's attempt to counter the alkalosis by slowing the breath and therefore increasing the levels of CO_2 and carbonic acid.
Respiratory acidosis in primary cause (usually accompanied by high blood pressure)	As blood pressure increases the aorta and carotid arteries carry more oxygenated blood past the chemoreceptors, which are stimulated and begin to lower the respiratory rate by changing rate and depth of breathing. This can result in respiratory acidosis.

Cardio-pulmonary disease, respiratory tract infections can interfere with the respiratory rate.

Urine pH, Saliva pH and Breath-Hold test can indicate acid/alkaline imbalances.

Metabolic pH Assessment

pH is the measurement of acidity and alkalinity. Some organs require an acid environment to work optimally (e.g. your stomach) while others require an alkaline environment (i.e. the small intestine). An optimal pH of the blood is needed for oxygen delivery to your cells and for the correct action of insulin to control blood sugar levels. The body uses chemical (bicarbonate) and mechanical (lungs) buffering systems to keep the pH within a normal and optimal range. These tests indicate if those regulatory mechanisms are functioning properly.

The two systems of regulation are the respiratory (lungs) and excretory systems (kidneys). They regulate the levels of acid and alkaline in your body. By measuring how long you can hold your breath, how many breaths you take in a minute, and your urine and salivary pH it can determine what areas of the body need support to bring the pH system into balance.

1. Breathe Hold Test
    a) This test is measurement of how long you can hold a deep breath. A digital clock or a watch with a second hand or a timer to time breathe holding.
    b) It is hard to time one's own breath-hold time, so it is best to have another person do the timing.
    c) You should be seated and should take a deep breath and hold it as long as you can. You should stop when it begins to feel uncomfortable or you feel as if you need to take another breath. This is not a test of endurance.
    d) When you can no longer hold your breath, let it out, and record the number of seconds the breath was held on the chart below.

2. Respiration Rate
    a) This is test is a measurement of how many breaths you take in a minute. This is your respiration rate. You will need a digital clock or a watch with a second hand, or a timer to time your respiration rate.
    b) It is difficult to tome one's respiration rate because you can alter your respiration rate if you are doing the timing. It is best to have another person to do the timing.
    c) You should be lying down when this test is performed and try to breathe as normally and unconsciously as possible.

2° Buffering Systems

1. Alkaline Minerals
The body uses the acidic and alkaline properties of minerals to help buffer the blood.

When the blood becomes too acidic, the other fluids, such as the lymphatic fluid, will move into a less optimal acidic range by releasing alkaline minerals to buffer the blood and bring it back into an alkaline range.

The mineral compounds that neutralize acids are the carbonic salts, symbolized as $AlkCO^3$ in the formula below.

Alk stands for any of the 4 alkaline or basic elements: Sodium (Na^+) Calcium (Ca^{2+}) Potassium (K^+) and Magnesium (Mg^{2+}).

When these carbonic salts meet with acids, the alkaline minerals making up the carbonic salts will combine with the acid to create a salt.

For example:
$AlkCO^3$ + H^2SO = $AlkSO4$ + H^2O + CO^2
Carbonic salt   Sulfuric acid   Sulfuric salt   Water   Carbon dioxide

This reaction has taken a strong acid and combined it with an alkaline salt to form a sulfuric salt, a compound excreted from the kidney without any harm.

2. The Liver and the Urea Cycle
The urea cycle of the liver combines carbon dioxide with ammonia (produced from the oxidation of the amino acid glutamine) and forms urea, which is excreted by the kidney.

3. The Digestive System
    a) Acid Blood:

- The digestive system buffers an acidic blood by supplying bicarbonate and other alkaline forming elements from the digestive enzymes systems of the small intestines to help buffer the acids.
- This leaves a more acidic condition in the small intestine causing the liver and pancreatic secretions of digestive enzymes to decrease function optimally resulting in digestion dysfunction.

  b) Alkaline Blood
  - The digestive system buffers an alkaline blood by supplying acidic elements from the stomach in order to buffer the alkalinity.
  - This causes more alkaline condition in the stomach,
  - This causes the digestion in the stomach to become weaken and a state of hypochlorohydria exists.

4. Ammonia
A method that the body can use in short-term situations is the release of alkaline ammonia. This method is used because there are less than optimal amounts of alkaline minerals in the body fluids, or to increase mineral levels in a short-term situation.

Assessment of 2° buffering systems
The assessment of the secondary buffering systems is performed by observing the buffering activity of the saliva in response to an acid challenge.

Oxidata Free Radical Test

Free radical molecules theory is about unpaired electrons. Unpaired electrons are by-products of normal metabolism and xenobiotics reaction. Free radicals are unstable, reactive with other molecules, help build energy by breaking down foods and can cause harm to tissue. Free radical reaction can multiply by chain reactions with cellular material. The chain reactions effect can cause cellular damage (i.e. cell membrane or DNA disruptions). Free radical or oxidative stress can cause an illness. High levels of free radicals exist in environmental pollutants, drugs, junk foods, inflammatory diseases and low antioxidant status. Oxidative stress destroys toxins, and fight disease etc. Abnormal decrease in oxidative stress causes problems.

Antioxidants nutrients such as Vitamin A, C, and E, lipoic acid and glutathione, can help to stop free radicals and protect the body from cellular damage. Antioxidants both treat and prevent oxidative damage.

The Oxidata Free Radical Test can determine the amount of free radical or oxidative stress and antioxidant status. The test measures the distal end of the polyunsaturated fat chain where aldehyde forms free radical reaction. Aldehypes are in body fluids such as serum, and blood etc. It is highest levels in urine. Urine aldehyde measurement is 50 times more sensitive than blood aldehyde levels.

This test is used:
1. To identify oxidative stress patterns in the body.
2. To indicate antioxidant status.

Directions:
Ideally all supplement use should stop two days prior to test. It is best to get the first morning urine and refrigerate the urine specimen in an airtight container. Urine should be at room temperature for the test.
1. Draw urine into the dropper supplied with the test kit.
2. Break open the top of the glass ampoule, which contains the reagent.
3. Place urine into the ampoule.
4. Wait five minutes, and then interpret the color change from the color metric chart and record result

Results

Pink color or +1	Optimal reading indicates optimum oxidation, healthy, and normal
Clear or 0	Abnormal reduced oxidation and low electron potential
Red +2	Moderate oxidation – level of free radical activity and oxidative stress is beginning to increase
Dark red +3	Heavy oxidation - levels of free radicals and oxidative stress are too high.

Low – Clear or 0

Implication	Information
Loss of energy electrons	A low redox indicates the loss of high-energy electrons in the urine causing a low electron potential. Electrons, produced by glycolosis and the Kreb's cycle, are not being used by the cell's mitochondria, because of mitochondrial membrane problems. This result in the inability to produce ATP and increase levels of fatigue. The electrons are excreted in the urine. This situation has been called Ox-phos derailment. The oxidative phosghorylation process has been derailed from the Kreb's cycle. This can indicate mitochondrial membrane dysfunction or a lack of ubiquinone or CoQ10, the last enzyme in the oxidative phosphorylation process, which "transports" energy intermediates through the enzymatic pathway.

High Increase In Oxidative Stress
+2 or Red color change

Implications	Information
Liver stress	The liver uses oxidation to perform its functions. Increasing oxidative stress puts more strain on the liver.
Kidney stress	The glomerulus of the kidney is sensitive to oxidative damage. Many of the xenotoxins that cause oxidative stress can damage the kidneys and block glomerular filtering function.
Pancreas stress digestive and blood sugar dysregulation	Increased oxidation stresses the pancreas, which impairs its function resulting in blood sugar problems and improper digestion.
Adrenal stress	Increased oxidation stresses the adrenal glands.
Lymphatic congestion	Increased lymphatic congestion can increase the levels of oxidation and decrease the body's ability to filter out waste.
Fatigue	There is a tendency of the decreased production of high-energy electron intermediates from the Kreb's cycle, which alters the cells ability to produce energy. As oxidation increase there is a reduced output of ATP from the mitochondria, resulting in fatigue. This process has been called a Kreb's cycle or Tri Carboxylic Acid (TCA) disruption.

+3 or Dark Red color change

Implications	Information
Lymphatic stress	The lymph system becomes impaired with the presence of pro-oxidative toxins, which increases oxidative stress
Xenotoxins	An increased tendency of the presence of xenotoxins in the body, which is increasing the oxidative stress
Greatly reduced ATP production	High oxidative stress decreases the production of high energy electron intermediates from the Kreb's cycles, which decreases the cell's ability to produce energy. As oxidation increases there is decreased output of ATP from the mitochondria, which causes fatigue and a slowing down of essential enzymatic pathways. This process has been called a Kreb's cycle or Tri Carboxylic Acid (TCA) disruption.
Maldigestion	The effect of increasing oxidative stress on the pancreas can weaken digestive enzyme production leading to maldigestion
Blood sugar dysregulation	The effect of increasing oxidative stress on the pancreas can impair the release of insulin from the beta islet cells.

Oxidative Stress and Free Radicals

Oxidative stress can cause an imbalance between the reactive oxygen species or free radicals and the antioxidant levels which result in an increase in species. Free radicals are reactive and unstable molecules. Free radicals unpaired electrons disrupt, disturb, and damage tissue. Molecules can have their electron orbitals occupied by paired electrons of opposite spin. This would be ideal and a stable state. The unpaired electron in the outer shell causes the instability and reactivity of all free radicals. Free radicals can be stopped by antioxidants, which can donate an electron and thus neutralize the problem and make the free radical stable and unharmful. This is the normal physiological activity that is used to neutralize toxins and harmful free radical molecules. Molecules become harmful if they are not immediately neutralized.

Free radicals are formed inside the body (endogenously) or from exposure to toxic chemicals outside the body (exogenous).

Endogenous causes of free radicals

1. The mitochondria, which is a source of endogenous free radicals formed by the enzymatically-controlled transfer of energized electrons for ATP generation in Oxidative phosphorylation.
2. The liver creates free radicals as part of the cytochrome P450 system of detoxification.
3. The Immune system uses oxidative species such as hypochlorite to neutralize microbes and their waste products.
4. The Immune, endocrine and neurological systems react to excessive stress via neurotransmitter activity that produces free radicals.

Exogenous causes of free radicals

1) The primary cause of increased free radicals is exposure to Xenobiotics, which causes the liver and adrenal cortex to produce free radicals. This depletes specific cellular antioxidants such as Glutathione, Vitamin C or Vitamin E. Xenobiotics that people are exposed to include:
   a. Pesticides and Herbicides
   b. Food additives, Junk Foods
   c. Household chemicals
   d. Industrial solvents
      Fuels and Fuel additives
   e. Synthetic Fertilizers
   f. Drugs (Proscription, legal and illegal)
   g. Air pollution
   h. Alcohol, cigarette and marijuana smoke

2) Exposure to radiation (cell phones, microwaves, LCD, plasma HDTV etc.)
3) Exposure to trauma, injuries
4) Exposure to cold

Free radical or oxidative stress can be a major factor in many chronic illnesses. Free radicals contribute to the following:

1) Diabetes and the destruction of pancreatic beta cells, which results in type 1 diabetes.
2) Tissue damage to colonic mucosal cells on ulcerative colitis and Inflammatory Bowel Disease.
3) Increased risk of breast and cervical cancer from increased levels of lipid peroxides, which are oxidized fats, in the tissue.
4) Damage to liver cell membranes, which result in impaired cellular transport, cell-to-cell communication and binding.
5) Damage to liver cells from junk food, drugs, sodas etc....
6) Disordered calcium, magnesium, and potassium cellular movement.
7) Interference in oxidative phosphorylation and the ability to convert the bi-products of the Kreb's cycle into ATP.
8) Oxidation of processed polyunsaturated and saturated fats, and increased risk of cardiovascular disease.
9) Cataract formation.
10) Decreased energy production, a cause of chronic fatigue.

11) Depressed immune function.
12) Alterations in the nucleic acids that make up the DNA, leading to increased cancer formation.
13) Rheumatoid arthritis, systemic lupus Erythematosus and glomerular diseases, which can increase levels of free radicals and lipid peroxides.
14) Systemic and local inflammation.

Assessment of Acid/Alkaline Imbalances

Assessment of acid/alkaline imbalances is evaluated by observing the patterns between the following:

1) Breath holding time
2) Respiration rate
3) Urine pH
4) Saliva pH

Breathe holding time and respiration rate

Breath holding time and respiration rate indicate the participation of the respiratory system in patterns of acid/alkaline imbalance in the bicarbonate buffering system,
The respiratory system maintains 50%-70% of pH compensation, the breath holding time and the respiration rate used to indicate the presence of an acidosis or alkalosis.

A normal breath hold time and respiration rate, it indicates no imbalances in the primary buffering system.

Urine pH and Salivary pH

The urine pH and salivary pH identify the type of acidosis or alkalosis, but not the presence of acidosis or alkalosis – only the breath hold time and respiration do that.

Breathe –Hold Test

The cardiovascular, pulmonary, or respiratory tract infections, breath – holding time can alter acid/alkaline pH balance. In acidosis there is high carbon dioxide and a decreased transport and uptake of oxygen by the body, causing a decreased breathe holding time. In alkalosis there is an increased uptake and transport of oxygen, as well as a compensatory suppression of the respiratory center, causing and increased inn the ability to hold ones breath.

This test is used to indicate acid/alkaline imbalance

Directions
This test is a measure of how long a person can hold a deep breath. When sitting, take a deep breath and hold it as long as you can. Use digital clock with a second hand to time the breath holding. When the breath can no longer held, record the seconds the breath was held on the results form.

Results: Normal 40 – 65

Increased Breath-Hold Time

Implication	Information
Metabolic alkalosis Respiratory alkalosis	Alkalosis causes an increase oxygen uptake and transport resulting in an increased ability to hold ones breath.
Metabolic acidosis Respiratory acidosis	In acidosis a decreased transport and uptake of oxygen by the body results in a decreased breath holding.
Anemia	Decreased oxygen carrying capacity of red blood cells caused by anemia may decrease breath hold time.
Other causes include	Antioxidant deficiency, emotional stress, anxiety

Directions for Test

Lingual Ascorbic Acid Test

1) Rinse the mouth thoroughly and the protruded tongue is grasped and held with a gauze pad.
2) With the mouth wide open, the anterior and middle third of the dorsum of the tongue may be observed.
3) Dry this area with a gauze pad being careful to stroke the papillae so that they stand erect.
4) Select an area with the papillae standing erect on the left or right of the midline of the tongue.
5) Drop 9 – 10 drops of the dye and begin timing immediately after the drop touches the tissue.
6) Continue timing until all the color has completely disappeared or 60 seconds has elapsed, and record the results in seconds.
7) Rinse the mouth thoroughly with water.

Dr. Bieler's Salivary pH Acid Challenge Test

1) Cut seven 2" strips of pH paper and lay out on paper towel.
2) Prepare lemon juice drink: 1 tablespoon of lemon juice and 1 tablespoon of water.
3) Make a pool of saliva in mouth and dip half of the strip, remove and measure pH. Record baseline.
4) Drink lemon juice, check pH and start timing.

Test and record pH every minute for 5 minutes

Zinc Taste Test

1) The mouth should be free of any strong tastes.
2) Hold 2 tablespoons of aqueous zinc in their mouth, sloshing it through the mouth.
3) Start timing and indicate when they taste the solution.
4) Swallow.
5) Describe the taste.

Record strength of taste and how many seconds it takes to taste the solution on the Functional Terrain Analysis Form.

Dr. Kane's Mineral Assessment Test

1) The mouth should be free of any strong tastes.
2) Pour a small amount of liquid in bottle #1 into a small cup.
3) Hold the solution in the mouth, sloshing it around their mouth.
4) Note the taste, if any, of the solution. Use the forms that come with the test to accurately document each response.
5) Continue with the other solution on the Functional Terrain Analysis Form.

Urine Specific Gravity Use Multistix 10 SG Test

1) Do not eat or drink any fluid for 1 to 2 hours then test.
2) For Multistix 10 SG test, dip Multistix in urine and take it out, then read results.

Urine Sediment Test

To determine the Total Urine Sediment:
CAUTION: Ferric Nitrate will stain yellow. Avoid contact with skin and clothing.

1) Add 10 ml of urine to a 15ml graduated centrifuge tube.
2) Add 4 droops of 50% Ferric Nitrate solution. Do not shake or mix.
3) Centrifuge the tube for 30 seconds.
4) Pour off the fluid away from the plug of solid matter.
5) Use the wooden end of a cotton applicator stick to level the sediment in the centrifuge tube.
6) Measure the amount (volume) of sediment in ml by visualizing where the sediment would level out rather than averaging the high and low points.
7) Record as total volume of the sediment on the Functional Terrain Analysis Form.

Calcium Phosphate Sediment

To determine sediment content:

1) Add enough 10% Acetic Acid to equal the amount of sediment shake or stir.
2) Fill to 10ml with Distilled Water.
3) Centrifuge tube at 3400 rpm for 30 seconds.
4) If sediment completely dissolves, record 100% Calcium Phosphate.
5) If sediment does not dissolve, pour off the fluid.
6) Measure the remaining sediment.
7) Subtract the remaining sediment measurement from the total sediment recorded above and record this number (in ml) as Calcium Phosphate on the Functional Terrain Analysis Form.

Total sediment - remaining sediment = Calcium Phosphate

Urine pH Using pH Meter

1) Remove protective cap on pH meter.
2) Insert pH meter into urine specimen.
3) Record digital reading.
4) Clean pH meter.
5) Calibration should take place after every 10 – 15 tests.

Urinary Adrenal Test For Urinary Chloride

1) Put 10 drops of urine into a small glass vial.
2) Add 1 drop of 20% Potassium Chromate – shake to mix.
3) Add 2.9% Silver Nitrate, one drop at a time – shake to mix.
4) Record the number of drops it takes to produce a deep brick red color --- no yellow remaining.

Urine Calcium Test

1) Put a dropper full of urine into a disposable glass test tube.
2) Add one dropper of Sulkowitch Reagent – shake to mix.
3) Wait 60 seconds.
4) Observe turbidity:
   - Record **Clear**... if there is little to no discernable fine white precipitate
   - Record **Light**... if you can see and read black type on a white page through the vial.
   - Record **Normal**... if the black type can be seen but not read through the vial.
   - Record **Heavy**... if the black type cannot be seen through the vial and precipitate rolls in the liquid.
   - Record **Milky**... if it looks like milk, which has been diluted with water.

Gastro Test For Determining Stomach pH

1) Eat protein rich meal 2 hours before test.
2) For an ambient pH, have the person fast for 8 – 10 hours.
3) Swallow a little water to lubricate the throat.
4) Swallow the capsule with a little water while the free end is held firmly outside the mouth.
5) After capsules has been swallowed, lay on left side or back on table for 10 minute.
6) After 10 minutes, sit up and with chin raised swiftly remove the string.
7) Lay string on paper and while the string is still moist, touch the pH stick to the string starting at the distal end.
8) The resultant colors are compared with the pH chart.

Uric Acid Sediment

1) Add enough 10% Sodium Hydroxide to equal the amount of sediment remaining in the test tube – stir well until color turns red.
2) Fill to 10ml with Distilled Water.
3) Centrifuge the tube for 30 seconds.
4) If sediment completely dissolves – record Uric Acid as the last amount (in ml) of sediments.
5) If sediment does not completely dissolve, pour off the fluid.
6) Measure the remaining sediment.
7) Subtract the remaining sediment from the previous remaining sediment calculated above and record this number (in ml) as Uric Acid on the Functional Terrain Assessment Form.

Calcium Oxalate Sediment

Record the sediment remaining in the test tube as Calcium Oxalate on the Functional Terrain Analysis Form.

Oxidata Free Radical Test

1) Draw urine into the dropper supplied with the test kit.
2) Break open the top of the glass ampoule, which contains the reagent.
3) Place urine into the ampoule.
4) Wait five minutes, then interpret the color change from the chart and record the result.

Iodine Patch

1) Paint a 2inch square patch of 2% solution of iodine onto the patient's abdomen.
2) Make sure it is dry before allowing it to come in contact with clothing, because it will stain.
3) Note the time of application and have the person record the time when they notice that it has disappeared.

Interpretations of Test Information

Metabolic pH Assessment

A balanced pH is important for bodily internal homeostatic mechanisms to function. The acidity in the stomach and alkalinity in the small intestine helps normal digestion. Other systems help with a balanced pH. The following is a list of the problems that can occur if the pH is out of balance:

1. Enzyme systems in the body fail to function.
2. The oxygen delivery mechanisms in the blood can be altered. The body stores excess acidity in the extracellular matrix (the spaces around the cells) of the tissue. The blood compensates for this, by increasing alkalinity. With increasing alkalinity, the red blood cells can saturate themselves in oxygen. Increasing oxygen saturation stops the red blood cells from releasing oxygen. If the blood cells do release oxygen, oxygen cannot get into the cells of the body causing tissue hypoxia and decreased production of ATP. Decreased oxygen content of cells can cause degenerative conditions.
3. Blood sugar dysregulation: the Insulin hormone facilitates the movement of glucose into the cell. The ability of the cells to recognize insulin is affected by pH fluctuations in the blood. The brain is one organ that relies on glucose and cannot store glucose and relies on the second to second supply of glucose from the bloodstream. pH fluctuations in the blood results in blood sugar problems and mood disorders.
4. Digestive function becomes impaired. Pancreatic insufficiency decreases the use of alkaline pancreatic fluids that buffer acidic blood. Hypochlohydria decreases the use of acidic stomach secretions that buffer an alkaline blood.
5. Electrolyte and mineral imbalance: Alkaline minerals and digestive fluid help to buffer the blood. The use of the digestive fluids to buffer the blood decreases and impairs digestion. This causes a negative effect on the digestion, absorption and assimilation of the alkaline minerals, which decreases the ability to use them to buffer the blood. The availability of there essential electrolytes and minerals is decreased, causing an electrolyte and mineral imbalance. Acids bind up the minerals in the buffering system and are no longer available to act as the co-factors for the mineral dependent enzyme reactions. An electrolyte imbalance decreases the ability of the extracellular fluid to carry nutrients and waste in and out to the cell, and the cell to carry on oxidation and other essential metabolic processes.
6. The electrical potential Theta of the cell begins to change. pH imbalances in the extracellular fluids interferes with the potential energy of the cell. The electrical cell potential is between 70 – 90mV, which is the optimal range for the movement of nutrients into the cell and waste products out the cell. Hyperacidity, heavy metals in the extracellular matrix and electromagnetic stress from microwaves, plasma HDTV's and cellular phones drop the voltage as low as 0mV. Under these circumstances, the cells cannot remove waste. Instead, they store waste, which reduces their function. As cellular function decreases, production of ATP decreases.

The body uses a number of complex buffering systems to keep pH within a normal and optimal range.

1° Buffering System	2°Buffering System
1. Bicarbonate buffering system(lungs and kidneys)	1. Alkaline minerals 2. Urea cycle (liver) and ammonia 3. Digestive system
The system used for about 90% of acid/alkaline buffering	The systems used for about 10% of acid/alkaline buffering

1°Buffering -- /the Bicarbonate Buffering System

The bicarbonate buffering system is the primary extracellular buffering system of the body. It maintains about 90% of the body's extracellular pH buffering. In this system, carbon dioxide, an acidic by-product of oxidative phosphorylation, combines with water using an enzyme called carbonic amhydrase, (an enzyme that needs the mineral zinc as a co-enzyme), to form carbonic acid. Carbonic acid is unstable in solution and will breakdown (dissociate) into its ionic form of bicarbonate ion and a hydrogen ion. The primary buffering system used is the kidney and respiratory systems to control acid/alkaline balance.

1. Respiratory system
   a. By altering the respiration rate and depth of breathing, the body can change the concentration of CO2 in the blood and control pH fluctuations.
   b. By increasing the respiration rate (hyperventilation) less CO2 is expelled from the body, which in turn raises the pH (more alkaline).
   c. By decreasing the respiration rate (hypoventilation) less CO2 is expelled from the body, which lowers the pH (more acidic)

2. The Kidney
   a. By altering the kidney's ability to reabsorb or excrete bicarbonate and H+ the body can change the concentration of bicarbonate of H in the Blood.
   b. Increased reabsorption of bicarbonate by the kidney in the descending loop of Henle will increase blood bicarbonate and raise the pH (more alkaline).
   c. Decreased reabsorption or increased excretion of bicarbonate will decrease blood bicarbonate and lower the pH (more acidic).

There are four main patterns of acid/alkaline imbalance that are outside of the body's control, which can alter the body's pH.

1. Metabolic acidosis 2. Metabolic alkalosis	1. Respiratory acidosis 2. Respiratory alkalosis
Two patterns of acid /base imbalance that are caused by alterations in bicarbonate (HCO^3) or H+ concentrations	Two patterns of acid based imbalance caused by alterations in CO^2 concentrations

In the above, the bicarbonate buffer begins to compensate:
1. The body starts to alter the respiration rate and depth of breathing in order to compensate by lowering or raising the amount of dissolved CO^2.
2. The body starts to alter the absorption or excretion of either bicarbonate (HCO3) or H+ via the renal tubules.

Determination of patterns of acid/alkaline imbalance
The evaluation of an acid/alkaline imbalance, requires measuring the body's compensatory mechanisms functions.

The below are factors:
When there is an acid/alkaline imbalance, the following are involved;
1. Acid/alkaline imbalance in the bicarbonate buffering system always involves the respiratory functions.
2. Acid/alkaline imbalances in the bicarbonate buffering system always involve the kidney.

An evaluation of imbalance determines whether the primary cause of the problem is the body's defense of compensation. This is seen in the respiratory system, which is involved in acidosis or alkalosis.

The respiratory system can cause the imbalance, or it can be the main defense in compensation for the imbalance. The respiratory system is always part of evaluating the patterns of acid/alkaline imbalance in the bicarbonate buffering system.

Respiratory system as a 1° cause of acid/alkaline imbalance		Respiratory system as a compensation for acid/alkaline imbalance	
Causative in respiratory acidosis and respiratory alkalosis		Compensatory in metabolic acidosis and metabolic alkalosis	
Respiratory acidosis	❖ Caused by hypoventilation ❖ CO_2 produced faster than it can be blown off ❖ ↑carbonic acid retention➔ acidosis	**Metabolic acidosis**	❖ Respiratory activity is increased ❖ CO_2 blown off to lower carbonic acid levels
Respiratory alkalosis	❖ Caused by hyperventilation ❖ CO_2 blown off faster than it can be produced ❖ ↓ carbonic acid levels➔ alkalosis	**Metabolic alkalosis**	❖ Respiratory activity slowed down. ❖ Retention of CO_2 in the form of carbonic acid to decrease the alkalosis.

1° Buffering System

The bicarbonate buffering system is one of the extracellular buffering systems of the body. Intracellular and plasma buffering is controlled by protein buffers.

The following is the chemical buffering:
The bicarbonate buffering system is the main extracellular buffer in the body. It accounts for about 90% of the body's extracellular pH buffering. In this system, carbon dioxide, an acidic acid by-product of oxidative phosphorylation, combines with water using an enzyme called carbonic anhydrase, (an enzyme that needs the mineral zinc as a co-enzyme), to form carbon acid. Carbonic acid is fairly unstable in solution and will dissociate into its ionic form of a bicarbonate ion and a hydrogen ion:

CO_2 + H_2O ⇔ H_2CO_3 ⇔ HCO_3 + H^+
Carbon   Water   Carbonic Acid   Bicarbonate ion   Hydrogen
Dioxide   ion

An increase in dissolves CO_2 An increase of bicarbonate ion
CO_2 will decrease the pH or   concentration will cause the pH
shift the acid/alkaline balance   to ride i.e. shift toward the alkaline.
toward acid.

The bicarbonate buffering systems help by physiological buffers because of losing CO_2 through respiration and bicarbonate and H+ through the kidneys. The body uses the respiratory and renal systems to control pH fluctuations.

A. <u>The Respiratory system: Alterations of the respiration rate and depth of breathing to control pH</u>

The body changes the respiration rate and depth of breathing to change the relative concentration of CO_2 in the blood and control pH fluctuations:

I. By increasing the respiration rate (hyperventilation) more CO_2 is expelled from the body, which in turns raises the pH (more alkaline)
II. By decreasing the respiration rate (hypoventilation) less CO_2 is expelled from the body, which lowers pH (more acidic)

The respiratory system helps to maintain 50%-70% of pH compensation, when the Bicarbonate buffering system is used.

B. <u>Renal system: Alterations in the kidneys ability to reabsorb or excrete bicarbonate and H+</u>

The kidneys function to reabsorb or excrete bicarbonate and H+ to change the relative concentration of bicarbonate or H+ in the blood. The kidneys, in collaboration with the liver, use the following mechanisms:
I. Increased reabsorption pH bicarbonate by using the kidney in the descending loop of henle will increase blood bicarbonate and thus raise the pH (more alkaline)
II. Decreased reabsorption or increased excretion of bicarbonate will decrease blood bicarbonate and thus lower the pH (more acidic)

The renal system helps to maintain 30%-50% of pH compensation, along with the bicarbonate buffering system is used.

Factors outside of the body can alter the body's pH. There are four main patterns of acid/alkaline imbalance that are seen when this happens:

1. Metabolic acidosis 2. Metabolic alkalosis	3. Respiratory acidosis 4. Respiratory alkalosis
Two patterns of acid/alkaline imbalance that are caused by alterations in bicarbonate (HCO^3) or H+ concentration	Two patterns of acid based imbalance caused by alteration in CO^3 concentrations

In the above, the bicarbonate buffer begins to compensate:
1. The body changes the respiration rate and depth of breathing in order to compensate by lowering or raising the amount of dissolved CO_2.
2. The body changes the reabsorption or excretion of either bicarbonate (HCO^3) or H+

Determination of Patterns of Acid/Alkaline Imbalance

The determination of an acid/alkaline imbalance includes the body's compensatory mechanism at work.

The following are factors:
1. Acid/alkaline imbalances in the bicarbonate buffering system always involve the respiratory functions.
2. Acid/alkaline imbalances in the bicarbonate buffering system always involve the kidneys.

Acid/alkaline imbalance, can be the primary cause of the problem or the body's defense or compensation. The respiratory system is always a factor in acidosis or alkalosis.

The respiratory system can be the main cause of the imbalance, or, it can be the primary defense in compensation for the imbalance. The respiratory system is part of evaluation the patterns of acid/alkaline imbalance in the bicarbonate buffering system.

Respiratory system as 1° cause of acid/alkaline imbalance		Respiratory system as a compensation for acid/alkaline imbalance	
Causative in respiratory acidosis and respiratory alkalosis		Compensatory in metabolic acidosis and metabolic alkalosis	
Respiratory acidosis	❖ Caused by hypoventilation ❖ CO_2 produced faster than it can be blown off ❖ ↑carbonic acid retention→acidosis	**Metabolic acidosis**	❖ Respiratory activity is increased ❖ CO_2 blown off to lower carbonic acid levels
Respiratory alkalosis	❖ Caused by hyperventilation ❖ CO_2 blown off faster than it can be produced ❖ ↓carbonic acid levels→alkalosis	**Metabolic alkalosis**	❖ Respiratory activity slowed down. ❖ Retention of CO_2 in the form of carbonic acid to decreased the alkalosis.

Acid/Alkaline Assessment

Pattern	Interpretation	Implication
↑ **Respiratory Rate** ↓ **Breath hold** ↓ **Urine pH** ↓ **Saliva pH**	**Metabolic Acidosis**	1. Alkaline saliva—the respiratory system kicks in by increasing the rate and depth of breathing to blow off as much CO_2 as possible. This will lower the carbonic acid levels in the body causing alkaline saliva. 2. Acid urine—this represents the kidney excreting H+ 3. Increased respiratory rate -- The body is attempting to blow off CO_2 to decrease carbonic acid levels. 4. Decreased breath holding time – acidosis causes a decreased oxygen transport and uptake, causing a decreased ability to hold ones breathe.
↑/↓ **Respiratory Rate** ↓ **Breath hold** ↓ **Urine pH** ↓ **Saliva pH**	**Respiratory Acidosis**	1. Acid saliva – due to the increased levels of CO_2 and carbonic acid 2. Acidic urine – due to the kidney excretion of H+ 3. Increased respiratory rate – The body is attempting to blow off CO_2 to decrease carbonic acid levels that have built up as a result of the hypoventilation, which causes respiratory acidosis. 4. Decreased breath holding time – acidosis causes a decreased oxygen transport and uptake, thus leading to decreased ability to hold ones breath

↑/↓ Respiratory Rate ↑ Breath hold ↑ Urine pH ↑ Saliva pH	**Respiratory Alkolisis** (known as stress or anxiety alkalosis)	1. Alkaline saliva – due to the increased loss of CO_2 and carbonic acid 2. Alkaline urine – due to the kidney retention of H+ 3. The respiratory rate may be increased or decreased – The body is attempting to blow off CO_2 to decreased the carbonic acid levels but the respiration patterns are often irregular 4. Increased breath holding time – alkalosis causes an increased oxygen transport and uptake, thus leading to an increased ability to hold ones breath
↓ Respiratory Rate ↑ Breath hold ↑ Urine pH ↓ Saliva pH	**Metabolic Alkalosis**	1. Acidic saliva – a slowing of the respiration will cause more carbonic acid in the extracellular fluids leading to an acidic saliva. 2. Alkaline urine – due to kidney excretion of bicarbonate and retention H+ 3. Decreased respiratory rate – as a result of the suppression of respiratory centers (the body is attempting to lessen the blow off CO_2 to increase carbonic acid levels.) 4. Increased breath holding time – alkalosis causes an increased ability to hold ones breath.

Assessment

PATTERN	INTERPRETATION	IMPLICATIONS
↑ Adrenal score ↓ Urine chloride ↑ Urine pH	**Excess alkaline reserves**	The extracellular fluid is alkaline. Large amounts of chloride are reabsorbed resulting in a decreased urine chloride. The renal tubules release bicarbonate and hold onto H+ in order to buffer the excess alkalinity
↓ Adrenal score ↑ Urine chloride ↓ Urine pH	**Excess acid reserves** **Electrolyte insufficiency**	The extracellular fluid is acidic causing the renal tubules to reabsorb bicarbonate in order to buffer the acidity. Urine becomes more acidic. Chloride ion reabsorption is decreased resulting in a high urine chloride and a low adrenal score. This is a normal variation.
↑ Adrenal score ↓ Urine chloride ↓ Urine pH	**Potassium deficiency** **Salt deficiency**	The blood is deficient in potassium, from junk foods, refined carbohydrates, sugar, or diuretic use, caues this pattern. The body is excreting H+ and retaining chloride, which leads to an acidic urine. In a low state pH state the body excretes ore potassium. If the pattern and urine output is low consider sodium deficiency because the body is retaining chloride and excreting H+.

PATTERN		
↓ Adrenal score ↑ Urine chloride ↑ Urine pH ↑ Calcium	Excess salt	This indicates the body is excreting bicarbonate, chloride, and calcium. This pattern indicates consumption of excess amounts of salt.
↓ Adrenal score ↑ Urine chloride ↑ Urine pH ↓ Calcium	Excess potassium	This is similar but different from the one above. This indicates the excretion of bicarbonate and chloride, and retention of calcium. This indicates salt deficient diets or too much potassium.

Calcium and Mineralization

PATTERN	INTERPRETATION	IMPLICATION
↓ Urine pH ↓ Calcium	Excess stomach acid	Excess stomach acid – possible causes are indicated with this pattern are: • Very high protein diet • Magnesium neutralizes HCl in the stomach • Medications • Taking Betaine HCl • Acid retention due to kidney disease • Ketosis from fasting or diabetes
↓ Urine pH ↑ Calcium	Complex carbohydrate deficiency Alkaline mineral deficiency	Complex carbohydrate deficiency associated with a junk food high in sugar and protein (↑sugar can cause ↑ calcium in the urine in the urine) Alkaline minerals are being depleting in order to alkalinize the cell. A pattern seen in respiratory conditions such as asthma and emphysema. This is seen after acute asthma attack.
↑ Urine pH ↓ Calcium	Hypochlorhydria	Hypochlorhydria can cause poor protein digestion resulting in low calcium levels because half of the calcium becomes bound to protein. It is suggestive of the following: • Poor protein and calcium digestion and transportation due to hypochlorhydria • Poor reserve levels of calcium in the bones • Fatty acid deficiency
↑ Urine pH ↑ Calcium	Protein deficiency	This indicates a protein deficiency caused by a low protein diet or poor protein absorption. Use of protease to increase absorption can be useful. The increase in calcium can be caused by the intake of non ionizing form of calcium.
N Urine pH ↓ Calcium	Low calcium levels in the body	Can be caused by insufficient intake of calcium or other factors that affect calcium digestion, absorption and utilization. The unabsorbed calcium will be excreted in the stool.

Macronutrient Improper Digestion Patterns

PATTERN	INTERPRETATION	IMPLICATIONS
↑ Adrenal score ↓ Urine chloride ↑ S.G	Protein maldigestion	This can indicate a difficulty in digesting protein either from a deficiency in protease enzyme or hypochlorhydria. This is indicated by a loss of muscle mass, poor recovery time after exercise, hypoglycemia/blood sugar dysregulation, and poor utilization of calcium and magnesium, which must bind with amino acids to be fully assimilated. This can indicate intestinal mucosal skin problems causing ileocecal valve problems, constipation and other lower bowel problems. This can be caused by glutamine deficiencies.
↑ Adrenal score ↓ Urine chloride ↓ S.G	Fat maldigestion	Indicates a difficulty digesting fats either from a deficiency in lipase enzymes or poor bile emulsification. It can be a fat intolerance. This indicates a deficiency in essential fatty acids, fat-soluble nutrient deficiencies and liver and/or gallbladder problems.
↓ Adrenal score ↑ Urine chloride	Fiber and carbohydrate maldigestion	Indicates fiber and carbohydrate maldigestion and metabolism, which can result from a deficiency in amylase or cellulose, or a high carbohydrate, low protein, low sodium, and low fat diet. This pattern can indicate irritable bowel type symptoms, such as diarrhea. With this combination the pituitary increases the stimulation of the ADH and GH to retain electrolytes. It can cause poor circulation, cold hands and feet, and a low sex drive.
↓ Adrenal score ↑ Urine chloride ↓ S.G	Sugar maldigestion	Indicates problems digesting metabolizing sugar. Indicates large amounts of refine carbohydrates and refine sugar intolerance. This pattern can indicate the following conditions: • Sugar handling difficulties • Malabsorption • Decreased cell permeability Sugar intolerance can cause depression, insomnia, emotional, and panic attacks.

Urine Bilirubin with Urine Urobilinogen levels

PATTERN	INTERPRETATION	IMPLICATION
↑ Bilirubin ↑ Urobilinogen	Liver dysfunction	Can indicate problems with the liver with possible hepatocellular dysfunction or partial obstruction.
↑ Bilirubin Neg Urobilinogen	Biliary Stasis	Indicates problems with the gallbladder or biliary stasis with congested bile or gallstone.
Neg Bilirubin ↑ Urobilinogen	Hemolytic in origin	There is an increase in red blood cell destruction caused by hemolytic anemia, oxidative stress ↑ Xenotoxins.

Other patterns:

Increased Oxidative Stress	↑ Oxidata test ↓ Lingual ascorbic acid test ↑ Urinary Urobilinogen ↑ Hemolyzed blood in urine

Acidic Urine – Urine pH < 6.4

Acidic urine indicates excess exogenously or endogenously produced acids, which are being excreted by the kidney.

Implication	Information
Alkalosis (respiratory or metabolic)	The body reacts to an acidosis by causing the kidneys to get rid of hydrogen and ammonia thus creating acidic urine.
Bacterial infection	This indicates consistent acid (below 6.4 pH) do not optimally digest carbohydrates and fats.

Alkaline Urine – Urine pH> 6.8

Implication	Information
Alkalosis (respiratory or metabolic)	The body reacts to an alkalosis by causing the kidney to both retain acid in the form of hydrogen and to excrete bicarbonate. Both of these will lead to alkaline urine.
Bacterial infection	Alkaline urine can cause a urinary tract bacterial infection. Need to rule this out first with the Multistix 10SG test for nitrites and leukocyte esterase. Common organisms include Proteus and Pseudomomas.

Results:
Normal: 7.1 – 7.4

Alkaline Saliva

Implication	Information
Metabolic Acidosis	The body responds to an acidosis by causing an increase in respiration to get rid of CO2 which will lower carbonic acid in the body, which causes a more alkaline salivary pH.
Respiratory Alkalosis	Extreme physiological stress can cause respiratory alkalosis. Too much CO2 is "blown off" from increased respirations or hyperventilation. This causes alkaline saliva.
Maldigestion	The more alkaline the saliva gets, the weaker the digestive juices in the stomach may become, causing maldigestion.
Hypochlorhdria	Alkaline saliva may indicate hypochlorhydria, which can upset the gastrointestinal equilibrium causing dysbiosis, yeast etc. that thrive in an abnormal digestive pH.
Sympathetic Dominance	Sympathetic dominance causes an increase excretion of potassium, which occurs with increased cellular acidity.
Dental Tartar	Alkaline saliva is one of the major causes of tartar buildup on the teeth.

Acidic Saliva

Implication	Information
Metabolic Alkalosis	The body reacts to an alkalosis by causing a compensatory suppression of the respiratory center in an attempt to retain CO2, causing increased levels of carbonic acid, and acid saliva.
Respiratory Acidosis	Respiratory acidosis is the result of insufficient respirations or air exchanges, which causes increased CO2 in the blood and concomitant acidic saliva.
Carbohydrate Maldigestion	Effective carbohydrate digestion depends upon the activation of alpha amylase in the saliva. A salivary pH below 7.1 will not provide the optimal pH for alpha amylase activity.
Pancreatic Insufficiency	Improper digestion caused by lack of enzymes can result on an increase in metabolic acid, which will cause acidity to build up in the interstitial fluids thus affecting salivary pH.
Essential Fatty Acid Deficiency	A salivary pH below 7.2 may indicate a deficiency in essential fatty acids.
Fat Digestion Problems	Excess dietary fats or an inability to completely metabolize fats will cause an increase in ketones, which will increase the acids present in the interstitium.
Dental Caries	Acidic saliva is a leading cause of dental caries and tooth decay.

Commonly Used Chemical Notations

Notation	Description
Na^+	The plus superscript indicates a positive ion.
Cl^-	The negative superscript indicates a negative ion.
$Na^+ + Cl^- \rightarrow NaCl$	The plus sign indicates synthesizing (combing) two particles. The right arrow indicates that a chemical reaction occurs towards a product.
$NaCl \rightarrow Na^+ + Cl^-$	Decomposing (breaking up) a molecule or chemical compound
$NaOH + HCl \rightarrow NaCl + H_2O$	Exchange reaction where a chemical compound is decomposed into its chemical elements are synthesized into o new compound. Here
$Na + Cl^- \rightleftarrows NaCl$	Reversible reaction is noted with a right arrow over a left arrow.
C - C	Single covalent bond.
C = C	Double covalent bond.
C ≡ C	Triple covalent bond.
H_2O	A subscript following a chemical symbol indicates the number of atoms (two hydrogen atoms). If no subscript is used, then it is implied there is one atom (here, one oxygen atom).

↑ = Increase

↓ = Decrease

> = More

< = Less

Common Signs and Symptoms of Acidosis and Alkalosis

ACIDOSIS	ALKALOSIS
1. Anxiety	1. Bad breath
2. Diarrhea	2. Cellulite
3. Poor digestion and assimilation of food	3. Constipation
4. Dilated pupils	4. Cold, clammy hands and feet
5. Fatigue, especially in early morning	5. Dizziness
6. Headaches, occipital to frontal	6. Fatigue in mornings, hard to arise from bed
7. High blood pressure and rapid heart beat	7. Headaches, side of head, temples (migraine)
8. Hyperactivity	8. Excitability of nervous system
9. Insomnia	9. Indigestion, fermentation
10. Nervousness	10. Introverted behavior, depression
11. Restless legs	11. Leg and muscle cramps, tetany
12. Shortness of breath	12. Low blood pressure
13. Warm, dry hands and feet	13. Paleness
14. Strong appetite	14. Slow pulse
15. Dry mouth	15. Sluggishness
16. Allergies	16. Poor digestion and assimilation of food due to decreased gastric secretion
17. Poor retention of important mineral nutrients	17. Joint and muscle pain
18. Inefficient function of kidneys, lungs and adrenal glands	18. Allergies – asthma
19. Inflammation	19. Poor retention of important mineral nutrients
20. Skin irritation 21. Arthritis	

Causes Of Respiratory Acidosis and Alkalosis

RESPIRATORY ACIDOSIS	RESPIRATORY ALKALOSIS
The cause of respiratory acidosis is hypoventilation; CO_2 is being blown off at a slower rate than it is being produced, which is usually caused by insufficient respirations or air exchange.	Respiratory alkalosis indicates stressor anxiety alkalosis because it can be caused by excessive physiological stress. Too much acid is "blown off" from increased respirations or hyperventilation. Some of the causes include:
1. Hypoventilation in compensation for metabolic alkalosis	1. Chronic and acute anxiety – respiratory alkalosis is called stress alkalosis
2. Acute respiratory acidosis can be seen in asthma	2. Low blood pressure causes a decreased flow of oxygenated blood through the aortic and carotid arteries, which stimulates the respiratory centers to increase respiratory rate.
3. High blood pressure: As blood pressure increases, the aorta and carotid arteries carry more oxygenated blood past the chemoreceptors, when stimulated the decrease respiratory rate by changing rate and depth of breathing. This results in respiratory acidosis.	3. Shock
4. A mild respiratory acidosis can occur at night because of a diminished respiration, which can cause acidic urine first thing in the morning.	4. Sepsis
5. Head injury (concussion) can damage the respiratory center in the Medulla Oblongata, which causes decreased respiration.	5. Head trauma (i.e. concussion) can damage the respiratory centers, which can cause hyperventilation.
6. Chest trauma can cause a compromised breathing rate and depth.	6. Psychoneurosis causing hyperventilation and an excess loss of CO_2. Hyperventilation of psychogenic or emotional origin, the increase in alkalosis causes the tingly sensation around the mouth and in the fingertips. Because of hyperventilation, blood is slowed to the brain, which stimulates the respiratory center to increase respirations. In psychogenic hyperventilation, the symptoms of tingling and feeling of smothering continue to worsen.
7. Respiratory diseases – Chronic respiratory acidosis can be caused by respiratory diseases such as emphysema and pneumonia, which have an increase in dead air space in the lungs and decreased pulmonary membrane surface area. This causes the lungs to malfunction. Acidosis develops slowly over a period of time.	7. High altitudes can cause a lowered concentration of oxygen, which triggers an increased respiration that lowers CO_2 concentration.
8. Obstruction to the respiratory passages	

Causes of Metabolic Acidosis and Alkalosis

METABOLIC ACIDOSIS	METABOLIC ALKALOSIS
1. Inefficient formation of ATP – an uncoupling of the Kreb's cycle from the oxidative phosphorylation system, caused by increasing oxidative stress will cause the creation and formation of organic acid metabolites in the cell.	**1. Use of diuretics** – Cause water, cation and chloride depletion, which bicarbonate ion is retained. Loss of $H+$, $K+$, and $Mg+$ exceeds loss of sodium.
2. The incomplete digestion / oxidation of proteins, fats and carbohydrates as a result of diminished or depleted enzymes or stomach acid can cause the build up of organic acids.	**2. Loss of acid** – loss of gastric fluid (Excessive vomiting), poor urinary retention of $H+$
3. Increasing kidney stress- Kidneys fail to process and eliminate $H+$.	**3. Chloride depletion-** adrenal fatigue, loss of gastric juice, poor retention of $Cl-$ and $K+$ ions
4. Anaerobic respiration causes a ↑production of lactic and pyruvic acids as a result of lack of oxygenation because of poor breathing techniques.	**4. Excess secretion of aldosterone** from the adrenal cortex- Causes a large amount of sodium to be re-absorbed and urinary loss of $H+$, $Cl-$ and $K+$ ions
5. Renal loss of bicarbonate, sodium and potassium	**5. Alkaline drugs-** e.g. the H^2 blockers of stomach acidity
6. Stress – excess stimulation of the sympathetic nervous system creates increased cellular metabolism and concentrations of acidic metabolites	**6. Excess consumption of bicarbonate-** Causes a decreased level of $H+$; anti-acids
7. A deficiency in vitamins and minerals used as buffers by the body	
8. Lack of exercise: muscles movement of the body fails to clean and filter lymph	
9. Liver dysfunction causes a failure of the liver dependent urea cycle to flush out acids	
10. Heavy metals and other oxidative catalysts	
11. Microbes- bacteria, funguses etc. produce acidic waste	
12. Consumption of organic acids: alcohol, sodas, coffee	
13. Drugs: both prescription and recreational	
14. Severe diarrhea and deep vomiting, which cause the loss excess bicarbonate.	

Salivary pH

Carbohydrate maldigestion	Effective carbohydrate digestion requires the activation of alpha amylase in the saliva. A salivary pH below 7.1 will not provide the optimum pH for alpha amylase activity, causing possible gas and bloating.
Pancreatic insufficiency	Improper digestion caused by a lack of enzymes can cause an increased in metabolic acids, which will cause acidity to build up in the interstitial fluids thus affecting salivary pH.
Essential fatty acid deficiency	A salivary pH below 7.2 can indicate a deficiency in essential fatty acids.
Fat digestion problems	Excess dietary cooked fats or an inability to completely metabolize fats will cause an increase in ketones, which will increase the acids present in the interstitium.
Alkaline mineral insufficiency	Alkaline or acidic saliva indicates that the alkaline mineral buffering reserves have been depleted and the body is being forced to compensate by other means.
Dental caries	Acidic saliva is one of the leading causes of dental caries and tooth decay.
Other conditions associated with acidic saliva	Anxiety, Chronic stress, Need of detoxification, Mental/emotional factors, Lack of exercise

Factors:

Falsely increased levels	Falsely decreased levels
• Exercise and perspiration increase saliva pH causing loss of acids through the skin • Increases during meals	• Smoking • Saliva pH decreases during sleep, after meals • Bacteria and microbes

Related Test:
Urine pH, breath-holding time, respiration rate

Findings in Patterns of Acidosis and Alkalosis

PATTERN	METABOLIC ACIDOSIS	METABOLIC ALKALOSIS
Discussion	A build – up of H+ in cellular fluids that leads to systemic acidosis	↑ Excretion of H+ or retention of HCO3→systemic alkalosis
Respiratory rate	**Increased** The respiratory system compensates by ↑the rate and depth of respiration to blow off CO^2 and ↓ carbonic acid levels	**Decreased** Suppression of respiratory centers causes ↓ rate and depth of respiration to retain CO^2 and ↑ ability to hold one's breath
Breath hold time	**Decreased** Acidosis cause ↓ O^2 transport and uptake leading to a ↓ ability to hold one's breath	**Increased** Alkalosis causes an ↑O^2 transport and uptake leading to a ↑ ability to hold one's breath
Urine pH	**Decreased** Acidic urine – kidneys compensate by excreting H+ in urine and retaining bicarbonate	**Increased** Alkaline urine – Kidneys compensate by retaining H+ and excreting bicarbonate in urine

Saliva pH	**Decreased** Acidic saliva - ↑ levels of CO_2 and carbonic acid due to hypoventilation	**Increased** Alkaline saliva- ↓ levels of CO_2 and carbonic acid due to hyperventilation

PATTERN	METABALIC ACIDOSIS	METABOLIC ALKALOSIS
Discussion	Retention of H+ due to ↓ excretion of CO_2 from lungs	↑Excretion of H+ or retention of HCO_3 → systemic alkalosis
Respiratory rate	**Decreased as a 1° cause** ↓Respiration rate (hypoventilation) is the primary cause of acidosis in respiratory acidosis. **Increased in compensation** The respiration rate is ↑in respiratory compensation for metabolic acidosis. Rate and depth of respiration is ↑ to blow off more CO_2 and ↓carbonic acid levels.	**Increased as a 1° cause** ↑Respiration rate (hyperventilation) is the primary cause of alkalosis in respiratory alkalosis. **Decreased in compensation** The respiration rate ↓ in respiratory compensation for metabolic alkalosis. Rate and depth of respiration is ↓ to retain more CO_2 and ↑ carbonic acid levels.
Breath hold time	**Decreased** Acidosis causes a ↓O_2 transport and uptake leading to a ↓ability to hold ones breath	**Increased** Alkalosis causes an ↑O_2 transport and uptake leading to a ↑ ability to hold one's breath
Urine pH	**Decreased** Acidic urine – kidneys compensate by excreting H+ in urine and retaining bicarbonate	**Increased** Alkaline urine – Kidneys compensate by retaining H+ and excreting bicarbonate in urine
Saliva pH	**Decreased** Acidic saliva - ↑ levels of CO_2 and carbonic acid due to hypoventilation	**Increased** Alkaline saliva- ↓ levels of CO_2 and carbonic acid due to hyperventilation

Urine pH: >6.8

Implication	Information
Bacterial infection	Alkaline urine can cause a urinary tract bacterial infection. Need to rule this out first with Multistix 10SG test for nitrites and leukocyte esterase. Common organisms include Proteus and Pseudomonas
Kidney stress	A symptom of an overly acidic body. The kidney is unable to keep up with the free unbuffered acids. It compensates by dumping the alkaline reserves.
Liver stress	Liver support is needed to enhance the urea cycle, which will increase the body's ability to remove excess acids and take the stress off of the kidneys.

Subsequent Urine Samples

<u>Optimum range:</u>
Subsequent samples: **6.4 – 6.8**
The value that should be used in the pH assessments patterns

Alkaline Urine – Urine pH: >6.8

Implication	Information
Bacterial infection	Alkaline urine can cause a urinary tract bacterial infection. Need to rule this our first with a Multistix 10SG test for nitrites and leukocyte esterase. Common organisms include Proteus and Pseudomonas
Susceptibility to virus and yeast	People who tend to have an alkaline pH can tend to have more susceptibility to viral conditions, chronic fatigue, Epstein Barr, and Candida (yeast overgrowth).
Protein maldigestion	A pH that is consistently above 6.7 poor digestion of proteins because of a protease deficiency
Alkalosis (respiratory or metabolic)	The body reacts to an alkalosis by causing the kidney to both retain acid in the form of hydrogen, and to excrete bicarbonate. Both of these can cause alkaline urine.
Other possible problems of urine pH increase.	1. Calcium metabolism problems 2. Anxiety 3. Immune dysfunction
These conditions may be associated with an alkaline urine	Pyloric obstruction, salicylate intoxication, renal tubular acidosis, chronic renal and/or, respiratory disease involving hyperventilation and of CO_2, vomiting, metabolic alkalosis

Urine pH: 5.65—6.8

Implication	Information
Increasing loss of buffer control	Inability to release stored acids indicates an increased difficulty in maintaining buffering control.

Acidic Urine – Urine pH<6.4

Acidic urine indicates an increase of exogenously or endogenously produced acids, which are being excreted by the kidney.

Implication	Information
Maldigestion	The incomplete oxidation of food causes an excess acid production in the tissues that are being excreted.
Carbohydrate and fat maldigestion	People who are consistently acidic (below 6.4 pH), do not adequately digest carbohydrate and fats.
Pancreatic insufficiency	Excess acid reserve indicates decreased alkalinity and an inability to activate pancreatic enzymes in the duodenum.
Acidosis (respiratory and metabolic)	The body responds to an acidosis by causing the kidneys to dump hydrogen and ammonia resulting in acidic urine.
Other problems of a urine pH decrease	Being more susceptible to acidic, hot, irritation conditions such as inflammation, degeneration, arthritis, and skin irritations.
These conditions may be associated with an acid pH	Metabolic and respiratory acidosis, uncontrolled diabetes, pulmonary emphysema, diarrhea, fasting and starvation, dehydration.

Factors

Falsely increased levels	Falsely decreased levels
• A urine sample that is left to stand, un-refrigerated will become alkaline because bacteria split the urea into ammonia (an alkaline base). Urine must be refrigerated if there is a delay between sample collection and testing.	• Consumption of cranberry juice may falsely acidify the urine • Ammonium chloride supplementation can cause acidity

Related Test:
Salivary pH, breath holding time, respiration rate, urinary calcium, urinary sediment, urinary chloride

Salivary pH

Saliva and lymph are formed from the interstitial fluid. It contains the following secretions:
- Ptyalin, an alpha amylase, which is a carbohydrate-digesting enzyme
- Mucin mucous secretions for lubrication
- Interstitial fluid contains alkaline minerals and bicarbonate. Salivary pH indicates the health of the extracellular fluids, their alkaline mineral reserves and, the results of the urine pH, breath holding time and respiration rate which can be used to assess the body's regulation for effective ptyalin activity, a pH dependent enzyme. A salivary pH between 7.1 and 7.4 usually is not deficient in essential fatty acids.

Salivary pH depends on other indications:

1. The main physiological indicator is the relative concentration of free CO2 and combined CO^2, in the form of carbonic acid (H^2CO^3). This buffering system will have the main effect on salivary pH.
    a) A high CO^2 concentration in the blood causes an increase in carbonic acid. This causes acidic saliva. Which indicates respiratory acidosis and metabolic alkalosis.
    b) A low CO2 concentration causes a decrease in carbonic acid, which can cause alkaline saliva. This indicates respiratory alkalosis and metabolic acidosis.
2. The ratio of metabolic acids and alkaline forming electrolytes in the lymph or interstitial fluid can alter salivary pH.
    a) The pH of your saliva fluctuates from low to high during the day and is relative to your diet, and how your body is compensating for acid and alkaline shifts and your respirations.
    b) Ideally the first morning salivary pH or random salivary pH as a reference to subsequent samples.

Alkaline Saliva

Implication	Information
Metabolic Acidosis	The reaction to acidosis causes an increase in respiration to blow off CO2 and which will carbonic aid in the body causing a more alkaline salivary pH.
Respiratory Alkalosis	Physiological stress can cause respiratory alkalosis. Too much CO2 is "blown off" from increased respirations or hyperventilation. This causes alkaline saliva.
Maldigestion	The more alkaline the saliva gets, the weaker the digestive juices in the stomach causing maldigestion.
Hypochlorhydria	Alkaline saliva can indicate hypochlorhydria, which can upset the gastrointestinal equilibrium causing dysbiosis, yeast etc. that increase in an abnormal digestive pH.
Sympathetic dominance	Sympathetic dominance causes an increase excretion of potassium, which occurs with increased cellular acidity.
Alkaline Mineral insufficiency	Acid or alkaline saliva indicates that alkaline mineral buffering reserves have been decreased and the body is being forced to compensate by other means.
Dental tartar	Alkaline saliva is the main cause of tartar build-up on the teeth.
Symptoms associated with ↑ saliva pH	Increased respiration, stiff joints, muscle cramps, calcium deposition in soft tissues, hypoglycemia, discomfort after eating, dysbiosis

Acid Saliva

Implication	Information
Metabolic Alkalosis	The reaction to alkalosis causes a compensatory suppression of the respiratory center in an attempt to retain CO2, which leads to increased levels of carbonic acid, and an acid saliva.
Respiratory Acidosis	Respiratory acidosis is due to insufficient respirations or air exchange, which causes increased CO2 in the blood and a concomitant acid saliva
Malabsorption	Can indicate a decreased bowel transit time as foods are moving too quickly through the digestive tract thus decreasing the absorptive time

Medical Astrology

How to Do Your Astrology Chart

There are many free online astrology companies that will provide a Natal Chart for free. The free Natal Charts are very accurate and tend to use ONLY the glyph symbols. They do not provide an interpretation of the Natal Chart.

Draw a circle 3 or more inches in diameter. Divide the circle into 12 equal sections (houses). Number the equal sections (houses) from 1 to 12 as indicated on the "Houses of the Zodiac" Chart. Write the name of each house or use the glyph symbol (see Zodiac Sign Symbols). Number 1 is the First house Aires, 2nd Taurus, continued numbering until the 12th house Pisces. Write the planet name or glyph (see Anagram of Planets) in the appropriate house. This completes your Chart.

There are two types of astrology charts used for Medical Astrology, the Natal Chart and Sun Chart. The Natal Chart is specific and requires location of birth, date and time of birth. If you do not know the time of birth use 12 noon (1200 hour).

List the names of the planets in each Element. Choose the element with the most planets. List the names of the planets in each Quality. Choose the Quality with the most planets. List the names of the planets in each Triplicity. Choose the Triplicity house with the most planets. List the names of the planets in each Quadruplicity. Choose the Quadruplicity house with the most planets. If there is a high amount of planets in the same Element, Quality, or houses of a Triplicity or Quadruplicity choose the one with the most Adverse Aspects. Use the Zodiac Profile to identify specific concerns of a Sign such as part of body, type of Flower, Trees, Stress, Color, Cell Salt etc. with an overview of all the information decide on the major health.

For each planet look up the planet in a sign, make a brief note of medical information. Then, look up your planet in a house; make a brief note of medical information. The organ and disease that appears the most in your chart is the primary focus for a treatment. There are many ways to interpret a chart. You should use an interpretation method that you feel is easy or comfortable for you. You can stay with your choice of method and/or add another method or use multiple methods. You have a variety of chart interpretation methods to select from such as element and quality evaluation, health house, glands, signs, rulers of houses, cadent, angular, succedent, and aspects etc.

Anagrams

Anagrams create a word, which is made by taking the first letters of another word (i.e. sign, planet). Then, the words are used to form a sentence. These Anagrams can be used to help to know the signs and planets. The words formed are in the order of the signs and planets.

Anagram of Zodiac Signs

A T the **G**em **C**an **L**eo **V**isit the **L**ibrary to see **S**corpio put a **S**ack on a **C A P**.

A. T. (Aries ♈, Taurus, ♉) the
Gem (Gemini, ♊)
Can (Cancer, ♋)
Leo, ♌
Visit (Virgo, ♍) the
Library (Libra, ♎) to see
Scorpio, ♏ put a
Sack (Sagittarius, ♐) on a
C. A. P. (Capricorn ♑, Aquarius ♒, Pisces ♓)

Anagram of Planets

My **V**ery **E**ducated **M**other **J**ust **S**erved **U**s **N**ine **P**izzas
 Sun ☉
 Moon, ☽
My = Mercury ☿
Very = Venus ♀
Educated = Earth ⊕
Mother = Mars ♂
Just = Jupiter ♃
Served = Saturn ♄
Us = Uranus ♅
Nine = Neptune ♆
Pizzas = Pluto ♇

Zodiac Signs and Symbols

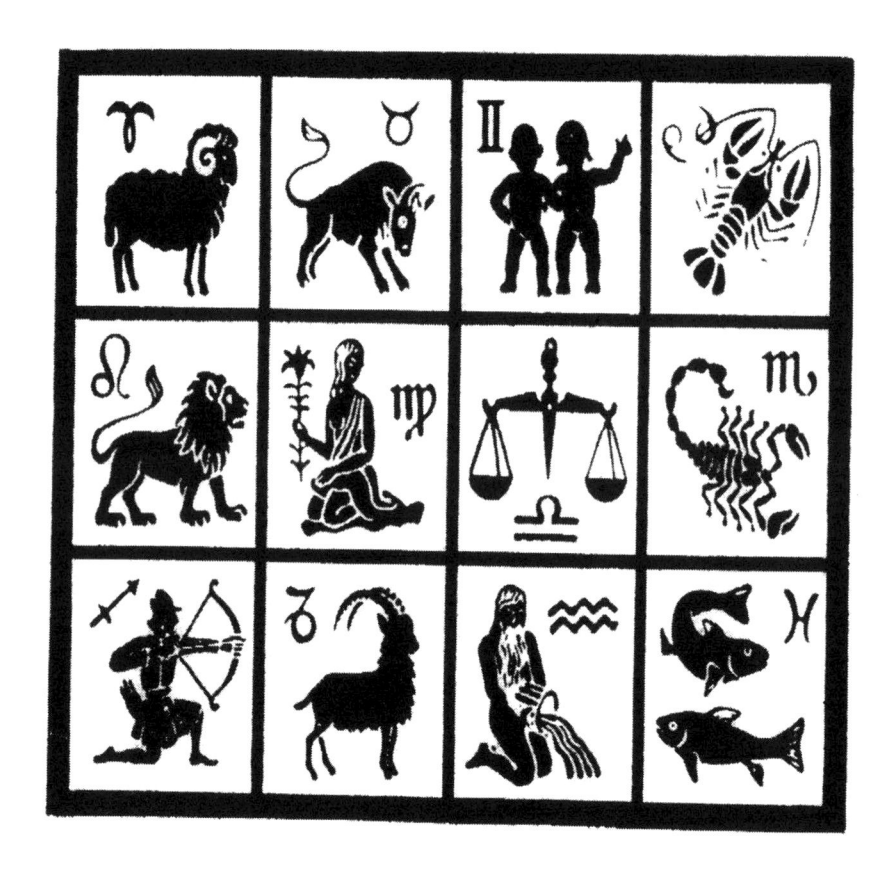

Zodiac Signs	*Egyptian Symbol*	*Modern Symbol*
Aires	Aries The Sheep	The Ram
Taurus	The Bull	The Bull
Gemini	Two Men Clasping Hands	The Twins
Cancer	The Scarab	The Crab
Leo	The Lion	The Lion
Virgo	The Maiden	The Virgin
Libra	The Horizon	The Scales
Scorpio	The Scorpion	The Scorpion
Sagittarius	He Who Draws a Bow	The Archer
Capricorn	The Goat	The Goat
Aquarius	The Water Man	The Water bearer
Pisces	The Fishes	The two Fishes

Element Evaluation

The Signs are classified as elements (Fire, Earth, Air, Water) and qualities (Cardinal, Fixed, Mutable), which can be used to understand the emotional problems a person, may have with a disease or disease treatment.

Fire
(Aires, Leo, Sagittarius)

Difficulties putting the treatment plan into action. Needs encouragement.

Earth
(Capricorn, Taurus, Virgo)

Finds it difficult to break bad health habits and lacks the ability to stay on treatment. Grows impatient with treatment protocol.

Air
(Libra, Aquarius, Gemini)

Tends to have problems understanding or accepting treatment. Usually is not interested in cause of disease and is only interested in the cure.

Water
(Pisces, Scorpio, Cancer)

Holds on to negative emotions, which can contribute to disease. Has problems expressing feelings about disease.

Quality Evaluation

Cardinal
(Activity, moveable= Aires, Cancer, Libra, Capricorn)

Open to many types of alternative disease treatments. Tends to have referred pain. Can be impatient. Usually has quick recovery from disease.

Fixed
(Rigid = Taurus, Leo, Scorpio, Aquarius)

Tends to lack endurance. Can be afraid of the treatment and may have weak immunity. Can have difficulties recuperating from disease.

Mutable
(Flexible = Gemini, Virgo, Sagittarius, Pisces)

Tends to start and stop treatment protocol. Usually is unable to accept responsibility for causing the disease and/or contributing to the wellness. Unstable and changeable disease condition. Tends to go from one healer to another healer.

Health House/ Planet Indicators

Health problems are indicated whenever Mars, Jupiter, Saturn, Uranus or Pluto form an adverse (negative) aspect such as a Square, Semi square, or Quincunx with a Sun Sign.

An aspect is the degrees apart between two planets. An aspect can be considered one planet "looking at" another planet. For example, if there is a Sun in Capricorn aspect then the Sun can be "looking at" Capricorn. This indicates that the Sun is placing its characteristics on Capricorn.

A square is two planets 90 degrees apart. It is an adverse (negative) aspect. This means that a disease can be stressful, cause physical, mental, and/or emotional difficulties, or challenges to health.

A semi square is two planets 45 degrees apart this is an Adverse aspect. This means that a mild disease challenges the health.

A Quincunx is two planets 150 degrees apart this is an Adverse aspect. This causes a disease to have unpredictable negative symptoms.

The combination of Aspects, Sun Sign, Planets, Houses etc. form a picture of a person's health.

Houses

5	Types of pregnancy, sex issues, drug use
6 (2, 10)	Sickness, acute disease, healing influences
1, 5, 9	Indicates disease and wellness state, has ability to follow protocol
8 (4, 12)	Indicates negative and/or positive types of transitions to wellness, addiction, and disease
12	Treatment facility, hospital and/or clinic, subjected to mental illness, chronic disease, diseases of long duration.

Barren Signs/Planets

Barren signs/planets means that the organ and/or organ system is non-functioning, malfunctioning decrease in function and/ or has a disease. Barren signs indicate that the part of the body ruled by the sign will have problems. A barren planet in a house indicates that the part of the body associated with the house will suffer disease, malfunction and/or degeneration.

Barren signs = Taurus, Gemini, Leo, Virgo
Barren Planets = Sun, Uranus, Saturn, Mars

Glands and Signs

Aires (Pituitary) – Secretes hormones that act on the reproductive organs, movement, growth of cells and tissue.
Taurus (Thyroid) – Thyroid hormone regulate metabolic functions, secretes thyroxin, thyrotropin, and uses iodine.
Gemini (Thymus) – Thymus hormones regulate immunity functions and maturation of T cell.
Libra (Adrenal) – Adrenal secrete hormones that stimulate metabolic functions, sympathetic and parasympathetic action, as well as epinephrine, norepinephrine and sex.
Scorpio (Gonads) – The ovaries and testicles gonads secrete hormones
Aquarius (Para-Thyroid) – Parathyroid hormones maintain mineral absorption and balance as well as calcium metabolism.
Pisces (Pineal) – Pineal hormones are the master hormones that regulate circadian cycles, growth, sleep, wake activities, and defend the health.

Rulers of the Houses

The twelve Houses are similar to the twelve Signs of the zodiac. The First House has the qualities of Aires the first sign of Zodiac; the Second House has qualities similar to the second sign of Taurus, and so on through the zodiac. The sign that corresponds to a House is the *natural ruler* of that House.

House	Zodiac Sign Ruler	Planet Ruler
First House is of the individual's health state	Aires	Mars
Second House indicates ability to possess wellness or disease	Taurus	Venus
Third House is to understand the various types of communication to self or others about health	Gemini	Mercury
Fourth House of home is the ability to have emotional peace or emotional conflicts which cause disease	Cancer	Moon
Fifth House is the ability to create wellness or illness	Leo	Sun
Sixth House is the ability to use the energy to serve wellness or illness	Virgo	Mercury
The Seventh House is impact of relationships upon wellness or illness	Libra	Venus
The Eighth House is the regeneration of wellness or generation of illness	Scorpio	Pluto
The Ninth House is the ability to explore health modalities or refusal to explore cause of disease	Sagittarius	Jupiter
The Tenth House is the impact of work on wellness or illness	Capricorn	Saturn
The Eleventh House is the emotional desire to be well and/or negative emotions causing illnesses	Aquarius	Saturn/Uranus
The Twelfth House is the sum total of mental or emotional or spiritual health causing deterioration, degeneration, or decline in health	Pisces	Neptune

Triplicities Kinds of Houses

The houses are divided in three groups (Triplicities), which have four houses in a group. These groups determined the overall picture of how Houses relate to health. There should be a planet or planets in each house in order for them to form angular, succedent and or cadent. The planets posited in a house have an effect on the illness or wellness.

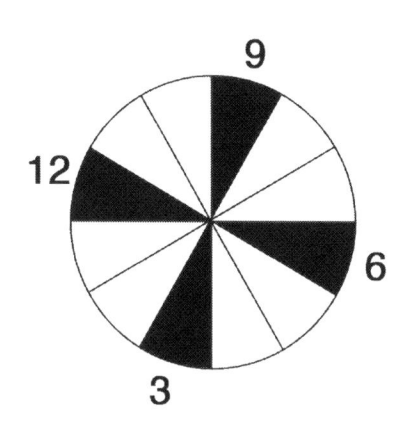

CADENT HOUSES (called Cadent because they "fall away" from the Angular and Succedent Houses. The word cadent comes from the Latin *cadere*, meaning, "to fall.") These are the Third, Sixth, Ninth and Twelfth Houses. Planets in these Houses indicate that you are mentally active and communicate your ideas.

ANGULAR HOUSES called Angular because they mark the four "Angles" of a chart. These are the First, Fourth, Seventh, and Tenth Houses. Planets in these Houses indicate that there is success in your health or there may be unsuccessful with remedies the medical sign and symptoms nature.

First House of self and (personality) of a disease

Fourth House inner emotions and spirit impact and the latter part of wellness.

Seventh House the future of disease treatment.

Tenth House of the level of wellness you will achieve.

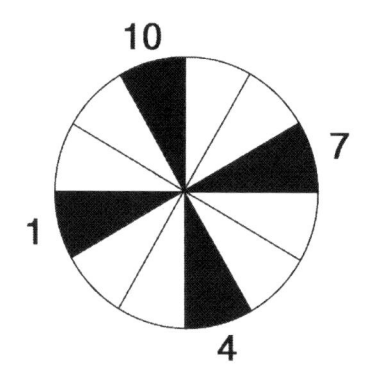

SUCCEDENT HOUSES (called Succedent because they "succeed" or follow the Angular Houses.) These are the Second, Fifth, Eighth, and Eleventh Houses. Planets in these Houses can indicate that you have stable wellness and desire for wellness or a disease that resisting treatment and the negative feeling can cause it to worsen.

Second House economic support of wellness or causing disease by putting money above wellness.

Fifth House of use of emotions or thoughts to create wellness or illness.

Eighth House of regeneration of health or generating of illness.

Eleventh House desires to achieve wellness or negative subconscious desire to be ill.

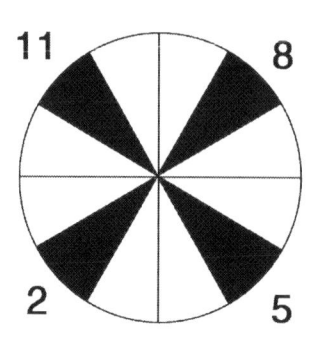

Quadruplicities Kinds of Houses

The houses are divided into four groups, which has three houses in a group.

HOUSES DIVIDED INTO FOUR GROUPS

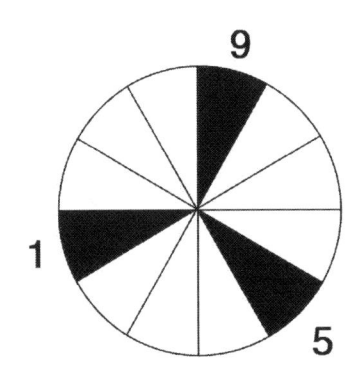

1) HOUSES OF LIFE - These are the First House of immunity, and vitality, the Fifth House creativity applied to treatments and healthy lifestyle and offspring, and the Ninth House of learning health concepts and conviction to treatment.

2) HOUSES OF WEALTH These are the Second House of personal ownership of preventive supplements, appliances for health, health treatments, the Sixth House of impact of work on wellness or illness, and the Tenth House impact of relationships on health and types of work that are morally emotionally and mentally good for wellness.

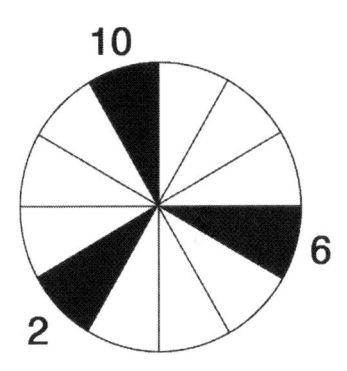

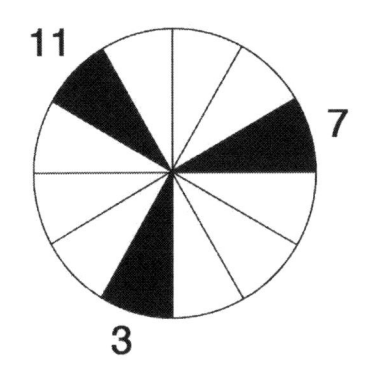

3) HOUSES OF RELATIONSHIPS These are the Third House impact of relationship of relatives and neighbors on wellness or illness, the Seventh House of partnership and marriage, and the Eleventh House of relationship friends and organizations on emotional and mental wellness or illness.

1) HOUSES OF ENDINGS These are the Fourth House of the wellness or illness in latter years of life, the Eighth House of degeneration and regeneration of wellness or illness, and the Twelfth House impact of the spirit on wellness or illness.

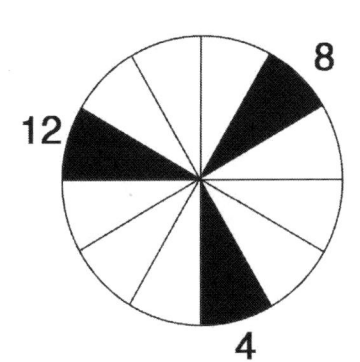

Aspects PLANETS DEGREES APART)

The degrees apart of two planets can contribute to the health can be positive, good effect, or a negative, bad effect toward an illness. Look at the chart and count how many bad and good effects the planets have. This can indicate whether an illness will have obstacles or be mild, severe or chronic. The planets have influences on wellness or illness.

Name of Aspect	Degrees Apart	Symbol	Meaning
CONJUNCTION	0° Two planets in the same sign (or within 10° of each other).	☌	A conjunction is the strongest aspect in astrology. It can be a beneficial influence on health. If the planets have other difficult aspects in the chart, a conjunction may worsen the health condition. A conjunction means the two planets involved have a strong influence on health, and are a focal point.
TRINE	120° Two planets for signs away from each other 120° apart (or within 9° either way of 120°).	△	Most harmonious. A trine is the most favorable aspect, bringing advantage and ease of a disease. Too many trines in a chart may make the health weak and lazy.
OPPOSITION	180° Two planets six signs away from each other, 180° apart	☍	Unharmonious. An opposition indicates wellness or illness can be a strain, discordance. Oppositions indicate as challenges to wellness or illness so there can be stimulating attraction between opposite to increase or decrease wellness or illness.
SEXTILE	60° Two planets two signs away from each other (60° either way).	✶	Emotionally and mentally harmonious and favorable toward wellness. A sextile brings opportunity. Unlike trines, sextiles require effort to overcome disease.
SQUARE	90° Two planets three signs away from each other 90° apart (or within 9° either way of 90°).	□	Challenging and stressful. A square places obstacles and health challenges and teaches lessons of wellness. This aspect indicates the challenges of overcoming a disease can develop strength of character.

QUINCUNX	150° Two planets 150° apart (or within 2° either way of 150°).	⚻	Its influence causes unpredictable health status. A quincunx indicates health problems.
SEMISQUARE	45° Two planets 45° apart (or within 2° either way of 45°)	∠	Mildly adverse. Brings anxiety and emotional tension that comes form stress of disease.
SESQUISQUARE	135° Two planets 135° apart (or within 2° either way of 135°).	⚼	Mildly adverse. Similar disease influence as a semisquare.
SEMISEXTILE	30° Two planets one sign away form each other, 30° apart (or within 2° either way of 30°).	⚺	Mildly beneficial to wellness. Brings wellness but is much less and influence than a sextile.

☉ Sun   ♃ Jupiter
☽ Moon   ♄ Saturn
☿ Mercury   ♅ Uranus
♀ Venus   ♆ Neptune
♂ Mars   ♇ Pluto

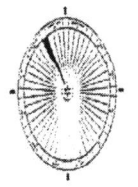

Conjunction: Two planets in the same Personology period

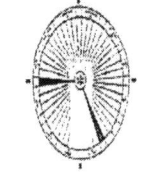

Trine: Two planets exactly four signs or cusps apart

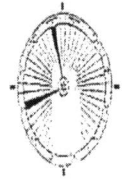

Square: Two planets exactly three signs or cusps apart

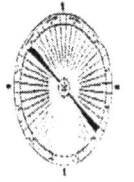

Opposition: Two planets 180 degrees--or directly-- opposite each other

Sun and Moon
Good Aspects
Healthy lifestyle: adaptable to alternative remedies and raw foods. Tends to have harmonious home life; recognizes and improves career and health.
Adverse Aspects: Inner emotional conflicts; lacks confidence about remedies. Can be emotionally overly sensitive which can often lead to disease.
Conjunction: Lifestyle is against wellness. This person is at times emotionally imbalanced or one-sided personality; deep-rooted emotional habits. Can be rigid and inflexible about changing health for the better.

Sun and Mercury
The Sun and Mercury are always within 28° of each other. Tend to form an aspect, which is a conjunction.
Conjunction: If 5° or less separate the Sun and Mercury, this person tends to be rigid and inflexible in accepting alternative health matters.

Sun and Venus
The Sun and Venus are usually no more than 48° apart, the only aspect is a conjunction.
Conjunction: A good aspect resulting in extroverted behavior, sociability, and temperament conducive for wellness.

Sun and Mars
Good Aspects: This person is self-motivated and assertive when focused on health, and their vitality is good. Can create good health plans
Adverse Aspects: They have a tendency to be emotionally negative, strong willed, and disruptive. Weak ability to follow treatment plans quickly follows diet fads.
Conjunction: Tends to be over reactive, hyperactive. Can work hard at being well.

Sun and Jupiter
Good Aspects: Has a positive outlook about health. Gravitates to beneficial health modalities and wellness.
Adverse Aspects: Emotionally over inflates their ability to be well and over inflates severity of disease. Indulges in emotional impulses and will not spend needed money for wellness.
Conjunction: A creative mind. Uses humor to support positive moods and behavior.

Sun and Saturn
Good Aspects: Self determine in health matters. Stays focus on health needs and organizes holistic lifestyle.
Adverse Aspects: Indicates emotional stress, obstacles, and problems achieving health. Subject must overcome self-defeating feelings of inadequacy and negative moods.
Conjunction: Understands the value of good lifestyle, self-determination and applies it to wellness.

Sun and Uranus
Good Aspects: Can initiate their own healing by seeking help. Intuitive ability helps with wellness.
Adverse Aspects: Relationship problems, stress and unstable emotion can cause illness.
Conjunction: Can be rigid in moving towards wellness. Tends to be introverted and independent, and can emotionally block out help.

Sun and Neptune
Good Aspects: Finds creative ways to use alternative treatments.
Adverse Aspects: Thoughts can be unfocused and vague. Emotional betrayal by others causes health and emotional problems.
Conjunction: Intuitive. Can feel the hidden meaning of others emotions. Creative ability is good.

Sun and Pluto
Good Aspects: Confident about achieving wellness. Easily dismisses negative thoughts and feelings. Can alter lifestyle to gain wellness.
Adverse Aspects: Introverted. Tends to stay away from people that have holistic health information that can help them with a disease.
Conjunction: Tends to want to control others. Feels that accepting other's wellness ideas is a threat to their ego or a loss of control.

Moon Aspects

Moon and Mercury
Good Aspects: Easily deciphers health concepts. Uses a common sense approach to wellness.
Adverse Aspects: Uses humor and emotions to achieve wellness. Emotionally vacillates.
Conjunction: Easily gets over stresses and can suffer from negative emotions that cause disease. Inclined to be very sensitive. Understand health and wellness concepts.

Moon and Venus
Uses emotions to stimulate their wellness
Good Aspects: Sees the beauty in health food dishes.
Adverse Aspects: Tends to let emotions to cause overeating.
Conjunction: Interpersonal relationships that are negative cause diseases. Can maintain harmonious life. Finds enjoyment is social activities that are good for health. Is creative with recipes.

Moon and Mars
Good Aspects: Good health, applies alternative remedies immediately, uses many holistic resources to gain wellness.
Adverse Aspects: Problems with health. Tends to have eating disorder, unstable moods, and defends unhealthy lifestyles.
Conjunction: Can focus on matters and dismiss obstructions to wellness. Energetic

Moon and Jupiter
Good Aspects: Enjoys reading about health matters. Has a positive outlook about overcoming disease. Can use emotions in a positive manner.
Adverse Aspect: Can have difficulty in overcoming disease. Emotions cause laziness and inability to maintain healthy lifestyle as well as follow healing remedies.
Conjunction: Changes to a healthy lifestyle is stimulating and challenging. Enjoys nurturing others and can be self conceded which can cause rigid emotions and illness.

Moon and Saturn
Good Aspects: Uses their understanding of natural remedies to overcome diseases. Their positive asset is their desire to be well and their patients.
Adverse Aspects: Emotional problems in intimate relationship can cause disease. Does not approach healing with confidence.
Conjunction: Emotionally stable. Follows health protocols to perfection. Tends to be too critical which can cause health problems.

Moon and Uranus
Good Aspects: Adjust to healthy lifestyle very easily. Intuition can guide to correct choices about health.
Adverse Aspects: Nervous tension. Unstable emotions and temperament causes diseases.
Conjunction: Will not conform or be restricted by a healthy lifestyle. Can use originality and creative personality to be well.

Moon and Neptune
Good Aspects: Can be inventive and creative and seek alternative health for healing. Has an interest in unusual health methods.
Adverse Aspects: Emotional problems with intimate relationships. Can have difficulties separating the real from the unreal, which causes illnesses.
Conjunction: Can be nurturing and sympathetic to others, which causes energy drain. Tends to be introverted.

Moon and Pluto
Good Aspects: Emotional and social changes have positive effects on health.
Adverse Aspects: Extreme mood swings cause health problems. Rigid negative feelings toward others cause disease.
Conjunction: Can make sudden changes in lifestyle, which can be good and/or bad. Tend to be emotionally impulsive.

Mercury Aspects

Mercury and Venus
Good Aspects: Enjoys reading about health. Tends to be creative in health pursuits and is in good humor.
Adverse Aspects: These two planets never form major aspects. Suppressed feelings can cause illness.
Conjunction: Emotional and mental balance can have positive effect on health.

Mercury and Mars
Good Aspects: Common sense approach to health. Can be emotionally determined to achieve wellness.
Adverse Aspects: Negative attitude, irritability and belligerence can cause diseases.
Conjunction: Intellectual ability makes understanding health and disease easy. Sense of humor contributes to wellness.

Mercury and Jupiter
Good Aspects: Does not need details about illness to be well. Uses good judgment and positive out look to achieve wellness.
Adverse Aspects: Skeptical about treatments. Easily makes mistakes in food choices. Emotions can cause problems with health.
Conjunction: Above-average intelligence. Optimistic about healing. Tends to be a nurturer.

Mercury and Saturn
Good Aspects: Takes practical and step-by-step approach to wellness. Can have a well discipline healthy lifestyle. Stays focus in defeating disease.
Adverse Aspects: Can be emotional rigid and afraid to change unhealthy lifestyle. Behavior can be abrupt.
Conjunction: Tendency to be depressed. Can endure severe illnesses can hold opinion about health that is unreasonable.

Mercury and Uranus
Good Aspects: Self motivated to be well. Good understanding of health and disease.
Adverse Aspects: Emotionally confused about what treatment is best. Can hold opinion contrary to wellness.
Conjunction: Understands the science connected to wellness. Tendency to be stubborn and does not change easily.

Mercury and Neptune
Good Aspects: Can use intuition and six sense to obtain wellness. Imagination and creativity helps with modifying treatments in a positive manner.
Adverse Aspects: Difficulty in concentrating on healing. Emotional negativity is harmful for health.
Conjunction: Explores spiritual wellness. Tends to be impulsive which can be a negative or positive attribute for healing.

Mercury and Pluto
Good Aspects: Able to adapt to alternative healing methods easily. Inner tension. Can have sudden changes in health.
Adverse Aspects: Tends to make emotional decisions about diet and health without considering the bad results. Anxiety and stress can cause health concerns.
Conjunction: Can have an in depth understanding of achieving wellness. Uses positive attitude to improve health, susceptible to anxiety and stress.

Venus Aspects

Venus and Mars
Good Aspects: Nurturing feelings helps to incubate healing. Is easily driven toward healing.
Adverse Aspects: Disturbed emotions, unsatisfied with self. Impulses lead to illness. Tends to have emotional stress from interpersonal relationships.
Conjunction: Emotionally balanced. Positive outlook about healing, can stress sex hormones.

Venus and Jupiter
Good Aspects: Easily expresses desire to nurture and be nurtured. Emotions influence health.
Adverse Aspects: Emotional extremes can cause numerous relationship problems. Excessive demands of affection cause betrayal and disease. Tends to have problems with weight.
Conjunction: Tends to require emotional attention from others. Uses sexuality to get attention.

Venus and Saturn
Good Aspects: Uses positive relationships to influence health. If emotionally attached to disease treatment will be serious and compliant.
Adverse Aspects: Tendency toward depression and loneliness. Negative emotions from others can cause illness.
Conjunction: Places material, worldly, and career success above health and emotional well-being. Can have a common sense approach to health.

Venus and Uranus
Good Aspects: Tends to use unusual treatment modalities and feels ancient remedies are best.
Adverse Aspects: Emotionally imbalanced. Dietary and behavioral choices cause disease.
Conjunction: Is lead by emotions. Easily excited which can cause problems.

Venus and Neptune
Good Aspects: Can use intuitive and creative ability to obtain wellness. Needs health matters explained clearly.
Adverse Aspects: Emotional disappointments and negative attitudes of others cause illness. Tends to be indecisive about choosing disease remedies.
Conjunction: Can be compatible, caring and sensitive in social relationships. Tends to have dietary, physical and/or emotional stress.

Venus and Pluto
Good Aspects: Sudden emotional changes that tend to improve health. Good stability.
Adverse Aspects: Emotional difficulties in relationships cause disease. Healing goes well then can reverse.
Conjunction: Stressful events can cause health problems. In depth understanding health and wellness.

Mars Aspects

Mars and Jupiter
Good Aspects: Positive outlook sustains good health. Confident about treatment success.
Adverse Aspects: Anxiety problem, misguided impulse behavior causes disease.
Conjunction: Good immunity. Tends to make quick decisions about illness.

Mars and Saturn
Good Aspects: Achieves wellness despite severity of disease. Endurance and immunity helps strengthen.
Adverse Aspects: Susceptible to injury and illnesses caused by emotional imbalance and weak health.
Conjunction: Can be susceptible to accidents. Tendency to neglect health. Emotional turbulent behavior causes illness.

Mars and Uranus
Good Aspects: Understands natural health alternatives for disease. Quick decisions help to overcome diseases but can sometimes cause harm. Tends to be knowledgeable about health options.
Adverse Aspects: Does not tolerate sickness and force self to take remedies. Suffers from stress and emotional problems, irritability, overly sensitive.
Conjunction: Good immunity. Can use principles of wellness but easily develops anxiety.

Mars and Neptune
Good Aspects: Desires to follow correct ideas about health. Emotionally stable. Uses creativity to be healthy.
Adverse Aspects: Wastes energy on unrealistic cures. Tendency to abuse drugs, alcohol, energy, and body building supplements.
Conjunction: Can use emotions to stimulate need for healthy lifestyle. Creative with remedies and wellness.

Mars and Pluto
Good Aspects: Good immunity. Self-confidence helps to overcome disease.
Adverse Aspects: Obsessive-compulsive behavior causes illness. Negative attitude causes disease. Tendency to reject healthy lifestyle.
Conjunction: Emotional explosiveness causes disease. Requires emotional stimulation.

Jupiter Aspects

Jupiter and Saturn
Good Aspects: Understands healing protocol and is able to maintain regiment, has persistence. Sustains emotional stability and patience with healing.
Adverse Aspects: Emotional problems present obstacles to wellness. Uncertain and pessimistic about recovery from illness. Problems feeling satisfied with treatment.
Conjunction: Can be emotionally discontented. Will accomplish wellness despite difficulties. Desires to be well.

Jupiter and Uranus
Good Aspects: Maintains emotional and mental balance. Enjoys being around health minded people. Is creative with healthy lifestyle.
Adverse Aspects: Absurd radical beliefs causes illnesses. Tends to defend negative ideas about health and healthy food.
Conjunction: Does not like restrictions of treatment protocol. Can have anxiety and/or mood problems.

Jupiter and Neptune
Good Aspects: Tends to be attracted to holistic and spiritual health. Good instinct for health concepts.
Adverse Aspects: Emotionally weak and can be oscillating in emotional extremes. Can deceive themselves to believe they are well.
Conjunction: Can be intuitive. Escapes into fantasy reality. Emotionally sensitive. Can be concern about health.

Jupiter and Pluto
Good Aspects: Seeks ideal health. Ability to change lifestyle to improve health. Understands holistic health concepts.
Adverse Aspects: Negative feelings can cause disease. Tends to emotionally abuse others.
Conjunction: Can be very forceful with others that will not accept healthy lifestyles. Has ability to make radical changes in lifestyle to obtain health.

Saturn Aspects

Saturn and Uranus
Good Aspects: Able to improve health and use creativity to make lifestyle changes. Can design a healing protocol with resourcefulness and efficiency.
Adverse Aspects: Does not accept health advice of others. Tendency to have anxiety and mood disorders that block health.
Conjunction: Good self-determination and self-control needed to be healthy. Communicates to others about healing.

Saturn and Neptune
Good Aspects: Uses a common sense approach to healing. Is creative with healing methods. Tends to be careful with diet and stays on guard about chemicals in food.
Adverse Aspects: Emotional problems, or paranoia, or tendency to be very introverted can block healing or cause illness. Many emotional and/or social obstacles cause disease reactions.
Conjunction: Strives to obtain ideal health and lifestyle. Emotionally stable. Tends to try to control others diet.

Saturn and Pluto
Good Aspects: Follows health diet principles. Understands the in depth degree of illness and wellness. Strong positive attitude.
Adverse Aspects: Tends to have unusual diseases. Emotionally unstable, can be obsessive compulsive.
Conjunction: Emotionally unpredictable and unstable. Can cope in a positive manner with emotional and/or social frustration, obstacles, and disappointments.

Uranus Aspects

Uranus and Neptune
Good Aspects: Inclined to be sensitive, intuitive and spiritual. Positive emotional attitude helps to maintain wellness.
Adverse Aspects: Easily is emotionally contrary to wellness. Can be swayed to go against wellness. Emotionally excitable.
Conjunction: Can be very creative in approach to healing and wellness. Intuitive ability can be positive and/or negative influence upon health.

Uranus and Pluto
Good Aspects: Can positively use emotions and lifestyle to become healthy. Tends to aim toward highest health principles.
Adverse Aspects: Emotionally troubled by others and/or vacillating and oscillating emotion. Stress and emotional outburst cause disease.
Conjunction: This generational influenced conjunction occurs every 115 years. Self motivated to achieve wellness. Emotions can be used negatively or positively, and have impact on health.

Neptune Aspects

Neptune and Pluto
Neptune spends 14 years in each sign and Pluto from 13 to 32 years in each sign. Any aspects formed has a long duration of time. Aspects are significant in an individual horoscope only if Neptune or Pluto is on the Ascendant, or Pisces or Scorpio is pronounced.
Good Aspects: Intuitive ability and inclination to new age remedies can be used to achieve wellness.
Adverse Aspects: Can be easily lead by impulses that can cause disease. Tends to be obsessive and compulsive
Conjunction: Good intuitive skills that can be used to improve health. Understands health and disease concepts.

Houses of Zodiac

Ruling Planets

The Natural order of the zodiac, beginning with Aries (Υ) on the ascendant. The ruling planet of each sign is in the Sign it rules. The influence of the Sign and Planet are nearly alike.

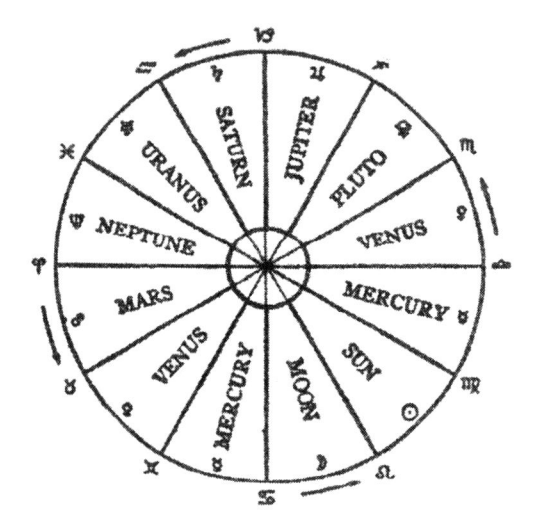

Houses indicate that you are emotionally and mentally active and can communicate your ideas to yourself as well as others.

Third House of day-to-day inner positive or negative talk to self that supports wellness or illness.
Sixth House impact of work on wellness or illness has ability to explore alternative health for wellness or Illness.
Ninth House of mental ability to explore alternative health for wellness or refusal to think positive about healing.
Twelfth House of the inner feelings about self and/or others that can have positive or negative impact on health.

House of Zodiac

When an individual is diseased they will subconsciously choose, or favor, or desire, or be prejudice towards a particular Zodiac Sign, Fragrance, Metal, Stone, Body section (injuries or diseases tend to occur in a section), Color, Number, or Music note problems.

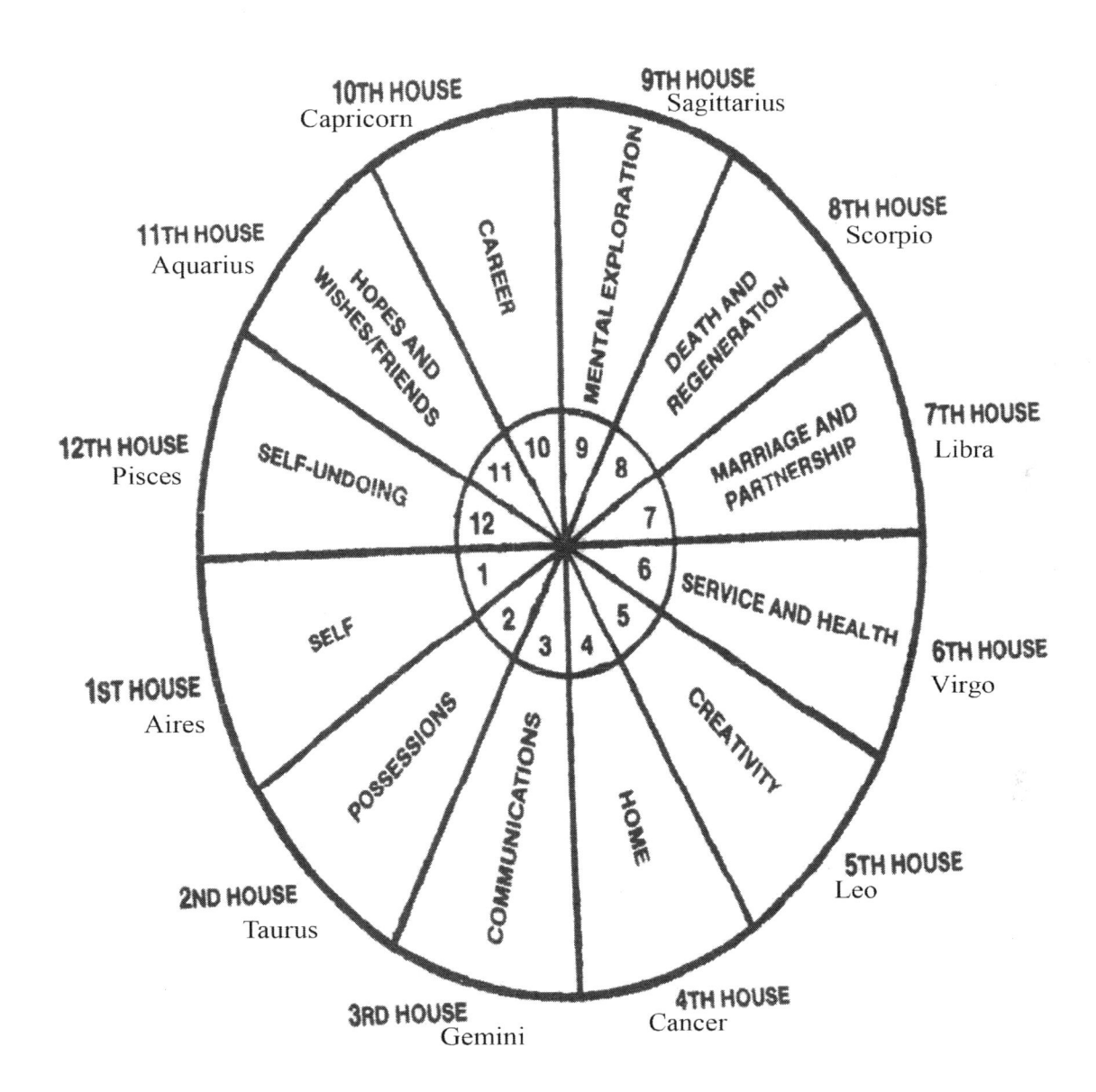

- 10TH HOUSE — Capricorn
- 9TH HOUSE — Sagittarius
- 11TH HOUSE — Aquarius
- 8TH HOUSE — Scorpio
- 12TH HOUSE — Pisces
- 7TH HOUSE — Libra
- 1ST HOUSE — Aires
- 6TH HOUSE — Virgo
- 2ND HOUSE — Taurus
- 5TH HOUSE — Leo
- 3RD HOUSE — Gemini
- 4TH HOUSE — Cancer

House themes: SELF, POSSESSIONS, COMMUNICATIONS, HOME, CREATIVITY, SERVICE AND HEALTH, MARRIAGE AND PARTNERSHIP, DEATH AND REGENERATION, MENTAL EXPLORATION, CAREER, HOPES AND WISHES/FRIENDS, SELF-UNDOING

Zodiac Profiles

Aries (Born between March 21 – April 19)

DUALTIY   Masculine
ELEMENT: Fire
QUALITY: Cardinal
ARIES: Tend to get into situations that can be dangerous, unhealthy and violently dangerous, likes diversity, new healing modalities, emotionally impulsive, energetic, active, and optimistic.
RULING PLANET: Mars: associated with extrovert behavior, accidents, aggression, tension, and conflict; it rules over danger.
SYMBOL: ♈ The Ram: acquires mobility around obstacles, assertive, and, emotionally passionate.
GLYPH (written symbol) pictograph is the symbol of the horns and long nose of the Ram. The symbolic picture of protection (eyebrow) of the sense (nose) of feeling rules the head. The symbolic glyph is two half moons joined by a straight line, which can indicate bonded to their emotions and idealism.
PART OF THE BODY RULED: Head brain and face Pituitary; illnesses such as headaches, skin eruptions, problems with ears, nose, and or accidents, injuries occur around the head and face.
HERBS: basil, catnip, nettle, wormwood, geranium, chervil
FLOWERS: Honeysuckle, Sweet Pea, Tulip, Calceolaria, Geranium, Daisy
TREES: All thorn-bearing trees
STRESS: Usually caused by impatience and frustration with self, or relationship or others, or events or situations.
STRESS REACTION: Emotionally uncontrollable explosive outburst, inflammations, headaches, migraines, stomach acidity.
DOMINANT KEYWORD: **I AM**
POLARITY: LIBRA
Aries is a "me-first" sign. Aries tendencies project their own personalities and can be selfish. Libra, Aries's opposite sign, is the sign of partnership. Natives of Libra feel incomplete without a relationship or partner or lover. They seek relationship happiness.
DAY: Tuesday
NUMBERS: 1 and 9
BIRTHSTONE Diamond: Can be a symbol of emotions, love, financial success and luck in new ventures. The diamond is particularly lucky for Aries people when worn on the left side of the body.
COLOR: Red: The color of fire and creating excitement.
METAL: Iron
CELL SALT: Kali, Phos.
FRAGRANCE: Basil
ETHIC: Will
MUSIC INSTRUMENT: Drum

Taurus (April 20 – May 20)

DUALITY: Feminine
ELEMENT: Earth
QUALITY: Fixed

TAURUS: Tends to be persistent, unyielding in maintaining goals and emotions, practical, stable, resistant to change of treatments, patient, quiet, and affectionate.

RULING PLANET: Venus: Get into chaotic and violent situations associated with emotions, creativity, arts, pleasure, and luxury.

SYMBOL: ♉ The Bull: gentle, unreasonably stubborn, pragmatic, emotionally strong, and fierce.

GLYPH (WRITTEN SYMBOL): this symbol is the horns and head of the bull. The symbolic glyph is a half-moon forming a cup that rests on the circle of the Sun. The cup represents the ability to receive and store emotions, ideas, wealth and power. The circle indicates a continuous line, and use of energy.

PART OF THE BODY RULED: Thyroid, neck, base of the skull and throat: Taurus tends to have a good voice and speech. They are susceptible problems in the neck, throat, thyroid, laryngitis, and skin problems on the neck.

HERBS: thyme, elderberry, primrose, marshmallow, catnip, rose, saffron, tansy, wormwood, yarrow, mint.

FLOWERS: Iris, Poppy, Lily of the Valley, Hydrangea, and Violet

TREES: Apple, Cypress

STRESS: caused by the lost good feeling, deviating, or gaining negative feeling, which is different from the original feeling/mood, situation, event, and/or relationship, sudden or planned changes in social life, economic, divorce, death, or conversation.

STRESS REACTION: Skin problems, neck pain, depression, sadness, anger, loss of esteem, diet becomes unstable.

DOMINANT KEYWORD: **I Have**

POLARITY: Scorpio

Taurus is the sign of property and money. They tend to hoard and cling and possessions. Scorpio, Taurus's opposite sign, is the sign of legacies and shared wealth. They nurture others spiritually and give to others in the form of writing, the healing arts and teaching.

DAY: Friday
NUMBERS: 6 and 4
BIRTHSTONE Emerald: Protects against infidelity and deceit, insures loyalty and improves memory.
COLORS: Pale blue and mauve: The soft colors of refinement and gentleness.
METAL: Copper
CELL SALT: Nat. Sulph.
FRAGRANCE: Rose
ETHIC: Creative
MUSIC INSTRUMENT: Harp, Guitar

Gemini (May 21 – June 20)

DUALITY: Masculine
ELEMENT: Air
QUALITY: Mutable

GEMINI: Is lively, energetic, versatile, and intellectual, they are usually thinkers and ignore emotions, and adaptable to new treatments. Their bipolar nature arouses unexpected anger in others. They tend to misjudge the emotional feelings of others.

RULING PLANET Mercury: This planet rules communication, the brain, nervous temperament, talking, and travel.

SYMBOL: ♊ The Twins: Positive and negative bipolar flexibility in communication (print, non-print, symbols), humanism, and versatility.

GLYPH: this indicates the bipolar dual symbol pictures the human arms, lungs and twins. The symbolic glyph is two upright lines bounded by top and bottom lines representing negative and positive logic, wisdom, learning behavior, spirituality, disease, and wellness.

DOMINANT PERSONALITY KEYWORD: **I THINK, I COMMUNICATE**

PART OF THE BODY RULED: Thymus, everything that is in sets of two such as arms, shoulders, lungs, as well as the wrist, nervous system, fingers and thyroid. Tends to have disease, and injuries involving arms, lungs, and hands.

HERBS: Anise, Lavender, Marjoram, Fennel, Oregano, Licorice, Dill, Horehound, Mint

FLOWERS   Lavender, Geranium, Alstromeria, Lily of the Valley, Rose

TREES: Nut-bearing trees

STRESS: loss of mental and/or emotional stimulation from random activities, conversation, relationship etc. activities and conversations that are not stimulating.

STRESS REACTION: respiratory problems, bronchitis, asthma, pneumonia, colds, cough, flu, frustration

POLARITY: Sagittarius

Gemini is the sign of positive and negative thoughts, communication, emotions, behavior, choices, and relationships. Natives of Gemini use bipolar self-expression, and try to manipulate others to accept their emotions and logic. Sagittarius, which is Gemini's opposite sign, is the sign governing the exploration of ideas, and adventures.

DAY: Wednesday
NUMBERS: 5 and 9
BIRTHSTONE Agate: translucent multicolor or pale blue or gray arranged in strips or blended clouds believed to protect from deceit, deception, falsehood, and indicates harmony in intimate and social relationships.
COLOR: Yellow: Enlighten, exposed change, or unusual
METAL: Mercury
CELL SALT: Kali. Mur.
FRAGRANCE: Lavender
ETHIC: Intellectual
MUSIC Instrument: Keyboards

Cancer (June 21 – July 22)

DUALITY Feminine
ELEMENT Water
QUALITY Cardinal

CANCER is emotional psychic receptive, sensitive, intuitive, kind, perceptive, clever, mischievous, abusive, intellectual, and sympathetic. They tend to become victims of accidents at home; they can be taken advantage (negatively manipulated).

RULING PLANET: The Moon governs emotions, intuitive behavior, fluctuates (waxes and wanes).

SYMBOL ♋ The Crab: hard exterior personality covering soft emotions inside. At the sign of danger, it withdraws into emotionalisms, and to the sea of emotions where it feels safe.

GLYPH (WRITTEN SYMBOL): Claws of the crab, the human breast, (the part of the anatomy that Cancer rules). Symbolic glyph is two circles of the Sun connected to two crescent Moons. The moons represent Cancer's ability to store emotional memories, possessions, and negative feelings; the circles tied to the moons represent the bipolar negative and positive emotional and ideas expressed through actions, imagination, feelings and spirit.

PART OF THE BODY RULED: Nurturing parts of the body stomach (helps nourish the body), ribs, the breast (makes milk). They tent to have digestion problems, or hormonal problems, and eating disorders.

HERBS: Mugwort, Aloe, Sage, Myrtle, Parsley, Bay Leaves, Cinnamon, Evening Primrose, Water Lily Flowers that bloom at night.

FLOWERS Acanthus, Gloxinia, Rose, Larkspur, Water Lily

TREES: Trees rich in sap

STRESS: Changes in ability to socialize, conflict with intimate groups, relationship, economics, emotions etc., negative domestic or family relationships

STRESS REACTION: Stomach problems, edema, eating disorder, hormonal problems, chemical sensitivity/ allergies.

DOMINANT KEYWORD: **I FEEL**

POLARITY Capricorn:

Cancer carry's it's feeling of home (shell) feelings and family life. Cancerians desire intimate personal relationships and are happiest in a family environment with those whom they love.

DAY Monday

NUMBERS 3 and 7

BIRTHSTONE Pearl: converts energy from disharmony to harmony or good, brings support in good or bad situations, or people.

COLORS Sea Green, Silver: Bringer of life, reflects or mirrors qualities.

METAL: Silver

CELL SALT: Calc. Flour

FRAGRANCE: Chamomile

ETHIC: Science

MUSIC INSTRUMENT: Horns

Leo (July 23 – August 22)

DUALITY   Masculine
ELEMENT   Fire
QUALITY   Fixed

LEO: Is powerful, enthusiastic, extravagant, expansive, dogmatic, creative, generous, and fixed in opinion. They challenge unknowingly others feelings and can provoke peoples emotional negativity. Their personality can cause their character to be assassinated.

RULING PLANET   The Sun: Leo tends to dominate and manipulate others for their own benefit. Enjoy the center of attention. The most powerful planetary influence, appropriating energy, immunity, and vitality can increase.

SYMBOL ♌ The Lion: attracts energy (mates with roar) and increasing the lost of energy (chasing away prey with roar)

GLYPH: two incomplete circles of the Sun joined by a crescent Moon, symbolizing power, reflecting of energy (reflects light) of emotions (moon) in a positive or negative manner.

PART OF THE BODY: Heart, back, spine, emotional, intellectual stress and strain, as well as physical overexertion causes health problems.

HERBS: Tarragon, Clove, Eyebright, Lemon balm, Frankincense, Sandalwood, Camphor

FLOWERS   Marigold, Carnation, Begonia, Sunflower, Gladiolus

TREES: All citrus trees

STRESS: Loss of ability to be the center of attention, creativity being blocked, issues with children.

STRESS REACTION: Fertility problems, heart problems, back and/or spine trouble.

DOMINANT PERSONALITY KEYWORD: **I WILL, I DEMONSTRATE**

POLARITY: Aquarius

Leo is the sign that governs pleasure and creativity. Natives of Leo look for what benefits their own life and tend to dominate others. Aquarius, Leo's opposite sign, is the sign of hopes and wishes and the higher aspirations of mankind. Aquarian are concerned with larger ideals, humanitarian concepts, and are more impersonal and aloof in their relationships.

DAY: Sunday

NUMBERS 8 and 9

BIRTHSTONE: Ruby (dark red): Believed to bestow serenity, faithfulness, protect against injury and disease.

COLORS: Gold, Orange: attracts and brings energy.

METAL: Gold

CELL SALT: Mag. Phos.

FRAGRANCE: Orange

ETHIC: Love

MUSIC INSTRUMENT: Woodwinds

Virgo (August 23 – September 22)

DUALITY   Feminine
ELEMENT   Earth
QUALITY   Mutable

VIRGO: Is analytical, practical, discriminating seeks understanding, industrious, reserved, modest, and their unemotional attitude caused criticism and negative feelings.

RULING PLANET Mercury: rules verbal, nonverbal communication, reason, commerce, intelligence, and tend to have a high level of sensitivity and irritability.

SYMBOL: ♍ The Virgin: modesty, industriousness, and unbiased service to others, purity, unspoiled, pristine.

GLYPH: It is a pictograph of the human reproductive organs closed and untouched. This is a straight line connected to two curved lines, one of which is crossed. This represents intelligence and emotions connected to wisdom, logic and unbiased truth.

PART OF THE BODY: The small and large intestines, nervous system
HERBS: Chervil, Marjoram, Dill, Caraway, Horehound, Lavender
FLOWERS: Pansy, Chrysanthemum, Gladiolus, Morning Glory, Aster
TREES: Nut-bearing trees
STRESS: Excessive exercise, or work, emotionally unfulfilling work or relationship, not feeling needed or wanted by others or a situation.
STRESS REACTION: Exhaustion, digestion problems, loss of ability to control appetite.
DOMINANT PERSONALITY KEYWORD: **I ANALYZE, I SERVE**
POLARITY: Pisces
Virgo is the sign of self-improvement and attempts to be a perfectionist who analyze emotions and facts to find the pure truth. Virgo's opposite sign is Pisces.
DAY: Wednesday
NUMBERS: 3 and 5
BIRTHSTONE: Sapphire (any color other than red): Protects against negativity, restores harmony
COLORS: Navy Blue, Gray: colors, art, spirituality, improve energy.
METAL: Mercury
CELL SALT: Kali. Mur.
FRAGRANCE: Lavender
ETHIC: Intellectual
MUSIC INSTRUMENT: Keyboards

Libra (September 23 – October 22)

DUALITY   Masculine
ELEMENT   Air
QUALITY   Cardinal

LIBRA: Are emotional, artistic, and diplomatic, adores beauty and harmony, peaceable, active, and sociable. They tend to be in love with love, arouse feeling of love. They oscillate and switch emotions off and on, and are under-decisive.

RULING PLANET   Venus: rules emotional pleasure, art, social pursuits, adornment, self-indulgence, and love of luxury

SYMBOL: ♎ The Scales: Signifying spiritual, emotional, physical, and/or intellectual, balance, equilibrium, order, justice, propriety, harmony, and reciprocity.

GLYPH: Ancient Egyptian symbol for the setting sun, the doorway between two worlds. The symbolic glyph is a crescent moon (emotions) connected to two straight lines (intellect) resting above a third line (spirituality). Emotion is controlled by bipolar logic and the line below represents partnership.

PART OF THE BODY RULED: Lower back, kidneys, buttocks, adrenal

HERBS: Elderberry, Lemon Balm, Thyme, St. Johns Wort, Catnip, Iris, Ivy, and Lillie's.

FLOWERS: Cosmos, Hydrangeas, Dahlia, Cyclamen, Rose

TREES Cypress, Ash, and Almond

STRESS: Unstable, loss and/or conflict in a relationship

STRESS REACTION: Kidney problems, skin disease, headaches, eyestrain, urinary tract infection.

DOMINANT PERSONALITY KEYWORD: **I BALANCE, I EQUALIZE**

POLARITY: Aries

Libra is the sign of social and intimate interpersonal relationships, partnership, and marriage. They function best within a relationship, can lose their positive attitude and equilibrium when forced to be alone. Aries is Libra's opposite sign.

DAY: Friday

NUMBERS: 6 and 9

BIRTHSTONE Opal (iridescent play of colors): Positive energy, insight, emotions, social change, protects against negativity.

COLORS: Blue, Lavender: Colors of art, right hemisphere of brain, refinement, and harmony.

METAL: Copper

CELL SALT: Nat. Sulph.

FRAGRANCE: Rose

ETHIC: Creative

MUSIC INSTRUMENT: Harp

Scorpio (October 23 – November 21)

DUALITY   Feminine
ELEMENT   Water
QUALITY   Fixed

SCORPIO: Is emotional, passionate, obstinate, imaginative, intense, perceptive, elusive, persistent, and rigid.

They are secretive and jealous which causes anger. Their emotions erupt and they can be emotionally abusive, verbally violent. Finds pleasure in dispensing emotions and thoughts to others, which is a sign of inheritance and legacies.

RULING PLANET Pluto: rules reproductive organs, glands, cyclic behavior, and emotions.

SYMBOL ♏ The Scorpion: A secretive, deadly creature, emotionally poisonous, penetrates deeply and cunning.

GLYPH: The curved lines and arrow directing emotions connected to a crafty ability to be intellectual and practically achieve objectives.

PART OF THE BODY RULED: sex organs and hormones, urinary system, rectum, vagina

HERBS: Sage, Catnip, Basil, Coriander, Nettle, Elder, Wormwood, Garlic, Catnip, Onions

FLOWERS: Rhododendron, African Violet, Gerbera, Chrysanthemum, Mum

TREES: bushy trees

STRESS: Conflict, worries and/or unstable economics, loss of attention in relationship, work and/or activities.

STRESS REACTION: Lower back problems, sex interest declines or increases excessively, constipation, sex organ problems, hormone imbalance

DOMINANT PERSONALITY KEYWORD: **I DESIRE**

POLARITY: Taurus: owning, collecting, and possessing emotions, objects, material, and thought.

DAY: Tuesday

NUMBERS 2 and 4

BIRTHSTONE Topaz (yellow to brownish yellow transparent): causes peace of mind, spiritual insights, protects against disease, and dysfunctional people.

COLORS: Purplish red, red, brownish red.

METAL: Plutonium

CELL SALT: Calc. Phos.

FRAGRANCE: Cypress

ETHIC: Commitment

MUSIC INSTRUMENT: Piano

Sagittarius (November 22 – December 21

DUALITY   Masculine
ELEMENT   Fire
QUALITY   Mutable
SAGITTARIUS: Is energetic, seek challenges, and enjoys freedom: ambitious, generous. In relationships and intimate relationships they have a desire for freedom, which can cause jealousy, avoidance in interpersonal relationships. They are influenced by others opinions and emotions.
RULING PLANET Jupiter: The planet of good, optimism, abundance, and fortune expansion.
SYMBOL ♐ The Archer: Exploring directness, high aims, physical activity.
GLYPH: glyph is the line of wisdom angled away from earth pointing to higher purpose, ideas, intellectual nature, concerns, philosophy, dislike of confinement of their broad ideas and physical activities.
PART OF THE BODY RULED: The thigh to the knees, hips, sciatic nerve, buttocks, and liver:
HERBS: Sage, Saffron, Basil, Clove, Borage, Chervil, and Nutmeg
FLOWERS: Holly, Dandelion, Azalea, Anemone, and Narcissus
TREES: Oak, Mulberry, and Birch
STRESS: Emotions, activities and/or social life becomes repetitious, exact with no new modification. Conversations that are routine and creates boredom, and being in one situation too long
STRESS REACTION: Infections, abuse of energy drinks, alcohol, liver problems, drugs and/or stimulants, skin rashes
DOMINANT KEYWORD: **I SEE, I KEEP THE TRUTH**
POLARITY: Gemini
This sign is of social and intimate interpersonal print, and non-print communication personal expression.
DAY: Thursday
NUMBERS: 5 and 7
BIRTHSTONE: Turquois, greenish blue, brings psychic ability, harmony, love, protects from harm.
COLOR: Purple, has affinity for art, esteem, and spirituality
METAL: Tin
CELL SALT: Lead
FRAGRANCE: Jasmine
ETHIC: Order
MUSIC INSTRUMENT: Strings

Capricorn (December 22 – January 19)

DUALITY   Feminine
ELEMENT   Earth
QUALITY   Cardinal
CAPRICORN is patient, discreet, frugal, quick to capture opportunity, acquisitive, determined, reserved, uses cunning instead of force, seeks security, concerned about reputation, career, image, and disciple. There past secrets are used by others to get revenge, can be aloofness, and reserve.
RULING PLANET   Saturn: represents, limitation, discipline, obstacles, and restriction.
SYMBOL ♑ The Goat: they overcome obstacles, reach for higher advantages, they emotionally and intellectually force its way through obstruction.
GLYPH: The pictograph indicates the V-shaped beard of the Goat and the curved tail of the Fish (the Sea-Goat, which was the ancient symbol for Capricorn). The symbolic glyph is two straight lines that are connected to a circle (spirituality) and a crescent (emotionally) combining authority and responsibility.
PART OF THE BODY RULED: Bones, joints, teeth, skin and knees: tend to have beautiful bone structure.
HERBS: Caraway, Tarragon, Dill, Rosemary, Marjoram, and Chamomile
FLOWERS: Ivy, Poinsettia, Chrysanthemum, and Carnation
TREES: Elm, Poplar, Pine
STRESS: Emotional negative or positive pressure from work, activities, and relationship: lack of stimulation from random activities or socializing.
STRESS REACTION: Knee, leg, and back problems, sleep disorder, arthritis, joint pain, teeth problems, orthopedic problems.
DOMINANT PERSONALITY KEYWORD: **I USE, I BRING THINGS TO ABUNDANT ACCOMPLISHMENT.**
POLARITY: Cancer
Capricorn's opposite sign is the sign of social, personal and interpersonal relationship and home life.
DAY: Saturday
NUMBERS: 2 and 8
BIRTHSTONE Garnet dark red, pomegranate-like color: Believed to enhance love, popularity, and high esteem.
COLORS: Dark Green and Brown: comforting colors of nature and the earth.
METAL: Lead
CELL SALT: Calc., Phos.
FRAGRANCE: Cypress
ETHIC: Commitment
MUSIC Instrument: Piano, Percussion

Aquarius (January 20 – February 18)

DUALITY   Masculine
ELEMENT   Air
QUALITY   Fixed

AQUARIUS: analytical, independent, inventive, progressive, original, firm, emotional, mental disposition, assertive, essentially an introvert but capable of being extrovert. Tends to get into social and or personal relationships with weird unusual people. Tends to be attacked by narrow-minded people because of eccentric behavior.

RULING PLANET: Uranus: The planet of the unexpected, modern science, change, progress, and invention.

SYMBOL: ♒ The Water bearer: Dispensing a gift that flows freely and equally to all; representing creation and the giving of life.

GLYPH: represents water, controlled and directed as it flows from the vessel of the Water bearer. This is the ridged unbroken line representing water/electric energy, the future, emotional flexibility, and universal thought.

PART OF THE BODY RULED: lower leg (tibia, fibula), calve muscles, circulatory system, ankles, and Parathyroid.

HERBS: Fennel, Mint, Valerian, Violet, Sage, Rosemary, Comfrey, and Wormwood

FLOWER: Primrose, Daffodil, Orchid, and Violet

TREES: Fruit trees

STRESS: Unsuccessful with social and /or emotional activities

STRESS REACTION: Exhaustion from self or others or activities, circulation problems, headaches, unusual disease or problem, heart problems, migraines, ankle sprains and breaks, varicose veins.

DOMINANT PERSONALITY KEYWORD: **I KNOW**

POLARITY: Leo

Opposite sign, is the sign of emotional diversity, love, self-centered, pleasure, and affection.

DAY: Wednesday

NUMBERS: 1 and 7

BIRTHSTONE: Amethyst: Clear purple, moderate purple, believed to help gain foresight, psychic ability, and faithfulness in relationship. Believed to bring faithfulness in love and bestows the gift of prescience.

COLOR: sky blue, bluish clear violet

METAL: Uranium

CELL SALT: Calc., Phos.

FRAGRANCE: Lavender

ETHIC: Progress

MUSIC INSTRUMENT: Piano

Pisces (February 19 – March 20)

DUALITY   Feminine
ELEMENT   Water
QUALITY   Mutable

PISCES: emotional intuitive, adaptive, mystical, imaginative, dreamer, changeable, intuition, romantic, receptive, and impressionable. Tendency to be emotionally unstable, drawn into toxic situations and have the ability to abuse alcohol and/or drugs.

RULING PLANET Neptune: planet of mystery, glamour, illusion, and deception.

SYMBOL: ♓ Two Fishes tied to one another and swimming in opposite directions: indicating, conflicting emotions, and changeable extremes of temperament.

GLYPH: This glyph is two crescent moons (bipolar emotions) connected by a straight line (intellect). Emotion and thoughts tied to economic, moral, and social limitations.

PART OF THE BODY RULED: Pineal Gland, feet and toes. They tend to have beautifully shaped, sensitive feet, bunions, and corns, ache problems, toenail problems.

HERBS: Clove, Nutmeg, Lemon Balm, Basil, Borage, Sage

FLOWERS: White Poppy, Jonquil, Cineraria, Freesia, Water Lily, and Daffodil

TREES: Fig, Willow

STRESS: Loss of direction for life, decrease or lack of emotional, spiritual, or reason for life.

STRESS REACTION: Chemical and/or impurities, of non-organic food causes sensitivity, abuse of alcohol, stimulants, and/or drugs

DOMINANT PERSONALITY KEYWORD: **I BELIVE**

POLARITY: Virgo

Opposite sign, is the sign of service to others, institutions, ideals, they are practical, like facts, strives to have achievements.

DAY: Friday

NUMBERS: 2 and 6

BIRTHSTONE: Aquamarine blue green, believe to bring serenity, secret knowledge, super natural and paranormal insights:

COLORS: Pale green and turquoise: The dreamy colors of the sea.

METAL: Platinum

CELL SALT: Calc., Phos.

FRAGRANCE: Mint

ETHIC: Adapt

MUSIC INSTRUMENT: Piano/Percussion

Planet and Herbs

Planet	Herbs
Venus	Bearberry, Cloves, Goldenrod, Sorrel, Marshmallow, Peppermint, Rose, Thyme, Yarrow, Elder, Burdock, Pennyroyal, Catnip, Colt's foot, Feverfew, Tansy, Motherwort, Mugwort, Raspberry Leaves, Plantain
Mars	Coriander, Gentian, Ginger, Horseradish, Hops, Butcher's Broom, Basil, Blessed Thistle, Nettle, Cayenne, Garlic, Hawthorn Berry, Wormwood, Tarragon
Sun	Angelica, Alum Root, Marigold, Chamomile, Rosemary, Lovage, St. John's Wort, Eyebright, Laurel, Bay
Moon	Violet, Hyssop, Iris, Seaweed, Clary, Sage, Purslain, White Willow, Chickweed, Cleavers, Wintergreen
Jupiter	Anise, Jasmine, Lemon Balm, Borage, Rhubarb, Myrrh, Dandelion Root, Bilberry, Melissa, Nutmeg
Saturn	Pansy, Rue, Senna, Hemlock, Mandrake, Comfrey, Shepherd's Purse
Mercury	Cascara Sagrada, Elecampane, Witch Hazel, Licorice, Fennel, Horehound, Fenugreek, Valerian, Parsely

Uranus, Neptune, and Pluto are second-octave planets their herbs are used more for spiritual and mental effect. There orbits are very slow and can spend 30-years in a house.
They have been recently discovered and have not had enough observation.

Medical Astrology Guidelines

Sun Health Profile

The Sun sign indicates a person's immune system, health and vitality. It rules the vital energy and corresponds with the spleen and heart. It rules chronic disease. When the Sun is posited above the horizon, strong vitality; and below the horizon, weak vitality.

It is an indicator of the natal health condition; the Sun shows the hereditary predisposition and, with other factors, indicates the health status. It points to the chronic and lasting bodily illnesses. A weak physical condition and afflicted Sun in a negative sign, weakens the health, and causes problems such as eye diseases, heart disease, palpitations and bone fractures. It affects the immune system and heart in both male and female. In a male chart, it has far greater effect health deterioration.

If the Sun is unafflicted and gets a good aspect from Jupiter, expect a healthy and long life. If badly placed and much afflicted, there will be many diseases. If a malefic elevated above the Sun afflicts, it injures the health more than if the Sun were the elevating planet.

BODY PARTS
The Sun rules the heart, liver's bile, skin, stomach, bone, right eye in males, left eye in females, abdomen, head and spinal cord. It rules the back, pituitary gland, and, to a lesser degree, the thyroid gland. It rules the general health of males.

DISEASES, WHEN AFFLICTED
Heart diseases, eye trouble, high fever, stomach and skin disease, nerve damage, head and brain trouble (including headaches), fainting, and bone injuries.

INFLUENCE
Because the Sun has a great influence in male charts, it indicates, through sign and house position, something about the male health status. When the Sun is badly afflicted, the health is weak. Consider health reinforced when well aspected. Favorable aspects from Venus and Jupiter indicate various types of addictions and self-indulgence not conducive to health. An absence of aspect from Mars weakens health in both male and female charts. Adverse aspects are better than none, imparting vitality. An afflicted Sun causes disease in a man's horoscope; especially if they have inadequate diets.

The health, according to position and aspects, indicates the health state, with males born under fire signs favored with the strongest vitality and having the best prospects for good health. There can be quick recuperation from severe illnesses.

Males born under air signs hold the next most desirable, health-influencing position. They can increase their health by avoiding emotional problems and nervous troubles. Males born under earth signs are able to endure stress, their illness is prolonged and their recuperation delayed. The least desirable influence of the sun is water sign birthdays. These males, with the exception of Scorpios, tend to have the weakest health.

Sun In Signs

SUN IN ARIES
Aries is the first Fire sign, cardinal and ruled by Mars. Arians tend to be hyperactive and over extend themselves. They have no patience with a treatment process or a disease. They desire fast recuperation and consider a day in bed as worse than the illness.

Aries state of health is suited for quick recovery. Aries recuperative ability is excellent. Any excitability, emotional or mental stress or insomnia, however tends to delay the recuperative process, so relaxation is necessary. Unexpressed inner emotional or mental stress can lead to high blood pressure, migraine headaches, stomach flu, ulcers and dizziness.

The head, face and teeth are the main areas of disease or injury. There is a tendency for a stroke resulting in paralysis and or impaired speech, sclerosed or ruptured brain blood vessels, cerebropathy, brain fever, cerebral anemia, congestion of the blood and fainting. Headaches caused by exhaustion and constipation, overindulgence, poor diet, or skipped meals. Avoiding alcoholic beverages is important for Aries. Aries should avoid excessive protein consumption and muscle building foods – these acidify the body and interfere with carbonization.

Amino Acid Glutamine; Vitamins B, C, and E; minerals, phosphorus, iodine and lecithin are needed by the brain for normal function. Lack of vitamins B and C is associated with neurasthenic headaches. Adequate sodium, choline, iron, magnesium, and iodine foods are needed.

Adequate sleep is required and simple food combinations and 70 to 80% raw foods.

The head should be protected from the Sun. Several planets in Aries tend to cause sinus problems.

SUN IN TAURUS

Taurus is the first earth sign, fixed and ruled by Venus. People born under this sign have good endurance and vitality if they eat adequate nutrition; otherwise they tend to chronic aliments.

Taurus has a good appetite and enjoys all the rich foods that are not good for them. They easily develop fixed habits and do not follow advice to change their bad habits.

They do not have the capacity to detox from conditions. They should follow the rules of good diet. They should fast periodically, drink plenty of water, and avoid heavy foods, junk foods and greasy foods.

They tend to eat too many cooked foods containing phosphorus and sulphur. They need these foods to be eaten raw.

Taureans tend to withstand high amounts of pain, instead of seeking natural remedies; they seek drugs to alleviate the suffering. They work excessively because Taureans endurance is high and inexhaustible. Taurus can resist disease. They are susceptible to heart problems. If there is a fatal disease, sudden death is a danger, check other factors including eighth house. Sudden collapse, strokes, and nerve damage are dangers of the sign.

The neck, throat, glands and tubes are weak points. Vocal chords are sensitive and infections of the throat can be a problem.

There is a tendency to obesity, diphtheria, tonsil abscess, and polypus of the nose. Afflictions in Taurus can indicate signs of fainting, strokes, nerve damage and convulsions. They are susceptible to digestive problems, enlargement of the liver, hoarseness, dry cough and inflammation of the throat, heart and kidney disease, and nasal catarrh. Overeating can cause gastrointestinal upsets, diabetes, liver problems, reflux and food addiction.

Many planets afflicted in Taurus point to trouble in the back of the head. Taurus sun square Leo, heart problems. Sun in Taurus square Jupiter in Leo, thyroid problems.

SUN IN GEMINI

Gemini is the first air sign, mutable and ruled by Mercury. Gemini's should use proper (sufficiently deep) breathing and exercise is important. Drugs affecting the respiratory system should be avoided.

There is a tendency toward lung problems, pneumonia, asthma, colds, pleurisy, hay fever, allergies, nervous disorders and headaches. Tuberculosis and lung cancer can be a part of chronic illnesses.

They often refuse treatment for illness because they do not want to rest. Gemini children will pretend to be well until they develop a high temperature, after which they gladly will go to bed and sleep right through meals to avoid the illness. Gemini is not compliant to treatments; instead, they just keep the disease.

Careless motion causes accidents. They have a hyperactive nervous system, requiring physical exercise. Some Gemini's will put all their energy into mental work.

Illness rarely gets a Gemini depressed. They tend to be cheerful whether they are sick or well.

The lungs need Vitamins A, B, C, and D; minerals, such as calcium, silicon, iron, and copper. Gemini's overeat carbohydrate foods, sugars and more raw fruits and vegetables. They should avoid high amounts of carbohydrates and eat plenty of raw foods containing sodium, potassium, magnesium and iron.

SUN IN CANCER

Cancer is the first water sign, Cardinal and ruled by the Moon. Afflictions in Cancer tends to have digestive problems, tumors, illnesses of the breast, arthritis and rheumatism, cancer, anemia, obesity, cataracts, edema, insulin resistance, hardening of arteries, reflux, nervous tension, malnutrition, anemia, and nerve damage.

The Sun in Cancer does not have good resistance to disease, tending to weaken the digestive organs. Cancerians may be so sick as to nearly die, but then recuperate.

Cancer's need digestive enzymes, which are essential to good digestion. There are enzymes in all raw foods, but cooking destroys them. Raw food at each meal would alleviate tendencies to have trouble with digestion. Cooked foods may require digestive enzyme supplements.

They should avoid overeating and should drink adequate fluids to cleanse the system. They need foods high in chlorine, silicon, and iodine.

Cancer can be emotionally upset and worry too much when they are sick, and fear the ailment itself. They are psychic and emotionally sensitive and absorb others illnesses and troubles. They have emotional overloads and need to learn how to protect themselves from other people's feelings.

SUN IN LEO

Leo is the second fire sign, fixed and ruled by the Sun. Afflictions in Leo include heart problems, heart disease, heart and muscle strain, obesity, backache, spleen disturbances, eye troubles, migraine headaches, and spinal problems. The Sun in Leo indicates good health with fewer ills than any other sign, because of quick healing and recuperative ability.

They tend towards heart disease and need to practice prevention. Vitamin E (as found in wheat germ, lettuce and raw peanuts) can strengthen the heart. Carotine and lecithin helps combat the destruction done by cooked cholesterol (Leo people like meat). Leo needs foods containing iron, sodium, choline, magnesium and iodine. They should avoid excessive protein and muscle building foods. They interfere with carbonization and cause sympathetic stress.

Sickness, for Leo, requires emotional nurturing, but boredom sets in if it lasts too long.

There is a tendency to high fevers. There is a tendency to fixed habits and Leo does not easily adapt to change.

SUN IN VIRGO

Virgo is the second earth sign, mutable and ruled by Mercury. They have fragile health and the bowels, and nervous system are weaker and the lung affected. Afflictions in Virgo tend to indicate digestive problems, constipation, colic, poor nutrient absorption, diarrhea, peritonitis, typhoid fever, weak muscles, nervousness and weak lungs.

Virgo is emotionally sensitive to suggestions of illness and tends to think their illness can make them a chronic invalid. They can become neurotic hypochondrias that enjoy sickness and wants sympathy. Attempts to treat them or cure the disease may cause resentment.

Once Virgo learns the true facts about their illness, diet and health, they become helpful. They tend to eat phosphorus containing foods, and cooked sulphur foods to excess. They require sulphur from raw foods. Sun in Virgo conjunct Mars and opposition Saturn in Pisces tend to nephritis. Virgo Sun square Gemini tends to weak lungs.

SUN IN LIBRA

Libra is the second air sign, cardinal and ruled by Venus. Afflictions tend to cause kidney diseases, Bright's disease, diabetes, headaches, head and stomach disorders, virus colds, rheumatic troubles, back trouble, leg pains and skin disease.

They tend to have good health and the ability to fight against functional disorders. The kidneys are the weakest organs. Libras are susceptible to developing illnesses from accidents and injuries. Libras can get ill from nervous stress. When Libras get emotionally upset, they may get indigestion, high blood pressure, nasal allergies, itchy skin eruptions and weak immunity. Libras require emotional stability. Libra can enjoy the emotional attention that they get when sick, especially if they get sympathy, gifts, and nurturing.

Vitamin A prevents the formation of stones and infection. Librans can procrastinate about following a treatment protocol until the problem escalates and severe treatment is needed. Libra's feel that what they do not know will not hurt them and seldom expects or desires treatment.

They have a natural desire to be healthy. Libra's eat excessive carbohydrate foods, sugars, and starches. They should eat foods, which contain sodium, potassium, magnesium and iron.

Sun in Libra conjunct, square or opposition Uranus tends to various anemia's.

SUN IN SCORPIO

Scorpio is the second water sign, fixed and ruled by Mars and Pluto. Scorpio natives should avoid junk foods and drugs which cause diseases. Addiction to alcohol, sex and drugs can become a problem. Scorpio has a need for chlorine, silicon and iodine containing foods(relatively organic, and free of toxins).

Afflictions in Scorpio tend to kidney disease, and stones, gallstones, uterine and ovarian problems, gout, fistula, appendicitis, inflammatory diseases affecting the throat and heart, stomach disorders, physical exhaustion, urinary infection, obesity, hemorrhoids and digestion problems.

The Sun here makes for a good health and immunity. Scorpio can adjust easily to drastic change and makes an excellent patient. They seek medical help early and follow protocols implicitly. Scorpio's distorted emotions cause a positive attitude toward pain, feeling that it will go away and its cause disappear. This causes illnesses to become chronic or fatal.

Sun in Scorpio square Leo tends to heart diseases. Opposition planets in Taurus, easily develops nose and throat problems.

SUN IN SAGITTARIUS

Sagittarius is the third fire sign, mutable and ruled by Jupiter. Afflictions in Sagittarius indicate sciatica, pulmonary and eye diseases, wounds through falling, muscle and ligament problems, sports, and stress problems. The circulatory and nervous systems are the weakest parts. They can have respiratory problems. Sagittarians tend to consume excessive amounts of, alcoholic beverages, sweets, caffeine and nicotine. Their addictive behavior is extremely difficult to break. Their imbalanced diet and malnutrition causes dental problems, bone disease, inflammation of tendons and arthritis. Sagittarius should not eat excessive amounts of protein and muscle building foods. Foods high in iodine, sodium, choline, and magnesium are needed. Sagittarians generally do not like to be sick and use preventive medicine to build immunity to many common diseases. Practicing moderation is a good asset.
They have excellent recuperative power. Sagittarius Sun opposition Gemini planets can cause lung problems.

SUN IN CAPRICORN

Capricorn is the third earth sign, cardinal and ruled by Saturn. Afflictions in Capricorn tend to be skin diseases, digestive troubles, constipation, sinus trouble, emotional illness, hypochondria, mood swings, edema, muscle problems, rheumatism, and susceptible to falls, colds, and bruises.
The Capricorn Sun tends to cause weak immunity. As an infant they were frail with good endurances. Capricorns, develop good health later in life. Self-preservation and moderation are natural to this sign. Capricornians need to keep warm because chills can cause problems. Capricorn tends to eat phosphorous foods and cooked sulphur foods to excess. They need phosphorus and sulphur raw foods.
Vitamins A, B, C, and D are needed for a good digestive system. The minerals sulphur, iron, sodium, potassium, and magnesium are needed for good health.
Capricorn can easily adapt behavior when health is involved. Self-discipline and self denial enable Capricorn to follow a strict health treatment protocol for quick recovery.
Sun in Capricorn conjunct, square or opposition Saturn or Uranus tends to gall and kidney stones. Capricorn Sun opposition planets in Cancer tend to digestion problems.

SUN IN AQUARIUS

Aquarius is the third air sign, fixed and ruled by Saturn and Uranus. Afflictions in Aquarius cause poor circulation, heart diseases, heartburn, anemia, headaches, migraine, bronchitis, allergies, eye problems and varicose veins.
The Sun in Aquarius causes good healing ability despite the fact that the native may seem frail and appear high strung. The primary health issue is poor circulation and nervous disorders.
Aquarius should avoid and prevent degenerative diseases because the Sun is in its detriment here and not an asset to health. Aquarius tends to neglect diet and skip some meals. There is an excessive amount of nervous energy in Aquarius, causing restlessness and changeability. An exercise routine begun early in life helps maintain and improve their health.
Generally Aquarius tends to like carbohydrates (sugars and starches). Aquarius should avoid overeating carbohydrates. They need foods containing sodium, magnesium, iron, and potassium.
Sun in Aquarius opposition Uranus in Leo tends to anemia. Sun conjunct, square or opposition Saturn or Uranus – gall and kidney stones.

SUN IN PISCES

Pisces is the third water sign, mutable and ruled by Jupiter and Neptune. The Sun in Pisces does not indicate good health or quick recuperation. The immunity is weak with low resistance to infectious disease.
Vitamin A and C are required to build resistance to disease. Pisces needs chlorine, iodine, and foods. Afflictions in Pisces causes intestinal troubles, stomach gas, dyspepsia, neurasthenia, typhoid fever, bunions, boils, nervous spasms, a tendency to perspiration, sweaty feet, poor muscle tone, colds, liver and pancreas problems and skin eruptions.
Pisceans can adjust to weak immunity by adopting good health preventive measures. Overeating causes diseases and more exercise may be needed. Pisces Sun square planets in Gemini – neurasthenia.

Sun in Houses

Sun In First House

Well aspected: This is an ideal house for good health and quick recuperation.
And sextile Saturn: Native is persistent, and stays on health treatment. Despite the challenges and discouragement involved, they and survive and recuperate.

In Cancer: The sight of the right eye is weak.
And Mars in first house: urinal diseases
And Saturn in fifth and Moon in eighth and Mars in ninth: bone fractures
Afflicted: cataract, eye problems
In Libra: night blindness
Aspected by Saturn: affects right eye
And Moon and Venus in first: dental problem
Square Moon: emotional problems and unstable feelings can cause chronic disease

Sun In Second House

And Moon in second: night blindness
Thinks positive about recovery

Sun In Third House

And Mars in third: Needs to protect hands against wounds
Afflicted: depression, psychotic episodes
Well aspected: ability to adjust; helps recovery
And Mars in the third house aspected by Saturn: broken bones

Sun In Fourth House

Well aspected: good resistance to disease
Emotionally upset until recovery from disease
And Jupiter in twelfth house: lung disease
Conjunct Mars in Capricorn in the fourth house: indicates digestive problems and feverish complaints
Weak immunity but sufficient resistance to combat disease
And Saturn in eighth house, and Moon in tenth: of bone fractures

Sun In Fifth House

Female chart: can indicate trouble during childbirth
And Moon, Mars and Saturn also in fifth: bone fractures
And Venus and Saturn in fifth house: urinal diseases
Well aspected: good immunity and outlook, when sick has a positive attitude towards healing

Sun In Sixth House

Unless well aspected the Sun here indicates many diseases, often a series of diseases causes a life of immunity problems.
Well aspected: indicates, practices disease prevention.
Sextile, trine or conjunction Mars or Jupiter: good health
Afflicted: chronic illness, emotional problems contribute to illnesses
Afflicted by Mars, Sun conjunct rulers of eighth and twelfth houses: heart disease
And Moon and Mars in sixth: boils, skin eruptions
Square or opposition Saturn or Uranus: the immunity and the recuperative ability are weak
And badly aspected Moon in sixth, eighth or twelfth house: causes harm to the respective eye ruled by them
And sixth in a dual sign: lung disease

Sun In Seventh House

Well aspected: An ideal house for the Sun causing good health. Good immunity and resistance to disease.
Afflicted: many diseases
And Mars in seventh aspected by a malefic: burns, skin problems

Sun In Eighth House

Conjunct Neptune in Gemini: Hemorrhage of lungs
And badly aspected Moon in eighth houses: harm to the respective eye ruled by them
And Moon in Eighth house: diarrhea, bladder, and liver problems
With malefic in eighth house: Diseases result from complications of other diseases, difficulty for early diagnosis.
And Mars and Venus in eighth: skin irritations
And Mars in eighth: abscesses, tumors and cysts, impure blood, and fevers.
And Venus and Mercury in eighth: When ill is tolerant and lets it take its course and makes no effort to fight the diseases.
And badly aspected Moon in sixth, eighth or twelfth houses: indicates harm to eyes.
And Mars in second, Saturn in twelfth, and Moon in sixth: eye problems
In Cancer, Scorpio or Pisces, and Sun aspecting malefics: Indicates lung disease. If Venus or Jupiter conjoins, increases severity of disease.
And Mars in eighth, aspected by malefic: burns.
And Mars in first, second, seventh or eighth house in Pisces: mental problems
And Moon, Saturn and Mars in eighth: Bone Fractures.
Afflicted: fistula, hemorrhoids.

Sun In Ninth House

Well aspected: good for health
And Moon in ninth: eye problems
And Moon, Mars and Saturn in ninth: bone fracture

Sun In Tenth House

Ideal house for the Sun; indicating good health. The Sun is accidentally dignified here, indicating good health and the ability to overcome most disease.
And Moon in second, and Mars in fourth: bone fracture

Sun In Eleventh House

No impact on health or disease

Sun In Twelfth House

Well aspected: good health
Afflicted: harms right eye
And if afflicted Moon in twelfth: eye diseases
And malefic in sixth, eighth or twelfth: problems with the respective eye ruled by them

Moon Health Profile

The Moon rules acute diseases. The Moon rules alkalinity. Its circadian cyclic activity correlates with ovulation, menstruation, daily rhythms, flow of blood, phases of childbirth and puberty. The Moon influences, more particularly, people born in water signs – Cancer, Scorpio, Pisces.

Body Parts Ruled

The Moon rules the, emotions, circulatory system, lungs, hormones, kidneys, heart, left eye in males, right eye in females, stomach, breasts, tear ducts, mucous membranes, lymphatic systems and body fluids. Toxins cause abscesses and boils.

The Moon rules by Venus and the thymus gland secondarily. It corresponds to the Parathyroid and its influence on calcium metabolism. Afflicted Moon and Venus have an effect on calcium absorption and deposits and arteriosclerosis.

The Moon indicates the emotional, psychic and instinctive functions, circadian cycles, hormone functions, sleep, and growth. Afflictions from Sun, Mars, or Uranus can cause insomnia. Diseases related to the moon's influence are emotional, periodic hormonal, glandular, and functional rather than organic. During a full moon, discharges and secretions increase, the emotions are sensitive and more aroused.

An afflicted Moon causes emotional problems in a female horoscope.

Moon in Saturn's house and hemmed in between malefics: burns, skin problems

And Mercury and ascendant all afflicted: weak emotions, nervous system and mentality. Emotional problems.

Critical time: is after the moon has moved around the entire horoscope and returns to its radical position. This is a crucial time for physical illnesses and emotional problems.

When the Moon is full: there is a hemorrhage tendency. Dysfunctional people have an increase emotional instability, and irritable. Mental and emotional illnesses and the epileptic problems can increase. Arthritis, asthma, neuritis and sinus patients have increased problems because of the positive ions in the air.

Operation: Do not select for the date of an operation, a day when the moon is in a sign ruling the part of the body to be operated on, the exact change in the Moon is not a good time to have an operation. When the moon is waxing (increase in size) is better.

During Waxing Moon: sedatives have a decreased effect and can need an increased dose.

During Waning (decrease in size) Moon: sedatives have an increased effect and the dosage may be decreased.

To judge the immunities functional ability, note house and sign of moon and aspects. Planets in favorable aspect increase health and immunity, aiding functional ability. Afflicting planets decrease the immunity's function, which indicates illness and emotional problems.

Moon In Signs

Moon In Aires

A sensitive part of the body is the head and face with its nerve pathways skeletal and muscular system, the cerebellum, upper jaw, and teeth. The moon influences circadian bodily energy and emotions, feelings, brain's hormonal and bodily function.

And conjunct, square, or opposition Jupiter or Saturn: Liver problems

Aspected by malefic and unaspected by benefic: kidney stones, hearing problems

Afflicted: wounds of head and face. Accidents, firearms, fire and electronics, headaches, baldness, insomnia, lethargy, weak eyes, colds, nerve damage and pain.

In Sixth house: stomach and nerve problems.

Habit of eating too fast, and inadequate chewing.

Natural inclination to infertility, and if Moon is afflicted by Uranus, Saturn, Mars or the Sun there is decrease infertility ability.

Tendency to have headaches caused by indigestion, insomnia, catarrh, eyestrain, emotional upsets, nerve damage and pain.

Other results of affliction: Nerve damage, stroke, problems with teeth, fevers, vertigo, and skin eruptions.

Violent emotional reactions cause heath problems.

Moon in Taurus

Good physical endurance, if well aspected.

Most vulnerable parts are ears, throat, neck, cerebellum, upper cervical vertebrae, Eustachian tubes, larynx, upper part of esophagus, lower jaw, upper back, cervical vertebrae, thyroid and tonsils.

Afflicted: Overeating can cause Illnesses. Tends to inflammation in throat and tonsils, tonsillitis, polypus, laryngitis, obesity, croup, thrush, gangrene, impaired circulation, venereal disease, heart trouble, edema of neck, stroke, thyroid problems and mucus congestion.

And square Jupiter in Leo: thyroid problems

Moon afflicted by Saturn, Mars, Uranus or Neptune: eye problems

Opposition Scorpio: sex and sex organ problems

In Sixth house: gall and kidney stones

Moon In Gemini

Needs mental stimulation for healthy nerves. Avoid living in or near damp, and/or cold places. Deep breathing is necessary. Requires more rest and sleep than others need, as well as outdoor exercise, bike riding, and long walks. Avoid smoking.
Sensitive parts: arms, inferior cervical ganglion, nerves, lungs, and hands
Afflicted: lung congestion, pneumonia, tubercular tendencies, asthma, emotional problems, rheumatic ailments, accidents to hands, arms and shoulders, nervous disorders, susceptibility to paralytic seizures, especially in cases when the nervous system was previously stressed
And square, opposition or conjunct Sun Mercury or Malefics: pleurisy, pneumonia, and asthma

Moon In Cancer

Well aspected: Favorable position for the Moon. It influences digestion. Cancer rules peristaltic action of the stomach, bodily fluids, blood, lymph and nutrition.
Most sensitive areas are: breasts, uterus, prostate, epigastric, thoracic duct, pancreas, diaphragm, upper lobes of the liver, and chest cavity.
Afflicted: Weakens health making it delicate. Tends to anemia, edema. Susceptible for digestive problems, tumors, inflammatory diseases, bronchial troubles, kidney problems, flatulence, adrenal exhaustion, epilepsy (square Aries), obesity, asthma, and excessive use of energy drinks and coffee.
Square Mars: weak digestion
And square Mercury: emotional problems disturb digestion. Unforgiving and doubts cause immunity problems.
And square Saturn: constipation
And conjunct, square or opposition Mars and other malefic: fistula, hemorrhoids
And ruler of Cancer in sixth house, and ruler aspected by any planet from any water sign: urinary tract diseases.

Moon In Leo

The health is good. The moon in this position indicates heart disease. The heart is the weakest part in the body. Avoid nervous stress, tension, avoid stimulating foods, drugs and alcohol. Needs adequate sleep and rest.
Afflicted: Aneurism, mood swings, convulsions, back pains, ailments caused by poor circulation, skin problems, vertebrae troubles, indigestion, angina pectoris, coronary thrombosis, inflammations, locomotor ataxia, spinal meningitis, sunstroke and heart disease.
And square Jupiter in Taurus: thyroid problems
And square to either light: heart problems requiring avoidance of stress.
Squared from Taurus: backaches
And Saturn in Leo: circulation problems.
In Sixth house: bronchitis, kidney and gallstones

Moon In Virgo

Good recuperative ability. May have tendency to abuse medicine.
Afflicted: weak intestines, diarrhea, constipation, colic, tumors in stomach and abdomen, peritonitis, gallstones, pneumonia, eczema and other skin eruptions, blockage in intestines, nervousness
And square Gemini: eczema, skin problems
When hemmed between malefics: skin and other diseases from liver and kidney problems
Square or opposition Mars: arthritis.
In sixth house: afflicts small intestines, poor absorption of nutrients which lowers energy.

Moon In Libra

Well aspected: Indicates good health and recuperative ability, responds well to treatment.
Afflicted: problems with ovaries, stomach, appendix, ureters, skin, Bright's disease, inflammation, headaches, abscess of kidneys, uremia, insomnia, diabetes, wounds of the hands and feet, kidney stones and problems, leg and back problems, as well as mood swings.
Afflicted in sixth house: decreases the function of the stomach and nerves
And Moon square Mars, Moon opposition Jupiter and Moon opposition Mercury: kidney problems

Opposition Jupiter: kidney problems
Square Mercury: decrease kidney function
Opposition Uranus, Mercury and Jupiter: urine secretion decreases, which increase toxins in the system. Need for emotional stability, rejects sympathy, anger and irritation increases and prolong health problems.
Afflicted by Venus, Mars, Jupiter, or Saturn: Bright's disease, diabetes, kidney troubles, back problems and kidney stones.

Moon In Scorpio

Even with good health disease can become a problem. Even well aspected makes for tendency to disorders of menstrual functions, urinary organs and can make menopause difficult, reproductive problems, uterine or prostate disease.
MALE: tends to prostate infection. Can have urethral stricture, which can be caused by earlier venereal infection.
Afflicted: rectal and venereal diseases, throat troubles, edema, bladder inflammation and weakness, hydrocele, various genito-urinary problems, tumors, lower bowel inflammation, prostate disease, fibroid tumors and ovarian cyst.
In sixth house: kidney and gallstones, respiratory problems.
And ruler of Scorpio in sixth house and aspected by any planet from a water sign: urinary diseases.
Conjunct, square or opposition Mars and aspected by other malefic: fistula, hemorrhoids
Moon afflicted by Venus, Saturn or Mars: especially for a male: kidney stones.

Moon In Sagittarius

Good health and immunity
Afflicted: effects blood, respiratory system, and nervous system. Sciatica, accidents and broken arms and legs, wounds from firearms or electronics, falls, blood diseases, asthma, weakness of hips and thighs, dislocation of hips, ataxia, exhaustion, and arthritis.
Square or opposition Sun: problems with eyes. Check for solar eclipse on afflicting planet for time of disease problems.
Afflicted by Sun, Mars, Uranus or Saturn: injuries from firearms, falls, electronics and electricity.

Moon In Capricorn

Emotionally obsess with negativity, worries about the future and creates problems to worry about which causes illness. Needs fiber to regulate bowels rather than a depend upon laxatives, drink sufficient water and avoid use of stimulants. Emotions tend to create an acid condition in the body. Needs emotional stability.
Afflicted: tendency for skin eruptions and skin ailments, digestive troubles, bone ailments, dental trouble, uricaria. rheumatism, cramps, eye problems and gouty arthritis
Opposition Saturn in Cancer: lung problems. Malefic aspects of Saturn, Mars or Neptune make the condition worse.

Moon In Aquarius
Good recuperative ability despite general health weakness.
Afflicted: heart and kidney problems, edema, tendency to varicose veins, anemia, ulcers of the leg, unstable moods and obesity tendency.
Hemmed in between malefics: bone fractures, especially legs

Moon In Pisces
Poor health, immunity and recuperative ability susceptibility to infectious diseases. Should slowly digest one meal before taking in another. Can have Eating Disorder.
Afflicted: tendency to abuse drugs, alcohol, caffeine and nicotine, abdominal disorders, pneumonia, bronchitis, colds, tuberculosis, corns, bunions, and mood swings.
And ruler of Pisces is in the sixth house, and is aspected by any planet from a water sign: urinary troubles.
And conjunct, square or opposition Mars: venereal disease
In sixth house: respiratory problems.
Afflicted by Saturn: eye problems

Moon In Houses

Moon In First House

Has a very strong influence on health. Female constitution depends on aspects to Moon.
Opposition Saturn and Mercury: Nerve damage and epilepsy tendency. Nervous System diseases predisposition is increased if Mars or Saturn in sign afflict Moon and Mercury ascendent
Conjunct malefic without benefic aspecting: poor immunity
And Saturn in the fourth house and Mars in tenth: bone injuries

Moon In Second House

In Water signs: skin diseases.
And Mars in second and both aspected by Saturn: skin diseases.
And Sun in second: eye problems
And Mars in fourth and Sun in tenth: bone problems

Moon In Third

Afflicted: hypochondria. Third house afflictions indicate emotional problems.

Moon In Fourth House

Afflicted and three malefics in first house: heart disease.

Moon In Fifth House

Conjunct, square or opposition Saturn: thyroid problems, tumors, and cancer

Moon In Sixth House

Well aspected: Changes and fluctuating emotional and social issues can cause diseases. Tendencies to illness are decreased through favorable aspects to the moon, but this is not a favorable position for good health. Well or adversely aspected there is a tendency for psychosomatic illness and indigestion.
Afflicted: Various illnesses in infancy. Health challenges, cyst and tumor problems, bowel disorders come later, and skin diseases. Tendency to cuts and wounds.
And Mars in sixth: liver problems; hepatitis and jaundice tendencies.
And Mars in sixth: bone problems
And Neptune, Pluto, Uranus or Mars in sixth, aspected by malefics: digestion problems, abdominal pains
Afflicted by Saturn or Mars: eye problems
And Mars in second, and Saturn in twelfth, and Sun in eighth: eye problems
And malefics in fourth and fifth house, without benefic aspect to any of them: eye problems
And Saturn in eighth, and Mars, Neptune, Uranus or Pluto in the twelfth, and ruler of the first house afflicted: nasal problems.
Afflicted in fixed signs: tendency to severe diseases.
Afflicted in the first half of dual signs: tends to severe ills.
And ruler of the sixth house is in the eighth and afflicted: heart trouble
And in water sign, and ruler of the sixth house is aspected by Mercury from a water sign: urinary disease.
In Gemini, Virgo, Sagittarius and Pisces: respiratory disease
In Taurus, Leo, Scorpio and Aquarius: kidney and gallstones, respiratory disease.
In Aries, Libra, Capricorn and Cancer: digestive problems and stressed nerves.
And Sun and Mars in sixth house: boils, skin eruptions
And Mars in sixth house: cuts, wounds
Square or opposition Sun or Uranus: digestion problems
Square or opposition Mars: inflammatory diseases
Square or opposition Saturn: chronic disease.
Health can deteriorate under adverse moon influences. Generally when planets afflict the Moon, the afflicting planet will indicate the disease.

Moon In Seventh House

Afflicted: tendency for many illnesses
Conjunct, square or opposition Saturn, or Mars: left eye problems
Weak and powerless Moon: infertility
Weak Moon conjunct square or opposition Saturn: lung diseases

Moon In Eighth House

Weak Moon and Saturn in eighth: edema
Weak or waning Moon in eighth, conjunct, square or opposition Saturn and Mars: fistula, hemorrhoids
Waning Moon in eighth with Saturn or Mars: ulcers, wounds, burns
Afflicted by Saturn and Mars: eyesight problems
Weak Moon conjunct, square or opposition strong Saturn: severe eye disease
And malefics posited in fourth and fifth houses and no benefic planet aspects any of them: eye problems
Afflicted by Mars: of immunity, problems and harmful disease
And Saturn in eighth: food poisoning
And Venus in eighth: diarrhea
And Mars in eighth: fistula, hemorrhoids
And Sun in first, and Saturn in fifth, and Mars in ninth: bone injuries
Afflicted generally: public attention due to injury or sickness

Moon In Ninth

Square or opposition Sun: emotional and or mental problems
And Sun in ninth: eye problems

Moon In Tenth House

And Sun in fourth, and Saturn in eighth: bone injuries

Moon In Eleventh House

Sun conjunct Saturn, square and opposition either an eighth house Neptune or Mars ruler of eighth house: severe illness

Moon In Twelfth House

Afflicted: left eye problem or harm and increases fatalistic emotions and fear of insecurity as well as insanity. Makes for tendency for illness of long duration.
And afflicted by either Saturn or Mars, both of which aspect each other: eyesight problems
And Saturn in tenth, fifth or ninth, and Sun in seventh or eighth: eye trouble
And Sun in twelfth: eye diseases and problems
And malefics in fourth and fifth, and no benefic planet aspects any of them: eye diseases and problems
Afflicted by malefic, and first house afflicted: arm and or leg problems

Mercury Health Profile

Since Mercury rules the nervous system, favorable aspects to Mercury are beneficial for healthy nerves. Unfavorable aspects can result in emotional and or mental problems, tension and irritability. To ascertain the health of the nervous system, see the health of Mercury's sign and house and aspects. Mercury governs the five sensors: smell, taste, touch, sight, and hearing. Mercury is the ruler of all sores and ulcers. Mercury is responsible for poliomyelitis and nerve inflammation. To see what part of the body will tend to paralysis, see what planet aspects Mercury. Paralysis in the part of the body ruled by that planet. Mercury rules the nerves, spinal cord, lungs, thyroid, chest, skin, nose, navel, and gall bladder. The thyroid regulates body metabolism, respiration, nerves of the brain that connect to hands, arms and torso.
Mercury, Uranus and Neptune are the main influences in mental illnesses and govern parathyroid glands.

Diseases: Afflictions to Mercury can cause diseases of the nerves, epilepsy, chickenpox, smallpox, high fevers, convulsions, sinus problems, hazards from poison, itches, typhoid, paralysis, bone fractures, gall bladder troubles, indigestion, ulcers, cholera, poliomyelitis, lung problems, COPD including emphysema and asthma. Mercury conjunct square or opposition Malefic and without benefic aspect: sinus problems.

Mercury In Signs

Mercury In Aires

Repetitive motion or, confining and boring activities can cause stress and nervous problems.
Afflicted: dizziness, vertigo, facial neuralgia, and insomnia after over exertion, back problems, kidney problems, and tension headaches
And conjunct, square or opposition Saturn: urinary tract disease

Mercury In Taurus

Well aspected or afflicted: Eating Disorder
Afflicted: throat disorders, difficulty swallowing, hoarseness, croup, genital and urinary problems, mental stress and/or convulsions in childhood

Mercury In Gemini

Deep breathing exercises are advisable.
Afflicted: nervous pain in shoulders, arms and hands, nervous pain in hips, intercostal neuralgia, defects in respiratory system, asthma, pleurisy, edema, bronchitis

Mercury In Cancer

Afflicted: stress, emotional anxiety, grief and sorrow can cause indigestion, mucus congestion, caffeine, nicotine, alcohol and/or drug abuse.

Mercury In Virgo

Sedentary lifestyles require mild exercises, take exercise breaks regularly and walk, Avoid being tensely bent forward
Afflicted: Stress, mood swings, palpitation and spasms of heart, convulsions, pains in spinal nerves, brain fatigue, back pain, fainting

Mercury In Virgo

Afflicted: diarrhea, digestion problems, nausea, stomach ache, spastic colon, flatulence, colic, itching of nose, constipation, shortness of breath, weak nerves.

Mercury In Scorpio

Afflicted: painful genitals, sexual troubles, hoarseness, neuralgia, inflammation of bladder, bladder pains, menstruation difficulties, reproductive problems, hearing problems.

Mercury In Sagittarius

Mercury in its detriment here indicates health problems.
Afflicted: sciatica, nervousness, weakness in hips and pelvis, asthma, paralysis, pleurisy, coughs, colds.
And conjunct, square or opposition Saturn, urinary tract disease

Mercury In Capricorn

Afflicted: back pain, skin diseases, gout, nervous indigestion, flatulence, itching, neurasthenia, rheumatism, mood swings, intestinal problems caused by negative emotions, fear and stress.
And conjunct, square or opposition Saturn, especially if Saturn occupies a cardinal sign: hearing problems

Mercury In Aquarius

Afflicted: Emotional problems, heart pain, shooting pains, mood swings, varicose veins, stress, and circulatory problems.
And in any aspect with Uranus: tendencies to vegetarianism.

Mercury In Pisces

Mercury here is in a sign of its detriment and can indicate harmful diseases.
Afflicted or otherwise: emotional problems, stress, caffeine, alcohol and or drug abuse, cramps in feet, feet sensitive to cold and tender, corns, bunions, tuberculosis, colic, gouty arthritis, hearing problems, moody and general weakness

Mercury In Houses

Mercury In First House

In Taurus and Capricorn: eating disorder tendency
Afflicted, with Sun and Moon also afflicted in first: nerve inflammation
Ninth house rules limbs. Afflictions to Sagittarius tends to indicate thigh and pelvis area problems.
And Sun and Saturn in sixth aspected by a malefix: heart disease

Mercury In Second House

Coughs, colds, indigestion
Square or opposition moon: skin diseases.

Mercury In Third House

In Cancer or Pisces: erratic, unstable and/or fluctuating moods, tendency to disobey treatment protocols
Afflicted: over exaggerate symptoms.

Mercury In Fourth House

Mood and emotional problems increases illness.

Mercury In Fifth House

Inclines to drink alcohol.

Mercury In Sixth House

Well aspected and especially occupying Virgo: Knowledgeable about health and hygiene
Afflicted: Feels disease will cause death. Do not talk too much about health. All diseases here are dangerous. Their mental and or emotional state can make disease worse. Social troubles can cause mental illness. Worry and anxiety come natural.
And conjunct, square or opposition Mars: problems with emotional illness. Over impulsive and lack emotional control
And square or opposition Saturn: mental stress caused by extreme anxiety. Tendency to develop a chronic illness with a gloomy, depressing outlook.

And square or opposition Uranus: Social problems can cause emotion disease. An affliction of Mercury and Uranus tends to cause a disease of the parathyroid glands.
And square or opposition Mars: can cause emotional injury from brooding over disease.
Especially when afflicted: emotions influence diet with a lack of commonsense regarding junk food diets and poor health

Mercury in Seventh House

Conjunct, square or opposition Mars, Pluto, Neptune, Saturn or Uranus: digestive problems and diseases

Mercury in Eighth House

Coughs and indigestion

Mercury in Ninth House

Tends to be non-compliant to health treatment
Afflicted: will not give treatment enough time to achieve wellness

Mercury in Tenth House

Will prevent disease and help speed recuperation if given all the facts about illness
Afflicted: hearing problems, especially square Uranus

Mercury in Eleventh House

May have doubts about natural treatments and recuperation

Mercury In Twelfth House

And Venus combust in twelfth: lack of mental and emotional stability, poor circulation. Hearing problems.
And conjunct Neptune, Mercury square Jupiter: poor circulation causes hearing problems
Square, opposition Mars or Uranus: tends to have emotionally driven outburst and negative behavior.
Conjunct, square, opposition Saturn: hearing problems, mood swings

Venus Health Profile

Venus and Jupiter have to do with cell reproduction. When well aspected, Venus increases immunity and health. Can influence weight gain. Good aspects to Venus stimulate immunity. When well placed, dignified or otherwise good, Venus stimulates anti-aging nutrients, which makes for youthful appearance in old age.
Venus rules: reproductive organs, circulation of blood and lymph, hormones, bladder, the face, eyesight, urine, kidneys, skin, hair, throat, chin, cheeks, glands, complexion; Thyroid gland (which is ruled by Mercury) is influenced by Venus; Venus regulates body metabolism. Thymus gland governed to a lesser degree by the Moon. It regulates parathyroid and calcium metabolism.
Afflicted: Salivary parotid gland problems, mumps, kidney and bladder disease, eye trouble, edema, throat trouble, indigestion, impotency, fever, glandular diseases, skin health, mood disorders, venereal disease, diabetes
In close aspect to ascendant or its ruler: improves health
Sun, Venus and Jupiter in one house: eye problems
Look to Sun and Mercury if Venus is afflicted impairs the heart's circulation into the right auricle and ventricle and lungs, toxic blood negatively affects heart and lungs.
Venus is dignified in Taurus and Libra, exalted in Pisces, improving health. Venus is weak and afflicted in Aries, Scorpio and Virgo, which can deteriorate health.
Venus square or opposition Moon: circulatory problems, arteriosclerosis.

Venus In Signs

Venus In Aires

Afflicted: Susceptibility to kidney problems, clogged sinus, colds, disorder of lachrymal glands, eczema, liver problems, skin troubles, allergic to cosmetics. A planet in a sign of its detriment can cause health problems.

Venus in Taurus

Afflicted: Thyroid problems, reproductive problems and diseases, headaches affecting occipital region, tumor in neck, mumps, glandular swellings in the throat, weak throat, inflammations of throat, pain in back of head, abscesses, tonsillitis.
Opposition Uranus in Scorpio: Venereal disease when the Moon conjunction of Venus or opposition of Uranus

Venus In Gemini

Respiratory and circulatory problems, sores, toxins
Afflicted: Tight clothing should be avoided

Venus in Cancer

Afflicted: Tendency to nausea, bloating and gastric tumors, enlarged stomach, weak stomach muscles, indigestion, vomiting, cysts of breast, periodic fluid discharge from uterus

Venus In Leo

Afflicted: heart problems, enlarged heart, backache, problems with the spinal cord, mood swings, blocked, and/or hard and diseases of arteries.

Venus In Virgo

Afflicted: parasites, worms, weaken peristaltic muscles of the intestines, tumors, Food Addiction, poor food combining, junk food diets, excessive amounts of cooked foods and or excessive cooked fructose, diarrhea.

Venus In Libra

Afflicted: kidney problems, polyuria, headaches, uric acid, uremia, reabsorption of urine-toxins into the blood, eczema, dry skin with eruptions, thirst, addiction to sweets and white sugar.
And conjunct, square or opposition Uranus: nephritis

Venus In Scorpio

A planet in its detriment can cause illnesses in the sign related to an organ. Caffeine, nicotine, sugars, and drugs over stimulate glands causing diseases.
Afflicted: ovarian disorders, throat problems, venereal disease, prolapsis of uterus, painful menstruation, cyst in ovaries, prostate disease, fluid on testicles, hernia, painful ovaries, tumors.

Venus In Sagittarius

Afflicted: sciatica, bronchial and pulmonary problems, pelvic and thigh problems, tumors
Opposition Gemini: excessive exercise and or sport activities can cause disease

Venus In Capricorn

Afflicted: edema in limbs, especially knees, bursitis, vomiting, stomach disturbances, skin diseases, worms, constipation, fluid on knee cap, digestion problems, gouty arthritis
Square Saturn: colds and diseases caused by depletion of energy and immunity, toxins cause negative emotions, weaken immunity.

Venus In Aquarius

Afflicted: heart trouble, anemia, swollen ankles, varicose veins, and unstable emotions

Venus In Pisces

Afflicted: feet problems, bunions, corns, gonorrhea, tumors, abdominal swellings, tumors, gouty arthritis, inflammation and swelling of feet and hands caused by over exposure to cold or hot weather

Venus In Houses

Venus In First House

Well aspected: good health
Afflicted: Life style and or job problems deteriorate health. In Aries, Gemini, Libra, Aquarius or Pisces best. In Virgo, Scorpio and Capricorn, alcohol, drugs, energy drinks and caffeine abuse
And sixth house ruler also in first house: urinary tract diseases

Venus In Second House

Afflicted: abuses health causing aging appearance
And Moon adversely aspected by a malefic: eye diseases

Venus In Third House

Well aspected: positive emotions and optimism creates good health
Conjunct, square, or opposition Saturn in the eleventh house: social relationships stress nervous system causing ill health

Venus In Fourth House

Well aspected: helps maintain good health in childhood and old age
Afflicted: Eating disorder

Venus In Fifth House

And Sun and Saturn in fifth house: urinary tract disease

Venus In Sixth House

Well aspected or not seriously afflicted: good effect on health. Health problems can develop into serious illness if there is a lack of self-control or abuse of caffeine, alcohol or drugs. The health is fragile and disease prevention is a must. Neglect of health can cause severe illness. Emotional nurturing helps to overcome disease and give health stability.
Afflicted: kidney problems, circulatory problems, throat and ear problems, and weakness

Venus In Seventh House

Ideal house for Venus good for health is.
Conjunct, square or opposition Saturn: backache
Conjunct Mars, Saturn, Uranus, Pluto or Neptune: diarrhea

Venus In Eighth

Afflicted: Harmed by junk foods, alcohol and/or drugs, harmed or by others, either accidentally or otherwise.
Conjunct Moon in eighth: diarrhea

Venus In Ninth House

Well aspected: a positive influence on health

Venus In Tenth House

Well aspected: influences good health
Aspected by Saturn, Mars, Pluto, Uranus, and Neptune without benefic aspect: fertility problems

Venus In Eleventh House

Well aspected: a positive influence on health

Venus In Twelfth House

Benefits from treatments whether well aspected or afflicted.
Afflicted: many diseases and poor health
Afflicted in Taurus or Scorpio: sexual excesses cause diseases
Afflicted, Saturn in first or seventh house: poor health, many diseases

Mars Health Profile

Mars rules the muscular system and inflammatory responses to disease. Where Mars is, there is an increased circulation. Aspects from Mercury to Mars tend toward strong muscles. Mars rules the body temperature. The action of Mars is centrifugal. Mars governs reproductive organs; harmonious aspects increase likelihood and number of children while conflicts do the reverse. In earth signs, Mars tends toward bodily injury. Mars causes all paralysis and strokes, is the ruling planet for types of injuries, cuts, cyst, and tumors, and is often involved in fatal diseases and accidents.
Body parts ruled: blood, muscular system, bone marrow, energy, vitality, genitals, rectum, liver, face, head, brain, nose, tongue. Mars has co-rulership with Saturn over primitive emotions, the medulla and adrenal cortex and their hormones, cortisol, noradrenaline and adrenaline, and rules male gonads.
Diseases: blood pressure, hypothyroidism, cuts, wounds, itches, cancer, neck problems, fatigue, sore eyes, strokes, bone marrow, bone fractures, female organ disease, menstrual problems, urinal disease, cysts, tumors, boils, ulcers, rectal diseases, diarrhea, and hemorrhoids.
Afflicted and strong: high blood pressure, skin eruptions, paralysis, accidents, and inflammation of organs
Afflicted and weak: anemia, leukemia, low blood pressure, ulcers, cyst, tumors, diseases of marrow, circulatory problems, skin eruptions, boils
Sun, Mars, Jupiter and Mercury in one house: eye problems
Square ascendant: arthritis

Mars In Signs

Mars In Aires

Drinks large amounts of liquid
Well aspected: desire for raw foods, enjoys exercise, good energy
Afflicted: delirium, pains in head, wounds in head, insomnia, strokes, ringworm, trouble with blood vessels, tendency to thickening of tubules of kidneys and bleeding of kidneys, smallpox, kidney stones, kidney disease, may need surgery, eye problems
Badly afflicted: mental illness can be a problem
Afflicted by Moon (ruling brain) points to brain damage

Mars In Taurus

A planet in a sign of its detriment may have a negative effect on health. Mars here strengthens the negative tendencies of Mars.
Well aspected or afflicted (worse if afflicted): back problems, gland problems, overeats foods, mumps, enlarged or inflamed tonsils, adenoids, diphtheria, thyroid problems, nosebleeds, suffocations, inflammation of larynx, swollen tonsils, polyps, boils, rheumatism in neck muscles, nasal catarrh, enlargement of prostate gland, kidney stones in bladder, venereal sores
Conjunct, square or opposition Saturn: neck and hearing problems
Conjunct Neptune: alcohol abuse. Sun in water sign increases tendency to abuse alcohol or drugs.
Opposition Moon or Venus in Scorpio: indications for tonsillitis.

Mars In Gemini

Afflicted: tendency for bleeding lungs, cough, pneumonia, pleurisy, bronchitis, lung cancer, fractures of hands arms and collarbone, wounds, fracture of hip and or thigh, sciatica, neuralgia, inflammation of nerves, fevers, bleeding stomach, diarrhea, liver complaints, COPD and severe lung diseases
Afflicted females: childbirth problems, natural or medically induced abortions

Mars in Cancer

Afflicted: indigestion, dry cough, inflammation, ulcers and bleeding of the stomach, vomiting of blood, dyspepsia, gallstones, vomiting of bile, fevers, and miscarriage. Delayed meals tend to cause pain. Vision troubles. Tendency to accidents by electronics, electricity, and/or fire. Acidosis, which affects eyes. liver stressed
And Mars square Venus: malnutrition
And Jupiter conjunct, square or opposition Mars: causes blood vessel problems affecting circulation

Mars In Leo

Afflicted: heart disease, endocarditis, heart enlargement, pericarditis, fainting, angina pectoris, heart pain, muscular rheumatism affecting back, suffocation, aneurysma of veins, strokes, malaria, herpes zoster, throat inflammation, aneurysms, pleurisy, indigestion, liver problems, paralysis, mental illness
And square Venus in Taurus: inflammatory problems in the nose, rectum and sex organs. Polypus, a growth from mucous membranes of nose, vagina or rectum. Respiratory problems can cause the closing of the nasal passages, particularly if they breathed through their mouth in childhood.
Square Sun in Taurus: wounds, fevers, inflammation, bleedings,
And Sun rising in Leo: heart problems

Mars In Virgo

Well aspected: Recuperate from disease quickly.
Afflicted: Eating Disorder, parasites, worms, colitis, cholera, peritonitis, typhoid, enteritis, diarrhea, ventral hernia, appendicitis, typhus, liability to accidents and sickness from stress, liver disease, weak immunity, and hypertension.
Configurated with Uranus, any aspect: susceptible to intestinal problems

And Moon afflicted by Mars: rheumatism, gland inflammation

Mars In Libra

Mars is in a sign of its detriment and so can become a detriment to the health.
Afflicted particularly: kidney problems, kidney stones, and back pain, nephritis, bleeding of kidneys, excess urine, and headache. Other people's behavior and feeling can have a negative effect on health.
Conjunct Uranus in Libra: susceptible to kidney problems

Mars In Scorpio

Afflicted: fibroid tumors or cyst on ovaries, vagina or prostate problems, scalding urine, renal stones, hemorrhoids, fistula, bladder diseases, gout, septic poisoning, abortions, coronary thrombosis, epilepsy, inflamed tonsils or larynx, nose bleed, throat and nose diseases, hernia, appendicitis, gall stones, enlarged prostate, varicocele, sores in sex organs, birthing problems, fallopian tube problems
And Jupiter ruler of eleventh house: birthing problems

Mars In Sagittarius

Afflicted: sciatica, dislocated femur, pelvic and thigh problems, fracture of thigh-bone, pneumonia, bronchitis, coughs, pneumonia, typhoid, boils, troubles with anus, accidents, trouble with eyes, inflammation of hip

Mars In Capricorn

Afflicted: skin eruptions, edema, inflamed skin, erysipelas, chicken pox, measles, smallpox, pimples, boils, rheumatism, stomach ulcers, inflammation of knee joint (gonitis), inflammation of mucous membrane of kneecap, rheumatic fever, rash, scabies, jaundice, abdominal ulcers, indigestion, arm and or leg accidents, arthritis of knee, paralysis can be a problem
Conjunct Sun in Capricorn: accidents involving the knee

Mars In Aquarius

Afflicted: fractures of legs, weak immunity, emotion and or mental problems, varicose veins, fainting, blood poisoning, fever, eye problems, sores on legs, skin eruptions, rashes, heart problems

Mars In Pisces

Afflicted: foot deformities or accidents to feet, diarrhea, caffeine, alcohol and or drug problems, poor circulation, bunions, corns, swelling of feet, perspiring feet, low energy, (hyperhidrosis) deformed feet, inflammation of bowels, respiratory problems, infectious problems, foot odor

Mars In Houses

Mars In First House

Well aspected: a good influence on the health, particularly in fire signs, Capricorn. Even in weak signs survives poor health in infancy and good health later.
Afflicted: takes good health for granted, neglects health, Eating Disorder, fevers and inflammatory disease, accidents, wounds, cuts, bruises, burns, scalds on face, brain, nose, tongue.
Square or opposition Sun: fevers and inflammations
Square or opposition Jupiter: broken bones. Susceptible to accidents when traveling or physical activities.
Conjunct, square or opposition Uranus or Saturn: bruises, accidental falls
Conjunct Sun in first house: urinary tract disease
And ruler of sixth house: debilitated, poor health
And ruler of sixth house in first: cuts, wounds
And Jupiter and Saturn in first house: wounds, cuts
And Sun in first, aspected by a malefic: burns

Mars In Second House

Check twelfth house. The Second house rules the nose, second rules one nostril and twelfth house rules the other
And Moon in second, both aspected by Saturn: skin diseases
Opposition Sun: boils, tumors, cyst, skin eruptions
And Saturn in second or conjunct second house ruler: eye diseases
And Saturn in twelfth, Moon in sixth, and Sun in eighth: tend to severe eye problems
Square, opposition Saturn or Uranus: danger of emotional and or physical violence and sudden illness
Conjunct, square or opposition Uranus: danger of emotional and mental disease with mental illness possible being hereditary.
Mars in Cancer or Pisces afflicted by square or oppositions: excessive sex weakens health, poor digestion,
And Moon in second, both Mars and Moon afflicted: injury and or fracture of bones
And Saturn and Jupiter in fourth house: heart disease
Afflicted generally: inflammatory diseases, accidents involving electronics, electricity, fire
And Sun in second, square, or opposition Saturn, Uranus, Pluto, or Neptune: nerve damage

Mars In Third House

Ideal Mars in Capricorn
Afflicted severe when Uranus afflicts Mars, Nerve Damage
In Cancer, Pisces, Scorpio, Emotional illness if Mars affects Mental Ruler
And Sun in third house: wounds to hands
Well aspected or afflicted: nerve damage

Mars In Fourth House

Well aspected: good health can continue in old age. Good digestion.
Afflicted: inflammatory diseases, fevers, susceptible to accidents involving electronics, electricity, and/or fire
And Saturn and Jupiter in fourth house: heart disease
If Mars is in Cancer or Pisces and afflicted by square or opposition: digestion problems, excessive sex weakens health.
Square or opposition Saturn or Uranus: danger of emotional and or physical violence and sudden illness
Square or opposition Mercury: negative feelings over things not connected with the disease, or grief, can cause disease to get worse
Ideal if Mars is in Aires, Leo, Capricorn
Conjunct Sun in first house: Urinary tract Infection
And ruler of Sixth house: weak, debilitated

Mars In Fifth House

Well aspected: consistent exercise (started while young) maintains good health
Afflicted: problems birthing, heart trouble, disease caused by emotional and or physical stress
Conjunct Saturn, Uranus, Pluto or Neptune, Mars: liver disease

Mars In Sixth House

Well aspected: increases good health, recuperating from illness can improve health
Afflicted: colitis, tends to have fever when ill, fevers can cause secondary illness, inflammation in the part of the body ruled by the sign Mars is posited. Work related injury. Scalds, burns, fevers, inflammatory diseases. Can have surgery. Eating disorder, sexual partner can give them a disease.
And Sun and Moon in sixth: skin eruptions, boils, and cyst
And Moon in sixth house: cuts, wounds
Square Sun or Jupiter: inflammatory complaints
Square or opposition Uranus: accident causes illnesses, susceptible to emotional and or mental illness
Conjunct Saturn in sixth house: eye problem
And Moon in sixth: vomiting, liver disease, bone fractures

Mars In Seventh House

And Saturn in eighth house: cyst, tumors, boils
Opposition Sun: tumors, cyst, and boils
And Saturn, Moon and Sun in first house: arm and or leg injury due to accident involving machines
And Saturn in first house: fistula, hemorrhoids
Conjunct, square or opposition Saturn, Neptune, Pluto or Uranus: urinal diseases, kidney stones
And Sun in seventh aspected by malefics: burns
Conjunct Saturn, Uranus, Pluto or Neptune: fistula, hemorrhoids

Mars In Eighth House

Afflicted: sudden and unexpected injury, cuts, wounds, accidents or fevers can cause severe illness. Sudden severe disease
Mars, ruler of sixth in eighth: high blood pressure
And opposition Sun: wounds, cuts, cyst, tumors, boils
And Saturn in eighth: eye problems
And Sun in eighth aspected by malefics: burns
Aspected by Saturn: fistula, hemorrhoids
And Moon in eighth: fistula, hemorrhoids

Mars In Ninth House

And Sun in first and Saturn in fifth and Moon in eighth: bones fractures

Mars In Tenth House

High energy level seems inexhaustible
Afflicted: susceptible to accidents
And Saturn in second, and Moon in fourth: bones fractures
Conjunct, square or opposition Saturn: urinary tract diseases

Mars In Eleventh House

Susceptible to disease and harm from or incidental to helping others

Mars In Twelfth House

Well aspected: institutional treatments of disease
Afflicted: affect the left eye. May be physically impaired in some way. Heart disease, wounds cuts.
Saturn, Mas, and ruler of first house in twelfth: fistula, hemorrhoids

Jupiter Health Profile

Jupiter is the planet of growth and expansion. Jupiter is concerned with cell reproduction and the Pituitary. Look to aspects between Jupiter and the Sun consider the circulatory system, heart and kidney
Body parts ruled: circulatory system, thigh, brain, kidneys, liver, right ear, tongue, cellular growth, spleen, Pituitary, pancreas, feet, hipbones, fat, lungs, memory.
Diseases: lung disease, pancreas disease (diabetes), painful feet, hepatitis, kidney problems, emphysema, memory problems, ear trouble, tongue ailments, edema, obesity, liver disease, arthritis, spleen problems, respiratory problems
With Sun and Venus in one house: eye problems

Jupiter In Signs

Jupiter In Aires

Afflicted: thrombosis, adrenal exhaustion, fainting, ulcerated gums of upper jaw, diabetes, mood swings, nerve damage, lethargic, dizziness

Jupiter In Taurus

Afflicted: gout, apoplexy, inflammation of throat, sores on lower jaw, ringworm, ulcerated gums of mandible, catarrh, nosebleed, Eating Disorder, skin eruptions
Square Sun or Moon in Leo: thyroid problems
Square or opposition Sun: smoking dietary extremes

Jupiter In Gemini

Jupiter is in a sign of detriment. Can have kidney problems
Afflicted: lung disease, pleurisy, lung congestion, bleeding of lungs, broken bones, fattening of the liver, arthritis, rheumatism
Conjunct, square or opposition Saturn or Uranus: obesity
Afflicted in sixth house: respiratory problems

Jupiter In Cancer

Well aspected: few health problems
Afflicted: Eating Disorder, diabetes, Liver problems, dropsy, rheumatism, flatulence, indigestion, skin diseases, skin eruptions, kidney problems, circulatory problems
On Ascendant: liver problems, eating disorder

Jupiter In Leo

Well aspected: good health and energy level
Afflicted: fatty degeneration of heart, heart disease, pleurisy, swollen ankles, poor circulation, paralysis,
Square Sun or Moon in eighth: thyroid problems

Jupiter In Virgo

Planet is in a sign of its detriment, which causes a negative effect on health, kidney problems
Afflicted: liver disease, poor digestion, intestinal problems, fattening of liver, abscess of liver, ulcerated liver, respiratory problems
Conjunct, square or opposition Saturn or Uranus: obesity
In sixth house: colon problems

Jupiter In Libra

Well aspected: a peaceful ending to the life, family and environment
Afflicted: kidney disease, weak adrenal glands, mood swings, poor circulations, skin eruptions, adrenal exhaustion, kidney abscesses, degeneration of kidneys, diabetes, renal abscess, pleurisy, coma, vertigo, dizziness, skin diseases

Jupiter In Scorpio

Afflicted: mucus discharge in urine, enlarged prostate, urethral problems, nosebleed, fistula, skin eruptions, heart troubles during old age, blood in urine, kidney problems, fibroid tumors, edema, paralysis, hemorrhoids
On Ascendant: circulatory system problems

Jupiter In Sagittarius

Afflicted: arthritis, rheumatism, poor circulation, pains and swelling in legs and hips, sciatica, bleeding of lungs (opposition Gemini), lung problems.
Square Venus in Pisces: tuberculosis, respiratory problems, poor circulation

Jupiter In Capricorn

Afflicted: Liver problems, eczema, psoriasis and other skin diseases, impaired digestion (opposition Cancer)
Conjunct Mars, ruler of eleventh house: problems giving birth
Conjunct, square or opposition Saturn or Uranus: obesity

Jupiter In Aquarius

Afflicted: hemorrhoids, heart problems (square Leo), blood vessel breakage, swollen ankles, edema of legs (opposition Leo), kidney problem, paralysis of legs

Jupiter In Pisces

Afflicted: enlarged liver, abdominal tumors, diseased intestines, jaundice, edema in feet, can have kidney problems, sweaty feet

Jupiter In Houses

Jupiter In First House

Health problems caused by emotional eating as a substitute for nurturing or to sooth, or ease painful feelings, disease occurs according to the sign where posited. Physically good health in middle age and after.
Afflicted: health suffers through impurities from non-organic foods and/or environment, liver diseases.
Health problems caused by toxins and or acidity
Conjunct Uranus: Excessive spices, and processed sugars
Afflicted in Cancer: Eating Disorder, stresses liver, pancreas and intestines problems, liver enlargement and serious illness
Afflicted in Pisces: addiction to caffeine, drugs, processed sugars, energy drinks, and /or alcohol

Jupiter In Second House

Tends to have a talent for recognizing and utilizing natural remedies for recuperating from diseases

Jupiter In Third House

And Saturn in ninth, both badly afflicted: diseases and problems with finger or fingers, hand or arm – especially on right hand or arm

Jupiter In Fourth House

Well aspected: tends to keep self-healthy throughout life
Square or opposition Mercury: sudden heart diseases
And Sun and Saturn in fourth: negative influence causing lung disease
And Saturn and Mars in fourth: heart disease

Jupiter In Fifth House

Heart problems caused by sudden blood overload into heart or, sudden fluctuation in blood pressure
Afflicted: emotions cause difficulty with self-control

Jupiter In Sixth House

Well aspected: good health. Applies positive emotions and thinking to health, exercise, diet, etc.
Afflicted and between two malefics: contributes to lung disease
Afflicted: Emotionally puts off or delays using natural remedies

Jupiter In The Seventh House

Well aspected: a positive influence on teeth and functions on the right side of body
Afflicted: has a negative effect on teeth and right side of body. See if Saturn afflicts the Sun – this increases the negative effect on teeth and right side of body

Jupiter In the Eighth House

Well aspected: good health in life. Stimulates positive behavior towards health.

Jupiter In The Ninth House

Well aspected: a positive influence on health, especially on the left side of the body
Afflicted: Protective and guarding self against negative influence on health, and mindful of health issues on the left side of the body

Jupiter In The Tenth House

Well aspected: stabilizes good health, health increases with natural remedies and outdoor activities and contact with nature's earth, air, water, sunshine
Afflicted: Uncontrolled emotions and or behavior can cause diseases

Jupiter In The Eleventh House

Well aspected: influences health on the left side of the body
Afflicted: has a negative effect on health on left side of body

Jupiter In The Twelfth House

Treatment facilitates can improve health
Well aspected: helps to overcome diseases, exercise self-control, and accept physical suffering.
Afflicted: disease of the spleen

Saturn Health Profile

Saturn influences the teeth, bones, and minerals and chronic diseases. Saturn makes all disease worse and is the ruling planet for all diseases.
RULES: skeletal system, teeth, bones, knees, liver, arms, legs, cartilages, muscles, hair, skin, spleen, adrenal medulla, adrenal gland hormones.
DISEASES: bone loss, osteoporosis, weak hip bones, deterioration of bones near knees, respiratory disease, loss or decay to teeth, hearing problems, skin diseases, leg problems, bone fractures, wounds, muscular pain, paralysis, ailments of connecting joints, anemia, stomach trouble, torn ligaments and tendons near bones, arthritis and rheumatism pain, hair loss, damage to bones
AFFLICTED: The part of the body, shown by the sign in which Saturn is posited, is the weakest and diseased. The part may be underdeveloped or deformed. Worse if Uranus also afflicts. Saturn obstructs, hampers and decreases the functions of the body, chronic and fatal disease, injury and or damage to organ if stressed
Afflicted in or from Pisces: diseases of feet
And Venus in one: eye problems
Semi square Ascendant: rheumatism
Saturn Occidental: severe illness
The particular disease is determined by ruler ship of afflicted and afflicting planets and houses. Saturn is involved in degenerative diseases, illnesses of long duration, weaken immunity, malnutrition, psychosomatic diseases, kidney disease, arthritis, rheumatism, blocked and obstructed arteries, poor circulation, high blood

pressure, deformity, weakness, arteriosclerosis. Part of the body indicated by the sign can suffer from severe chills, diseases, injuries and accidents to the head and parts in and on the head.

Saturn In Signs

Saturn In Aires

Teeth problems, colds, tooth decay, eye and hearing problems, headaches, mood swings, arthritis, fainting, fits, chills, meningitis, allergies, sinus problems, mental problems, renal disorders, near sightedness, stomach disorders (square Cancer), kidney disease, and kidney problem (opposition Libra).
And Jupiter square Mercury in Taurus: eye and ear problems, and poor circulation
And Mercury afflicted: mood and thought disorders

Saturn In Taurus

Disease and or injury to throat, lower jaw and neck, chronic problems with the throat, croup, tendency to phlegm, choking, decay of lower teeth, larynxgitis, whooping cough, diphtheria, mumps, pyorrhea, decayed teeth, constipation, poor peristalsis, myocarditis, colds, nasal passage congestion, ear problems, blocked and or clogged colon, inflamed throat
Conjunct Neptune: thyroid problems
And Neptune in Taurus: reproductive organ problems

Saturn In Gemini

One of the two least adverse places for Saturn. Pains in shoulders, arms and hands, dislocation of arm or shoulder, respiratory problems, bronchitis, asthma, acute pneumonia, general weakness, sciatica (opposition Sagittarius), hip problems, digestion problems (square Virgo), job related illnesses, rheumatism pain in shoulders, nerve damage, numbness and trembling in arms, hands, feet and legs.
Much afflicted: Emotional problems caused by relatives or opponents. Social problems caused by others. Dry climate is best, avoid damp climate, damp home and living near water. Deep breathing is best for health.

Saturn In Cancer

Poor absorption of nutrients, poor digestion, lack of appetite, arthritis, stiff knee joints, eye troubles, anemia, gall stones, cancer, breast and stomach disease, kidney problems, liver and pancreas disease. Avoid chronic indigestion, avoid eating habitually, masticate food well and eat regularly. Avoid over consumption of meat or spices.

Saturn in Leo

Heart disease, psychosomatic diseases, avoid stress, weak back, poor circulation, edema in ankles, arteriosclerosis, meningitis, curvature of the spine, calcification of blood vessels, sclerosis of the spinal cord, liver disease, heart smaller than average. Saturn here is in a sign of its detriment and has a negative effect on health.
And Moon in Leo: circulation problems, obstructed of blood vessels
And Saturn in first house: gastric reflux
Square or opposition Sun: heart afflicted from birth by hereditary problems. Damage or malfunction of organs follow eventually
Square or opposition Moon: poor nutrition, negative emotions, and heart problems
Opposition Mercury: contraction of heart valves
Opposition Mercury in fixed signs: heart problems
Cardiac remedies are more effective: when increasing Moon conjoins, or trines or sextiles radical Jupiter or Venus
When waning Moon squares or opposes radical Jupiter or Venus avoid stimulants

Saturn in Virgo

Poor absorption of nutrients, indigestion, liver problems, colic, weak intestines, colon obstructions, appendicitis, headaches, mental disease, hypochondria, poor growth during childhood, over active pancreas (hyper-insulin), sclerosis.

Saturn In Libra

Kidney problems, urine retention, infertility problems, Bright's Disease, anuria, nephritis, locomotor ataxia, malnutrition, headache (opposition Aries), toothache, back pain, kidney stones, gall stones, edema, arthritis caused by toxins related to kidney problems.
And conjunct Venus in Libra: kidney problems

Saturn in Scorpio

Constipation, weaker in legs, sudden disease, nasal bone loss, menstruation problems, arthritis, hemorrhoids, fistula, nasal catarrh, phlegm and other throat problems, hoarseness (opposition Taurus), weak in large intestine, myocarditis (square Leo), hernia, degeneration
Conjunct Uranus in Scorpio: anus problems
Conjunct Mercury in Scorpio: negative emotions, depression
And Neptune in Scorpio: sex organs problems
And Jupiter square Mercury, and Jupiter square Saturn: constipation, hemorrhoids. Circulation problems.

Saturn In Sagittarius

One of the two least adverse places for Saturn. Tendency for degenerative diseases. Can have kidney problems, hips and thighs can be out of alignment, meningitis, sciatica, bronchitis, tuberculosis (opposition Gemini), arthritis, problems with pelvic area and thigh, rheumatism in thighs
Conjunct, square or opposition Mars or Uranus: paralysis in hips, pelvis, thigh and leg areas

Saturn In Capricorn

Tendency for depression in late adulthood, painful emotions about past, arthritis, and liver problems. gall stones, skin eruptions, and diseases including cancer of the skin, eczema and psoriasis, constipation, headaches, fevers, weakness in knees, indigestion
And in mutual aspect with Mercury and Sun when they are rulers of eighth and sixth houses: bone problems and fractures

Sun In Aquarius

Well aspected: Good nutrition helps to avoid diseases.
Foot deformity, ankle weakness, sprained ankles, and poor circulation, below the knee leg problems, diseases of spine, heart disease, illness of the spinal cord, cataracts, fatigue, bone marrow problems

Saturn In Pisces

Foot problems, bunions, fallen arches, and cold feet, intestinal obstructions, rheumatism, neuritis, respiratory disease (square Gemini), swollen lymph glands, edema, colds.

Saturn In Houses

Saturn In First House
Causes diseases and poor health.
Conjunct ascendant: accident or a broken limb
Conjunct Sun in first house: skin disease
Conjunct, square or opposition Mars: skin disease
Opposition Mars in seventh house: fistula, hemorrhoids

Saturn In Second House

Problems with right eye, teeth crooked, out of alignment, uneven growth and or gaps
Many planets in second conjoining or semisextile Saturn: vision problems
And Mars in second: eye diseases
Conjunct, square or opposition Mars, Uranus, Neptune or Pluto: tumors, cyst, boils, and skin eruptions
And Moon in fourth, and Mars in tenth: bone fractures

Saturn In Third House

Bronchitis tends to be caused by Saturn Venus afflictions involving the third house either by occupancy or rulership. Saturn, conjunct, square or opposition Mars: skin diseases, eruptions on skin, itchy skin

Saturn In Fourth House

And Sun and Jupiter in fourth: can cause lung disease
Saturn, Mars and Jupiter in fourth: heart disease
And north node and Moon in seventh: heart disease

Saturn In Fifth House

Heart problems
And Sun in first, and Moon in eighth, and Mars in ninth: bone fractures
Sun, Venus and Saturn in fifth: urinary tract disease
In mutual aspect with Mars, and further aspected by sixth house ruler: abdominal pain

Saturn In Sixth House

Poor health, immunity, and energy. Many diseases during life. Degenerative diseases from inadequate nutrition and processed foods, poor health can be caused by over exposure to cold. Injury from accidental falls and or hit by falling objects. Lack good digestion. Tends to have periods of good health but eventually deteriorates temporarily or permanently because of Saturn Malefic effect.
Afflicted: Illnesses caused by ignoring emotional need to socialize with others or by emotional or social conditions that they have no control over. Tend to use excuses to neglect self.
And Saturn in Virgo or Pisces, and Moon afflicted: appendicitis
Or Saturn ruling sixth: Influenced by observing others eating. Eating disorder triggered by eating with others. Becomes emotionally misguided.
And Mars in sixth: Saturn and or Mars conjunct, square and a weak ruler of first house: chronic illnesses, degenerative diseases
And Mars in sixth: eye problem
And Sun in sixth: Sun or Saturn conjunct, square or opposition Mars, Uranus, Pluto or Neptune and Mercury in first: heart disease
In Taurus, Leo, Scorpio or Aquarius: lung problems, bronchitis, heart disease, and throat infections, and problems
In Gemini, Virgo, Sagittarius, and Pisces: severe colds, kidney problems, asthma, cancer, leg problems, colon problems, and respiratory problems
In Aries, Libra, Cancer and Capricorn: arthritis, weak stomach, and respiratory problems
In Libra: liver problems or diseases
Conjunct, square or opposition Sun or Moon: chronic ill health

Saturn in Seventh House

Afflicted: influences health negatively, urinary tract disease
And Moon between two malefics: boils, abscesses, cyst, and skin eruptions
And Mars without strength or afflicted by conjunction, square: abnormalities of arms and legs, toxic blood

Saturn In Eighth House

Well aspected in Capricorn or Libra: long life; Free of many diseases
Afflicted: hearting problems, hearing loss
Afflicted in Cancer: an addiction to sweets causes poor health
And Mars in eighth: eye problems
Aspected by Mars: cyst, tumors, boils, abscesses, skin eruptions
Conjunct, square or opposition Mars, Neptune, Pluto or Uranus and without benefic aspect: infertility problems
And Sun in fourth and Moon in tenth: bone fractures
And Mars in seventh: cyst, tumors, boils
And Jupiter in twelfth: both very severely afflicted: injury of finger, hands, or fingers
And other malefic severely aspects eighth: emotional illness, or paralysis
Afflicted in Aries or Cancer: degenerative disease
Two or more malefics in eighth or aspecting eighth: many diseases, eye problems
And Moon in sixth, and Mars, Uranus, Neptune or Pluto in twelfth and ruler of first afflicted: nasal and respiratory problems
Conjunct Mars, Pluto, Neptune or Uranus: factor in lung disease
And Moon in eighth: digestion problems
And Sun in fourth and Moon in tenth, both without strength: injuries, wounds, and cuts

Saturn In Ninth House

And Jupiter in third, both very severely afflicted: injury of a finger or fingers or hand
Square or opposition Uranus: emotional problems, mental illness

Saturn In Tenth House

Painful teeth
Aspected by malefics and without benefic aspect: infertility problems

Saturn In Eleventh House

May have fear, emotional insecurity, and or stubbornness about taking natural remedies. Need to be emotionally acceptable to others or not seem odd or conspicuous when trying remedies

Saturn In Twelfth House

Afflicted: can have deformities of arms, hands, legs or feet, fear of death and/or the future and thinking the worst outcome causes emotional problems
And Mars in second, Moon in sixth, Sun in eighth: can cause vision problems
And Jupiter in eighth: damage of finger to fingers or hand.
And Mars and ruler of First in twelfth: fistula, hemorrhoids

Uranus Health Profile

Uranus is the planet of irregularity. It influences of the nervous system, emotions, and psychosomatic illnesses. It rules the nervous system, spinal cord, cerebral spinal fluid, and membranes of the brain. Under favorable aspects, Uranus can bring seemingly miraculously quick recuperation from disease. With Mercury, Uranus rules the nervous system. Uranus governs the sudden and unexpected outcomes of illness, recuperation or sudden return of disease.
Afflicted: sudden illnesses, cramps, spasms, mental illness, mood swings, accidents from electricity, electronics, and/or explosions, convulsions, sudden falls from great height, appendicitis, ruptures, paroxysm, sudden return of a disease or sudden new disease.

Uranus In Signs

Uranus In Aires

Afflicted: disease and or injury to head, face, ears, eyes, nose, mouth, or facial muscle cramp, paralysis of facial nerves, spasmodic, headaches, meningitis; mental stress and or overexertion can cause illness

Uranus In Taurus

Afflicted: pituitary stress, inadequate hormone secretion of pituitary, temporal mandibular jaw dysfunction, abnormality in growth, difficulty with vocal chords, frequent and sudden attacks of laryngitis, nerve damage, strain to voice

Uranus In Gemini

Afflicted: respiratory problems, asthma attacks, coughs, colds, dry cough, cramps in arms and shoulders, lung problems,

Uranus In Cancer

Afflicted: gastric reflux, stomach gas, nerve damage, cramps, tendency to hiccough, anemia, and stomach indigestion

Uranus In Leo

Uranus is in a sign of its detriment causing, heath deterioration and illness
Afflicted: heart disease, spinal meningitis, infantile paralysis, heart problems, and accidental injuries
In Sixth house: heart disease
In female chart: childbirth problems and or possible injury of child by accident
Opposition Moon and Saturn: heart disease, heart problems
Opposition Saturn and Moon: In fixed signs worse, vision problems

Uranus In Virgo

Afflicted: digestion problems of intestine, flatulence, nerve damage, and colon problem

Uranus In Libra

Afflicted: sudden severe headaches, shooting sharp pains in head (opposition Aries), kidney problem or failure, mental illness, neck cramp, venereal disease, muscle cramps
And Mars in Libra: kidney problems

Uranus In Scorpio

Afflicted: reproductive problems, birth problems, miscarriage, abortions, venereal disease, accidents or sudden illness or injury through explosions, electricity, airplanes, electronics, sex organ problems, bladder cramps
In Fifth house: birthing problems painful, difficulty in childbirth with electronics or of instruments needed or computers used causing injury to child
Square Mars in Aquarius: gallstones

Uranus In Sagittarius

Afflicted: cramps and or injury to hips and thighs, sports injuries or injuries doing exercise

Uranus In Capricorn

Afflicted: injury or deformity of knees, accident to knees or legs

Uranus In Aquarius

Afflicted: injury or cramp in ankles and calf of leg
With unfavorable direction susceptible to accidents, nervous afflictions to ankles, knee and calf of leg

Uranus In Pisces

Afflicted: aches, numbness, tingling, pain or cramps in feet and toes, blockage and spasms of colon

Uranus In Houses

Uranus In First House

Afflicted: Accidents and or injuries to head, particularly the right side of head, and right side of body in whatever part is ruled by the sign in which Uranus is posited

Uranus In Second House

Sharp pains connect to the respiratory system particularly when breathing
Afflicted: avoid straining the voice. Accident to right eye. Often has laryngitis
And affliction to second house ruler: dental problems

Uranus In Third House

Accident or injury to right hand, right side of body

Uranus In Forth House

Afflicted: sudden injury or accident, especially on the right side of the body
Note sign Uranus is in. Later in adulthood injury or accident on right side of the body. Sudden accident.

Uranus In Fifth House

Afflicted: childbirth problems. Accident to right side of body. Birthing difficulties, miscarriage.

Uranus In Sixth House

Well aspected: Beneficial treatments of disease with massage, acupuncture, hypnotism, and alternative medicine
Afflicted: degenerative diseases. Obsessive thoughts and behaviors, mood and thought disorders, most diseases related to nerve damage and or nervous system. Uranus rules immunity. Neurodermatisis, rheumatic fevers, epilepsy, allergies, accidents and illness through sudden shock. Respiratory trauma, mental illness, environmental, factory and workplace related diseases, nervous twitch, and hormonal imbalance during puberty

Uranus In Seventh House

Afflicted: back injury or spinal problems caused by accident.
Afflicted without benefic aspect: problems with teeth

Uranus In Eighth House

Abrupt degenerative disease related to accident or paralysis
Afflicted: emotional and or physical violence can contribute to degeneration

Uranus In Ninth House

Afflicted: sudden disease or injury on the left side of body

Uranus In Tenth House

Afflicted: sudden accidents and or disease involving left side for the body or the organs on the left side

Uranus In Eleventh House

Afflicted: sudden disease or accidents involving the left hand or the left side of body

Uranus In Twelfth House

Afflicted: accidents, injuries and diseases with the left leg and the left side of the body
Conjunct Sun: right eye accident, injury or harm
Conjunct Moon: left eye accident, injury or harm

Neptune Health Profile

Neptune rules emotional and mental illnesses, hallucinations, delusions, neuroses, psychosis, anxiety and panic attacks, caffeine, steroid and drug addictions, depression, and nerve and brain tissue damage. Neptune causes susceptibility to suffocation and drowning. Neptune has a predominate effect on the parathyroid (mineral loss), cerebral spinal fluid, brain, ears and eyes. It influences bodily deformities and malfunctions, leukemia and other type cancers. Neptune adverse Mercury it influences neurotic, thoughts, moods and behaviors causing susceptibility to suicide ideation or abnormal behavior. Neptune diseases tend to be misdiagnosis, or have unexpected diagnosis, obscure factors and hidden causes. Neptune can cause obsessive behavior and or thoughts, comas, sleep walking, and nerve disorders.

Neptune In Signs

Neptune In Aires

Afflicted: Brain tissue and nerve damage, eye problems, and head and face deformity. Uncontrolled use of caffeine, steroids, energy drinks, stimulants, nicotine, sex drugs, depressants. Can have wide mood swings and neurotic thoughts and abnormal behaviors

Neptune In Taurus

Afflicted: abuse of caffeine, nicotine, energy drinks, steroids, sex enhancement drugs and or stimulants. Desires to overeat or have an Eating Disorder behavior. Tendency to neglect, cleanliness care of the body, disorganized surroundings, room, house, work place etc. Throat problems and or inflammation.
Opposition Moon in Scorpio: neurotic sex thoughts and obsessions
And Mars in Taurus: Sun in Cancer, Scorpio, or Pisces increases tendency. Alcohol, drug, steroid, energy drinks, caffeine and stimulant abuse excess drug and alcohol use

Neptune In Gemini

Afflicted: respiratory problems, bronchitis, asthma, and hay fever
Afflicted Venus and Jupiter: aggravates tendencies to asthma
Square Venus in Virgo: blocked or obstructs blood vessels to lungs. (If Sun squares Mars the condition increases in severity)

Neptune In Cancer

Much afflicted: digestion problems, stomach disorder, malformed stomach, ovarian cysts and fibroid tumors, sinus problems. Strange exotic appetites and tastes can lead to digestive system problems and Eating Disorder.
Negative emotions, moods and thoughts, stress, anxiety and panic can cause diseased digestive system

Neptune In Leo

Afflicted: heart weakness, heart problems caused by processed foods, white sugar, artificial sweeteners, fast foods. Back misaligned and weakness.

Neptune In Virgo

Neptune here is in sign of its detriment can cause diseases or poor health.
Afflicted: obsessive thoughts and or behaviors, colon problems, hypochondriac tendencies, delusional thoughts

Neptune In Libra

Afflicted: kidney problems, kidney failure, caffeine, drugs, energy drinks, stimulants, and/or mind-altering drugs abuse

Neptune In Scorpio

Afflicted: obsessive desire for alcohol or drugs, tendency to abuse and self. Injury caused drowning either by accident or design
Afflicted, and Venus and Mars afflicted: venereal disease

Neptune In Sagittarius

Afflicted: loss of decision-making ability, accidents

Neptune In Capricorn

Afflicted: injury or accidents can harm or deform knees, harm from synthetic chemicals in cosmetics

Neptune In Aquarius

Afflicted: psychotic and chaotic imagination, disturb sleep and dreams

Neptune In Pisces

Afflicted: malformation of feet and toes, edema, danger from hypnosis, coffee and tea in excess, energy drinks, alcohol, drugs, and/or addiction

Neptune In Houses

Neptune In First House

Premature deterioration of health and skin aging with wrinkles
Afflicted: causes loss, drain and or depletion of physical, mental and emotional energy

Neptune In Second House

Afflicted: premature deterioration of health and skin wrinkling with loss of radiance
Square or opposition Mercury: nasal problems
Afflicted, and Uranus on second cusp and afflicted: disease of the mouth
Conjunct, square or opposition Saturn: vision problems

Neptune In Third House

Afflicted: injury or disease on the right side of the body

Neptune In Fourth House

Afflicted: Remain in places or situation that drain energy and weakens immunity, and live in restraining condition in the latter portion of life
Afflicted by Sun and Moon: poor suffers
Square or opposition Mercury: mood and thought disorders

Neptune In Fifth House

Afflicted: heart problems caused by drugs or smoking, alcoholism

Neptune In Sixth House

Well aspected: good health but has tendency for peculiar disorders resulting from possession by distorted moods and thoughts or unseen entities. Diagnosed only with difficulty.
Afflicted: very unfavorable for health, for atrophy, incurable and hereditary diseases, made worse by sexual activities. Chronic, degenerative diseases, deformity, ptomaine and other forms of poisoning. Alcohol, drugs, sex stimulant, energy drink, and smoking abuse

Neptune In Seventh House

Afflicted: alcohol abuse tendencies
Afflicted without benefic aspects: teeth problems, dental diseases
And Sun in seventh conjunct Saturn and Neptune: affects right eye

Neptune In Eighth House

Afflicted: degenerative diseases ruled by Neptune. Disease slowly gets worst. See planets aspecting ruler of the eighth for factors, which contribute to the disease severity. Possible of harm to the right eye.
Afflicted and Venus and Jupiter afflicted: symptoms from other diseases contribute to diabetes
And Moon and Jupiter afflicted: influences from other diseases cause diabetes
And heavily aspected especially by Jupiter, Venus, and Moon and not necessarily afflicted: mucus congestion of the lungs.
Uranus stimulates self destructive behavior, moods and thoughts, suicide tendency, severe afflictions to Sun or Moon, ruler of third house; Mercy Saturn afflictions, and Jupiter adversely aspecting Saturn, or Jupiter in Capricorn

Neptune In Ninth House

Afflicted: phobic or constant thoughts about being in accidents. Accident, injury and diseases to the left side of the body.

Neptune In Tenth House

Afflicted: diseases tend to be on the left side of the body

Neptune In Eleventh House

Afflicted: diseases tend to be on the left side of the body

Neptune In Twelfth House
Afflicted: neurosis, respiratory disease, and left lung affected most
And heavily aspected especially by Jupiter, Venus or Moon, not necessarily afflicted: mucous congestion of lungs
Opposition Mercury: mood and thought disorders, may need institutional treatment

Pluto Health Profile

The information on Pluto's relationship to health is insufficient. Pluto tends to influence emotional and mental illnesses, anxiety and panic attacks, attention deficit, seizures, convulsions, epilepsy, and nerve damage. It rules aerobic and anaerobic digestion of food, and the liver, pancreas and stomach enzymes. Influences are diverticulosis, intestinal obstruction, bloating, blockages, intestinal problems, and leaking gut. Also, deep seated emotional problems.
Afflicted in First house: disease onset is quick, unexpected, and severe, which can alter the lifestyle.
Well aspected or afflicted in second house: disease treatment can have a positive effect
Afflicted in sixth house: Excess radiation or use of x-rays or electronic devices can cause diseases.
Well aspected or afflicted in eighth house: painless degeneration and terminal illness, which can start suddenly.

Oriental Planets

Planets posited on the left half of the natal chart signify quick, short, sudden, sharp onset of disease

Occidental Planets

Planets posited on the right half of natal chart produce chronic illnesses, degenerative diseases of long duration

General House Health

Angular houses: 1, 4, 7, and 10 ability to resist disease
Succedent houses: 2, 5, 8 and 11
Cadent houses: 3, 6, 9, 12 Majority of planets in cadent houses health deterioration and immunity depleted, unstable health condition

The House of Endings: 4, 8, and 12

Fourth: terminal illness
Eighth: degenerative and terminal disease
Twelfth: the effects of lifestyle, diet and diseases on the health

Planets In First House

Rule right side of body.

Planets In Second House

Rule right side of body, head, skull, face, ear, cheek, lip, teeth, mouth, nose, right leg, torso and foot. Afflictions cause escalated early degeneration of health. Second House rules disease to the internal and external right side of head, neck and body, diseases of the head, scalp, ears, eyes, nose, throat, mouth, face, or right nostril, right leg, teeth deformities and problems
Mercury is ruling planet for nose.
Second House afflicted by sixth ruled Jupiter: nasal and sinus cavities diseases. The right eye is ruled by second house and Sun. See twelfth house for left eye. Many planets in second house afflicted by Saturn: vision defect

Planets In Third House

Rules, right side of body and right hand

Planets In Fourth House

Rules right side of body

Planets In Fifth House

Rules right side of body

Planets In Sixth House

Rules right side of body.
Malefics in sixth: physical harm or injury to the right eye.
Any planet in sixth, between two malefics or conjunct, square or opposition a malefic: respiratory problems
For key to health condition, see sixth house, its ruler, see what sign and house placed, what part of body ruled and what planet aspect the sixth house ruler

Planets In Seventh House

Rule right side of body, dental diseases, spinal cord, injury or disease,
Malefic in seventh without benefic: causes dental problems
Sun in seventh conjunct Saturn: right eye problems

Planets In Eighth House

Rules left side of body
Malefics in eighth physical injury harm to the right eye
Malefic in eighth, and Venus and Jupiter afflicted: disease can contribute to diabetes
Malefic in eighth and Moon and Jupiter afflicted: indicates susceptibility to diabetes
Afflictions in eighth: emotional and mental problems, self destructive behavior can lead to suicidal tendencies

Planets In Ninth House

Rules left side of body

Planets In Tenth House

Rules left side of body

Planets In Eleventh House

Rules left side of body and left hand

Planets In Twelfth House

Rules left side of body. Left leg.
Left eye is ruled by twelfth house and Moon.
When the twelfth house is badly afflicted see if the second house is too, see if their rulers are afflicted or badly placed. See if Sun, Moon and Venus are afflicted or badly placed. See if Sun, Moon and Venus are afflicted or badly placed. These afflictions can indicate eyesight problems
Positive influences can eradicate negative influences
Sun in twelfth: harms right eye
Moon in twelfth: harms left eye
Twelfth rules left nostril (second house rules right one)
Respiratory diseases see twelfth house and rulers and expect this disease to involve mutable signs.
Afflictions of twelfth, being the house of self-undoing, treatment in facility for physical, emotional or mental problems

Planets Afflicting Ascendant

Sun: Illnesses, which begin with cold or flu
Moon: functional disorders, irregularities in system
Mercury: emotional or mental illnesses, anxiety or panic attacks
Venus: ignoring health, abuse of body
Mars: accidents, inflammatory disease
Jupiter: circulatory system problems, illnesses resulting from overeating or other excesses, such as work, drugs, alcohol, exercise, sex
Saturn: degenerative disease, chronic diseases, illnesses, colds, stress, malnutrition, poor diet, fast food diet. If in addition, ruler of eighth house afflicts the ascendant, heart disease
Uranus: degenerative disease, immune deficiency, accidents, stress
Neptune: illness resulting from drugs, steroids, caffeine, sex enhancers, body building supplements, sport performance enhancing drugs

Very Poor Health Indications

Ruler of ascendant in the sixth house and afflicted by the ruler of the eighth without favorable aspects from benefics indicates escalating aging process
A planet rising which is afflicted by the ruler of the eighth house, particularly if it be a malefic planet that is rising – possibility of degenerated health
Either Sun or Moon in an angle and conjunct, square or opposition
Mars, Saturn, Pluto, Neptune or Uranus without good aspects from Venus or Jupiter: possibility of early degeneration
Ruler of ascendant in the sixth house, ruler of ascendant afflicted by eighth house ruler, with no benefic aspects from benefics: indication of early degeneration
Malefics afflicting Sun or Moon, or Mars, Pluto, Neptune, Uranus or Saturn in any adverse aspect to both luminaries: indication of early degeneration
Any two malefics in opposition to each other and square the Sun and Moon; and the Sun and Moon in adverse aspect to each other: susceptible to early degeneration
Ascendant and luminaries in adverse aspect to each other, malefics angular, and no benefic aspects from Jupiter or Venus: indicates early degeneration
Sun or Moon angular and conjunct Mars, Saturn, Pluto, Uranus or Neptune, and this planet being of the same longitudinal distance from either luminary and no benefic aspecting them: degenerative or terminal disease early in childhood
Treatments afflicting individual Sun, Saturn, Mars, or Ascendant, practitioners should not treat if Saturn in their own sixth: sedatives given when moon is increasing in light (waxing); stimulants given when moon is decreasing in light (waning).
Operations performed during dark of Moon, immunity weak

Signs of Long And Short Illness

Long Illness

Common signs: Gemini, Virgo, Sagittarius, and Pisces disease duration lasting a few weeks
Long Illness: Ruler of the first, sixth or the moon in Taurus, Leo Scorpio or Aquarius tends to have disease of long increased duration and duration if these rulers afflict each other.
The Moon is in adverse aspect to the ruler of the first house.
The sixth house ruler conjoins the Sun or in his fall, or is posited in the eighth house and conjunct, square, sesquisquare, or opposition Uranus or Saturn or Mars – this can cause a degenerative or terminal disease.
Malefic planets in sixth house, ruler of sixth afflicted in the sixth, eighth or twelfth houses.
The Sun and Moon in cadent houses, their disposers with first house ruler and afflicted.
Ruler of first in sixth, and ruler of sixth in first.

Short Illness

Ruler of the first and sixth house is in Aries, Caner, Libra or Capricorn.
Venus or Jupiter is in sixth house in Libra, Pisces or Sagittarius.
Rulers of the sixth, or first house or the Moon in harmonious aspect with each other.

Ascendant And Descendant Health Profile

Note ruler of ascendant. Afflictions involving this planet tend to cause diseases of long duration. See how many planets, if any, are in the same sign as the ascendant. The more planets there are in that sign, the more tendencies for the body to target those parts of the body ruled by that sign. Note whether these planets are well or badly aspected.
Childbirth problems, traumas or injury results from aspect to the ascendant.

Aries Ascendant   Libra Descendant

Physical health and immunity good and has good recuperative ability. Mars becomes important in the chart. Check its sign, house, aspects etc. If afflicted it will cause disease, deformity or injury to the parts ruled by Aries, which are the head, brain etc., and by reflex action (opposition Libra) the kidneys tend to be diseased or malfunction, and perhaps the stomach. There can be unstable emotional states and stress, diabetes, uremia, head colds, nervousness as a result of disharmony in social life. Requires rest at the start of stressors. Dislikes following treatment plan, especially following them to the last detail. If they take herbs, supplements or other medicines they are emotionally impulsive and prone to overdose.
If no mole or mark on any part of head or face, scar may later appear.
And Sun opposition Moon: vision problems, eyestrain, weak eyesight, and sore eyes
And Sun or Moon afflicted by Mars or Saturn: eye problems, weak eyes, sore eyes, and eyestrain
And Saturn in Virgo: susceptible to emotional and mental problems
And malefic on ascendant or aspecting Aries: dental problems
Temperature rises several degrees higher than that of most people, and may even thin hair or cause balding, but endures fevers that harm others.
Accidents from fire, burns, cuts, electronics, radiation.
Skin eruptions on face.

Taurus Ascendant   Scorpio Descendant

Body structure built short, solid and without excess flesh, muscular, and good endurance.
Note Venus in chart, its aspect, house position, where posited.
As ruler of Taurus, Venus becomes very important to the health.
Blemishes, moles, marks or scars on ears, neck and throat.
Problems with throat, glands of neck, lower jaw, heart, kidney problems and/or lumbar region of spine.
Susceptible to paralysis, insomnia, laryngitis, fistula, hernia, hemorrhoids, appendicitis, kidney stones, gall stones, excretory system, sex organs, pelvic region, heart disease, throat, and/or feverish complaints. In accidents protect head and face.
Develops strict routines and habits, which can cause boredom.

Gemini Ascendant   Sagittarius Descendant

Lean, hyperactive, always finds activities to think about or do, good health with rapid disease recuperation while staying active and excited which drains emotional, mental and physical energy. This tends to weaken immunity, emotion obsessiveness with thoughts that lead nowhere and go nowhere causing anxiety, panics and restlessness and stress. Accidents through travel, sports, exercise. Blemishes, moles, or marks on arms, hands or shoulders or expect a scar.
Gemini rules arms, shoulders, lungs, chest, nervous system and mind and these are susceptible to diseases and to problems especially if you find many planets in Gemini. Hips, thighs, liver, lungs are susceptible to problems. Tendency to respiratory diseases, COPD, bronchitis, and circulatory problems.

Cancer Ascendant   Capricorn Descendant

Cancer tends to have a life of long duration. Their life begins with some health problems, but there is a tendency to develop stable health with age. They are full body particularly in later life. Eating disorders cause problems with the liver, pancreas, and digestive system. The upper body, chest, bones, knees, and joints may present problems. Falls and objects or debris falling can cause physical harm.
Susceptible to blemishes, moles, or marks on breast, stomach or epigastric area or can expect scar on areas.
And Sun and Mars, or Mars close to ascendant: Social activities and emotions contribute to digestion problems.
Rheumatism, cancer, hypochondria, swollen glands, edema, sleepwalking, digestive problems, diabetic problems.

Leo Ascendant   Aquarius Descendant

Good energy and strength. Muscular with large body and excellent immunity. Good recuperation from disease. Develops routines and sticks to them. Tendency to have back pain, digestion problems, severe and violent type diseases, heart diseases, heart weakness, eye, leg, ankle and circulatory problems, aneurisms, syncope, spinal meningitis, varicose veins, colds, chills, ear problems. Should maintain proper elimination and good circulation.

Virgo Ascendant   Pisces Descendant

A slender, short, solid angular body in youth, which thickens in the middle in later years. Use early treatments for disease before they develop into a chronic condition. Can have emotional and mental problems (psychosomatic), which causes illnesses. Health problems from travelling short or long distances or to work, only drink distilled spring water or spring water. Tendency to have respiratory problems, constipation, diarrhea, colon problems, back injuries, problems and or complaints, digestive problems that can cause debility, sensitive feet, glands and mucus membranes. Must maintain personal hygiene for good health.
Blemishes, moles, rash, skin eruptions, scars, marks on abdomen or colon areas.
Conjunct, square or opposition Saturn, Pluto or Mars: hernia.
And Saturn in ascendant: emotional and mental illnesses
And Mercury conjunct Saturn in twelfth, both adverse Mars that rules brain: nerve damage, epilepsy

Libra Ascendant   Aires Descendant

Venus and Saturn are important in the chart; note their aspects
Adverse aspects of these planets can deteriorate health.
Disease Recuperation generally good in finely built, well formed body. Sustains healthy and excellent vitality
Libra rules kidneys, lymph nodes, spleen, and lumbar region—there can be disease and weakness here, especially if rulers are afflicted.
Kidney disease, Bright's disease, nephritis, back pain, urine retention problems, skin disorders, eczema, circulatory problems, nerve damage, malfunction of brain nerve tissue, digestion problems, diabetes, insomnia, fevers, influenza, typhoid, malaria, problems with head. Accidents, injuries, cuts, wounds and illnesses, which effect head and face. Should avoid emotional and physical stress and strain.
Blemishes, scars, marks, rashes, or moles on the inguinal (groin) or lowest lateral region of the abdomen.

Scorpio Ascendant   Taurus Descendant

Very good health sustaining ability, muscular strength, endurance and disease resistance. Diseases can be severe when it occurs. Can eat too much and if process foods are eaten, the health deteriorates, the system becomes toxic which weakens health and immunity.
Blemishes, rashes, sores, marks, or moles on genitalia.
Body heavier after middle age.
See if Mars is well aspected or otherwise. Note its sign and house. Mars becomes an influence on the condition of health.
Excretory system and sex organs disease tendencies, heart, throat, eyes, ears and/ or neck problems, Eustachian tubes, esophagus, tonsils, larynx, kidneys, lumbar region and occipital cortex of brain. There can be ruptures, fistula, fevers, infections, cuts, wounds, burns, heart, and throat problems.

Sagittarius Ascendant   Gemini Descendant

Lean, angular body and can be skinny but strong. Good disease recuperative ability but lack of resistance to respiratory diseases, pneumonia, bronchitis, asthma and pleurisy. Emotional and mental stress and strain resulting in weakness if the diet is processed foods or the air is polluted or insufficient nourishment and rest. Skin problems, scars, moles, or marks on hips or thighs.
Weak parts: legs from hips to knees, arms, chest, and nerves. Tendency for rheumatism in hips and thighs, sciatica, bone fractures, arthritis, feverish ailments, wounds, cuts, dislocation of hip, respiratory disease, bronchial disorders and tuberculosis. Diseases caused by circulatory problems. Check Jupiter's aspects, sign, house position.
Jupiter influences health.

Capricorn Ascendant   Cancer Descendant

Capricorn rules diseases of long duration. Lean body can be thin, out of proportion with a good structure. Note Saturn's position and aspects in chart. Saturn influences immunity.
Diseases early in childhood tend to be of long duration. Good immunity and vitality in advanced age. Weak mental and physical condition improves with aging.
Skin problems, scars, marks, or moles on knees, or buttocks.
Emotional, social and personal relationship stress has a negative effect on health. Diseases problems in the sternum, chest cavity, and abdominal areas. Cartilage and tendon problems. Tendency for skin diseases, hives, eczema, psoriasis, impetigo. Susceptible to mucus congestion of the respiratory system, phlegm discharges (i.e. runny nose), dry cough and digestive organ problems. Accidents and injury from exercise, sports, or while traveling short and long distances.
Capricorn rules the tissue and bone building and rebuilding processes. If healing is hampered or slowed down, the body deteriorates and ages.

Aquarius Ascendant   Leo Descendant

Large, muscular, sturdy body, physical strength; In illness the disease is severe with speedy recovery. Excessive stress weakens the heart, circulation and back. Tendency to colds, inflammation of heart and nerve damage. Heat and cold drains energy.
Skin problems, rashes, scar, mark or mole on legs or ankles.
And Sun conjunct or opposition Saturn: vision problems
Rules legs from knee to ankle, and circulatory system. Spine and heart can have problems. Susceptible to calves and ankles sprained, broken legs, emotional and nervous disorders, cramps and eye problems. Susceptible to rare diseases.
Note Uranus in chart for this planet is influential on health and to those with this sign rising.

Pisces Ascendant   Virgo Descendant

Deteriorating health, becoming obese by middle age with decreased immunity, physical resistance or disease recuperation. Mental strain causes illness.
Pisces rules the feet and mucous membranes, problems with toes and feet, gout, arthritis, colon problems, cyst, tumors, edema, fevers, colitis, bacterial and viral diseases.
Skin problems blemishes, scars, bunions, corns, moles or marks on toes and feet.

Sun Sextile Trine Moon

This causes a mild stimulus to good health. Indicates energetic ability to recover from fatigue and physical and emotional energy loss.

Sun Conjunct Moon

In a female chart, poor health results from too acidic or alkaline body fluids. Avoid excessive emotional, mental or physical stress during menstruation.
And aspecting Mars or Saturn: rheumatic fever
And conjunct, square or opposition Mars: health deteriorates quickly. Babies born at the new moon are susceptible to traumas, sudden infant crib death, failure to thrive and or terminal diseases.

In twelfth house: strong tendency to abuse caffeine, alcohol and drugs. If a solar eclipse and child survives, this will be so throughout life
Excessive emotional or physical or mental stress not recommended at any time.

Sun Square, Opposition Moon

Susceptible to diseases, colds, flus with recuperation slow from any disease. Weak immunity with decreased energy. Seldom has a long life span. Unequal sight in two eyes. Nerves damage can decrease maintenance of healthy organs. System affected by cold. Excessive emotional and physical stress should be avoided.
And Saturn afflicted Sun or Moon: disease of long duration
From Sixth to twelfth: Tends to deplete energy and strength. Will not conform to health treatment if it is felt to cause restriction on lifestyle.
From Pisces to Sagittarius: respiratory diseases, pneumonia or congestion of lungs
In water signs generally: have negative effect on health, causes emotional unrest, lowers energy and stimulates anxiety and nervousness.
Eyes suffer.
And in affliction with two malefics in opposition to each other: escalates degenerative and terminal diseases

Sun Conjunct Mercury

Possible mental disorders. Mercury afflicting Sun and Moon is an indication of accelerated degenerative and or terminal diseases.

Sun Conjunct Venus

Improves health.

Sun Semisquare, Sesquisquare Venus

Excessive emotional, mental and physical activities cause mild diseases

Sun Without Aspect To Mars

In a child's horoscope, tendency to have many childhood diseases. Tendency to lack emotional concern about self, feels dejection, depression and has no interest in life. There are occasional exceptions to this, for example if Mars is strong and well aspected on the ascendant.

Sun Sextile, Trine Mars

Extremely energetic, active and healthy throughout lifetime.

Sun Conjunct Mars

Good health and a high capacity for work and activities. Slight tendency to fever and can endure high temperatures. Slight danger of physical injury, to heart and susceptible to diseases. Body thin, lean. Excess emotional, mental and physical stress influences health.
And Mars afflicting Sun and Moon: indication of terminal illness
In Capricorn: accidents and injury to knees
Sun, Mars and Saturn in one house in aspect to second house ruler of Mercury: nasal and sinus diseases
Can become thin because of rapid loss of bodily heat and an overactive thyroid disease. Should eat more frequently.

Sun Square, Opposition Mars

Inadequate oxygen absorption – causing respiratory problems after middle age and after trips from low to high altitudes. Any aspect of Mars to the Sun, however, including this one, tends to increase immunity.
Sun conjunct, square, opposition Mars and Saturn: inflammatory disease, rheumatic fever,
And in either one in first, second, seventh or eighth: cyst, tumors, skin eruptions, tendency for injury and accidents from electronics, knife wounds, electricity, burns, scalds, excessive work, and heart problems.
And Mars conjunct, square, opposition Uranus, or mental rulers and Moon.

Sun and Moon afflicted by Saturn and or Mars: eye injury or harm to eyes.
One in first, second, seventh or eighth: cuts, wounds. Fevers, cold, chill. Very negative influence for females.
Mars afflicting Sun and Moon: indication of early health deterioration and or terminal illness
And Jupiter square Mars: appendicitis
In mutable signs: damage nervous system, convulsions
Either Angular, or Mars elevated above Sun: severe inflammatory diseases, injury and accidents, very sudden health deterioration

Sun Sextile, Trine Jupiter

Resistance to illness and immunity is increased by positive thinking, which improves recuperative ability.

Sun Conjunct Jupiter

Excellent immunity, good health, energy and endurance, quick disease recovery. And Aries, tendency to stroke, nerve damage and paralysis.

Sun Square, Opposition Jupiter

Increased appetite, which causes eating disorder, sex addiction. Diseases during latter part of life. Tends to have obesity, poor circulation, stroke, nerve damage, high blood pressure, respiratory disease, liver disease, gouty arthritis, toxemia, and weakened immunity. Eats too many processed foods, fried foods, pastries, rare meats, pizzas. Tendency to form addictions and every (on or around the) tenth year of life has health problems.

Sun Sextile Trine Saturn

Eating at least 70% or more raw foods extends life and health to old age. Exercises self control prevents accidents.
In mutual reception (Saturn in a sign ruled by Sun and Sun in a sign ruled by Saturn) there is a deep basic reason for disease. If planets in angles and in fixed signs, severe, chronic or fatal disease

Sun Conjunct Saturn

Debilitating chronic disease gradually causes dependence upon others for care in latter years.
Immunity is too weak to throw off disease. Poor circulation. All treatment modalities must have the added focus of improving circulation to be of benefit. Diseases can be in areas of the body shown by the signs in which the Sun and Saturn are posited. Avoid stressful, heavy physical labor. Teeth should be cared for or else serious trouble.
And Saturn also afflicting Moon: early deterioration of health.
Sun, Mars and Saturn in one house in aspect to second house ruler or Mercury: sinus and nasal disease
On ascendant: skin diseases
In Gemini or Sagittarius: tendency to respiratory disease
In fixed signs: does less damage. Resistance to disease and recuperation is very slow.

Sun Square Opposition Saturn

Poor circulation. Avoid processed foods, which cause slow digestion with fermentation in the intestines. Decreased energy and disease resistance affects health. Avoid allowing body to be weakened by excess exercise. Use good tooth care (this aspect usually means dental trouble).
The parts of the body indicated by the signs in which the Sun and Saturn are posited can be poorly developed and should not be stressed or strained. There is slow metabolism, lack of appetite.
Saturn otherwise afflicting Sun and Moon: early deterioration of health or terminal disease
Saturn square Sun and Neptune opposition Jupiter: accident-involving water,
Saturn opposition Sun: myocarditis, heart disease
Female chart: reproductive and fertility problems
If Mars and Uranus both mingle aspect with this: severe dental problems
In fixed signs: least damage. Resistance is good. However, disease can be chronic and recuperation slow
Especially when either planet is occidental: poor health, severe illness of long duration

Sun opposition Saturn and square Uranus: poor immunity and poor physical stamina causes diseases.
And Mars afflicting Sun: Even the affliction is a benefit. The Saturn aspect means a loss of energy. The Mars aspect increases energy. However see Mars-Sun.
And Sun in Cancer, male chart: arthritis, chronic disorders, enlarged prostate, tumors, and cyst

Sun Sextile, Trine Uranus

Exercises good self-control. The temperament is high strung.
Sun trine Uranus and sextile Pluto: indication of long duration of life, good physical health, immunity and energy

Sun Conjunct Uranus

Emotionally unstable, can be out of control, gets moody, panic and, anxiety attacks. Tendency for childbirth problems and/or miscarriage. Predisposition for disease of nervous system, damaged nerves, anxiety and panic attacks, and lack of coordination, epilepsy. Accidents resulting from electronics, and electricity.
And Jupiter prominent: rheumatic fever
In Gemini: Labored breathing and respiratory problems
And Sun angular: life shortened, health deteriorates
Uranus afflicting both Sun and Moon: indication of early health deterioration, terminal disease, and inflammatory disease
If Mars is not afflicted in natal chart use a Mars hour to treat the native during the illness

Sun Square Opposition Uranus

Rare diseases, nerve damage, anemia, epilepsy, other nervous system disorders, injuries and accidents from electronics and electricity, and suicides tendency.
And Jupiter prominent: inflammatory diseases, rheumatic fever
Female chart: childbirth problems
Planets in Libra or Aquarius: predispose to pernicious anemia
Uranus afflicting Sun and Moon: indication of early health deterioration
If Mars not afflicted in natal chart: when ill-use Mars hour to treat diseases

Sun Sextile, Trine Neptune

Outdoor exercise improves health. Easily adapts to natural foods and health protocols that contribute to wellness.

Sun Conjunct Neptune
Caffeine, sexual enhancement drugs, steroids, energy drinks, stimulants, alcohol and or drug addiction can cause obsessive behavior
In Water sign: tendency for alcohol abuse and nerve damage
In eighth in Gemini: hemorrhage of lungs
In eighth: accident or injury, tendency for water accidents
Especially in sixth: overdoses of medicine should be avoided
Ptomaine food poisoning if not cautious in the use of seafood.
And Sun angular: health deterioration can shorten life
Neptune afflicted Sun and Moon: terminal disease or rapid deterioration

Sun Square, Opposition Neptune
Susceptible for addiction to drugs, alcohol, caffeine, steroids, and stimulants. Allergies to synthetic fibers, animal fur and many ordinary items of food, allergy can be unknown for long periods.
Emotional problems, psychic ability mixed with mental illness causes the mind to misinterpret thinking and creates delusional ideas attributed to conspiracy, fraud and hatred
In Water sign: increases problem with illusion of people, and delirium episodes, sees drug and or alcohol delirium as real. Illness is difficult to diagnose.
Neptune afflicting Sun and Moon: indication of early deterioration

Moon Sextile, Trine Mercury

Healthy mental and physical condition. Has the ability to cooperate with the health practitioner, particularly when planets are on positive angles and exalted.
And Moon or Mercury in sixth: good for health develops habits, conducive for health.

Moon Conjunct Mercury

Improves health and nervous system. Tends to be careful regarding hygiene.

Moon Square, Opposition Mercury

Tends to be emotionally explosive, and neurotic. If too many fixed signs, causes obsession about condition of health, will not change behavior to improve health. Cannot be motivated to improve health. Tends to be moody, emotionally unstable, with neurotic episodes. Can develop paralysis.
And Moon square Mercury and Conjunct Mars: phobias about animals, falling, heights, darkness, suffocation, colors, smells, shapes
Opposition in female chart: can have health crisis in infant
And Saturn conjunct, square or opposition to either: very moody, depressed
And Mercury afflicting Sun and Moon: degenerative or terminal diseases may occur later in life
And prominent, afflicted Mercury and Moon: poor memory, nerve damage

Moon Sextile, Trine Venus

Generally strengthens immunity, digestion and circulation.
And Moon trine Sun in Cancer: tendency to overeat, mild eating disorder

Moon Conjunct Venus

Eating disorder with desire for sweets, liquids, pastry, abnormal food cravings.
If Moon in Pisces liquids are alcoholic. To some extent an alcoholic if Moon is in Cancer or Scorpio

Moon Square Opposition Venus

If Saturn squares or opposes Venus menstruation will be painful, irregular and perhaps entirely suppressed, or prostate problems.
If Venus squares or opposes Moon and Venus is in the sign of Saturn and the Moon is in Venus's sign, susceptibility to the menstruation never occurring and barrenness. When pregnant she should consult midwife or health practitioner in order to detect problems early enough for it to be overcome. Prostate and fertility problems
Whether male or female: weakens immunity and health condition

Moon Sextile, Trine Mars

Above average endurance, good health, and immunity. Overcome health disease traumas to health. Stimulants have a strong effect on health. Menopause is mild and does not have traumatic effect. Good hormonal balance and physical health.

Moon Conjunct Mars

If the moon is well aspected, this increases quality of immunity and health, particularly in the horoscope of a woman.
In water signs: susceptible to abuse alcohol, coffee, energy and performance drinks
Stimulants have dramatic effect; should be very careful when using them. A minimum dose may be excessive.
And Mars afflicting Sun: early deterioration of health
In Scorpio: sex addiction or too much sexual intercourse can weaken health of sex organs and have an effect on colon
Afflicted Moon – Afflicted Mars: injury or problems with head, eyes, breasts and digestive system. Tendency to have degenerative diseases, harmful injury or disease, rupture blood vessels, surgery, fevers, wounds.

Accidents involving fire, scalding, electronics, and or water. Emotionally compelled to take risk for adrenaline rush. Has psychic ability, can be inspired to use it; however, can be spiritually possessed which can be detrimental or helpful.

Moon Square, Opposition Mars

Health challenges, diseases and problems. Tendency to have poor circulation, diseases of the stomach, breast, sex organs, ear, nose, sinus, skin and hair of head. Susceptible to accidents with disease treatments, and or surgery on parts of the body shown by sign and house that planet is posited. Possibility of accidents, injury and or disease from electronics, fire, hot water, articles made from metal, defective, or malfunctioning of old devices or machinery. Tendency to abuse caffeine, sports drinks, sex and muscle enhancement drugs and or alcohol. Many diseases can cause a life of short duration.
And Moon conjunct, square, opposition Saturn: inflammatory diseases, rheumatic fever
And Mars affects mental rulers and Sun and Uranus: emotional and mental illness
In Virgo: arthritis
If opposition in twelfth and sixth houses: heart and circulatory diseases, stressed nerves, ulcers (Mars square Uranus makes ulcers worse)
And Mars in seventh: danger of easily provoked terminal illness.
And Uranus square: respiratory diseases
And Mars afflicting Sun and Moon: early deterioration from diseases
And if either planet in water sign, particularly Pisces: alcoholism
Health problems can be caused by electronics, operations, fevers, accidents, ruptured blood vessels and water.
And Mars afflicting both Sun and Moon: easily becomes too anxious about illness, needs emotional support
And Uranus afflicts this combination: nerve damage
And Mars prominent: eye problems

Moon Conjunct, Sextile, Trine Jupiter

Good health and emotional personality that can be used to heal self or others.

Moon Square, Opposition Jupiter

A negative impact on health can result in eating disorder, digestive system diseases, pancreas, and liver disease. Can have cyst, tumors, periodic illnesses, burns, scalds, wounds that bleed, damage from toxins and or free radicals

Moon Sextile, Trine Saturn

Good health and self-control. Maintains health, which can contribute to longevity. Self-denial, which is an asset to health.

Moon Conjunct Saturn

Emotional illness, which can lead to depression, hypochondria, mood swings, neurosis, feeling rejected and helpless, tends to hold on to feelings and troubles.
Stimulants have very little effect, poor circulation. Constantly pays attention to their disease, troubles and depression in an introverted, egocentric manner.
And Saturn afflicting Moon and Sun: indication of early health deterioration. Subject to poor circulation; may become neurotic, self-possessed.
In Leo: problems with back, decreased synovial fluid to lubricate vertebrae of spine and weak ligaments, which connect spinal bones
In Aquarius: poor circulation especially in lower limbs

Moon Square, Opposition Saturn

Poor health, weak immunity, chronic ailments, aggravated by poor circulation, has a feeling of dejection and hopelessness. Part of body shown by Saturn's position in body's weak area and can be underdeveloped. Aspects from Uranus influences deformity of the part. If a vital organ, it should not be overstrained or deterioration will result. Infant with this aspect needs nurturing and good nutrition—first few years health is challenged.
And Saturn afflicting Mono and Sun: indication of early health deterioration
Opposition: colon and kidney diseases, colitis, nephritis, Bright's disease.
Expect temporary health challenges and diseases, colds, falls, injuries, accidents. Good muscle development and strength can cause over exercising, and weaken immunity. Healthful moderate exercise is good.
And Sun afflicted by malefics, and Moon and Sun are seventh and eighth house rulers: kidney stones and stones in urinal passage

Moon Sextile, Trine Uranus

Motivated to use natural remedies eat raw food and drink raw juices for disease and results are positive. Will use holistic practitioners, acupuncturists and chiropractors as well as colonics, fasting and alternative remedies.

Moon Conjunct Uranus

Tends to have strain, sensitive and stressed nervous system with nervous spasmodic action in the part of the body ruled by the sign the conjunction is in.
Conjunction in Cancer: indigestion influenced by emotions, nervousness and stress
In Leo: heart problems, irregular heartbeat, which can become dangerously spasmodic. This, with other, indications can prove chronic or fatal.
In Sagittarius: lung problems
Opposition Saturn: emotionally triggered psychotic episode can become a mental illness
And Moon in Virgo: food absorption problems, intestinal problems
And Uranus afflicting Sun: indication of early health deterioration can become a terminal disease

Moon Square, Opposition Uranus

Digestive system problems.
And Jupiter afflicting either planet: eating disorder and overeating of snack and junk foods
And Saturn afflicting either planet: eating disorder and weak digestion
And Mars afflicting either planet: too much highly spiced food eaten
And Neptune afflicting either planet: alcohol, caffeine, stimulants or drugs can be a problem
Opposition: a disease in life of infant female can become a traumatic effect.
And Uranus afflicting Sun: indication of early degenerative diseases

Moon Sextile Trine Neptune

Emotionally needs to contact those that were helpful in the past with health problems, regardless of money or distance.

Moon Conjunct Neptune

Lymph vessels circulation blocked or clogged can be to lack of exercise. Meningitis.
And square Uranus: possession by unseen entities, paranoia emotions attached to feelings of non-self
And square Mercury: symptom of emotional and mental illness, paranoia (possession of unseen entities)
And Moon conjunct Uranus opposition Saturn: emotional and mental illness, psychotic episode
And Neptune afflicting Moon: indication of early deterioration, of health

Moon Square, Opposition Neptune

Tendency to water accidents, possession by emotions attached unseen entities to non-self, emotions controlled by spirits (psychic) or spirit possession, latent danger of degenerative disease, meningitis. Seafood can cause ptomaine food poisoning, especially if sixth house is not well tenanted.
Either planet in a water sign: trauma or injury to health
Affects mental health or nervous system through physical disorder. Note signs occupied.
And in common signs: nerve tissue, brain and nervous system become affected
And in fixed signs: glandular system and secretory glands processes become affected
And in cardinal signs: circulatory system and digestion metabolism become affected.
Desire to eat to satisfy emotions, rather than eat for nutrition can causes to injury of health, especially if either planet is in a water sign
And Neptune afflicting Sun: indication of early deterioration and degeneration

Mercury Sextile, Trine Mars

Healthy nervous system uses knowledge of natural remedies when diseased and accepts illness as a challenge to immunity and knowledge of health. Illness is overcome with good humor and resourcefulness.

Mercury Conjunct Mars

Liver problems, gouty arthritis, inflammatory diseases, meningitis, metabolic changes, dyspepsia, arteriosclerosis, overeating processed foods, animal flesh and animal fats, cooked oils as well as rich foods cause health problems.
And Moon square or opposition Mercury: emotional illness, trauma, injury and phobias, which can degenerate the health.

Mercury Square, Opposition Mars

Inflammatory diseases, neuritis, meningitis, mental stress and strain, excessive work, unresolved anger, unhealthy attachment to stimulating activities causing emotional and mental overexcitement can lead to possession by unseen spirit entities. Problems or diseases caused from wounds, from surgical operations, tools, instruments, devices, equipment, drugs, electricity, electronic devices, Cataracts, violent delusions or manias, insomnia, migraines, peritonitis, nerve pain, suicidal attempts, and malaria. Accident or disease or malformation, of part of body shown by sign
In mutable signs: nervous system disorder, convulsions

Mercury Sextile, Trine Jupiter

Applies patience, understanding, and optimism to disease recovery. Denies self of pleasures for the sake of health. Excellent health.

Mercury Conjunct Jupiter

Compliance with treatment protocols and concentration on treatment bring recovery. Excellent health.

Mercury Square, Opposition Jupiter

Suffers from tension headaches, painful throbbing headaches, mental confusion and dizziness. Can be doubtful about disease treatment. Emotions block accepting advice. Step by step approach to giving advice or written health treatment instruction should be given.
And Jupiter conjunct Saturn in Virgo: hypochondria

Mercury Sextile, Trine Saturn

Health problems and remedies must be explained to understand. Tends to be complaint with treatment and does not mind time spent for recuperation.

Mercury Conjunct Saturn

Tends to procrastinate about taking remedies for disease. However understands disease diagnosis. Follows the remedies to regain wellness with positive, and optimistic emotions. Emotional dysfunction can cause the need to escape problems, which can result in suicidal tendencies. Health practitioner's confrontation about emotional problems causes them to rationalize and justify behavior before accepting problems. Timidity and embarrassment over exposure of emotional faults causes rejection of remedies.

Mercury Square, Opposition Saturn

Mucus congestion of sinus, nasal passage, nasal discharge (running nose) colds, flu, headaches, sinus headache, dull head pain. Negative thoughts can cause worry, mood swings, emotional outburst, and delay of treatment and or surgery because of fear. Circulatory problems, poor digestion, intestinal disease and or obstruction, constipation and tooth decay. Sad depressive mood slows down recuperation.
Injured emotions or nerve damage in part of body shown by Saturn's position causes weakened condition. And Mercury in Capricorn conjunct, square or opposition Saturn, and Saturn in a cardinal sign: increases tendency for hearing problems
In mutable signs: nervous system problems, convulsions

Mercury Sextile, Trine Uranus

Will try natural remedies and new treatment modalities if there is positive testimonials and science validation.

Mercury Conjunct Uranus

Nervous system problems, nerves sensitive. Nervous irritation, neuritis. See square and opposition.

Mercury Square, Opposition Uranus

Weak nervous system and or diseases, neuritis, excessive emotional, mental and or physical stress and strain can cause psychotic episodes and or mood swings, foggy feelings, respiratory problems, asthma, sudden sharp pains that leave quickly, tendency to hearing problems. These planets rule the nervous system. When afflicted, strange emotional, mental and nervous problems. Eye disease or problems, cataract, squinting.

Mercury Sextile, Trine Neptune

Uses many treatment modalities because of anger and resentment for having illness. Should follow inspirations regarding health treatments. Meningitis.

Mercury Conjunct Neptune

Emotional unbalance, delusions, palsy, paralysis, and meningitis. Accepts facts not as they are, but as they dream them to be. Susceptible to emotional and unseen spirit entities that control health. Follows emotions and unseen spirit entities guidance remedies.
In fifth house: difficult health problems in childbirth

Mercury Square, Opposition Neptune

Health problems and diseases caused by nicotine, caffeine, energy drinks, muscle building supplement, sex enhancement drugs, alcohol, legal and/or illegal drug abuse. Tendency to have paralysis, cataract, nerve damage, eye problems, squinting, meningitis.
And if either planet in third, and both planets without good aspect, and other adverse influence operating: emotional and mental problems. Abstinence from processed foods, flesh foods and liquor can be helpful.
Opposition involving sixth and twelfth houses: mental illness
Either planet in sixth: obscure nervous system problems, difficult to diagnose

Venus Sextile, Trine Jupiter

Very good influence for health. Promotes ability to sustain good health and longevity.

Venus Conjunct Jupiter

And Jupiter opposition Moon: diet of excess process foods, snacks and wrong food combing. Tendency for mucus congestion, inflammation in digestive tract, influenza, and enteritis.

Venus Square, Opposition Jupiter

Free radical damage as a result of excesses in eating and drinking of processed foods. These foods satisfy dysfunctional emotions and are contrary to good health. Disease or weakness of parts of the body are determined by signs the planets are posited in.
And planets in Pisces: tendency to use stimulants, steroids, sex and performance enhancer drugs, caffeine, energy drinks, alcohol.

Venus Sextile, Trine Mars

Health tends to be good with good energy level. Willingly changes diet or activities for health reasons.

Venus Conjunct Mars

Stress and overstrain to nervous system, constantly fluctuating emotionally and switching from one health practitioner to another. Obsessed with dysfunctional emotions, worries too much, depression, grief, fears, regrets and sorrow that is unresolved.

Venus Square, Opposition

Dysfunctional emotions cause health to deteriorate.
And Mars in Leo, and Venus in Taurus: nasal inflammation, sex organs or rectum problems. Polypus, which closes nasal passages, causing breathing difficulty, can grow in vagina or rectum.
And Venus in fire sign: tendency for accidents and or danger from fire or electronics
And Venus square or opposition Moon: female, painful menstruation, hormonal imbalance, excessive menstruation flow, mood swings, and irritability, males prostate problems, hormone imbalance
And Pluto aspect involving Venus or Mars: acne, skin problems
Self-indulgent goes to extremes

Venus Sextile, Trine Saturn

Balances energy level and conserves energy. Can influence good health.

Venus Conjunct Saturn

Kidney disease, blood in urine
In one house: vision problems
And Saturn afflicted by Jupiter and Uranus: can be suicidal. Emotionally unable to overcome emotional problems, or stress of disease. Can overcome crisis with emotional support and nurturing.

Venus Square, Opposition Saturn

Disease is emotionally draining, dysfunctional emotions, depression, and self-pity, despondent, loneliness. Stress from work can cause illness. Tendency for vision problems, or disease or deformity.
Opposition Aries Libra axis: skin eruptions, abscess, toxins and free radical damage
And one planet in seventh house: back pain, disorder and disease to spine
And either planet in sixth house: work related disease
And Capricorn on fourth: suicide tendency. Check Mars in chart injury from, violent injury, accident, trauma and (Mars-Saturn) accidental falls.

Venus Sextile Trine Uranus

Frequently and unexpectedly is given emotional support for good health by friends.

Venus Conjunct Uranus

Physical risks, danger of violence, attacks, accidents, reckless behavior or problems with emotions cause injury. Tendency for circulatory problems, varicose veins.

Venus Square, Opposition Uranus

Mental problems and or disease, neurosis, psychosis, nervousness, suicidal tendency

Venus Sextile, Trine Neptune

Fragile health, susceptibility to diseases

Venus Conjunct Neptune

Weak nervous system, fragile health, fistula, tends to exaggerates aches, pains and physical problems

Venus Square, Opposition Neptune

Tendency to abuse drugs, narcotics, caffeine, stimulants, energy drinks, or sex stimulants. Sensitivity to drugs, therefore a minimal dose can be excessive.
Knowledge about health and nutrition can cause diet of health foods (unprocessed) and or vegetarianism.

Mars Sextile, Trine Jupiter

Good health, immunity, endurance and energy level. Emotionally positive and optimistic about recuperation from disease.

Mars Conjunct Jupiter

Strengthens and increases health and immunity but has little effect on anemia, leukemia.
In water sign, especially Pisces: tends to abuse drugs and alcohol

Mars Square Opposition and Sesquisquare Jupiter

Tends to have problems with circulation, liver disease, contagious disease, paralysis, anemia, leukemia, colds, flu, and eating disorder tendency
Square or opposition with planet in water sign, especially Pisces: alcohol abuse
Sesquisquare can be more malignant in effect than Mars square Sun
And Mars powerless, and sixth house lord conjunct a malefic, and the Sun in Scorpio, Taurus or Leo: heart disease
And Jupiter ruler of sixth and aspected by a malefic Mars: colon problems and or intestine pain

Mars Sextile Saturn

Calmness and courage to fight disease
And Mars afflicted in Leo: abdominal pain
Good health, muscular or strong physique

Mars Conjunct Saturn

Unusual physical suffering from disease, injury, emotional stress and or accident, skin injury. See Saturn for place on the body for skin problems, cuts, stabs, severe burns, violence, chronic irritation, wounds, blows, falls
In Aquarius square Mercury: nerve inflammation, nerve damage, neurasthenia, and meningitis
Conjunction in Virgo: eczema, arthritis, and chronic irritation
And ruler of first in twelfth house: fistula, hemorrhoids
And Mars conjunct Moon: obsessive compulsive, emotionally dysfunctional

Mars Square, Opposition Saturn

Teeth malformation, misaligned, gaps, crooked, defective or without proper hygiene consistency and neglect tooth care is detrimental to health. Dental hygiene is important. Meningitis. If in mutual reception or one disposes the other health condition is worse
Sign Saturn occupies: indicates problems with part of body, weakness or underdevelopment of part
Anger, dysfunctional emotions, embitterment may cause digestion problems, liver disease, elimination problems.
And Saturn in a fixed sign: susceptible to serious accident or injury.
And aspecting planets in water signs: cramps while bathing or in shower, possible injury, and problems associated with water,
And aspecting planets in air signs: air travel problems
And aspecting planets in earth signs: mines, quarries, and excavations dangers to safety. Susceptible to falls in muddy or rocky places
Opposition: accidents, and with injuries, related to falls, falling debris. See houses and signs. The opposition is very disease, injury, or accident causing but less so in fire signs.
And Mars in Aquarius square Saturn: circulation blockage and or obstruction in lower limbs and varicose veins. Excessive stress or strain to body organs and muscles can cause disease to strict behavior or physical activities.
Square: accidents, injuries burns, scalds, anemia, loss of energy, stiffness in muscles or immobility of muscles, skeletal system problems, problems with skin, fever, teeth, cartilage, lower jaw, can be physically harmed by others.
Opposition from Taurus to Scorpio: thyroid disease
Excessive exercise can cause permanent injury. Tendency to be emotionally abused by others.

Mars Sextile, Trine Uranus

Abundance of energy, can be hyperactive and any adverse aspect to this combination will increase it. Tension can cause accidents. Compliant to health treatments and good coping ability with disease, makes disease recuperation a primary concern. Capable of following health regiment for extended periods of time, and with good results.

Mars Conjunct Uranus

Tends to be prone to accidents while traveling short or long distances. Emotional problems, stress and strain on nerves, physical defects.
And Mars in Virgo: intestinal and colon problems

Mars Square, Opposition Uranus

Emotional problems cause inability to cope with irritation and frustration, emotional upsets cause explosive temper. Endocrine gland problems, peptic ulcers, severe wounds and sores cause problems. There is danger from electronics, electricity from short circuits, overloaded wiring, damaged wiring insulation, electric devices, appliances, automobiles, planes. May get severe or fatal wounds in physical conflicts or combat (see fourth and eighth houses).

And in air signs: danger from synthetic chemicals or explosives
And in fire signs: danger from synthetic chemicals or motors
And Mars in Virgo: colon and or intestines problems
And either planet afflicted by Saturn: mental illness caused by spirit possession

And Virgo or Scorpio involved
Opposition: and either planet square Sun and Moon which are in affliction with each other: early in life health deterioration and or degenerative disease or terminal illness

Mars Sextile, Trine Neptune

Knowledgeable about health. Able to exercise self-control. Habit of cleanliness, tends to drink adequate amount of water

Mars Conjunct Neptune

The conjunction if Mars and Neptune are both well aspected is an asset in sound judgment in health matters or illnesses. Emotionally dysfunctional about feelings, Medicates emotional problems with drugs.

Mars Square Opposition Neptune

Tends to get emotionally unstable. Health degeneration and diseases caused by emotional problems, recreational use of drugs, synthetic chemicals, polluted water, anesthetics, narcotics, overdoses of medicine, misdiagnosis, socializes with emotionally abusive people, prescription drug abuse, health problems caused by wrong medicines or errors in medical treatment. Can be manipulative.
Opposition: and Neptune square Sun and Moon which afflict each other: early degeneration or terminal illness, caffeine, nicotine, energy drinks, sex enhancement drugs, cause disease.
Psychosomatic diseases. Burns from hot liquids. Illness from environmental chemicals and or consumption of synthetic chemicals

Jupiter Sextile, Trine Saturn

Has ability to exercise self-control over emotions and avoidance of detriments to health. Health can improve with maturity.

Jupiter Conjunct Saturn

Lacks ability to control health unless both planets are very well aspected. Tends to accept disease as fate, Tendency for kidney disease, headaches, obesity, emotional problems, and hardening of arteries.

Jupiter Square, Opposition Saturn

Lacks the emotional ability to control health, obesity, and arteriosclerosis. Headaches, kidney disease, arteriosclerosis, emotional problems, self-hatred can cause suicidal tendency
Opposition: infantile paralysis
Square involving Mars and Venus: diarrhea, digestion problems, gripping, colon and intestine disease, and metabolism and circulation problems
Opposition involving the Moon and Mars: injury or accidents causing burns, scalds, which can be severe or fatal
And Saturn strongly aspected: liver disease, hepatitis

Jupiter Sextile, Trine Uranus

Has will power to exercise self-control, apply long-term efforts to regain or maintain health
Will try health alternative remedies to achieve wellness

Jupiter Conjunct Uranus

Can have some physical abnormality and or deformity. Emotional injury and dysfunctions cause ability to maintain long-term treatment needed to regain health. Obesity problem.
On ascendant: eating disorder, over season food, eats for emotional reasons. Overeats to medicate resentment of self.

Jupiter Square, Opposition Uranus

Eating disorder, overeats rich foods, frequently goes on health food and/or weight loss diets and fails to continue, indigestion, intestinal blockage or clogged, obstructive, irritated colon, intestinal disorder that becomes inflammatory. Obesity problem.
And Moon opposition Mars: obsessive-compulsive behavior, mental imbalance, is in denial, has addictive behavior, resents health and emotional advice, and violates treatments

Jupiter Sextile, Trine Neptune

Understands health is body, mind and spirit wellness and will maintain wellness.
And Jupiter out of dignity: poor eyesight, nervous system weakness, and nerve damage

Jupiter Conjunct Neptune

Fistula, mucus congestion

Jupiter Square, Opposition Neptune

Emotional illness, mood swings, hysterical episodes, avoids and evades emotional problems, does not seek treatments, accidents with gas or fumes, Abuses caffeine, drugs, chemicals, opiates, narcotics, sex stimulants, and energy drinks.
Opposition: digestive weakness, fevers

Saturn Sextile, Trine Neptune

Ability to maintain good health. Will follow treatment regiments and uses alternative modalities for healing body, music, art, color, dance.

Saturn Conjunct Neptune

In Taurus or Scorpio: painful hemorrhoids, menstruation problems, inflamed tonsils, sex organ disease, deformity and malformation of sex organs, thyroid disease, nose, and throat problems

Saturn Square, Opposition Neptune

Emotionally injured, mildly neurotic, emotions block and distort reality, obsess with negative thoughts and feelings. Poor diet influenced by emotions, worries about past and future. Seafood may cause ptomaine poisoning. Can be sensitive to fluoridation and other synthetic chemicals
Opposition from Taurus-Scorpio: sex organs under develop, severe and/or painful childbirth.
Opposition in Gemini and Sagittarius in sixth and twelfth: spinal problems. For details on obstruction see Saturn.
Square involving Jupiter: mental illness

Saturn Sextile Trine Uranus

Abundance of patience and inspiration for maintaining and regaining health. Will try alternative disease treatments.

Saturn Conjunct Uranus

Good health and immunity, susceptible to injuries, accidents, harm caused by physical violence, mental retardation problem
In Scorpio: see Saturn in Scorpio
And Mars square Saturn: seeks mental help after they emotionally distort of reality. Feels that they deserve their illness or that it is fate. Trouble in bony structure of body, tendons, cartilages, and teeth.

Saturn Square, Opposition Uranus

Mistrustful of health practitioners, and does not follow any treatment unless it is felt that the creation of a treatment protocol was by there own design. Injuries and or accidents from fall, explosives, electronics, transportation vehicles, planes, trains, bus, boats.
Saturn's position shows which organs are underdeveloped or out of place and will not take stress or strain
And either afflicting the Sun: kidney and or gallstones
Opposition with Moon conjunct Uranus: possession
Saturn in Cancer square Uranus in Libra: kidney stones and or gallstones

Saturn Sextile, Trine Pluto

Capable of self control and self-denial. Takes extreme treatments to achieve wellness. Follows treatment protocols.

Saturn Conjunct, Square, Opposition Pluto

Injuries to skeletal system or bones can cause malformation and deformity

Uranus Square, Opposition Neptune

Tense nerve, nerve damage or disease

PLANET	RULER	EXALTED IN	ALSO IN HARMONY	IN FALL
Sun	Leo	Aries	Sagittarius	Libra
Moon	Cancer	Taurus	Pisces	Scorpio
Mercury	Gemini & Virgo	Aquarius	Scorpio	Leo
Venus	Libra & Taurus	Pisces	Aquarius	Virgo
Mars	Aries & Scorpio	Capricorn	Leo	Cancer
Jupiter	Sagittarius & Pisces	Cancer	Taurus	Capricorn
Saturn	Capricorn & Aquarius	Libra	Virgo	Aries
Neptune	Pisces	Sagittarius	Cancer	Gemini
Pluto	Scorpio	Leo	Aries	Aquarius

PLANET	IN DETRIMENT	ALSO IN HARMONY IN
Sun	Aquarius	Gemini
Moon	Capricorn	Virgo
Mercury	Sagittarius & Pisces	Taurus
Venus	Aries & Scorpio	Leo
Mars	Libra & Taurus	Aquarius
Jupiter	Gemini & Virgo	Scorpio
Saturn	Cancer & Leo	Pisces
Uranus	Leo	Aries
Neptune	Virgo	Capricorn
Pluto	Taurus	Libra

Under favorable aspects, planets in exaltation or harmony are indication of good health.

Under unfavorable aspect, those in fall or detriment or disharmony indicate health problems

Medical Abbreviations

Medical Abbreviations

ABBREVIATION	WORD	ABBREVIATION	WORD
a	artery	CO	Cardiac Output
A	Anterior	C/O	complains of
abd	Abdomen	comp.	complication
ABE	Acute Bacterial Endocarditis	COPD	Chronic Obstructive Pulmonary
abn	abnormal	CP	Cor Pulmonaic
ACh	Acetylcholine	CRF	Corticotrophin Releasing Hormone
ADH	Antidiuretic Hormone	CT	Computerized Axial Tomography
AGN	Acute Glomerulonephritis	CT	Connective Tissue
ALS	Amyotrophic Lateral Scelorosis	CV	Cardiovascular
APB	Atrial Premature Best	CVA	Cardiovascular accident
ARDS	Acute-Respiratory Disease Syn.	CVD	Cardiovascular disease
ASD	Atrial Septal Defect	cx	Cervix
ASA	acetyisalicylic acid (aspirin)	d/c	discharge
assoc.	associated	D&C	Dilation & Curitage
asymp.	asymptomatic	D&E	Dilation& Evacuation
a/v	artery/vein	DES	diethylstilbestrol
BBT	Basal Body Temperature	Decr. Or ↓	decrease
BC	Birth Control	def.	deficiency
BCP	Birth Control Pills	devel.	developing
bid	two times a day	DIC	Disscrolusted Intravascular Coagulation
Intravascularbilat.	bilateral	DIP	Distal-Interphalanges
Botan	Botanicals	DISH	Diffused Idiopathic Skeletal Hyperostosis
BM	Bowel Movement	DM	Diabetes Mellitis
BP	Blood Pressure	DMSO	Dimethyl Sulfoxide
BS	Blood Sugar	d/o('s)	disorder(s)
bx	biopsy	DOE	Dyspties On Exertion
CA	Cancer or Carcinoma	d/t or dt	due to
CAD	Coronary Artery Dz	DTR	Deep Tendon Reflex
Cap(s)	capsule(s)	DUB	Dysfunctional Uterine Bleeding
CBC	Complete Blood Count	Ddx	Differential Diagnosis
cc	cubic centimeter	Dx	Diagnosis
CHD	Congestive Heart Dz.	DVT	Deep Vein Thrombosis
CHF	Congestive Heart Failure	dz	disease
chol	Cholesterol	E.	Estrogen
CN	Cranial Nerve	EAB	Elective Abortion
CNS	Central Nervous System	ECM	Erythema Chronicum Migrainea
ABBREVIATION	WORD	ABBREVIATION	WORD
EEG	Electroencephalogram	HPV	Human Papilloma Virus
EENT	eye, ears, nose, throat	hr	hour
EKG	electrocardiogram	HR	Heart Rate
enz	enzyme	HSV	Herpes Simplex Virus
EO's	Eosinophil's	Ht	height
EOM	Extra Ocular Muscles	HTH	Hypothalamus
ERT	Estrogen Replacement Therapy		
ESR	Erythrocyte Sedimentation Therapy	HTN	hypertension
ET	Eustachian Tube	Hx	History
EOH	ethyl alcohol	IBD	Irritable Bowel Disease

eval	evaluation or evaluate	IBS	Irritable Bowel Syndrome
F.	Female	IDDM	Insulin Dependent Diabetes Mellitus
FBS	Fasting Blood Sugar	IM	Intramuscular
FH	Family History	Incr. OR ↑	Increase
FSH	Follicle Stimulating Hormone	Inflame	inflammation
f/u	follow-up	Infx	infection
GABA	Gamma- Amino Butyric Acid	ITP	Idiopathic Thrombocytopenic Parpura
GB	Gall Bladder	IUD	Intrauterine device
GERD	Gastro- Esophageal Reflex Disorder	IV	Intravenous
GFR	Glomerular Filtration Rate	IVP	Inter-Vascular Pressure or Intravenous Pyelography
GI	Gastrointestinal	Jt(s)	Joint(s)
GC	Ghonorrhea Culture	KOH	potassium hydroxide
GnRH	Gonadotropin Releasing Hormone	→	leads to
gr.	grain	LAL	Left Arm Lying
git	drop	LAS	Left Arm Sitting
GTT	Glucose Tolerance Test	LDH	Lactic Dehydrogenase
GU	Genital Urinary	LES	Lower Esophageal Sphincter
h/a	headache	L or lt	left
HBP	High Blood Pressure	LH	Luteinizing Hormone
HBV	Hepatitis B Virus	LLQ	Left Lower Quadrant
HCG	Human Chorionic Gonadotropin	LOC	Loss of Consciousness
Hct	Hematocrit	LPF	Lower Power Field
Hep	Hepatitis	LUQ	Left Upper Quadrant
----	----	LMP	Last Menstrual Period
----	----	----	-----
ABBREVIATION	**WORD**	**ABBREVIATION**	**WORD**
MVS	Mitral Valve Stenosis	PIE	Pulmonary Infiltrate w
M	Male	PMH	Past Medical History
m	muscle	PMN	polymorphonuclencytes
m/b or mb	maybe	PMP	Previous Menstrual Period
mcg	microgram	PMS	Premenstrual Syndrome
MCL	Mid Clavicular Line	PND	Paroxysmal Nocturnal Dyspnea
med	medication	pos	positive
mets	melastatic	poss	possible
mg	milligram	preg.	Pregnancy
MI	Myocardial infarction	PSA	Prostate Specific Antigen
mi	milliliter	PT	patient
mm	millimeter	P.T.	Physical Therapy
mod.	moderate	PTH	Para-Thyroid Hormone
MRI	Magnetic Resonance Imaging	PUD	Peptic Ulcer Dz
MS	Myocardial infarction	R. or RT	Right
MVP	Mitral Valve Prolapse	RA	Rheumatoid Arthritis
NSU	Non-specific urethritis	RAL	Right Arm Lying
N.	nerve	RAS	Right Arm Sitting
N	normal	RBC	Red Blood Cell
neg	negative	RE:	regarding
NIDDM	Non-Insulin Dependent	REGURG.	regurgitation

Abbreviation	Word	Abbreviation	Word
	Diabetes Mellitus		
Lv	Liver	PIP	Proximal Phalanges
L.V.	Left ventricle	Pit	Pituitary
nullip	nulliparous	RIND	Reversible Ischemic Neurological Deficit
N/V	Obstetrics	RLQ	Right Lower Quadrant
N/V/D	Nausea/ Vomiting	ROM	Range of Motion
OB	Nausea/ Vomiting/ Diarrhea	RUQ	Right Upper Quadrant
OC	Oral Contraceptive	R/O	Rule Out
OM	Otitis Media	ROS	Review of Systems
OTC	Over the Counter	SA	Sinostrial
oz	ounce	SAB	Spontaneous Abortion
P	Plan	SBE	Subacute Bacterial Endocarditis
P.	Progesterone or Posterior	SGOT	Serum Glutamic Oxalacetic Trans aminase
P&A	Percussion & Ausculation	SH	Social History
para	number of pregnancies	sig	instruction for prescription
NSR	Normal Sinus Rhythm	----	-----
ABBREVIATION	**WORD**	**ABBREVIATION**	**WORD**
PAT	Paroxysmal Atrial Tachycardia	VDRL	Venereal Disease Research Lab
PDA	Patent Ductus Anterious	VMA	Vanilly Mandelic Acid
PE	Physical Exam	VPB	Ventricle Prmature Beat
perm	permanent	VSD	Ventrical Septal Defect
PFT	Pulmonary Function Test	w/	with
PID	Pelvic Infammatory Disease	w/i	within
R/I	Rule In	w/o	without
RF	Rheumatic Fever	WBC	White Blood Cell
SLE	Systemic Lupus Erythema	wk	week
slt	slight	WNL	Within Normal Limits
sm.	small	wt.	weight
SOB	Shortness of Breath	x	times
STD	Sexually Transmitted disease	y.o.	year old
Sx	Symptom	yr.(s)	year(s)
TB	Tuberculosis		
TG's	triglycerides		
TIA	Transient Ischemic Attack		
tid	three times a day		
TMJ	Templemandibular Joint		
TNTC	Too Numerous To Count		
tr.	trace		
TRH	Thyroid Releasing Hormone		
Trich	Trichomonas		
TTp	Thrombotic ?		
Tx	Treatment		
UA	Urinalysis		
U.C.	Ulcerative Colitis		
UGI	Upper Gastrointestinal series		
unilat	unilateral		
URI	Upper Respiratory		

		Infection		
U/S		ultra sound		
usu.		usually		
UT		Urinary Tract		
UTI		Urinary Tract Infection		
v.		vein		
Vac.		Vaccine or Vaccination		
vag.		Vaginal or Vagina		
vas.		vasectomy		
VD		Venereal Disease		

Systems and Diseases

System & Diagnosis

Blood/ Peripheral vascular	
Symptom	Diagnosis
Anemia	Aplastic Iron deficiency Hemolytic Megaloblastic Pernicious
Cold hands and feet	Connective tissue disease Vasospastic disorder Diabetes Cold Exposure Decreased cardiac output
Deep leg pain	claudication
Easy bleeding or bruising	Hemophilis
Thrombophlebitis	IV drug users Buerger's disease Varicose veins Injury to veins
Varicose veins	Obesity Hormonal changes -menopause -pregnancy standing too long
Cardiac	
Symptom	Diagnosis
Blood Clots	Insufficient Vit. K ↑ coagulation factors w/ pregnancy BCP'S Liver disease
Chest pain/ Angina	Cardiac: -angina -aortic dissection -coronary artery disease -hypertrophic cardiomyopathy -MI -pericarditis -valvular heart disease GI: -esophageal reflux or spasm Mental/Emotional -anxiety -depression -panic attack Pulmonary -bronchitis -lung cancer -pleurisy -pneumonia -pulmonary embolism Others: -herpes zoster (w/or w/out eruptions) -costochondritis

Cyanosis:
Bluish color of skin & mucous membranes
  A. Central:
    Arterial hypoxemia d/t right to left cardiac shunt, pulmonary AV fistula, pulmonary dz
      ▪ Best visualized around mouth.
  B. Peripheral:
    Stagnant circulation d/t cold or anxiety w/ normal 02 saturation
	Central:
	-congenital heart disease
	-pulmonary disease
	-hemoglobin abnormalities
	Peripheral:
	-cold exposure (Raynaud's)
	-nervous tension
	-reduced cardiac output
	-vascular obstruction

Dizziness on rising	Transient ischemic attack Drug induced (antihypertensive) tiredness stress anemia heart block hypoglycemia subdural hemorrhage hematoma
Dyspnea (shortness of breath) -Orthopnea (shortness of breath while lying down) -Paraxysmal nocturnal dyspnea (PND) -SOB Waking person (aka Cardiac Asthma)	Anemia Aortic dissection Asthma Chest deformities CHF Emphysema Fibrosis GERD High altitude d/t arterial hypoxia Hyperventilation syndrome Pneumonia Pulmonary disease Pulmonary edema d/t CHF Rib fracture
Edema, leg	Cellulitis CHF Cirrhosis Cushing's disease DM Lymphatic obstruction Nephritis Pregnancy Protein def. Salty overload Tuberculosis Thrombosis Thyroid disease Tumor Varicose veins
Fainting	Vasovagal attack due to: -severe pain -fear -prolonged cough -straining to defecate, urinate -stuffy room, little 02 -standing still too long standing up suddenly

	DM
	Drug induced (antihypertensives)
	Vertebrobasilar insufficiency
	TIA
	Stroke- Adams syndrome
	Arrhythmia- heart block
High Blood Pressure	Pregnancy
	BCP'S
	Kidney disease
	Adrenal gland disorder's
	Coarctation of the aorta
	Atherosclerosis
	Arterial sclerosis
	Associated w/ DM
	Alcoholism
	Obesity
	Smoking
	stress
Low blood pressure	Drug induced (antidepressants)
	DM
	Injury- heavy blood loss
	Anemia
	MI
	Adrenal failure
Murmurs	Normal: softer sounds, S4 sound,
Heart sounds	S3 sound is abnormal in elderly
	Split S2: possible right BB Block if < with Inspiration
	Systolic ejection murmurs:
	-benign if grade 1-2, short, on rad
	-aortic valve stenosis
	-hypertrophic obstructive cardiomopathy
Palpitations	Allergies
	Anemia
	Aneurysm
	Angina
	Anxity
	Bradycardia
	Cardiomegaly
	Coffee
	Drugs
	Emotional stress
	Exercise
	Fever
	Heart block
	Hypoglycemia
	Hypokalemia
	Hypomagnesemis
	Hypoxia
	Menopause
	MI
	Migraine
	Myocardial Ischemia
	Pericarditis
	Poor conduction
	Pregnancy
	Stenosis
	Stress
	Tachycardia

	Valvular heart disease
...is	Inflammation of the veins
...umatic fever	Follow strep Infection autoimmune
Swollen ankles	Heart disease Trauma to ankles
Syncope (loss of consciousness)	A fib. Aortic stenosis Arrhythmias Bradycardia Carotid sinus syndrome Electrolyte imbalance Heart block Hemorrhage Hypoxia Inner ear disorder Micturition syndrome Orthostatic hypotension Pulmonary embolus Pulmonary Hypertension/thrombosis Seizures Tachycardia Vertebral artery compression

Dermatology

Symptoms	Diagnosis
Acne	Hormonal reaction Dietary problems Sebaceous over activity Poor hygiene Acne rosacea Primary bacterial folliculitis Steroid use Topical irritants Tinea Flourinated toothpaste Perioral derm Staphylococcal folliculitis Milaria Pityrosporum folliculitis
Boils	Irritation Moisture Poor hygiene DM Staph aureus Pseudomonas Herpes simplex Epidermal inclusion cyst Sporotrichosis Blastomycosis Hydradenitis suppurativa
Bruising/blood vessels	Trauma Hematoma Arteritis Vasculitis Toxic erythematous disorders Drugs/chemo/transplant reaction Urticaris

		Purpura
		Skin infarcts
		Vasooccluseive disease
		varicosities
Burning		Neuritis
		Fever
		Infection
		Circulatory changes
Color Changes		Infection
		Cancer
		trauma
Cracking		Fissures
		Infections dermatitis
		Eczema
		Fungal infections
		Dehydrations
		malnutrition
Dryness		Dehydration
		Decreased circulation
		Absence of skin lipids (topical soaps astringents)
		Malnutrition
		Dry environment
Eczematous Eruptions		Atopic eczematous dermatitis
		Nummular eczimaluos dermatitis
		Stasis derm
		Dyshidrotic ecematous derm
		Lichen simplex chronicus
		Contact derm syndrome
		Seborheic derm syndrome
		Erythroderma syndrome
Fungus		Ringworm
		tinea
		dysbiosis
		immune dysfunction
		poor hygeine
Hair loss		Genetics
		N aging
		Local disease or infection
		Systemic diseases or infection
		Toxic alopecia (following febrile diseases such as scaly fever or myxedema)
		Hypopituitarism
		Early syphilis
		Drug/vit. A reaction
		Autoimmune
		Neurotic habit
Itching		Anemia
		Cancer
		Chemical irritants
		Depression
		Dermatitis
		Drugs
		Flea bites
		Healing process
		Hypercalcemia
		Infections
		Insect bites or stings
		Iron deficiency

		Lice
		Lichen planus
		Medications
		MS
		Obstructive biliary disease
		Pemphigus
		pityriacis
		polycythemia
		pregnancy
		psoriasis
		psychogenic
		scabies
		stress
		stroke
		sunburn
		thyroid disease
		uremia
		xerosis (dry skin)
Lumps		Tumor (lipoma cancer neuroma) wart
		Mole
		Fibroma
		Trigger point
		Cyst
		Furuncle/carbuncle
		Lymphoma
		LA
		Erythema nodosum
Nails brittle		Nutritional deficiency, topical irritants, vascular or neurologic disorders, trauma, genetic, hypothyroid, low HCL, low protein, mineral deficiencies
Pain		Neuritis
		Cellulitis
		Erysipelas
		Infections
		Burns
		Bites
		Trauma
		Growths
		sunburn
		ulcers
		drug reactions
		parasites
		cysts
		bullous diseases
		pressure sores

Female Reproduction

Symptom	Disease
Amenorrhea	Absent ovaries, uterus, or vagina
	Adrenal abnormalities
	Anorexia nervosa
	Cervical or uterine adhesions
	chromosomal abnormalities
	crash diets
	Cushing's disease
	Depression
	Drugs: (barbiturates, opiates, steroids, phenothiazine's, reserpine, progestin's)
	Emotional or environmental conflicts

		Hyperthyroidism
		Hypothyroidism
		HTH-Pit failure
		Malignancies
		Menopause
		Obesity
		Ovarian dysfunction (↓LH/↑FSH w/ o ↓estrogen)
		Ovarian tumor
		Physiological delay
		Pituitary malfunction
		Pituitary tumor
		Polycystic ovaries (↑androgens)
		Pregnancy
		Serious systemic illness
		Sheehan's syndrome
		Stress
		Thyroid dysfunction
Breast lumps		Fibrocystic disease
		Mastitis
		Fibrosdenoma
		Breast cancer
		Lipoma
		Intraductal papilloma
		Cystosarcoma phylloides
Breast pain/tenderness		PMS
		Hormonal changes
Dysfunctional Uterine Bleeding (DUB)		Anticoagulants
		BCP'S
		Blood or marrow dysplasias
		Cervical erosion
		Cervicitis
		CHF
		Hormonal imbalance
		HTN
		Liver disease
		Polycystic ovaries
		Psychological factors
		Tumor
		unopposed estrogen stimulation
Dysmenorrhea		Adenomyosis
		Adhesions
		Congenital malformation
		Ectopic preg
		Endometriosis
		Fibroids
		Infection
		IUD
		Ovarian cyst
		Pedunculated cervical polyps
		PID, acute & chronic
		tight cervical openining
		tumors
Fibroids		Adherent adnexa
		Benign hypertrophy
		Congenital anomaly
		Malignancy
		Pregnancy
		sarcoma

...charge	Addison's disease
	Breast cancer
	Drugs: (OC, tricyclics, antidepressants, tranquilizers, cannabis)
	Hypothyroid
	Intraductal papilloma
	Lung cancer
	Mammary dysplasia
	Nipple inflammation
	Pituitary tumors (prolactin)
	Polycystic ovaries
	Pregnancy, normal
	Renal or liver failure
	Thyroid disease
Ovarian failure	Adrenal hormone excess
	Adrenal hyperplasia
	Hermaphroditer
	Pure gonadal dysgenisis
	Testicular feminization
	Tumer's syndrome
Pelvic Pain	Adhesions
	Adnecal torsion
	Appendicitis
	Diverticulitis
	Ectopic pregnancy
	Endometriosis
	Hernia, inguinal or abdominal
	Herniated disc
	IBD/ IBS
	Mittelschmitz
	Ovarian cyst
	PID
	Pregnancy
	Renal stones
	Sexual abuse
	Tumor
	UTI
PMS	Endorphins
	Estrogen excess
	Life style
	Oxytocin effects
	Progesterone defects
	Vasopressin
Vaginal Bleeding	Abnormal hormonal stimulation
	Anemia
	Diet (iron def.,vit C. def.)
	DM
	Follicular cystitis
	Hepatic disease
	Infections
	Medications
	Obesity
	OC
	Polyps
	Pregnancy
	Renal disease
	Thyroid dysfunction
	Trauma (foreign body, sexual abuse)
	Tumor urethral prolapse

	vulvovaginitis
Vaginal discharge	B-strep Allergies Candida Chlamydia Douches E. coli GC Herpes Hormonal HPV Infections Mycoplasma Perfumed feminine products Pinworms Trichomonas vaginosis

Valvar itching	Candida
	Dermatitis
	    - contact
	    - seborrheic
	DM
	Drug
	Gardnella
	Gout
	Hepatic disease
	HPV
	Infections
	Leukemia
	Lichen
	 -simplex
	 -plants
	 -sclerosis
	lymphoma
	parasites
	pellagra
	pregnancy
	psoriasis
	renal disease
	Sjogren's
	Trichomonas
	Tumor
	UTI

URINARY	
Symptoms	Disease
Bed Wetting	Idiopathic UTI Polyuria Sexual abuse Fecal withholding DM Chronic renal failure Diabetes insipidus Renal tubular acidosis Ectopic ureter Sickle cell anemia
Frequency	Cystitis Anxiety

		Stones in bladder Enlarge prostate Bladder tumor Renal failure
	Hemataria	Acute leukemia BPH Cystitis Diet (beets, blackberries) Drugs Endometriosis HTN Neoplasm Nephrolithiasis Nephrosclerosis Obstruction Papillary necrosis Polycystic kidney Prostatitis Pyelonephritis Renal infarction Renal vein thrombosis Trauma Urethritis
	Incontinence	Anxiety Delirium Dementia Depression Infection Inflammation Medication CHF Polyuria BPH Lax muscle tone, prolapse (uterine, vaginal, etc.) Stones in bladder
	Oligaris/ Anuris Retention	Obstruction Prostatitis Stones in bladder Enlarge prostate Bladder tumor Uterine fibroids Nerve injury Surgery Drugs
	Pain in urination	UTI Vulvovaginitis STD Chemical irritation Allergies Prostatitis Urine obstruction Tumor Postmenopausal atrophic -vaginitis sexual abuse Reiter's syndrome
	Urgency	Infection

| | Stones in bladder |
| | Bladder tumor |

Respiratory Symptoms

Symptom	Disease
Sputum	URI (pneumonia, rhinitis)
	Allergic reaction
	Inhaling irritant (smoke, dust)
Hemoptysis (expectorate w/blood)	Alcoholic-esophageal
	Varies
	Bronchiectasis
	Bronchitis
	CHF
	Fungal infection
	Lung abscess
	Pneumonia, necrotizing
	TB
	tumor
Wheezing	Asthma
	Bronchitis
	Pulmonary edema
	Foreign object
Asthma	Extrinsic
	- allergies
	- resp. infection
	- smoke
	- exercise
	Intrinsic
	- emotions
	- stress
	- anxiety
Bronchitis	Bacterial infection
	↑ risk w/ smoking, immune compromised
URI	Allergic rhinitis
	Atypical pneumonia
	Bronchitis
	Croup
	Epiglottitis
	Foreign body
	Group A strep
	Influenza
	Mononucleosis
	Otitis media
	sinusitis
Pleurisy	Lung infection
	Pulmonary embolism
	Lung cancer
	Rheumatoid arthritis
Pain of breathing Chest pain	Lung causes
	- pleurisy
	- bronchitis
	- pneumonia
	- embolism
	- Malignant tumor
	- Acid reflux
	- Hiatal hernia
	- Strained or bruised muscle
	- Broken rib
	- Nerve compression

	- Injury to vertebrae - Disc prolapse - Osteoarthritis - Shingles - Tietze's syndrome
Dyspnea (SOB)	Anemia Aortic dissection Asthma Atelectasis Chest deformities CHF Emphysema Fibrosis High altitudes d/t arterial Hypoxia Rib fracture

Reproduction

Symptom	Disease
Discharge	See penile and vaginal Discharge below
Pain on intercourse	Anxiety, emotional disorder, vaginismus, vulvovaginitis, vaginal, atrophy, tumors, cervicitis, yeast infection, genital lesions (STD), trauma, too much sex
Sexual difficulty	Emotional disorders, impotence, antidepressants, antihypertensives, low libido, dyspareunia
Sores	Herpes, cancroid, condyloma accurninata, chancre, granuloma inguinal, scabies

Male Reproduction

Symptom	Disease
Impotence	Anxiety, emotional disorders, androgen deficiency, testicular disease, hormonal deficiency, hypertensive medications, neurologic disorders, cardiovascular disease, surgery, diabetes, prostate disorders, antidepressants, trauma
Penile discharge	Neissiria gonorrhea Chlamydia trachomatis Ureaplasma urcalyticus Reiter's syndrome B-strep
Scrotal Pain/Mass	Aortic aneurysm henochschnlein purpura Appendicitis Epididymitis Hernia, inguinal Hydrocele Renal colic Trauma Tumor Viral orchitis

Disease Analysis Charts

Cardiovascular Disorders

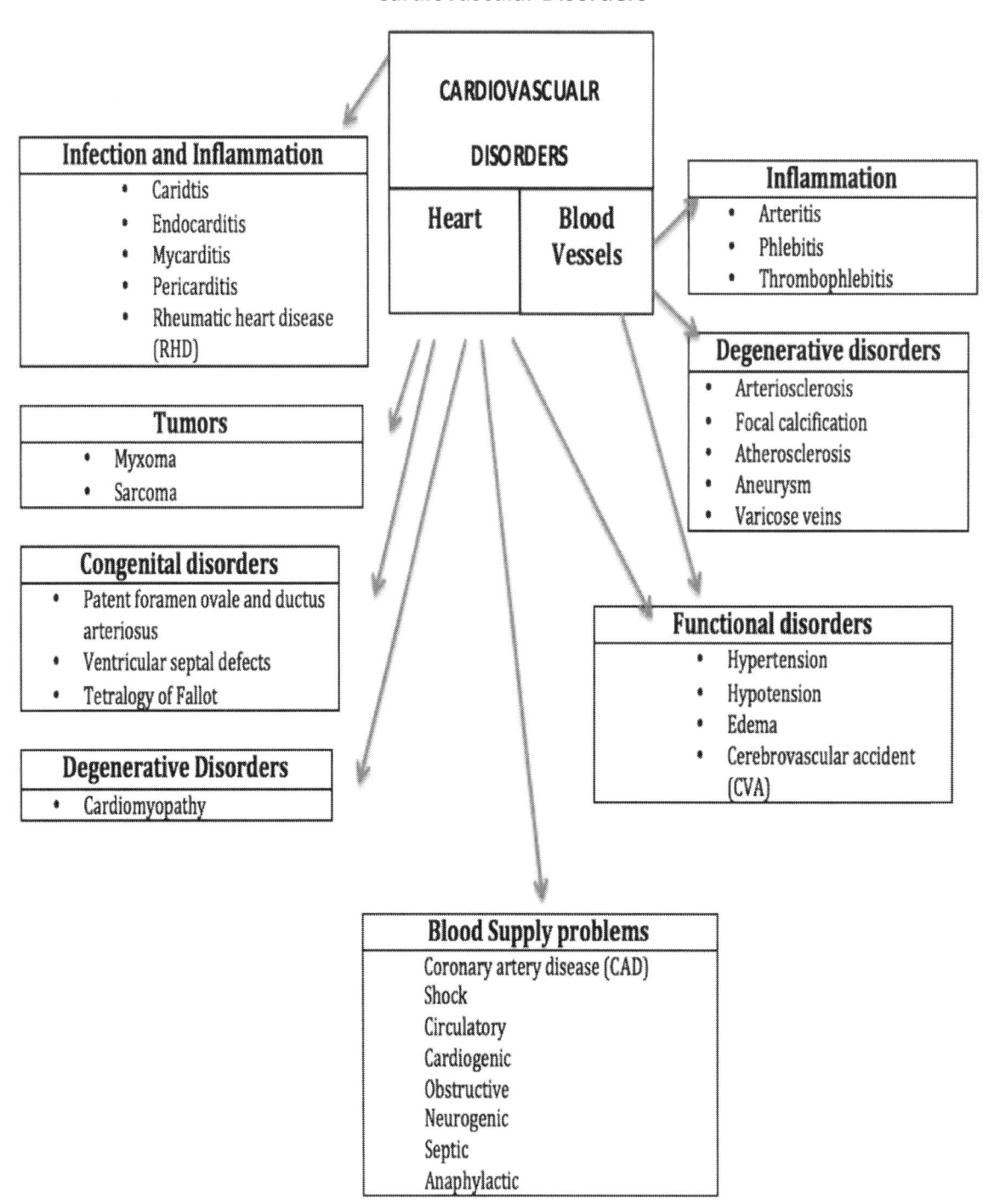

CARDIOVASCUALR DISORDERS
- Heart
- Blood Vessels

Infection and Inflammation
- Caridtis
- Endocarditis
- Mycarditis
- Pericarditis
- Rheumatic heart disease (RHD)

Tumors
- Myxoma
- Sarcoma

Congenital disorders
- Patent foramen ovale and ductus arteriosus
- Ventricular septal defects
- Tetralogy of Fallot

Degenerative Disorders
- Cardiomyopathy

Inflammation
- Arteritis
- Phlebitis
- Thrombophlebitis

Degenerative disorders
- Arteriosclerosis
- Focal calcification
- Atherosclerosis
- Aneurysm
- Varicose veins

Functional disorders
- Hypertension
- Hypotension
- Edema
- Cerebrovascular accident (CVA)

Blood Supply problems
Coronary artery disease (CAD)
Shock
Circulatory
Cardiogenic
Obstructive
Neurogenic
Septic
Anaphylactic

Blood Disorders

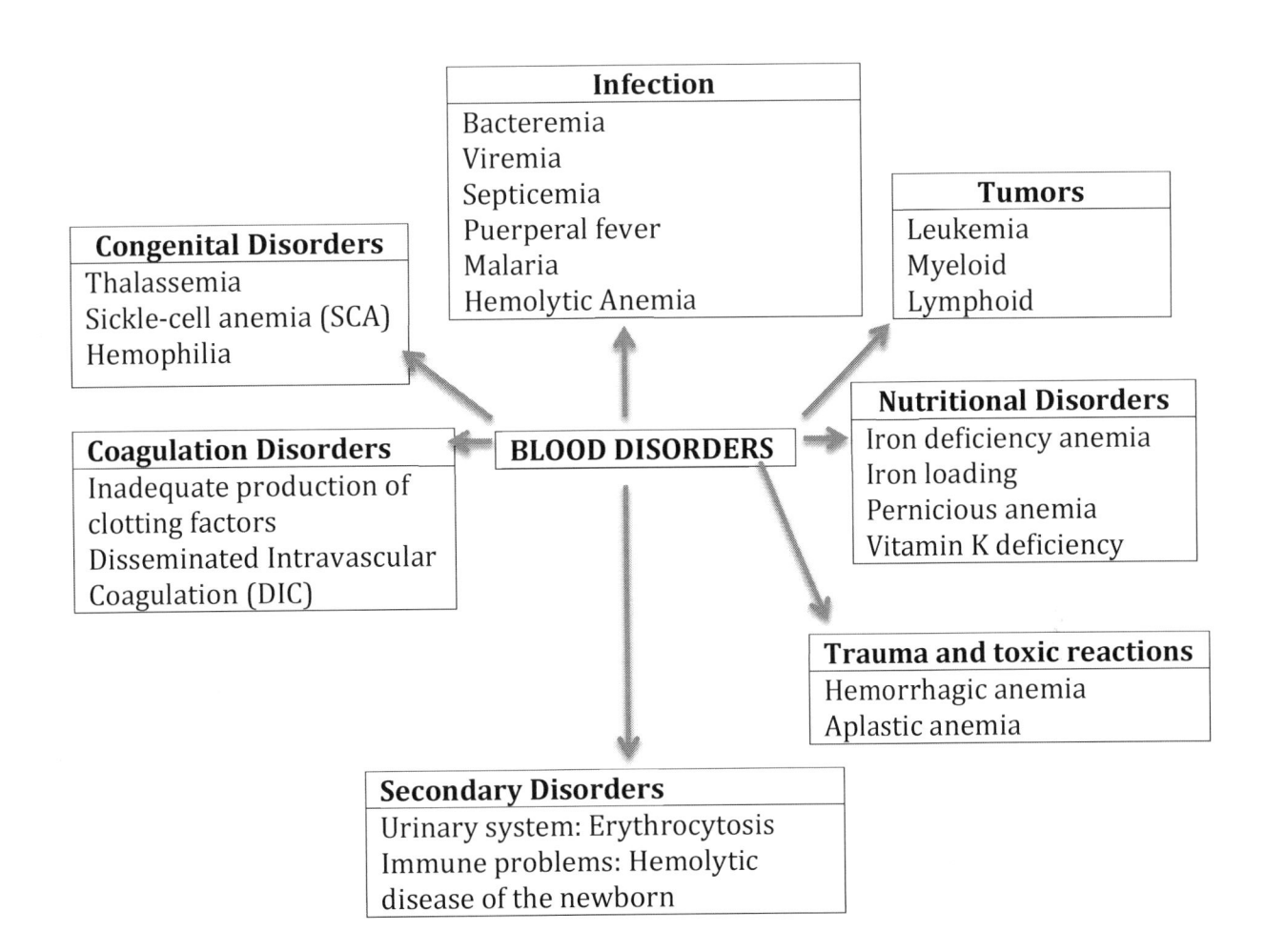

Infection
- Bacteremia
- Viremia
- Septicemia
- Puerperal fever
- Malaria
- Hemolytic Anemia

Tumors
- Leukemia
- Myeloid
- Lymphoid

Congenital Disorders
- Thalassemia
- Sickle-cell anemia (SCA)
- Hemophilia

Nutritional Disorders
- Iron deficiency anemia
- Iron loading
- Pernicious anemia
- Vitamin K deficiency

Coagulation Disorders
- Inadequate production of clotting factors
- Disseminated Intravascular Coagulation (DIC)

BLOOD DISORDERS

Trauma and toxic reactions
- Hemorrhagic anemia
- Aplastic anemia

Secondary Disorders
- Urinary system: Erythrocytosis
- Immune problems: Hemolytic disease of the newborn

ENDOCRINE DISORDERS

Primary Effects on Metabolism
- Glucose Metabolism
  - Addison's disease
  - Cushing's disease
  - Diabetes mellitus
- Metabolic rate abnormalities
  - Hyperthyroidism
  - Hypothyroidism
  - Cretinism

Primary Effects on Fluid and Electrolyte Balance
- Addison's disease
- Hypoaldosteronism
- Diabetes insipidus
- Syndrome of inappropriate ADH secretion (SIADH)
- Hyperparathyroidism
- Hypoparathyroidism

Primary Effects On Reproductive Function
- Precocious puberty
- Adrenogenital syndrome
- Gynecomastia

Primary Effects On Growth
- Gigantism
- Acromegaly
- Pituitary growth failure

Effects On Cardiovascular Function
- Addison's disease (produces hypotension)
- Hyperthyroidism (increases heart rate; arrhythmias)
- Pheocromocytoma (produces hypertension)
- Diabetes mellitus

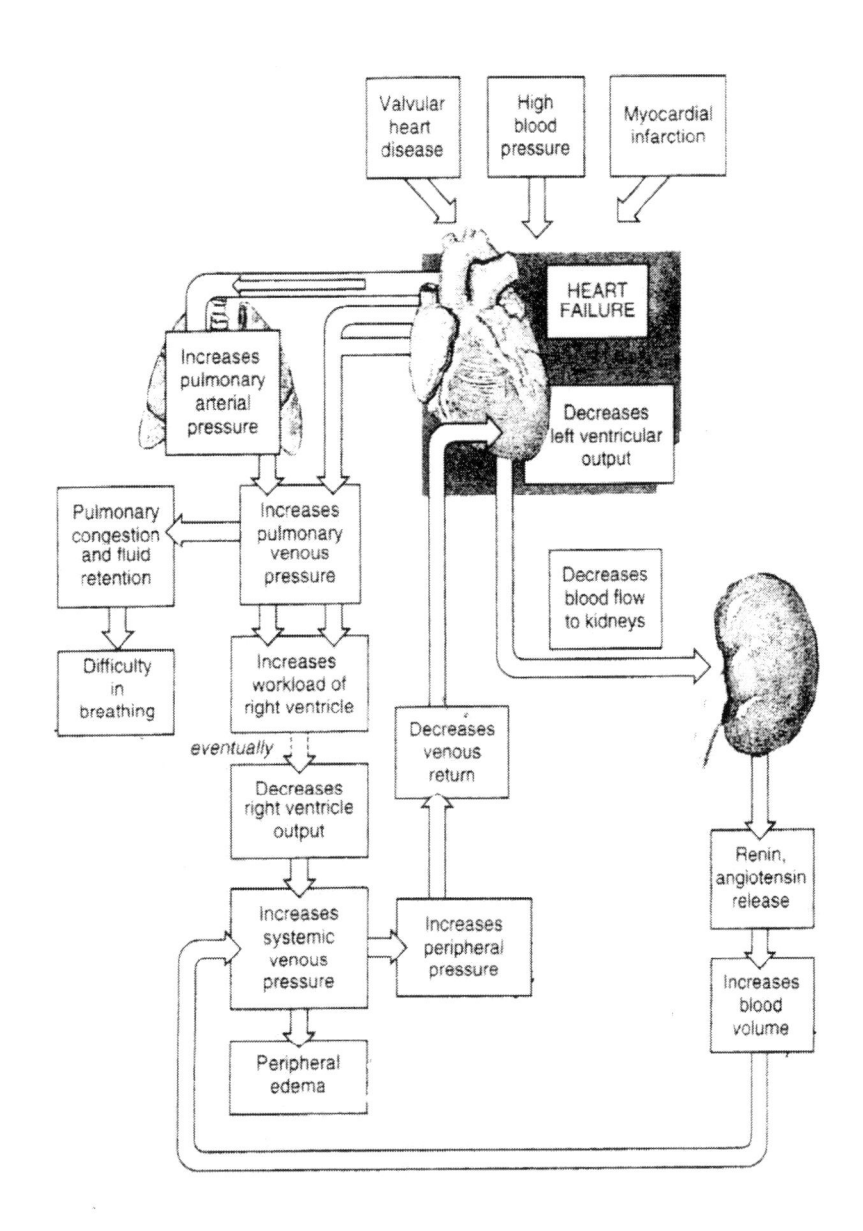

Heart Failure

Valvular heart disease → **HEART FAILURE**
High blood pressure → **HEART FAILURE**
Myocardial infarction → **HEART FAILURE**

- Increases pulmonary arterial pressure
- Decreases left ventricular output
- Increases pulmonary venous pressure
- Pulmonary congestion and fluid retention
  - Difficulty in breathing
- Increases workload of right ventricle
- *eventually* Decreases right ventricle output
- Increases systemic venous pressure
  - Peripheral edema
- Increases peripheral pressure
- Decreases venous return
- Decreases blood flow to kidneys
  - Renin, angiotensin release
  - Increases blood volume

Joint Disorders

JOINT DISORDERS

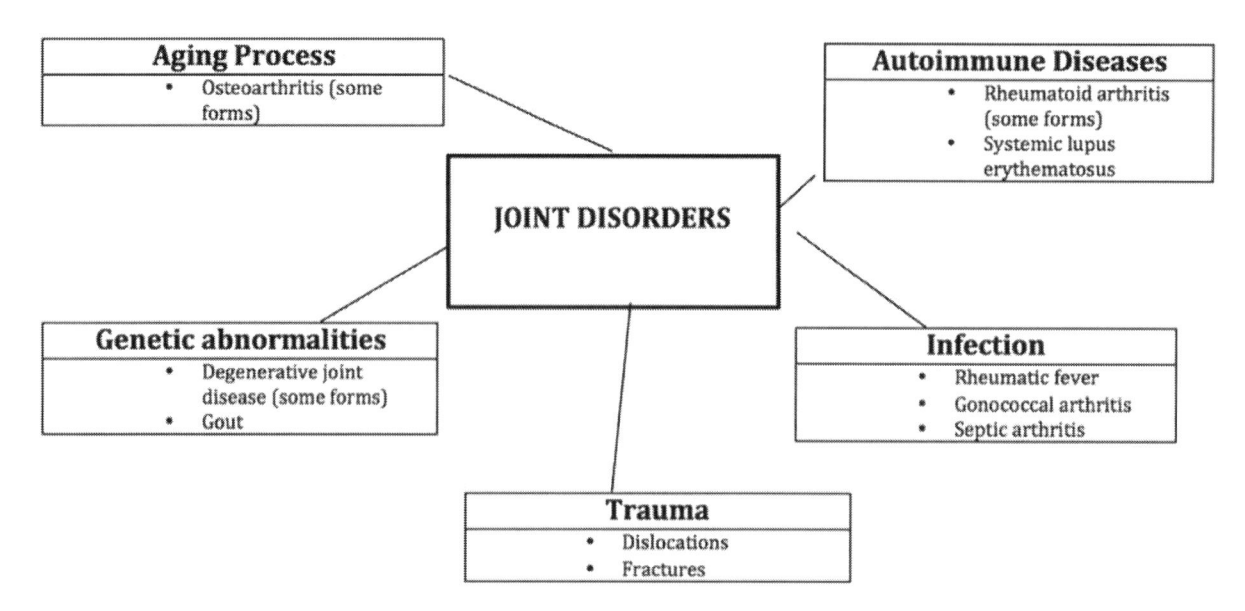

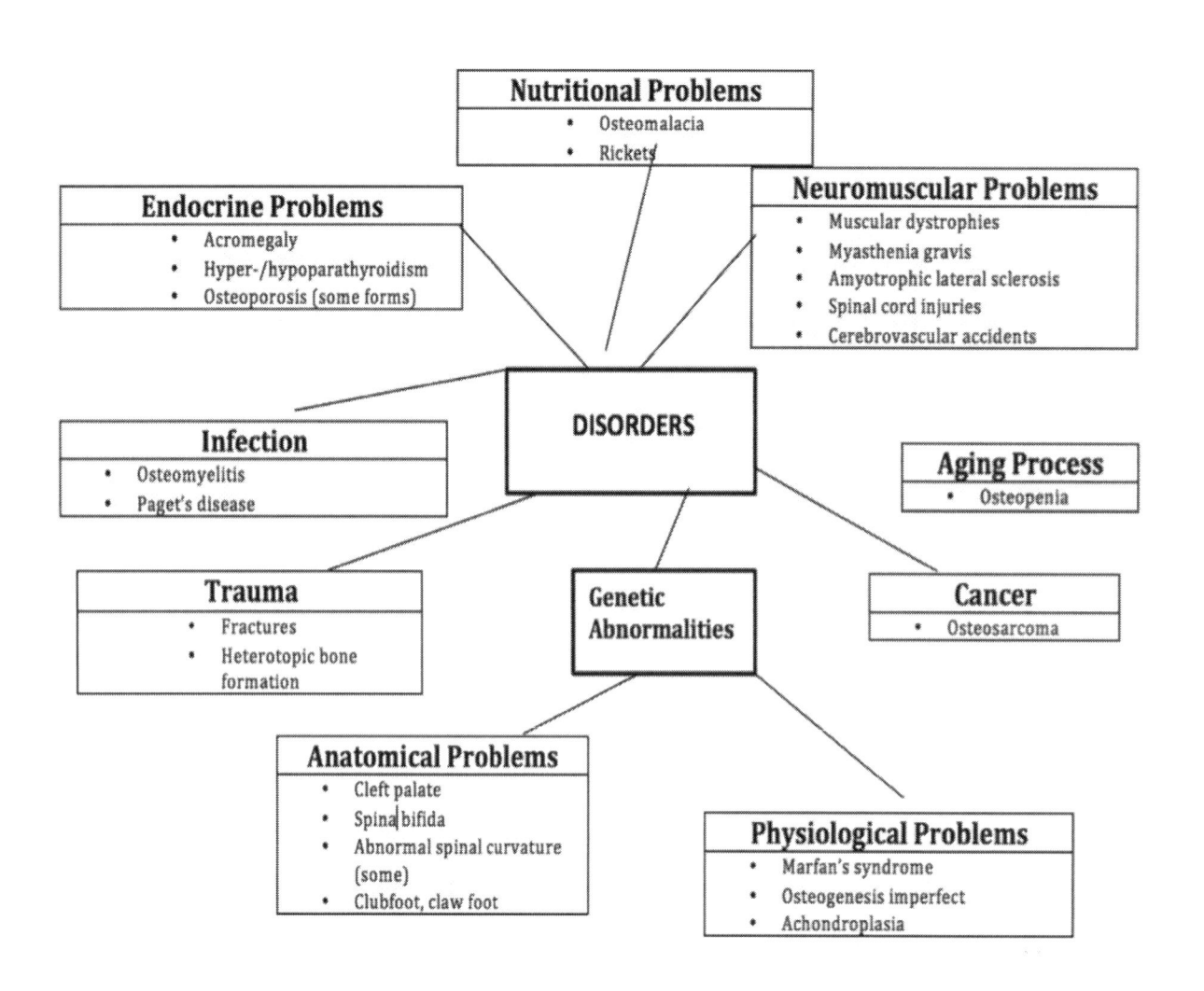

Aging Process
- Osteoarthritis (some forms)

Autoimmune Diseases
- Rheumatoid arthritis (some forms)
- Systemic lupus erythematosus

Genetic abnormalities
- Degenerative joint disease (some forms)
- Gout

Infection
- Rheumatic fever
- Gonococcal arthritis
- Septic arthritis

Trauma
- Dislocations
- Fractures

DISORDERS

Nutritional Problems
- Osteomalacia
- Rickets

Endocrine Problems
- Acromegaly
- Hyper-/hypoparathyroidism
- Osteoporosis (some forms)

Neuromuscular Problems
- Muscular dystrophies
- Myasthenia gravis
- Amyotrophic lateral sclerosis
- Spinal cord injuries
- Cerebrovascular accidents

Infection
- Osteomyelitis
- Paget's disease

Aging Process
- Osteopenia

Trauma
- Fractures
- Heterotopic bone formation

Cancer
- Osteosarcoma

Genetic Abnormalities

Anatomical Problems
- Cleft palate
- Spina bifida
- Abnormal spinal curvature (some)
- Clubfoot, claw foot

Physiological Problems
- Marfan's syndrome
- Osteogenesis imperfect
- Achondroplasia

Muscle Disorders

Infection
Myositis
Necrotizing fasciitis
Tetanus
Trichinosis
Fibromyalgia

Trauma
• Hernias
• Compartment syndrome
• Bruises and tears
• Carpal tunnel syndrome

MUSCLE DISORDERS

Inherited Disorders
Muscular dystrophy
Duchenne's muscular Dystrophy

Tumors
• Myomas
• Sarcomas

Secondary Disorders

Nervous System:	**Immune**
• Botulism	• Myasthenia gravis
• Poliomyelitis	
Cardiovascular System:	**Metabolic Problems:**
• Anemia	• Hypercalcemia
• Heart failure	• Hypocalcemia

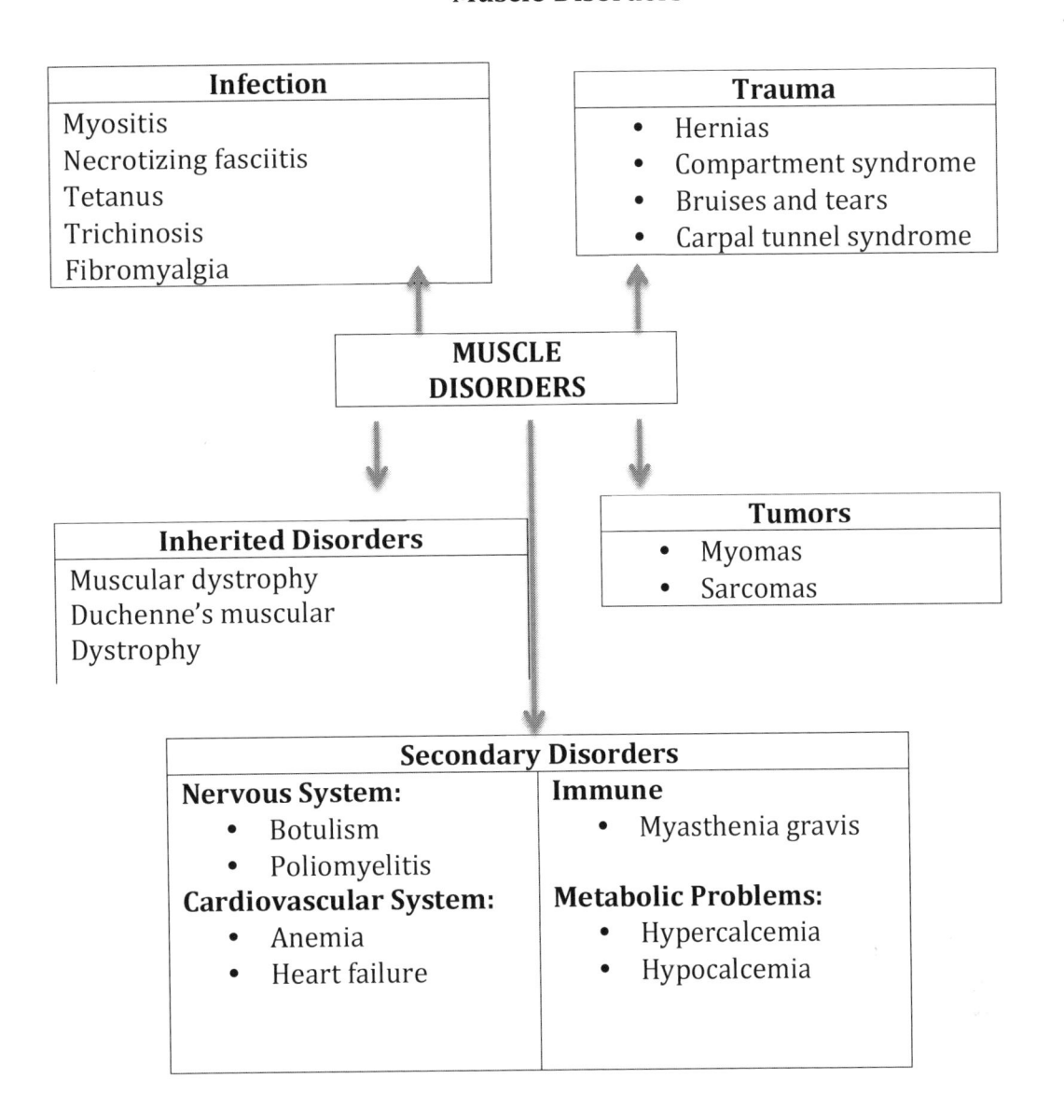

Disorders of the Respiratory System

Inflammation and Infection
Rhinitis
Common Cold
Sinusitis
Pharyngitis
Laryngitis
Epiglottitis
Bronchitis
Diptheria
Pertussis
Pneumonia
Tuberculosis
Influenza
Adult Respiratory Distress Syndrome (ARDS)

Congenital
Cystic fibrosis
Neonatal respiratory distress Syndrome (NRDS)

Degenerative
Emphysema
Chronic Obstructive Pulmonary Disease (COPD)

Cardiovascular Disorder
Pulmonary hypertension
Pulmonary embolism

DISORDERS OF THE RESPIRATORY SYSTEM

Tumors
Lung cancer

Immune Disorder
Asthma

Trauma
Nosebleeds
Pneumothorax

Nervous System Disorders

Nervous System Disorders

Infection
- Diptheria
- Neuritis
- Shingles
- Hansen's Disease
- Polio
- Meningitis
- Rabies
- Encephalitis
- African sleeping sickness

Congenital Disorders
- Tay-Sachs disease
- Spina bifida
- Huntington
- Hydrocephalus
- Cerebral palsy

Degenerative Disorders
- Parkinson
- Alzheimer

Tumors
- Neuromas
- Gliomas
- Neuroblastomas
- Meningiomas

Trauma
- Spinal cord injuries
- Peripheral nerve Palsies
- Cranial injuries
  - Epidural and subdural
  - Hemorrages, Concussions, Contusions
  - Lacerations

Secondary Disorders
- Cardiovascular System
  - Cerebrovascular Disease
  - Cerebrovascular Accident (CVA) or stroke
  - Aphasia
- Immune problems
  - Multiple Sclerosis

Disorders of the Urinary System

Inflammation and Infection
Urinary tract infections (UTIs)
Kidney
  Nephritis
  Pyelitis
  Pyelonephritis
  Leptospirosis
  Ureteritis
Urinary bladder
  Cystitis
Urethra
  Urethtitis

Congenital Disorders
Polycystic kidney disease
Tubular function disorders
  Renal glycosuria
  Aminoaciduria
  Cystinuria

Urinary System Disorders

Tumors
Kidney
  Renal cell carcinoma
  Nephroblastoma
Urinary bladder

Immune Disorders
Glomerulonephritis

Degenerative Disorders
Incontinence
Renal failure
  Acute renal failure
  Chronic renal failure

Disorders of Renal Function
Fluid imbalances
  Edema
Electrolyte imbalances
  Hypernatremia
  Hyponatremia
  Hyperkalemia
  Hypolakemia
  Hypercalcemia
  Hypocalcemia
Acid-base imbalances
  Respiratory acidosis
  Respiratory alkalosis
  Metabolic acidosis
  Metabolic alkalosis

Digestive System Disorders

Malabsorption disorders
Biliary obstruction
Pancreatic obstruction
Lactose intolerance

Congenital disorders
Cleft palate
Pyloric stenosis
Intestinal atresia, stenosis volvulus, or
Meconium obstruction

Tumors
Leukoplakia
Pharyngeal cancer
Esophageal cancer
Stomach cancer
Colorectal cancer
Pancreatic cancer
Liver cancer
 Hepatoma
Gallbladder cancer

Oral cavity
Dental caries
Pulpitis
Gingivitis
Vincent's disease
Periodontitis
Mumps
Stomatitis
Thrush

Esophagus
Esophagitis

Digestive System Disorders

Stomach
Gastritis
Peptic ulcer
 Gastric ulcer
 Duodenal ulcer

Accessory Organs
Pancreatitis
Hepatitis
 Cirrhosis
 Viral hepatitis
Sheep liver fluke
Cholecystitis

Intestines
Enteritis
Dysentery
Gastroenteritis
Traveler's diarrhea
Typhoid
Cholera
Viral enteritis
Giardiasis
Amebiasis
 Amoebic dysentery
Ascariasis
Colitis
 Irritable Bowel Syndrome
 Inflammatory bowel syndrome
Diverticulitis

Nutritional and Metabolic Disorders

Eating Disorders
Inadequate food intake
 Anorexia/Bulimia
Excessive food intake
 Obesity

Thermoregulatory Disorders
Elevated body temperatures
 Fever
 Heat exhaustion
 Heat stroke
 Hyperthermia
Lowered body temperature
 Accidental hypothermia
 Induced hypothermia

Nutritional and Metabolic Disorders

Metabolic Disorders
Catabolic problems
 Ketosis
Congenital disorders
 Phenylketonuria (PKU)
Protein deficiency disease
 Marasmus
 Kwashiorkor
Mineral disorders
 Deficiencies
 Excessive
Vitamin disorders
 Hypervitaminosis
 Avitaminosis
Water balance disorders
 Dehydration
  Over hydration
   Water intoxication

Normal Child

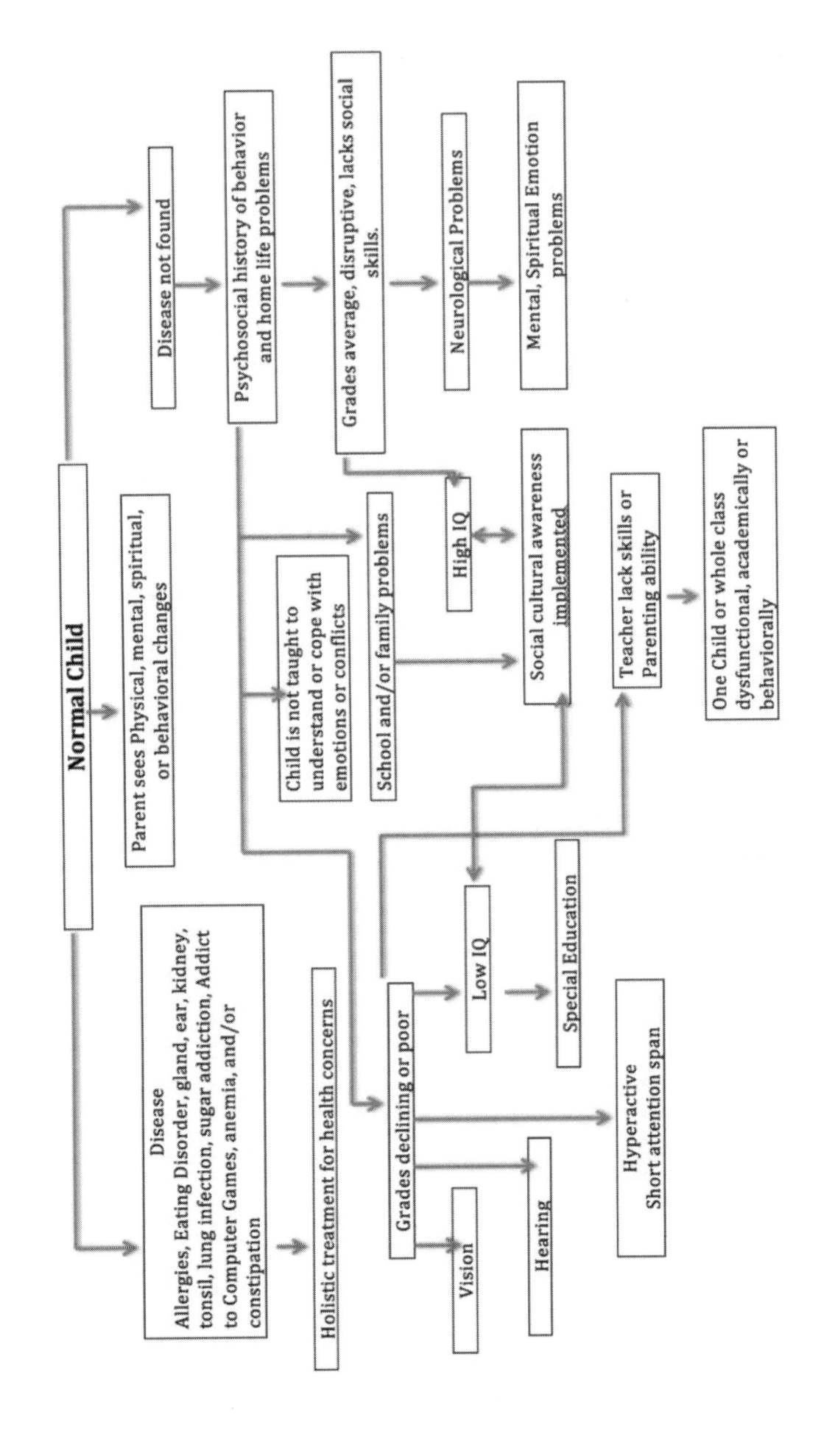

Parent sees Physical, mental, spiritual, or behavioral changes

Branch 1: Disease not found
- Psychosocial history of behavior and home life problems
  - Grades average, disruptive, lacks social skills
    - Neurological Problems
      - Mental, Spiritual Emotion problems
  - Child is not taught to understand or cope with emotions or conflicts
    - High IQ
  - School and/or family problems
    - Social cultural awareness implemented
      - Teacher lack skills or Parenting ability
        - One Child or whole class dysfunctional, academically or behaviorally

Branch 2: Disease
Allergies, Eating Disorder, gland, ear, kidney, tonsil, lung infection, sugar addiction, Addict to Computer Games, anemia, and/or constipation

- Holistic treatment for health concerns
- Grades declining or poor
  - Low IQ
    - Special Education
  - Vision
  - Hearing
  - Hyperactive / Short attention span

565

Diarrhea

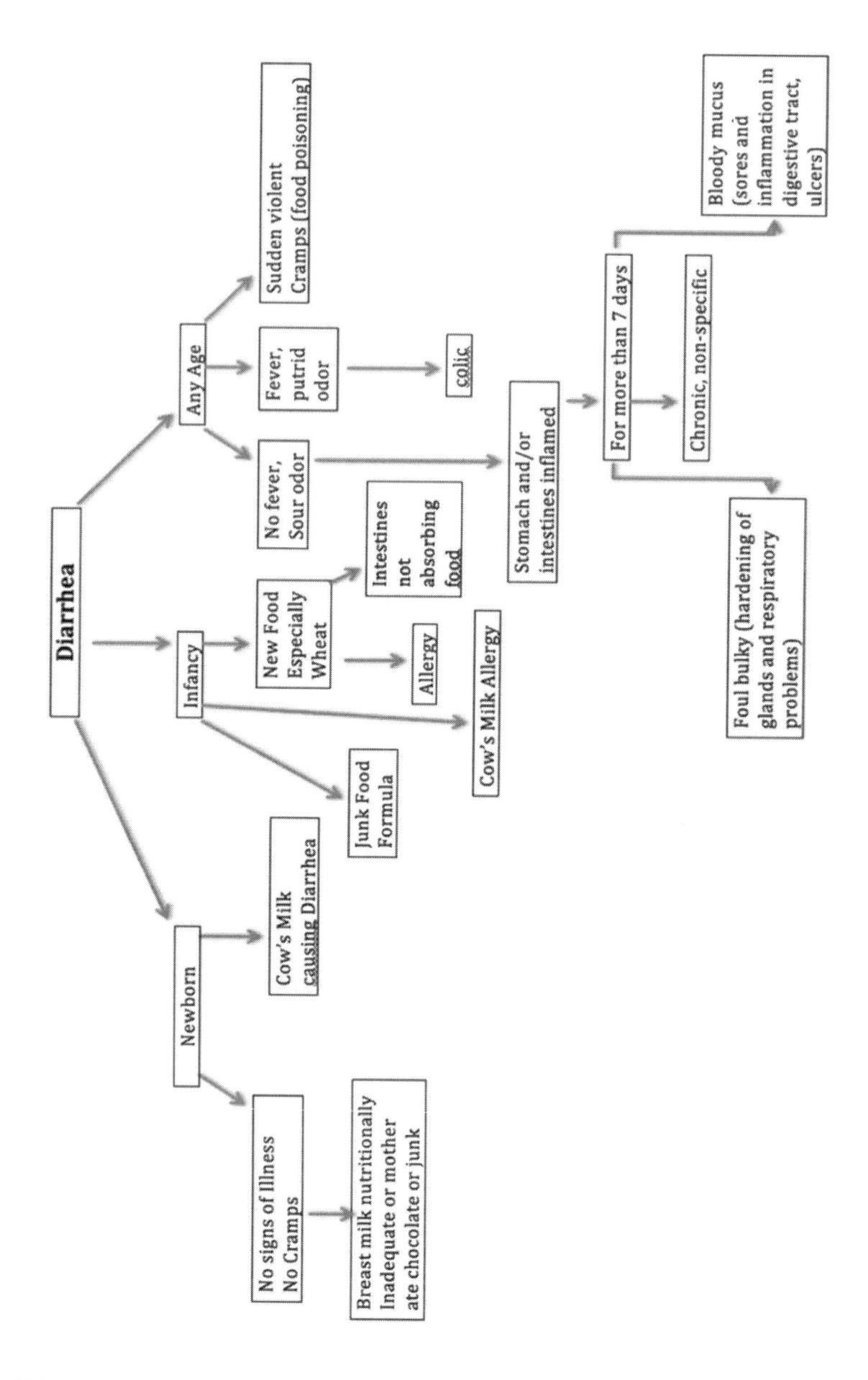

Newborn
- No signs of Illness, No Cramps → Breast milk nutritionally Inadequate or mother ate chocolate or junk
- Cow's Milk causing Diarrhea

Infancy
- Junk Food Formula
- Cow's Milk Allergy
- New Food Especially Wheat → Allergy
- New Food Especially Wheat → Intestines not absorbing food

Any Age
- Sudden violent Cramps (food poisoning)
- Fever, putrid odor → colic
- No fever, Sour odor → Stomach and/or intestines inflamed

Stomach and/or intestines inflamed → For more than 7 days
- Chronic, non-specific
- Bloody mucus (sores and inflammation in digestive tract, ulcers)
- Foul bulky (hardening of glands and respiratory problems)

Fever and Rash

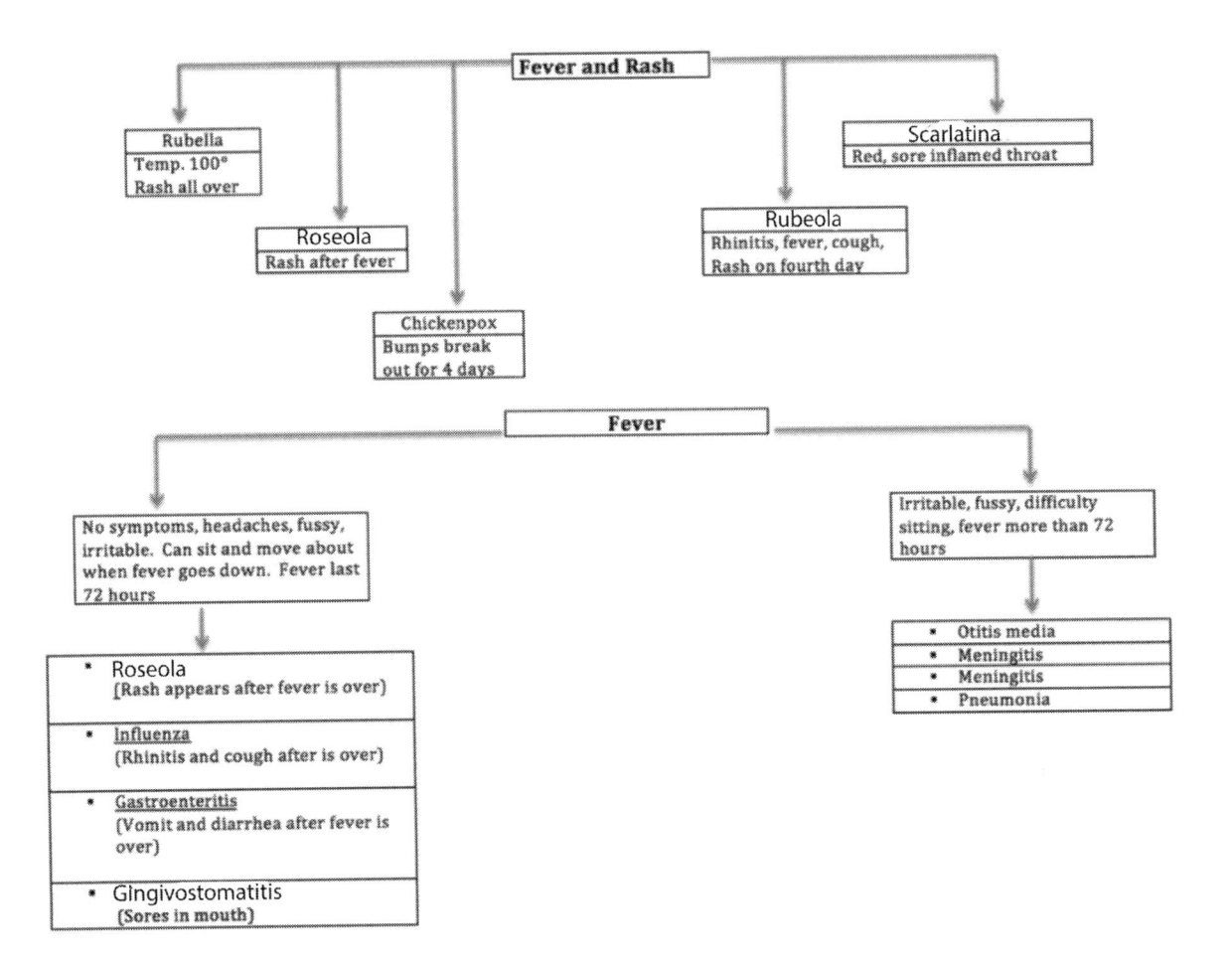

- **Rubella** — Temp. 100°, Rash all over
- **Roseola** — Rash after fever
- **Chickenpox** — Bumps break out for 4 days
- **Rubeola** — Rhinitis, fever, cough, Rash on fourth day
- **Scarlatina** — Red, sore inflamed throat

Fever

No symptoms, headaches, fussy, irritable. Can sit and move about when fever goes down. Fever last 72 hours

- Roseola (Rash appears after fever is over)
- Influenza (Rhinitis and cough after is over)
- Gastroenteritis (Vomit and diarrhea after fever is over)
- Gingivostomatitis (Sores in mouth)

Irritable, fussy, difficulty sitting, fever more than 72 hours

- Otitis media
- Meningitis
- Meningitis
- Pneumonia

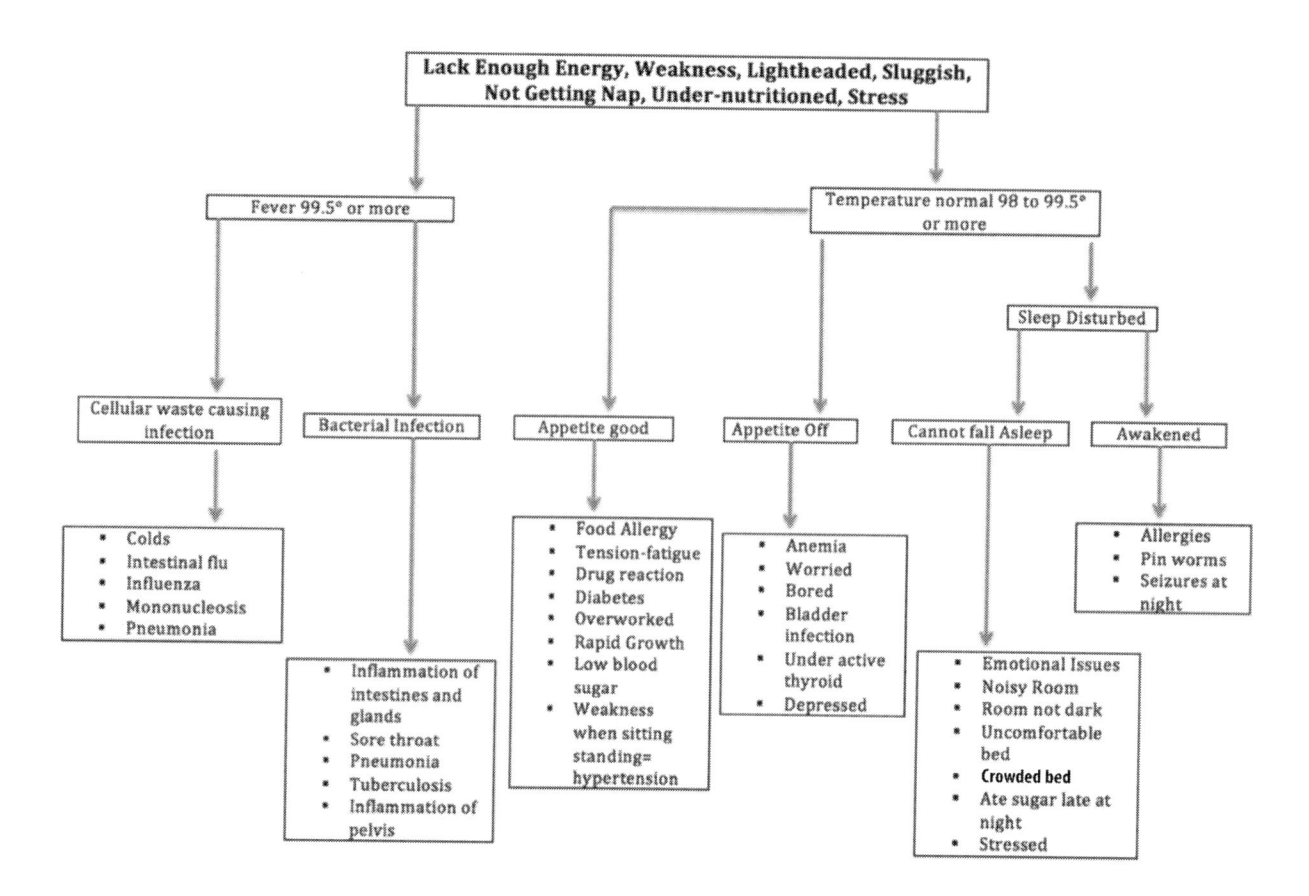

```
Lack Enough Energy, Weakness, Lightheaded, Sluggish,
Not Getting Nap, Under-nutritioned, Stress
```

- **Fever 99.5° or more**
  - **Cellular waste causing infection**
    - Colds
    - Intestinal flu
    - Influenza
    - Mononucleosis
    - Pneumonia
  - **Bacterial Infection**
    - Inflammation of intestines and glands
    - Sore throat
    - Pneumonia
    - Tuberculosis
    - Inflammation of pelvis

- **Temperature normal 98 to 99.5° or more**
  - **Appetite good**
    - Food Allergy
    - Tension-fatigue
    - Drug reaction
    - Diabetes
    - Overworked
    - Rapid Growth
    - Low blood sugar
    - Weakness when sitting standing= hypertension
  - **Appetite Off**
    - Anemia
    - Worried
    - Bored
    - Bladder infection
    - Under active thyroid
    - Depressed
  - **Sleep Disturbed**
    - **Cannot fall Asleep**
      - Emotional Issues
      - Noisy Room
      - Room not dark
      - Uncomfortable bed
      - **Crowded bed**
      - Ate sugar late at night
      - Stressed
    - **Awakened**
      - Allergies
      - Pin worms
      - Seizures at night

Pus in Eye

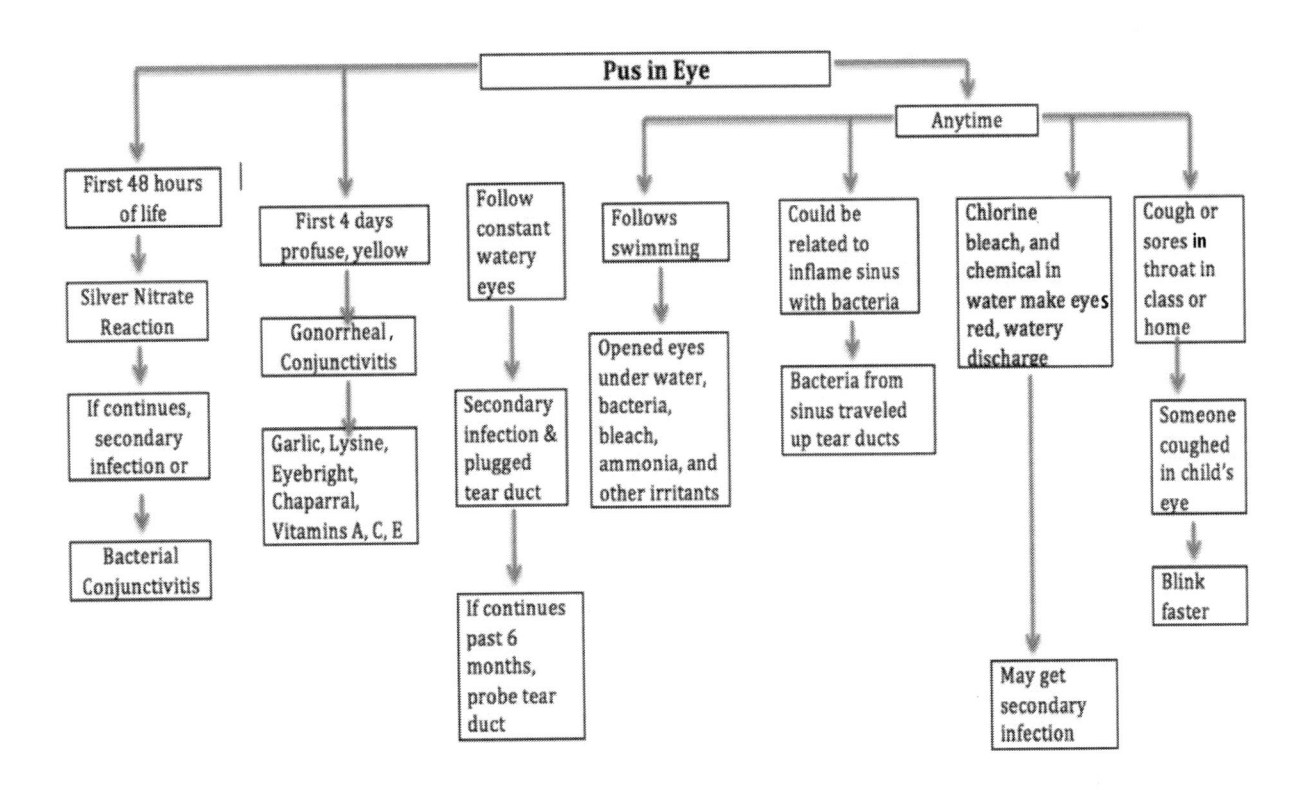

First 48 hours of life
- Silver Nitrate Reaction
- If continues, secondary infection or
- Bacterial Conjunctivitis

First 4 days profuse, yellow
- Gonorrheal, Conjunctivitis
- Garlic, Lysine, Eyebright, Chaparral, Vitamins A, C, E

Follow constant watery eyes
- Secondary infection & plugged tear duct
- If continues past 6 months, probe tear duct

Anytime

Follows swimming
- Opened eyes under water, bacteria, bleach, ammonia, and other irritants

Could be related to inflame sinus with bacteria
- Bacteria from sinus traveled up tear ducts

Chlorine bleach, and chemical in water make eyes red, watery discharge
- May get secondary infection

Cough or sores in throat in class or home
- Someone coughed in child's eye
- Blink faster

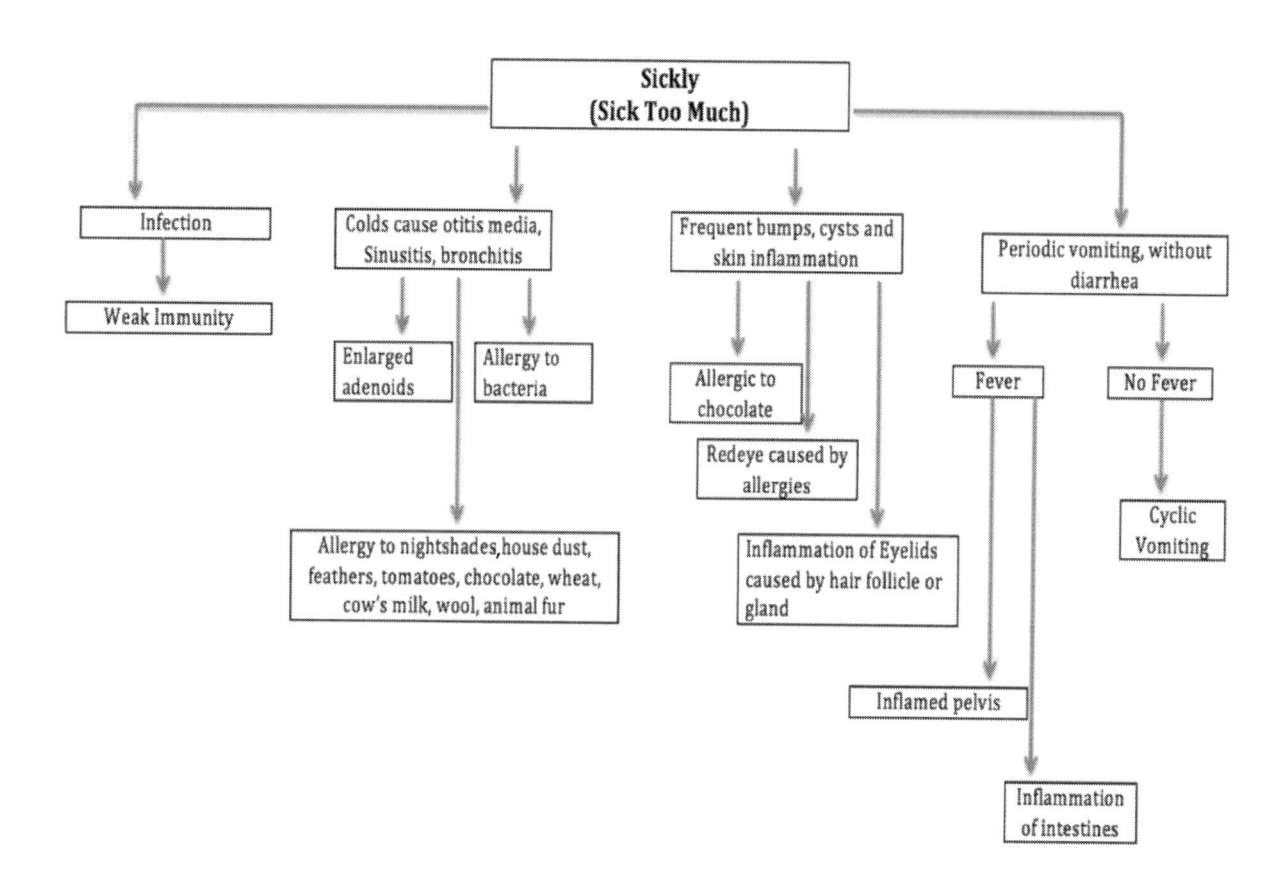

```
                        ┌─────────────────────┐
                        │       Sickly        │
                        │  (Sick Too Much)    │
                        └─────────────────────┘
         ┌──────────────┬──────────┴──────────┬──────────────┐
         ▼              ▼                     ▼              ▼
   ┌──────────┐  ┌──────────────┐   ┌──────────────┐  ┌──────────────┐
   │ Infection│  │ Colds cause  │   │Frequent bumps│  │Periodic      │
   │          │  │ otitis media,│   │cysts and     │  │vomiting,     │
   │          │  │ Sinusitis,   │   │skin          │  │without       │
   │          │  │ bronchitis   │   │inflammation  │  │diarrhea      │
   └──────────┘  └──────────────┘   └──────────────┘  └──────────────┘
         │         │         │         │       │         │        │
         ▼         ▼         ▼         ▼       ▼         ▼        ▼
   ┌────────┐ ┌────────┐ ┌────────┐┌────────┐          ┌─────┐ ┌────────┐
   │ Weak   │ │Enlarged│ │Allergy ││Allergic│          │Fever│ │No Fever│
   │Immunity│ │adenoids│ │to      ││to      │          └─────┘ └────────┘
   └────────┘ └────────┘ │bacteria││chocolate│                      │
                         └────────┘└────────┘                       ▼
                              │                               ┌─────────┐
                              ▼          ┌────────────┐       │ Cyclic  │
              ┌──────────────────────┐   │Redeye      │       │Vomiting │
              │Allergy to nightshades│   │caused by   │       └─────────┘
              │house dust, feathers, │   │allergies   │
              │tomatoes, chocolate,  │   └────────────┘
              │wheat, cow's milk,    │         │
              │wool, animal fur      │         ▼
              └──────────────────────┘   ┌────────────┐
                                         │Inflammation│
                                         │of Eyelids  │
                                         │caused by   │
                                         │hair follicle│
                                         │or gland    │
                                         └────────────┘
                                                │
                                                ▼
                                         ┌────────────┐
                                         │  Inflamed  │
                                         │   pelvis   │
                                         └────────────┘
                                                │
                                                ▼
                                         ┌────────────┐
                                         │Inflammation│
                                         │of intestines│
                                         └────────────┘
```

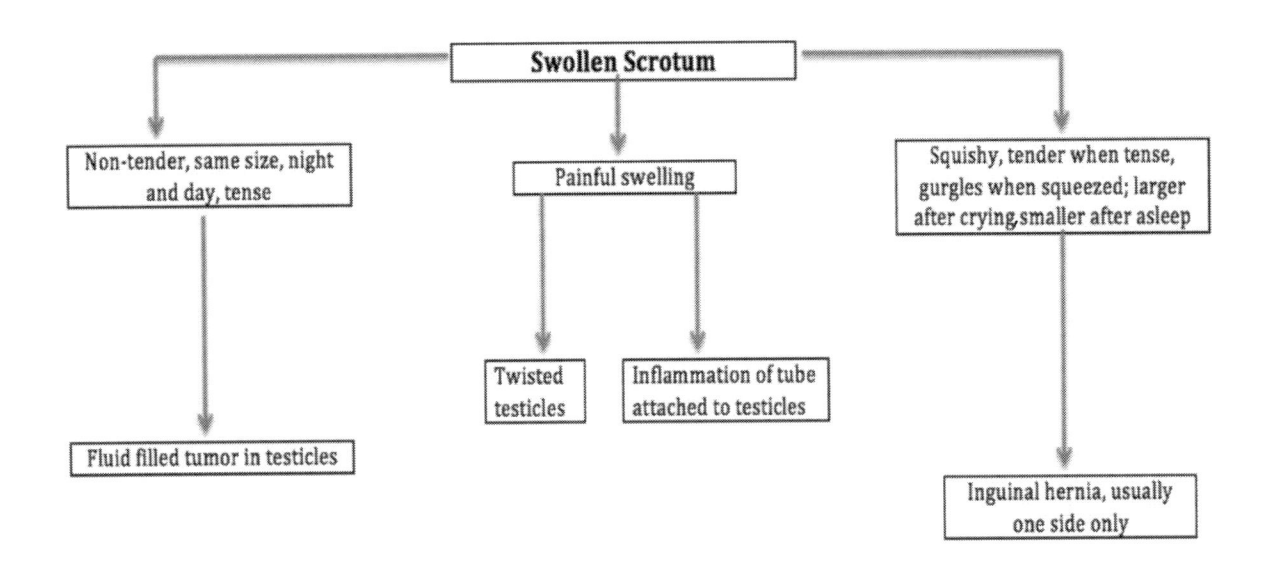

```
                          ┌──────────────────┐
                          │  Swollen Scrotum │
                          └──────────────────┘
           ┌─────────────────────┼─────────────────────────┐
           ▼                     ▼                         ▼
┌──────────────────────┐  ┌──────────────┐   ┌──────────────────────────────┐
│ Non-tender, same     │  │  Painful     │   │ Squishy, tender when tense,  │
│ size, night and day, │  │  swelling    │   │ gurgles when squeezed; larger│
│ tense                │  │              │   │ after crying, smaller after  │
└──────────────────────┘  └──────────────┘   │ asleep                       │
           │              ┌───────┴────────┐ └──────────────────────────────┘
           ▼              ▼                ▼                 │
┌──────────────────────┐ ┌─────────┐ ┌──────────────────┐    ▼
│ Fluid filled tumor   │ │ Twisted │ │ Inflammation of  │  ┌─────────────────────┐
│ in testicles         │ │testicles│ │ tube attached    │  │ Inguinal hernia,    │
└──────────────────────┘ └─────────┘ │ to testicles     │  │ usually one side only│
                                     └──────────────────┘  └─────────────────────┘
```

```
                          ┌─────────────────┐
                          │    Earache      │
                          └─────────────────┘
                  ↙                              ↘
        ┌──────────────┐                  ┌──────────────────┐
        │   No Fever   │                  │ Fever (100° to 104°) │
        └──────────────┘                  └──────────────────┘
                ↓                           ↓              ↓
```

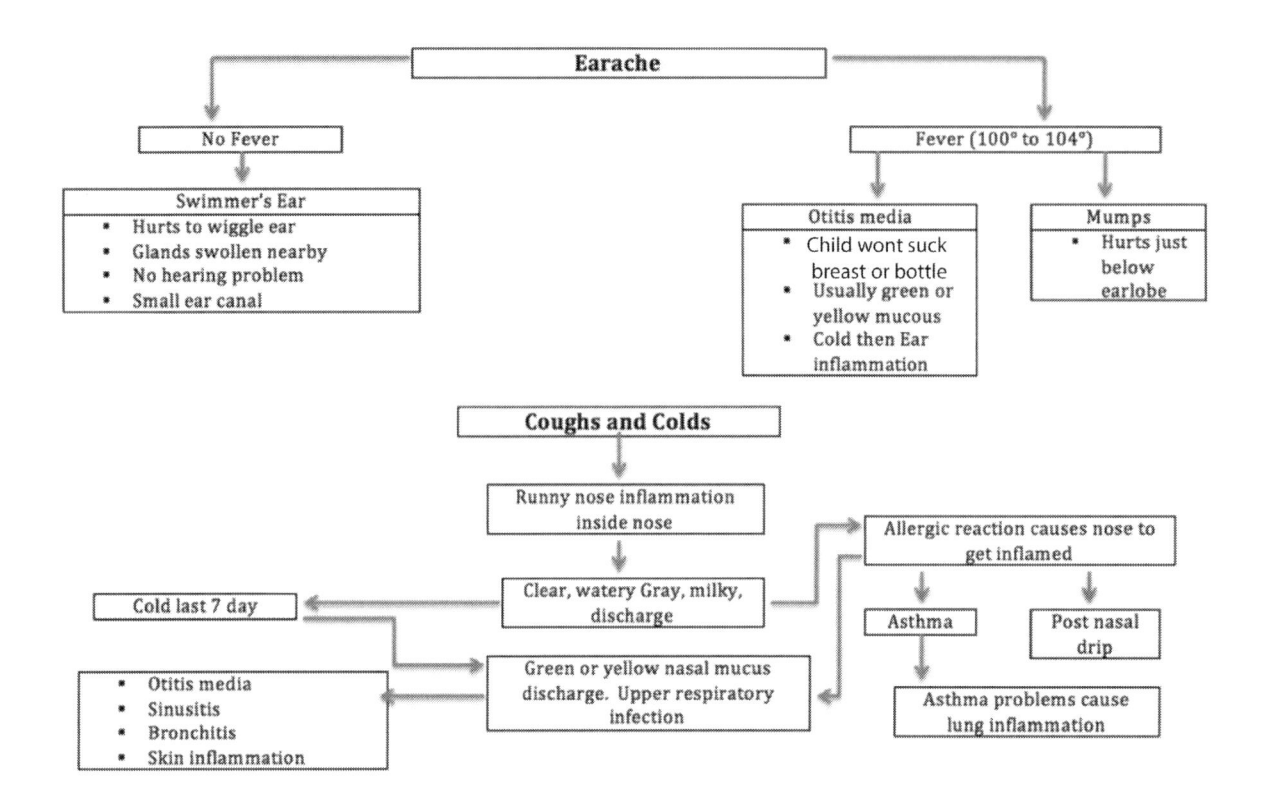

Swimmer's Ear
- Hurts to wiggle ear
- Glands swollen nearby
- No hearing problem
- Small ear canal

Otitis media
- Child wont suck breast or bottle
- Usually green or yellow mucous
- Cold then Ear inflammation

Mumps
- Hurts just below earlobe

Coughs and Colds

↓

Runny nose inflammation inside nose

↓

Clear, watery Gray, milky, discharge → Allergic reaction causes nose to get inflamed

← Cold last 7 day

↓   ↓   ↓
Green or yellow nasal mucus discharge. Upper respiratory infection   Asthma   Post nasal drip

↓
Asthma problems cause lung inflammation

- Otitis media
- Sinusitis
- Bronchitis
- Skin inflammation

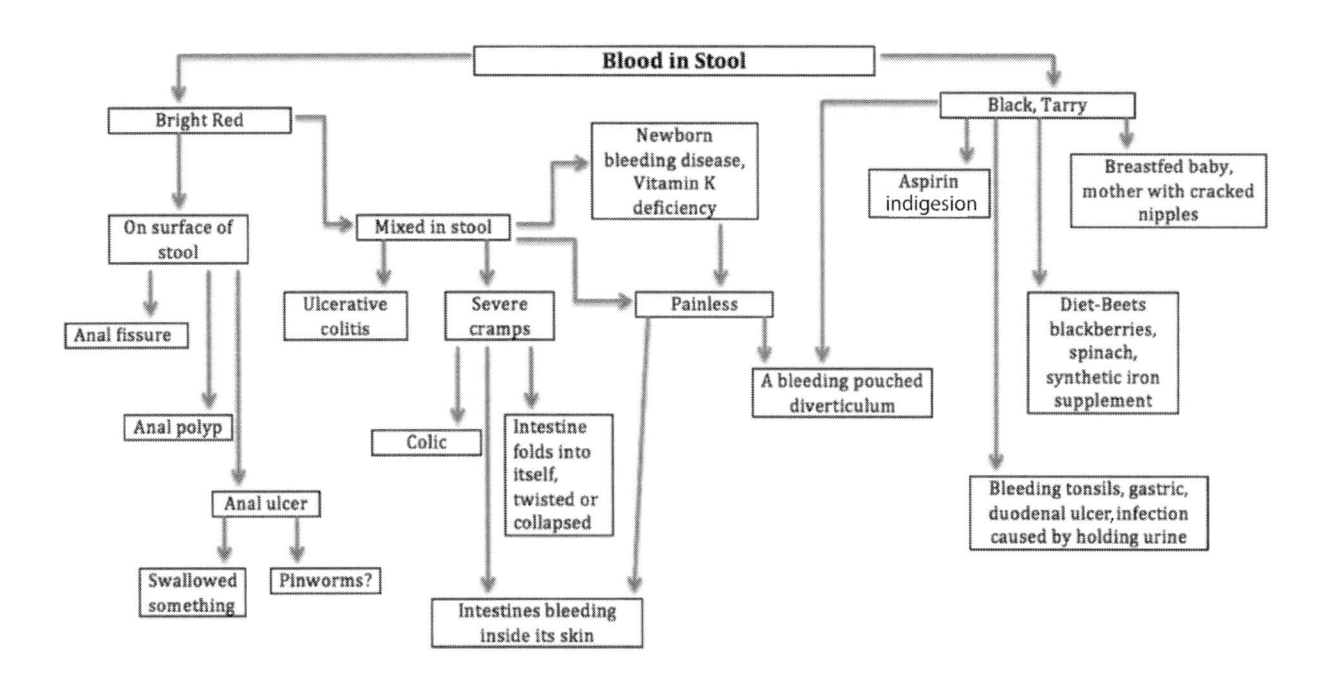

```
                                    Blood in Stool
                                          │
      ┌───────────────────────────────────┼───────────────────────────────┐
      ▼                                                                    ▼
  Bright Red                                                         Black, Tarry
      │                                                    ┌──────────┬──────┴──────────┐
      ▼                                                    ▼          ▼                 ▼
  ┌─────────────┐         ┌──────────────┐           Aspirin    Breastfed baby,
  │ On surface  │         │ Mixed in     │──▶ Newborn          indigestion    mother with cracked
  │ of stool    │         │ stool        │    bleeding disease,                      nipples
  └─────────────┘         └──────────────┘    Vitamin K
      │                    │     │    │       deficiency
      ▼                    ▼     ▼    ▼           │
  Anal fissure         Ulcerative Severe Painless │        Diet-Beets
                        colitis   cramps    │     │        blackberries,
      │                           │  │  │   │     │        spinach,
      ▼                           ▼  ▼  ▼   ▼     │        synthetic iron
  Anal polyp                   Colic Intestine  A bleeding  supplement
                                     folds into pouched
      │                              itself,    diverticulum
      ▼                              twisted or
  Anal ulcer                         collapsed         Bleeding tonsils, gastric,
   │       │                              │            duodenal ulcer, infection
   ▼       ▼                              ▼            caused by holding urine
Swallowed Pinworms?                 Intestines bleeding
something                           inside its skin
```

573

Blood in Urine

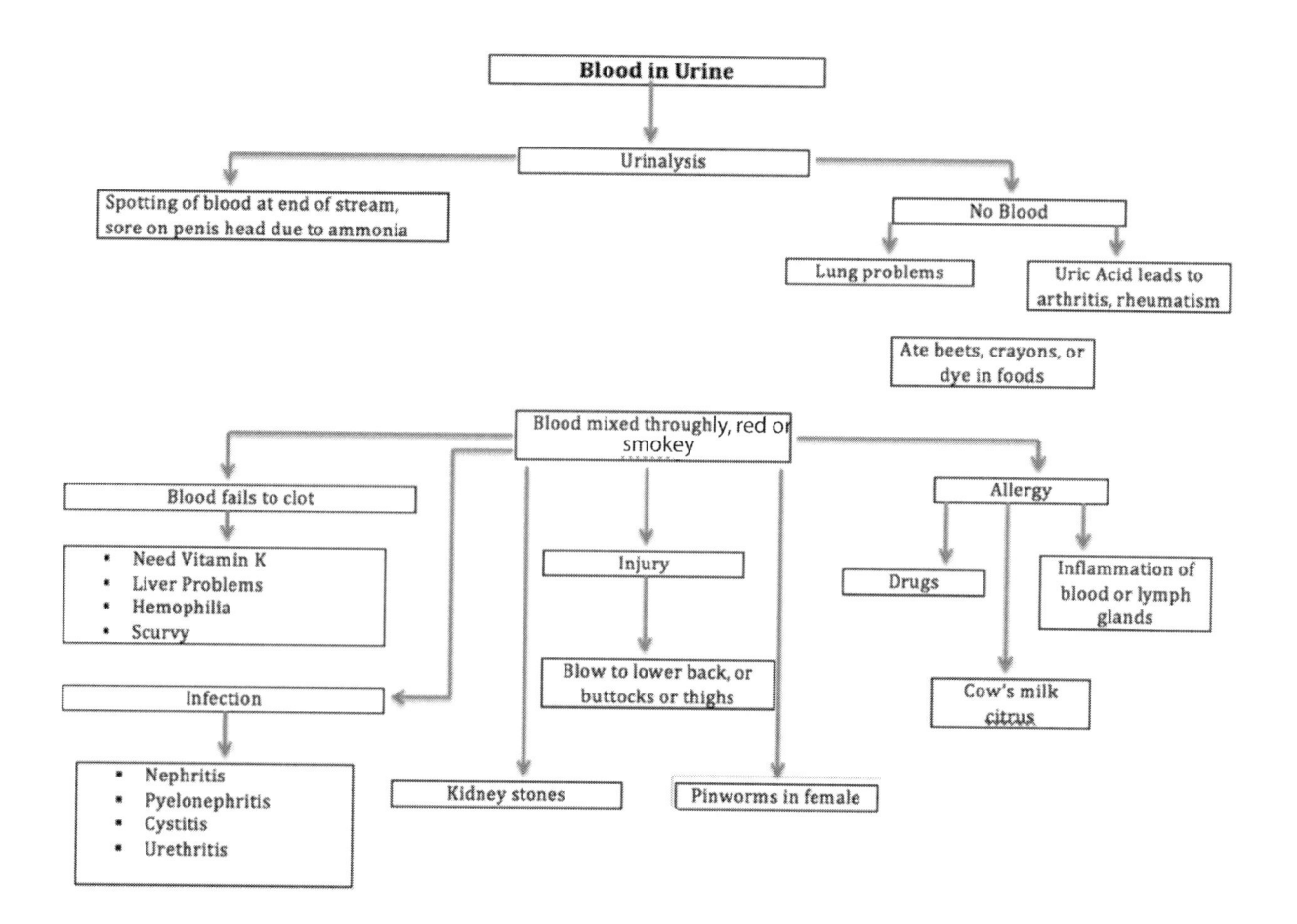

Urinalysis

- Spotting of blood at end of stream, sore on penis head due to ammonia
- No Blood
  - Lung problems
  - Uric Acid leads to arthritis, rheumatism
- Ate beets, crayons, or dye in foods

Blood mixed throughly, red or smokey

- **Blood fails to clot**
  - Need Vitamin K
  - Liver Problems
  - Hemophilia
  - Scurvy
- **Infection**
  - Nephritis
  - Pyelonephritis
  - Cystitis
  - Urethritis
- **Injury** — Blow to lower back, or buttocks or thighs
- Kidney stones
- Pinworms in female
- **Allergy**
  - Drugs
  - Inflammation of blood or lymph glands
  - Cow's milk, citrus

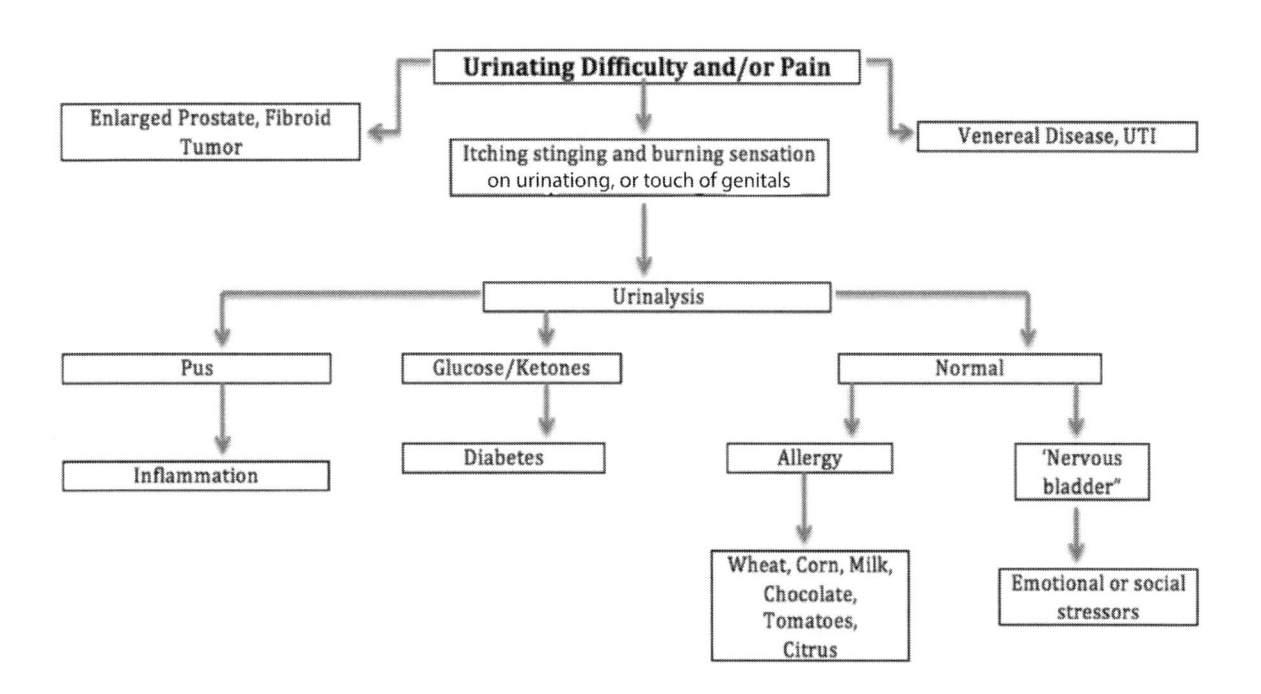

```
                    ┌─────────────────────────────────┐
Enlarged Prostate,  │  Urinating Difficulty and/or Pain │   Venereal Disease, UTI
Fibroid Tumor   ←───┤                                 ├───→
                    └─────────────────────────────────┘
                                    ↓
                    ┌─────────────────────────────────┐
                    │ Itching stinging and burning    │
                    │ sensation on urinationg, or     │
                    │ touch of genitals               │
                    └─────────────────────────────────┘
                                    ↓
                    ┌─────────────────────────────────┐
                    │           Urinalysis            │
                    └─────────────────────────────────┘
           ↓                        ↓                         ↓
        ┌──────┐           ┌────────────────┐            ┌────────┐
        │ Pus  │           │ Glucose/Ketones│            │ Normal │
        └──────┘           └────────────────┘            └────────┘
           ↓                        ↓                   ↓         ↓
     ┌────────────┐            ┌──────────┐       ┌─────────┐  ┌──────────┐
     │Inflammation│            │ Diabetes │       │ Allergy │  │'Nervous  │
     └────────────┘            └──────────┘       └─────────┘  │ bladder" │
                                                       ↓       └──────────┘
                                              ┌──────────────┐      ↓
                                              │Wheat, Corn,  │ ┌──────────────┐
                                              │Milk,Chocolate│ │Emotional or  │
                                              │Tomatoes,     │ │social        │
                                              │Citrus        │ │stressors     │
                                              └──────────────┘ └──────────────┘
```

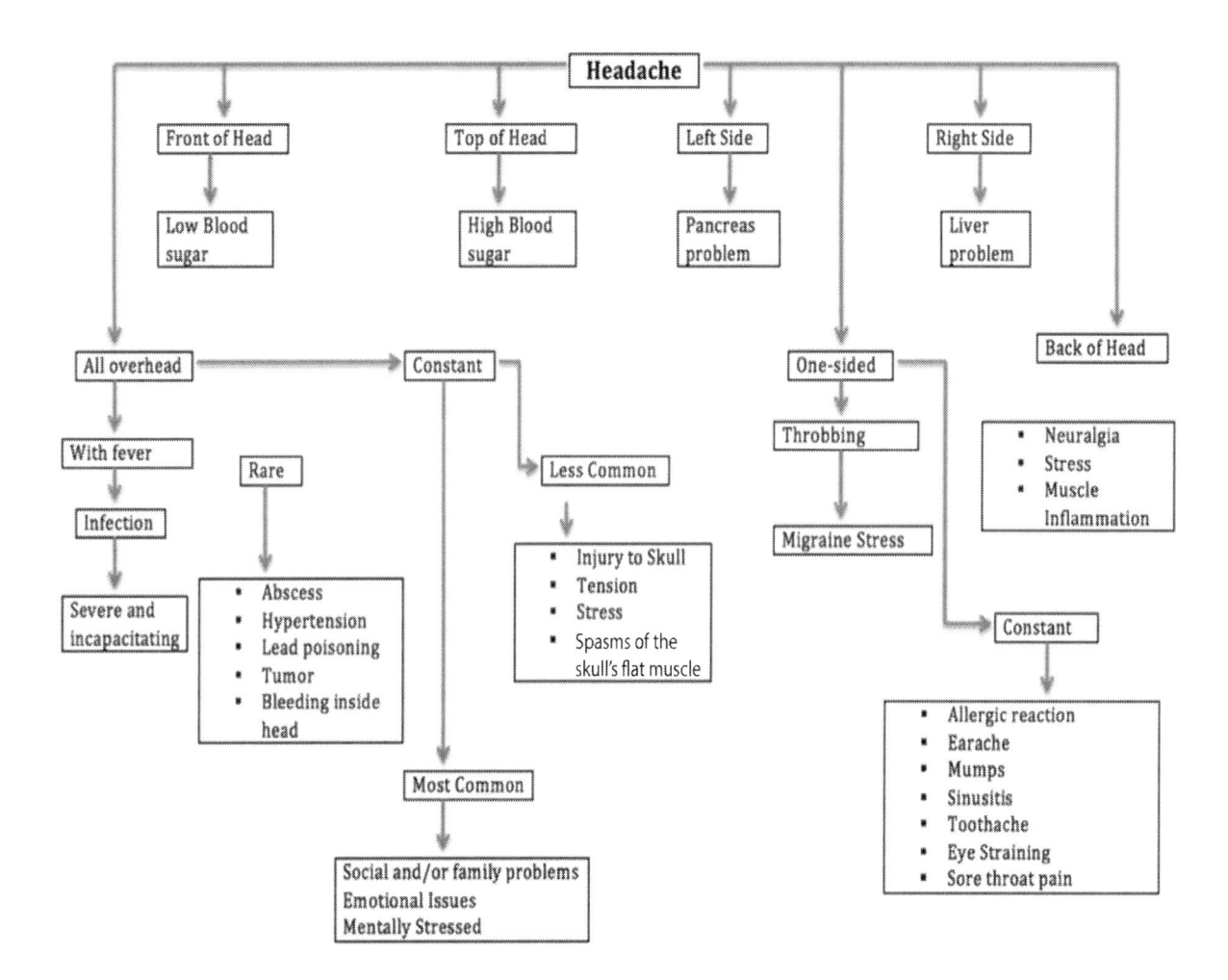

```
Headache
├── Front of Head → Low Blood sugar
├── Top of Head → High Blood sugar
├── Left Side → Pancreas problem
├── Right Side → Liver problem
├── All overhead
│   ├── With fever → Infection → Severe and incapacitating
│   └── Constant
│       ├── Rare
│       │   • Abscess
│       │   • Hypertension
│       │   • Lead poisoning
│       │   • Tumor
│       │   • Bleeding inside head
│       ├── Less Common
│       │   • Injury to Skull
│       │   • Tension
│       │   • Stress
│       │   • Spasms of the skull's flat muscle
│       └── Most Common
│           Social and/or family problems
│           Emotional Issues
│           Mentally Stressed
├── One-sided
│   ├── Throbbing → Migraine Stress
│   └── Constant
│       • Allergic reaction
│       • Earache
│       • Mumps
│       • Sinusitis
│       • Toothache
│       • Eye Straining
│       • Sore throat pain
└── Back of Head
    • Neuralgia
    • Stress
    • Muscle Inflammation
```

Supplies

Urine reagents needed to do the Functional Urinalysis Testing

Reagent	Amount
Chemstrips (100)	100 test strips
Ferric acid	2 ounce bottle
Acetic acid	2 ounce bottle
Sodium hydroxide	2 ounce bottle
Potassium chromate	1 ounce bottle
Silver nitrate	2 ounce bottle
Sulkowitch reagent	4 ounces bottle

The above reagents can be ordered from the following company:
Rocky Mountain Reagents Inc.
3207 West Hampden Avenue, Englewood, CO 80110
(303) 762-0800
They may require a copy of your professional license Equipment for Test

Equipment	Quantity Needed
Centrifuge	1
pH Meter or pH paper	1
Test tubes (box of 250)	1 box
Applicator sticks (box of 1000)	100 individual applicator sticks
Safety glasses	1
Urinometer (float and jar)	1
Graduated cylinders	4
Graduated cylinders brush	1
Test tube racks	1
Wash bottles	1
Funnels	1
Glass droppers	6
Beakers	2
Iodine patch test	1 bottle
Zinc tally	1 bottle
pH paper	1 roll
Dr. Kane's mineral assessment tests	1 test kit
Lingual ascorbic acid test	1 box
Gastro string test	5 test
Oral Thermometers	5 to loan to patients
Multistix 10SG	1 container

Resources
Gastro Test

The Gastro – Test is manufactured in the US by HDC Corporation.

Mailing Address	Telephone	Web
628 Gibraltar Court, Milpitas, CA 95035	408-942-7340 or 800-227-8162	http://www.hdccorp.com

Kanes Mineral Assessment Test

The Kane Mineral Assessment Test are manufactured in the US by E-Lyte, INC

Mailing Address	Telephone & Fax	Web
45 Reese Road Millville, NJ 08332	888-320-8338 (in US) 856-825-8338 (Outside the US)	http://www.e-lyte.com

Oxidata Test

The Oxidata test is manufactured in the US by Apex.

Mailing Address	Telephone & Fax	Web
1701 E. Edinger Ave, Suite A-4, Santa Ana, CA 92705	714-973-7733 800-736-4381 Fax: 714-973-2238	www.oxidata.com ww.apexenergetics.com

Apex Energetics also retails salivary pH paper and urine dipstick kits (Chemstrip 10)

Zinc Taste Test

The Zinc Taste test we recommend is manufactured in the US by Biotics Research Corporation.

Mailing Address	Telephone & Fax	Web
6801 Biotics Research Drive, Rosenburg, TX 77471	800-231-5777 Fax: 281-344-0725	

Lingual Ascorbic Acid Test, Iodine Patch Test, pH Paper

The Lingual Ascorbic Acid test, Iodine for the Iodine Patch Test, and salivary pH paper can be ordered from Nutritional Therapy Association.

Mailing Address	Telephone & Fax	Web
P.O Box 354 Olympia, WA 98507	800-918-9798	www.NutritionalTherapy.com

Places to obtain Equipment:
Centrifuge: You can buy one from second hand medical suppliers or get one from your testing lab.

pH Meter: You can search on the Internet. Hanna instruments make a very reasonable pH meter, or use pH paper.

Test tubes, finger cots etc.: Rocky Mountain Reagents is a one-stop resource for all of the equipment you need to set up a Functional Lab. Their address and phone numbers are:

Rocky Mountain Reagents Inc.
3207 West Hampden Avenue, Englewood, CO 80110
(303) 762-0800

pikeagri.com pH paper, pH meters, chemistry equipment etc.
biousa.com- Multistix 10SG, pH paper etc.
privatemdlabs.com- does all type of blood test for less the Doctor visit go to lab for test

Ovuscope: ovuscope.com
Early PregnancyTest.com
Fairhaven.com

Contact medical supply companies for supplies.

Index

A

Abdomen 233, 331, 332, 333, 334, 352, 536
acid. 15, 19, 20, 40, 42, 66, 140, 142, 212, 224, 317, 365, 366, 372, 374, 376, 380, 381, 383, 384, 386, 389, 390, 391, 392, 393, 397, 399, 400, 401, 402, 404, 405, 406, 407, 408, 411, 412, 413, 414, 415, 416, 419, 425, 426, 427, 428, 429, 430, 431, 433, 434, 436, 437, 438, 439, 440, 441, 442, 536, 578
Acne 75, 544
acupuncture 9, 44, 176, 232, 334
acupuncture meridian 44
addiction 56, 195, 448
adhesions 546
alkaline ... 15, 40, 317, 374, 376, 380, 382, 383, 389, 391, 397, 399, 400, 412, 414, 415, 416, 419, 425, 426, 427, 428, 429, 430, 433, 438, 439, 440, 441, 442
Amino Acid 224
Amylase 3, 319, 320
Anabolic 16
Anaerobic 16, 437
Anagrams 445
anemia 48, 54, 55, 110, 123, 142, 159, 271, 275, 381, 383, 384, 386, 387, 388, 391, 392, 393, 397, 406, 419, 432, 542, 549
ANGULAR HOUSES 450
Antioxidant 16, 397, 419
Aquarius 91, 166, 257, 445, 447, 471, 477
arch 124, 298, 335, 337
Areola 257
Aries 81, 166, 445, 449, 467, 473
Arthritis 19, 112, 155, 198, 357, 366, 374, 435, 537
Astrology 444

B

Barren 448
benign 543
Bilirubin 375, 376, 432
binding 387, 394, 418
Birth 64, 536
bleach 381
Bleeding 19
blockages 352
Blood .. 4, 15, 23, 107, 114, 132, 195, 228, 243, 273, 319, 320, 326, 327, 352, 368, 372, 373, 375, 376, 377, 379, 381, 390, 391, 400, 412, 413, 415, 416, 417, 425, 426, 536, 537, 538, 541, 543, 547
Blood Pressure 4, 23, 195, 228, 273, 319, 320, 373, 536, 537, 543
Boils 544
Bonding 3
Bone 19, 74, 275, 383
Botanicals 536
Bowel 20, 22, 317, 320, 410, 411, 418, 536, 537
Brain 3, 23, 110, 317, 324
Breast 112, 113, 166, 247, 256, 257, 258, 317, 319, 360, 547, 548
Bronchitis 551
Bruising 544
bulging 98, 263, 333, 337
burning 15, 361, 406, 407
buttocks 11, 107, 290, 328, 359, 363, 364, 473, 475

C

Callouses 212
Cancer ... 84, 166, 257, 445, 447, 470, 476, 536, 545
Candida 440, 549
Capricorn 90, 166, 257, 445, 447, 470, 476
Cataracts 110, 319
cervical 3, 112, 113, 363, 418, 547
Cervix 112, 113, 247, 536
chest 20, 22, 107, 112, 113, 257, 287, 291, 328, 352, 357, 360, 364, 400, 406
chin .. 72, 81, 83, 84, 85, 90, 92, 95, 98, 99, 100, 364, 422
Chlamydia 549, 552
Chronic fatigue 270
Circulation 10, 231
Cirrhosis 319, 385, 542
cleansing 12
CONJUNCTION 452
Cramps 19, 155, 365
Cyanosis 542
cyst 1, 99, 142, 210, 544, 547, 548

D

Dandruff 19, 155
deficiency 48, 49, 144, 160, 224, 370, 376, 380, 383, 384, 385, 386, 387, 388, 389, 391, 392, 393, 397, 401, 402, 403, 404, 405, 408, 419, 430, 431, 432, 434, 437, 438, 440, 536, 541, 545, 546, 552
Dementia 550
Depression 319, 330, 545, 546, 550
Dermatitis 19, 545, 549
deterioration .. 56, 57, 110, 112, 117, 124, 142, 161, 265, 275, 328, 357, 358, 370, 372, 402, 449
Diabetes 23, 376, 380, 381, 383, 389, 418, 536, 537, 541, 549
Diarrhea 16, 19, 320, 374, 406, 435, 538
Dietary 401, 410, 457, 544
Digestion. 3, 28, 31, 38, 79, 136, 228, 326, 401, 434
discharge 362, 536, 548, 549, 552
Disease. 71, 121, 154, 155, 215, 235, 236, 243, 319, 320, 326, 351, 357, 361, 374, 378, 380, 381, 382, 383, 384, 385, 386, 387, 388, 389, 390, 391, 392, 393, 394, 395, 418, 536, 538, 539, 546, 549, 551, 552, 553
Disease Analysis Chart 553

Digestive System Disorders 563
Disorders of the Urinary System......................562
Endocrine Disorders 556
Heart Failure..557
Nervous System Disorders 561
Disorders..562
Displacement..288, 295
Douches 549
Ducts 17, 242
duodenum.......32, 59, 107, 213, 229, 328, 406, 412, 440
Dyspnea 537, 542, 552

E

ear................. 132, 136, 138, 235, 281, 364, 370, 544
earth 475, 476
ectoderm 7
Ejaculatory...242
ELEMENT.. 467, 468, 469, 470, 471, 472, 473, 474, 475, 476, 477, 478
Elimination 38, 410
embryo..8, 9, 62
Endoderm... **7**
Endorphins...548
Energy 9, 10, 19, 20, 40, 223, 230, 231, 233, 243, 264, 326, 374
Enzymatic 228
Enzyme... **3**, 43, 193, 425
Epididymitis...552
Erect 247
Exam............ 257, 352, 360, 363, 364, 367, 368, 538
excretory 49, 56, 57, 73, 106, 123, 136, 142, 158, 164, 173, 197, 211, 213, 214
eye.. 1, 20, 70, 83, 91, 108, 110, 113, 119, 120, 123, 127, 129, 138, 250, 326, 353, 355, 356, 357, 365, 366, 368, 371, 536
eyes . 1, 20, 22, 23, 43, 70, 73, 81, 82, 84, 85, 89, 90, 91, 92, 94, 97, 100, 101, 102, 105, 106, 113, 119, 125, 127, 129, 248, 257, 267, 294, 326, 353, 354, 355, 356, 357, 364, 365, 366, 367, 368, 370, 371, 403

F

fallopian 83, 166, 257, 268
fatigue.. 19, 109, 164, 197, 210, 211, 357, 365, 370, 394, 401, 406, 417, 418, 437, 440
feet .22, 92, 119, 193, 277, 286, 287, 299, 319, 326, 327, 328, 353, 354, 357, 358, 364, 367, 432, 435, 478, 541
Female Principle 8, 10, 14, 15, 16, 17, 18, 19, 20, 23, 62, 102, 106, 108, 123, 127, 132, 157, 176, 300, 373
fertilize 268
fetus 263
fibroid tumor...250
Fibrosis 542, 552
Fingernail..160, 163
Flexibility Test 364

Fluid.. 23
Foods..38, 398, 418
Fracture...357
fruit 144, 407
Fungus 206, 545

G

G.l17
Gemini................ 83, 257, 445, 447, 448, 469, 475
genitals 23
Gingivitis.. 19
GLANDS..323
Globulin 384, 385
Glucagon... 16, 23
Glucose...17, 375, 376, 380, 537
glycogen..17, 268, 380, 383
GLYPH467, 468, 469, 470, 471, 472, 473, 474, 475, 476, 477, 478
goiter 17, 370, 402
gonads... 166, 257, 448
Gout 23, 383, 549
Gravity 15, 280, 375
groin 327, 364
Grounding 287
gums 19, 20, 144, 151, 361, 401

H

hair 1, 19, 22, 43, 82, 94, 101, 102, 132, 173, 226, 233, 234, 235, 248, 255, 257, 326, 332, 370
hand.........45, 52, 129, 157, 158, 172, 174, 248, 257, 326, 334, 336, 337, 352, 357, 363, 366, 367, 371, 400, 401, 414, 415, 419, 579
Hay fever 19
HDL..389
Headaches...19, 319, 326, 435
HEALING...269
Hearing..113, 132, 136, 320, 330, 361
Hemolyzed 15, 16, 377, 433
hepatitis 89, 198, 376, 385, 386, 388, 391
Hernia 19, 34, 263, 548, 552
hip...281, 363, 366, 367
Histamine... 17, 20
hormone .15, 57, 142, 253, 268, 271, 370, 371, 384, 393, 394, 402, 403, 405, 408, 425, 448, 474, 548
HPV 536, 549
Hydrogen... 15, 427
hypoactive...334
Hypoglossal 362
Hypothalamus 17, 536

I

Illiocecal..328
illness 3, 39, 95, 97, 100, 101, 102, 179, 328, 357, 416, 449, 450, 451, 452, 454, 455, 456, 457, 458, 459, 460, 464, 546
immune system 109, 267
Incisors 16, 148

581

Indigestion 17, 435
infection 17, 23, 36, 87, 109, 112, 113, 142, 198, 206, 364, 367, 369, 376, 377, 382, 383, 385, 386, 387, 390, 391, 392, 402, 408, 411, 412, 433, 439, 440, 473, 537, 545, 551, 552
injury 3, 243, 326, 357, 360, 364, 365, 458, 471, 550
insomnia 17, 164, 197, 381, 406, 432
insulin 15, 393, 414, 417, 425
Intestine 10, 132, 155, 166, 231, 243, 334, 363, 367
Iodine 41, 228, 402, 403, 404, 409, 578, 579
ionic 425, 427
Iron 40, 41, 228, 387, 388, 391, 393, 467, 541, 545
irritation 17, 112, 113, 231, 368, 370, 403, 407, 410, 412, 413, 435, 440, 550

J

joints 90, 162, 163, 176, 267, 281, 286, 357, 366, 367, 401, 442, 476
Jupiter .. 99, 158, 178, 198, 445, 448, 449, 454, 455, 456, 457, 458, 459, 475, 479

L

Labia 243, 247
Lacrimal 17
Lashes 110
lead 383, 389, 392, 408, 433, 454, 457, 462
Leg ulcer 20
Leo 85, 166, 257, 445, 446, 447, 448, 471, 477
Leukocytes 375, 377
Libra 87, 166, 445, 447, 467, 473
Lice 545
Lipase 3, 319, 320
LIPS 53
Liver 3, **7**, 10, 17, 109, 113, 132, 136, 151, 155, 171, 196, 198, 209, 228, 231, 235, 243, 317, 326, 328, 330, 363, 374, 380, 384, 386, 388, 395, 415, 417, 432, 437, 439, 538, 541, 547
Liver disease 541, 547
lumbar 3, 112, 113, 358, 363, 364
Lumps 319, 546
Lungs 10, 132, 155, 157, 228, 231, 243, 317, 328, 330
Lymph 228, 364, 367

M

malnutrition 124, 383, 384, 385, 387, 388, 393, 394
Malocclusion 364
Mars 97, 198, 445, 448, 449, 454, 455, 456, 457, 458, 467, 479
Massage 52, 79, 126, 128, 144, 146, 233
melanin 7
menopause 268, 360, 372, 387, 388, 541, 543, 546
mental illness 448
Mercury 96, 184, 198, 445, 449, 454, 455, 456, 469, 472, 479
Moon 95, 110, 198, 445, 449, 455, 470, 471, 479
mouth 7, 10, 17, 22, 23, 35, 56, 57, 58, 59, 70, 81, 83, 85, 86, 87, 90, 91, 100, 138, 144, 155, 248, 257, 267, 326, 330, 356, 357, 362, 364, 365, 366, 368, 369, 370, 398, 401, 404, 408, 410, 421, 422, 435, 436, 542
Muscle 21, 23, 222, 231, 232, 233, 243, 315, 316, 357, 360, 365, 374
Myocardium 17

N

nausea 155, 326, 327, 405
Neck 78, 166, 228, 257, 292, 294, 319, 364, 468
Neptune 102, 445, 449, 454, 455, 456, 457, 458, 459, 460, 461, 462, 478, 479
Neutrophils 390
nipple 257, 363, 367, 368
Nodes 364
Non-hemolyzed 16
nose 44, 47, 48, 49, 50, 51, 52, 70, 81, 82, 86, 88, 89, 90, 95, 96, 99, 100, 101, 108, 120, 129, 138, 155, 257, 265, 326, 357, 362, 368, 369, 370, 371, 403, 467, 536

O

occipital 64, 435
oiliness 43, 72, 332
OPPOSITION 452
oral 408, 409, 410
Organ 6, 12, 155, 223, 229, 233, 234, 254, 259, 326
ossification 64
Osteoarthritis 366, 551
ovaries 117, 125, 142, 164, 215, 229, 360, 448, 546, 547, 548
overactive 150, 157, 169, 197, 366, 370
Oxidant 16

P

parasites 109, 161, 390, 391, 406, 546, 549
parasympathetic nervous system 15
parathyroid 91, 257, 384
Parotid 17, 228
Penis 16, 17, 247, 259, 260, 317
Phlebitis 20, 356, 544
Pineal 17, 228, 243, 267, 378
Pisces 92, 166, 257, 445, 447, 472, 478
Pluto .. 445, 448, 449, 454, 455, 456, 457, 458, 459, 460, 461, 462, 474, 479
poison 20, 101
POLARITY .. 467, 468, 469, 470, 471, 472, 473, 474, 475, 476, 477, 478
Polyuria 17, 549, 550
Potassium 17, 41, 110, 193, 194, 228, 380, 415, 422, 430, 578
Progesterone 17, 378, 538, 548
Protein 150, 228, 375, 377, 387, 431, 432, 440, 542
PSA 537
Pulse **4**, 17, 373, 378, 397, 398

R

rectal 112, 113, 412
Renal 381, 382, 428, 437, 548, 549, 550, 552

respiratory......... 10, 48, 52, 56, 73, 83, 96, 106, 117, 120, 142, 157, 158, 163, 172, 173, 198, 211, 364, 372, 389, 391, 397, 399, 400, 414, 415, 419, 425, 426, 427, 428, 429, 430, 431, 433, 434, 436, 438, 439, 440, 441, 442, 469
Round worms 161

S

Sagittarius 89, 166, 445, 447, 469, 475
salty 20, 125
Saturn 100, 180, 198, 445, 448, 449, 454, 455, 456, 457, 458, 459, 460, 476, 479
science 15
Scoliosis 358
Scorpio 88, 166, 257, 445, 447, 468
SEX 231, 240, 269
SEXTILE 452
Skeletal 21, 107, 536
skin 1, 6, 7, 20, 22, 23, 36, 43, 54, 58, 65, 66, 67, 68, 72, 73, 84, 100, 123, 125, 142, 150, 158, 167, 191, 192, 198, 206, 210, 214, 222, 223, 224, 226, 231, 233, 234, 235, 254, 255, 257, 259, 260, 271, 290, 326, 332, 334, 357, 358, 360, 362, 364, 366, 368, 369, 370, 371, 372, 381, 387, 391, 393, 402, 403, 404, 405, 406, 407, 421, 432, 438, 440, 542, 545
Skin eruptions 142
Sodium 17, 41, 110, 228, 264, 380, 415, 423, 578
Spinal 109, 329, 367
Square. 56, 160, 164, 167, 184, 186, 188, 189, 300, 448
stagnation 142, 195
stress ... 15, 49, 54, 68, 72, 75, 86, 95, 109, 110, 112, 123, 124, 129, 142, 144, 158, 164, 198, 211, 243, 268, 272, 285, 288, 326, 334, 372, 373, 374, 376, 377, 378, 390, 393, 397, 400, 401, 402, 406, 411, 412, 414, 416, 417, 418, 419, 425, 430, 432, 433, 436, 437, 438, 439, 442, 453, 454, 456, 457, 458, 471, 542, 543, 545, 551
Stroke 357, 368, 542
Sun 94, 182, 198, 445, 448, 449, 454, 468, 470, 471, 479
sunburn 545, 546
Swollen. 49, 55, 56, 59, 75, 142, 155, 172, 327, 357, 364, 544
SYMBOL 467, 468, 469, 470, 471, 472, 473, 474, 475, 476, 477, 478
sympathetic. 15, 105, 109, 142, 164, 243, 268, 334, 378, 397, 400, 406, 412, 414, 437, 448, 455, 470
sympathetic nervous system 15, 142, 397, 437
systolic 15, 17, 373, 378

T

Taurus ... 82, 166, 257, 445, 447, 448, 449, 468, 474
Tendon 536
testicles 83, 113, 229, 242, 263, 367, 448

throat 82, 97, 198, 257, 326, 327, 361, 366, 368, 369, 401, 422, 468, 536
Thrombosis 536, 542, 544, 550
Thymus 17, 243, 327, 448
Thyroid 17, 36, 79, 109, 110, 193, 194, 198, 228, 231, 243, 317, 319, 320, 326, 366, 370, 384, 393, 394, 395, 448, 537, 538, 542, 546, 548
Tissue 401, 405, 418, 536
Tongue 144, 149, 150, 153, 248, 326, 330, 362, 368
Tonsils 368
tooth ... 144, 147, 357, 361, 364, 365, 370, 434, 438
Transverse Colon 112, 113, 363
Triglycerides 388
Trimester 6, 68
TRINE 452
Tryptophan 45
Tumor 384, 542, 546, 547, 548, 549, 550, 552

U

Ulcer 33, 55, 319, 537
ultra sound 539
Upper jaw 16
Uranus 101, 445, 448, 449, 454, 455, 456, 457, 458, 459, 460, 461, 477, 479
Uric Acid 383, 423
Urinary incontinence 20, 327
uterus 49, 84, 117, 215, 229, 247, 253, 257, 268, 328, 412, 546

V

Vagina 16, 17, 243, 247, 254, 255, 317, 539
Vagus Nerve 366
varicose 91, 356, 365, 477
Vas Deferentia 242
vasectomy 539
Venus 97, 198, 445, 449, 454, 455, 456, 457, 468, 473, 479
Virgo 86, 166, 257, 445, 447, 448, 472, 478
Vitamin 20
Vitamin E 20, 228
vocal cords 82, 257, 330
voice 82, 151, 468
Vomiting 33, 538

W

Warts 20, 150
watermelon 38
Webbed Fingers 174
Weight 319
wheat germ 38
white blood cells 20, 318, 377, 390, 397
wrinkles 54, 57, 73, 100, 142, 150, 192, 206, 332

Y

Yeast 228

Z

zinc 20, 385, 404, 405, 408, 421, 425, 427

Zodiac Sign..93, 257, 449, 465

Suggested Reading

A Bipolar Theory of Living Process, George Crile

Applied Kinesiology, David Walther
African Holistic Health, Llaila Afrika
Asian Medical Systems, Charles Leslie
Assessment Made Incredibly Easy, Springhouse Corporation
A Text Book of Materia Medica, Samuel Hahnemann
Ayurvedic for Health and Long Life, Dr. D. K Garde
Boulek Paprus
The Biology of Transcendence, Joseph Chilton Pearce
Biocircuits, Leslie Patten
Bedside Diagnostic Examination, Richard De Gowin
Clinical Autonomic Disorders, Phillip A. Low
The Canon of Medicine, Avicenna (Hakim Ibn Sina)
Collins Dictionary of Human Biology, Robert Youngson
Discovery in the Realm of Nature and Art of Healing, Ignatz Von Peckzely
The Elements, Theodore Gray
Eber's Papyrus
Essentials of Medical Astrology, Dr. KS Charack
Fluids and Electrolytes Demystified, Joyce Johnson
Greek Medicine, Being Extracts Illustrative of Medical Writers from Hippocrates to Galen, Arthur Brook
Iridology, Farida Sharon
Handbook of Iridiagnosis and Rational Therapy, Robert Wilborn
Immaculate Deception: A New Look at Women and Childbirth in America, Suzanne Arms
The Language of Mathematics, Keith Devlin
Music, Physics, and Engineering, Harry F. Olson
The Merck Manual of Diagnosis and Therapy, David Holvey
Mobsy's Manual of Diagnostic and Laboratory Test, K.D. Pagana
New Concepts in Diagnosis and Treatments, Albert Abrams
Periodic Tables, Hugh Aldersey-Williams
Practical Acupuncture, Clausen Torben
Pulse Diagnosis, Reuben Amber and Baboy Brooke
Raising Black Children, Llaila Afrika
Standardized Naturopathy, Dr. Paul Wendel
Quiet: The Power of Introverts in a World that Can't Stop Talking, Susan Cain
The Yellow Emperors Classic of Internal Medicine, Llza Vieth
Your Health in Your Horoscope, Stefan Stenudd

Made in the USA
Columbia, SC
07 March 2021